016.61073

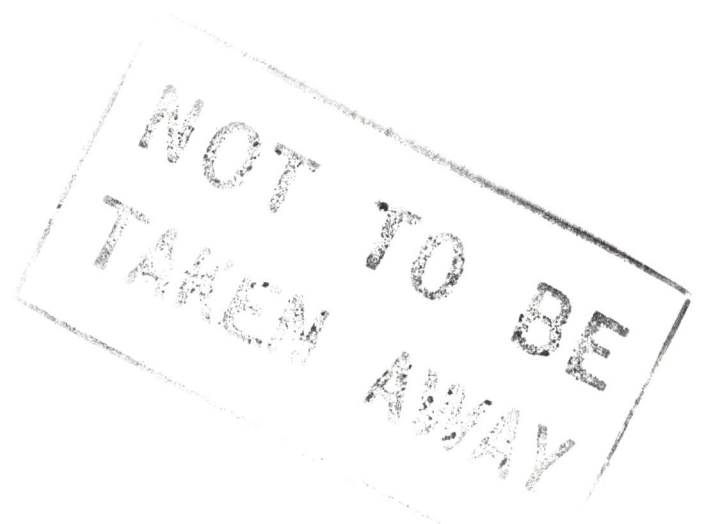

CLASSIFICATION No.	ACCESSION No.
REF DB	~~002456~~ 002457

W06839

A BIBLIOGRAPHY OF NURSING LITERATURE
1961-1970

A BIBLIOGRAPHY OF NURSING LITERATURE
1961-1970

Edited and Compiled by
ALICE M. C. THOMPSON, F.L.A.

LONDON
THE LIBRARY ASSOCIATION
THE ROYAL COLLEGE OF NURSING
AND NATIONAL COUNCIL OF NURSES OF THE UNITED KINGDOM
IN ASSOCIATION WITH
KING EDWARD'S HOSPITAL FUND FOR LONDON

1974

SOUTH BANK UNIVERSITY LIBRARY

Published by
The Library Association
7 Ridgmount Street, London WCIE 7AE
for
The Royal College of Nursing
Henrietta Place, Cavendish Square, W.1

© 1974 The Royal College of Nursing

ISBN: 0 85365 316 X

This work forms a supplement to
*A Bibliography of nursing literature,
1859-1960*, published in 1968.
(SBN: 85365 470 0)

Text set in 8 point Times New Roman,
'Monotype' Series 327

Printed and bound in England by
STAPLES PRINTERS LIMITED
at The Stanhope Press, Rochester, Kent

ACKNOWLEDGMENTS

THANKS must again be given to the King Edward's Hospital Fund for London, which, having already made a generous grant for the original volume of this bibliography, extended the grant for the compilation of this supplement.

I am much indebted to Miss Frances Walsh, Librarian, Library of Nursing and the library staff for the help given in so many ways and to Mrs. Sheila Harvey who again gave invaluable help in proof reading. Special thanks must be given to Miss Anne Kenney for her clerical assistance.

Finally I must thank the Council of the Royal College of Nursing and National Council of Nurses of the United Kingdom, not only for inviting me to compile the supplement, but also for the generous support given.

ALICE M. C. THOMPSON

Pinner, Middlesex

May 1973

CONTENTS LIST

Acknowledgments v

Preface xi

Introduction xiii

HISTORY OF NURSING

GENERAL WORKS. 1

NURSING IN OTHER COUNTRIES 1

HISTORY—SPECIAL ASPECTS 2
    Air-Force Nursing 2
    Army Nursing. 2
    Domiciliary Nursing 2
    Naval Nursing. 2
    Practical Nursing 2
    Occupational Health Nursing 2
    Red Cross and the Order of St. John of Jerusalem . . 2
    Uniforms 3

WAR NURSING 3

BIOGRAPHY

COLLECTIVE BIOGRAPHY 4

INDIVIDUAL BIOGRAPHY 4

NURSING AS A PROFESSION

GENERAL WORKS. 6

MALE NURSES 11

NURSING IN INDIVIDUAL COUNTRIES 12

ASSOCIATIONS AND ORGANIZATIONS 15

NURSING JOURNALS 18

NURSING LEGISLATION 19

SALARIES AND CONDITIONS OF WORK 19

HEALTH AND WELFARE 21
    Accommodation 21
    Sickness 22

RECRUITMENT AND WASTAGE 22
    Part-Time Staff 28

APTITUDE AND PERSONALITY TESTS 28

EDUCATION AND TRAINING 29
    Basic Training—General Works 29
        Associate Degree Programmes 39
        Bibliographies 39
        Careers in Nursing 39
        Collegiate Schools 40

EDUCATION AND TRAINING—*continued*
    Curricula and Syllabus 40
    Dictionaries, Glossaries, Year Books, Directories 41
    Diploma Schools 41
    Examinations 41
    In-Service Education 42
    Integrated Courses 43
    Pre-nursing Courses 43
    Student Status 44
    Evaluation of Students 45
    Teaching and Learning 45
    Teaching Machines and Programmed Learning 47
    Visual Aids 48
    University Courses 49
  Libraries 50
  Post-basic Education 52
  Training Schools 54

NURSING RESEARCH 55
  Operational Research 59
  The Patient—research 59
  The Work of the Nurse—research 59

NURSING ETHICS 60
  Nurse-Patient Relationship 60
  Professional Staff Relationships 62

WORK OF THE NURSE 63
  General Works 63
  Administration 67
    General Works 67
    Automation 73
    Communication 74
    Job Analysis 75
    Nursing Service Organization 76
    Staffing 77
  Aero-space Nursing 79
  Auxiliaries 80
  Clinical Nurse Specialist 81
  Enrolled Nurse (including the Practical Nurse) 81
  Prison Nursing 83
  Private Nursing 84

TECHNIQUES OF NURSING 84
  General Works 84
  Intensive Care 85
    Pain 87
  Monitoring 87
  Patient Care 88
  Progressive Patient Care 92
  Quality of Care 93
  Team Nursing 95
  War and Disaster Nursing 95

SPECIALITIES OF KNOWLEDGE AND PRACTICE

ALLERGIES 96

ANATOMY AND PHYSIOLOGY 96

ARITHMETIC 97

BACTERIOLOGY	97
BIOLOGY AND GENETICS	98
CANCER NURSING	98
CARDIAC NURSING	99
CHEMISTRY	102
CIRCULATORY DISEASES	102
DENTAL NURSING	103
DERMATOLOGY	103
DIABETES	104
DIAGNOSIS AND DIAGNOSTIC TECHNIQUES	105
DIGESTIVE SYSTEM	105
EAR, NOSE AND THROAT	106
ENDOCRINE, METABOLIC AND NUTRITIONAL DISEASES	107
GENITO-URINARY SYSTEM	107
GERIATRICS	109
GYNAECOLOGY	113
INFECTIOUS AND PARASITIC DISEASES	113
Leprosy	113
Poliomyelitis	113
Typhoid	114
LOCOMOTOR SYSTEM	114
MEDICINE	114
First-aid and Domestic Medicine	115
Tropical Medicine	115
MENTAL HEALTH	115
MENTAL SUBNORMALITY	116
NEUROLOGY	118
Speech Disorders	119
OBSTETRICS	119
OCCUPATIONAL HEALTH NURSING	121
General Works	121
Administration	125
Education	127
Special Occupational Health Services	128
OPHTHALMIC NURSING	129
PAEDIATRIC NURSING	129
Children in Hospital	131
Handicapped Children	133
Maternal and Child Health	133
Premature and New-Born Babies	133
PHYSICS	134
PSYCHIATRIC NURSING	134
Administration	141
After-Care	141
Education and Training	142
Psychiatry in the General Hospital	144
Research	144

PSYCHOLOGY	144
PUBLIC HEALTH NURSING	145
General Works	145
Administration	148
District Nursing	150
General Works	150
Administration	150
Education	151
Health Visiting	151
General Works	151
Administration	153
Education	153
Health Visiting and General Practice	154
School Nursing	156
RESPIRATORY SYSTEM	157
SOCIAL PROBLEMS AND NURSING	158
General Works	158
Abortion	158
Alcoholism	158
Drug Addiction	158
Family Planning	159
Problem Families	159
SURGERY	159
General Works	159
Accidents and Burns	161
Orthopaedics	162
Surgical Nursing	163
Central Sterile Supply Departments	166
Infection Control Sister	167
Transplants, Skin Grafts, Plastic Surgery	168
THERAPEUTICS	168
Anaesthetics	168
Dietetics and Nutrition	170
Music and Art Therapy	170
Oxygen Therapy	170
Pharmacology	171
Physical Medicine	173
Rehabilitation Nursing	174
TUBERCULOSIS NURSING	175
VENEREAL DISEASE NURSING	176

HOSPITALS

GENERAL WORKS	177
ADMINISTRATION	177
Staff	178
Ward Clerks and Hotel Services	179
PLANNING	179
Equipment	180
HISTORY OF HOSPITALS	181
General Works	181
History of Individual Hospitals	181
SPECIAL DEPARTMENTS AND UNITS	182

PREFACE

THE original volume of this bibliography covered the period 1859–1960. The volume, in the same format as this present one, ran to 132 pages. The supplement, covering the ten years from 1961–1970, fills an additional 50 pages.

Comparison between the original volume and the supplement gives an indication of the rapid growth and development of the nursing profession during the years 1961–1970. In the century which followed the publication in 1859 of Florence Nightingale's *Notes on nursing, what it is and what it is not*, 123 publications on the basic training of the nurse and 13 on university courses for nurses were recorded. In the ten years covered by the present volume the figures are 375 and 46 respectively.

Nursing research has expanded quickly, with 83 entries in the original volume and 181 for the years 1961–1970, and the increasing awareness of the value of libraries in nursing education is shown by the comparative figures of 31 and 76.

The number of entries under the heading "nurse-patient relationships" may give the reader pause. There are 70 entries in the first volume and 58 in the supplement.

The obsession with administration is emphasised by a comparison of 67 entries with 233.

The supplement provides a comment on the changing pattern of disease. Entries for cardiac conditions and cancer have risen sharply with 10 entries against 97 for cardiac conditions and 19 against 48 for cancer. As might be expected entries for infectious diseases generally have dwindled from 37 entries to 12, but the entries for tuberculosis are, surprisingly, only two less for the years 1961–1970 than the total for the previous century.

Increasing concern for the care and welfare of the elderly is shown by the increase from a mere 17 entries to 151.

The growth of a profession is indeed reflected in its literature.

INTRODUCTION

AFTER the successful publication of Miss Alice Thompson's *A Bibliography of nursing literature 1859–1960* in 1968, the Rcn has always hoped and intended that it should be followed as soon as possible by a supplement covering the next decade. That this hope has been fulfilled is due in no small measure to the generous support of the King Edward's Hospital Fund for London, which, as Chairman of the Library Committee of the College, it gives me great pleasure to acknowledge. I would also like to pay a warm tribute to the work of Miss Thompson. The College is fortunate in having been able to retain her services as Editor, although she has retired from her post as Librarian at the College.

The Editor in her introduction comments on the fact that the supplement is larger than the original volume, although the period it covers is but one tenth of that covered by the original volume. While she sees this as an index of the progress of the profession, it also reflects the growth of the literature; whereas the original volume had something like 4,600 entries, the number in the supplement must be approaching 7,000. They include both books and articles in journals, the latter having been selected from a more widely based card index maintained in the Library of Nursing at the College. In addition, an author index has been included which covers the entries in both the original *Bibliography* and the supplement. This has been compiled by the staff of the Library.

In January 1972 the first issue of the Rcn *Bibliography of nursing* appeared. This monthly publication and Miss Thompson's two volumes provide essential tools for those wishing to find their way about the literature of nursing past and present.

LEONARD M. PAYNE
Chairman
Rcn Library Committee

HISTORY OF NURSING

GENERAL WORKS

BROCKBANK, WILLIAM
The history of nursing at the M[anchester] R[oyal] I[nfirmary], 1752-1929. Manchester, University Press, 1970.

BULLOUGH, BONNIE, and BULLOUGH, VERN L.
The emergence of modern nursing. New York, Macmillan, 1964.
2nd edn., 1969.

BULLOUGH, V., and BULLOUGH, B.
Nursing and history. *Nursing Outlook*, Oct. 1964, p. 27-9.

DIETZ, LENA DIXON
History and modern nursing. Philadelphia, Davis, 1963.

EDWARDS, M. M.
Nurses and the National Health Service. *Nursing Times*, Aug. 9, 1963, p. 998-9.

EDWARDS-REES, DÉSIRÉE
The story of nursing. Constable Young, 1965.

MORRISON, A. A.
The sociological history of nursing. *The Australian Nurses' Journal*, May 1965, p. 106-113.

NAIMAN, H. L.
Nursing in Jewish law. *American Journal of Nursing*, Nov. 1970, p. 2378-9.

NIGHTINGALE, FLORENCE
Florence Nightingale at Harley Street: her reports to the Governors of her Nursing Home, 1853-1854. Introduction by Sir Harry Verney, Dent, 1970.

PELLEY, THELMA
Nursing: its history, trends, philosophy, ethics and ethos. Philadelphia, Saunders, 1964.

ST. THOMAS'S HOSPITAL, LONDON
The doctors versus the nurses: correspondence from the archives.... *Nursing Times*, June 15, 1962, p. 783-4.

STEWART, ISABEL MAITLAND, and AUSTIN, ANNE L.
A history of nursing from ancient to modern times: a world view.
5th edn., New York Putnam, 1962.
[Earlier editions published as "A short history of nursing" by Lavinia L. Dock and Isabel Maitland Stewart.]

DOLAN, J.
Nursing leadership—1895. *Nursing Science*, Aug.-Sept. 1963, p. 224-8.

TAYONA, SINFOROSO
A brief history of psychiatric nursing in the Philippines. *The Philippine Journal of Nursing*, Jan.-Feb. 1964, p. 12-22, and 32.

NURSING IN OTHER COUNTRIES

AFRICA

NIGERIA

DUKE, E. O.
History of nursing in Nigeria. *The Australian Nurses' Journal*, Feb. 1967, p. 34-6.

SOUTH AFRICA

HARRISON, P. H.
Coloured nursing progress in South Africa 1944-1969. *South African Nursing Journal*, Nov. 1969, p. 27 and 26.

M.A.M.E.
An outline of the development of the Bantu Nurse in South Africa. *South African Nursing Journal*, Nov. 1969, p. 25-6.

PASK, M. M. F.
"Marie". Reminiscences of a pioneer South African nurse. *South African Nursing Journal*, Sept. 1969, p. 7-11; Oct. 1969, p. 35-6 and 40; Nov. 1969, p. 29-31; Jan. 1970, p. 17-19 and 22; Feb. 1970, p. 29-30 and 35; Mar. 1970, p. 30-1.

SEARLE, CHARLOTTE
Episodes in our nursing history. 1. Contribution from Natal to the Nightingale Fund, 1856. *South African Nursing Journal*, Oct. 1963, p. 11.

SEARLE, CHARLOTTE
Fifty years of nursing service in South Africa 1914-1964. *South African Nursing Journal*, Nov. 1964, p. 32-55.

SEARLE, CHARLOTTE
The history of the development of nursing in South Africa 1652-1960: (a socio-historical survey). Cape Town, Struik, 1965.

AUSTRALIA

BOWE, E. J.
The story of nursing in Australia since foundation day. (New South Wales College of Nursing. 8th annual oration, 8th September 1960). *UNA Nursing Journal*, Mar. 1961, p. 75-89.

BRODSKY, ISADORE
Sydney's nurse crusaders. Sydney, Old Sydney Free Press, 1968.

KETTLE, E. S.
Development of rural health services in the Northern Territory. *The Tasmanian Nurse*, Dec. 1969, p. 12-14.

CANADA

CASHMAN, TONY
Heritage of service: the history of nursing in Alberta. Edmonton, the Alberta Association of Registered Nurses, 1966.

CHITTICK, R.
Our anabasis. [Development of nursing in Canada and U.S.]. *Australian Nurses' Journal*, Mar. 1969, p. 58-67.

SEARLE, CHARLOTTE
A review of nursing in Canada. *South African Nursing Journal*, Dec. 1962, p. 25-7; Jan. 1963, p. 22-4.

CARIBBEAN

LUTY, E.
The role of the nurse in the past—flash back—with special reference to nursing in Montserrat, St. Croix, Dominica and Jamaica. *The Jamaican Nurse*, Sept. 1968, p. 10-11.

JAPAN

ACHIWA, G.
Linda Richards in Japan. *American Journal of Nursing*, Aug. 1968, p. 1716-19.

UNITED STATES OF AMERICA

BULLOUGH, B., and BULLOUGH, V.
The origins of modern American nursing. The civil war era. *Nursing Forum*, vol. II, no. 2, 1963, p. 12-27.

SHIELDS, HAZEL P., *compiler*
White caps in the desert: a history of nursing in Arizona: golden anniversary Arizona State Nurses' Association 1919-1969. Arizona, The Association, [1969].

SPECIAL ASPECTS

AIR FORCE

BOORER, D.
Life in Princess Mary's. [Royal Air Force Nursing Service]. *Nursing Times*, Aug. 25, 1967, p. 1133-6.

NELSON, RICHARD
Nursing in the Royal Air Force. Part I. *Nursing Mirror*, Oct. 22, 1965, p. 178-80.

NELSON, RICHARD
Nursing in the Royal Air Force. Part II. *Nursing Mirror*, Oct. 29, 1965, p. 207-10.

ARMY NURSING

AMERICAN JOURNAL OF NURSING
The army nurse. *American Journal of Nursing*, Feb. 1966, p. 290-2.

AMERICAN JOURNAL OF NURSING
Men nurses are there in the military services. In Air Evac, by Gordon C. Fosberg. In refugee camps, by Karen J. Kelly. *American Journal of Nursing*, Feb. 1969, p. 310-15.

SHORT, D. P.
The New Zealand surgical team in Vietnam 1966-1967. *International Journal of Nursing Studies*, Sept. 1968, p. 163-71.

STRATFORD, D. O.
Canadian Associations with the South African Military Nursing Service. *South African Nursing Journal*, Mar. 1969, p. 33-5.

STRATFORD, D. O.
Nursing in the Zulu War, 1877-1879. *South African Nursing Journal*, Nov. 1967, p. 34-5.

STRATFORD, D. O.
Nursing in East and Central Africa—World War 1. *South African Nursing Journal*, Oct. 1965, p. 22-4.

STRATFORD, D. O.
On active service in East Africa. *South African Nursing Journal*, Oct. 1966, p. 27-9.

STRATFORD, D. O.
Women in uniform—IV. A brief account of nursing in the Crimea giving details of uniform worn. *South African Nursing Journal*, Jan. 1961, p. 26-7.

STRATFORD, D. O.
Women in uniform—V. A. history of early army nursing describing nurses' duties and required standard of conduct. *South African Nursing Journal*, Mar. 1961, p. 33-4.

STRATFORD, D. O.
Women in uniform—VI. (Decorations: The Royal Red Cross; the Victoria Cross; The Florence Nightingale Medal). *South African Nursing Journal*, Sept. 1961, p. 28-30.

STRATFORD, D. O.
Women in uniform—VII. (Decorations cont.: Florence Nightingale Jewel.) *South African Nursing Journal*, Oct. 1961, p. 24-36.

STRATFORD, D. O.
Women in uniform—VIII. *South African Nursing Journal*, Feb. 1962, p. 14-16.

STRATFORD, D. O.
Women in uniform—IX. *South African Nursing Journal*, Sept. 1962, p. 33-5.

STRATFORD, D. O.
Women in uniform—X. *South African Nursing Journal*, Dec. 1962, p. 33-5 and 49.

DOMICILIARY NURSING

DONNAN, S. G.
Looking back. Early experiences of a health visitor. *South African Nursing Journal*, Nov. 1963, p. 13 and 16.

EAST LONDON NURSING SOCIETY
East London Nursing Society, 1868-1968: the history of a hundred years. [Compiled by Edith Ramsay.] [The Society, 1968.]

MANCHESTER DISTRICT NURSING SERVICE
Centenary of district nursing, Manchester. *Nursing Times*, Dec. 18, 1964, p. 1667 and 1670.

NAVAL NURSING

QUEEN ALEXANDRA'S ROYAL NAVAL NURSING SERVICE
Nursing in the Navy. Queen Alexandra's Royal Naval Nursing Service past and present. The Service, 1961.

QUEEN ALEXANDRA'S ROYAL NAVAL NURSING SERVICE
Nursing with the Navy. *Nursing Times*, Oct. 19, 1962, p. 1317.

WIRTH, A.
Caring for the sick and wounded sailor. An account of the development of Sickberth Staff in the Royal Navy. *Nursing Mirror*, Sept. 14, 1962, p. v-vi.

PRACTICAL NURSING

JOHNSTON, DOROTHY F.
History and trends of practical nursing. St. Louis, Mosby, 1966.

OCCUPATIONAL HEALTH NURSING

ARMS, F. C.
The first industrial nurse in the U.S. was a Vermonter. *American Association of Industrial Nurses Journal*, Oct. 1962, p. 20.

OBUCHOWSKI, MARY, *compiler*
The industrial nurse in New England: from the horse-and-buggy days to the atomic age. New England Association of Industrial Nurses, 1963.

WILLIAMS, M.
Industrial nursing during the first world war. Personal recollections of Mrs. Mercy Evelyn Owen. *Nursing Mirror*, Nov. 16, 1962, p. xi.

WOODARD, E.
Industrial nursing in South Carolina: its history and growth. *American Association of Industrial Nurses Journal*, June 1965, p. 29.

RED CROSS & THE ORDER OF ST. JOHN OF JERUSALEM

BRITISH RED CROSS SOCIETY
One hundred years of Red Cross. *British Hospital Journal and Social Service Review*, July 24, 1970, p. 1437-9; July 31, 1970, p. 1484-5.

BRITISH RED CROSS SOCIETY
The proudest badge: the story of the Red Cross. 5th edn. The Society, 1966.

CLAPPISON, GLADYS BONNER
[Vassar's rainbow division 1918]. The training camp for nurses at Vassar College under the auspices of the National Council of Defence and the American Red Cross, June 24 to September 13, Poughkeepsie, N.Y., 1918. Iowa, the Graphic Publishing Co., 1964.

CLIFFORD, JOAN
A good uniform: the St. John story. Hale, 1967.

HEALTH
A century of service. British Red Cross Society 1870-1970. *Health*, Aug. 1970, p. 28-33.

INTERNATIONAL RED CROSS
The ceaseless challenge: souvenir of the Red Cross centenary, 1863-1963. Interspan Press Services, Ltd., 1963.

LEAGUE OF RED CROSS SOCIETIES
(Collected papers relating to the League, 1863-1963.) Geneva, the League, 1963.

HISTORY OF NURSING

LEAGUE OF RED CROSS SOCIETIES
Important dates in the history of the League of Red Cross Societies. [Geneva], the League, 1963.

LEAGUE OF RED CROSS SOCIETIES
Red Cross nursing around the world. Geneva, the League, 1963.

NEW ZEALAND RED CROSS SOCIETY
Refugee welfare in South Vietnam. A programme completed. *New Zealand Nursing Journal*, Jan. 1970, p. 13-16.

OLIVER, BERYL
The British Red Cross in action. Faber, 1966.

PEACEY, BELINDA
The story of the Red Cross. Revised edn. Muller, 1969.

UNIFORMS

DISTRICT NURSING
The history of Queen's uniform and badges. *District Nursing*, May 1961, p. 36.

GETTINGS, B.
Is nurses' uniform really necessary? *Nursing Mirror*, Oct. 24, 1969, p. 44-6.

HOPKINS, T. D.
Are uniforms in hospital really necessary? *Nursing Mirror*, Nov. 29, 1968, p. 12-13.

HOWE, J.
What's all this about colored uniforms? *American Journal of Nursing*, Aug. 1969, p. 1665-7.

LOVELL, H.
Nurses' uniform—for and against [Uniforms of domiciliary nursing staff in Ealing]. *Nursing Mirror*, Oct. 24, 1969, p. 40-4.

MACLEOD, E. B., *and* BAUMGART, A. J.
Is "capping" really outdated? *The Canadian Nurse*, June 1965, p. 462-4.

MINISTRY OF HEALTH AND SCOTTISH HOME AND HEALTH DEPARTMENT
Those national uniforms! 1. The Falkirk Experiment [Trials of the proposed new nurses' uniforms]. *Nursing Mirror*, May 3, 1968, p. 12-15.

MINISTRY OF HEALTH AND DEPARTMENT OF HEALTH FOR SCOTLAND
Those national uniforms! 2. Shotley Bridge experiment. *Nursing Mirror*, May 10, 1968, p. 44-9.

MINISTRY OF HEALTH AND SCOTTISH HOME AND HEALTH DEPARTMENT
Why a national uniform for nurses? *Nursing Mirror*, April 12, 1968, p. 12-14.

NURSING JOURNAL OF INDIA
The cap. *Nursing Journal of India*, June 1969, p. 195 and 203.

REES, S. A. H.
Staff uniforms. *Hospital and Health Management*, Jan. 1964, p. 58-60.

SIEGEL, H.
The nurse's uniform: symbolic or sacrosanct? *Nursing Forum*, vol. VII, no. 3, 1968, p. 314-23.

WATKIN, B. V.
The story of nurses' uniform. *Nursing Times*, Oct. 11, 1963, p. 1279-83.

YATES, E. L.
The apron story. *Nursing Mirror*, June 10, 1966, p. xii-xiii.

WAR NURSING

BOLSTER, EVELYN
The sisters of mercy in the Crimean war. Cork, Mercier Press, 1964.

GUYOT, H.
The nurse in civil war literature. *Nursing Outlook*, May 1962, p. 311-4.

HACKER, C.
The bluebirds who went over [Canadian nurses in World War I in Cairo, Salonika and the Isle of Lemnos]. *The Canadian Nurse*, Nov. 1969, p. 31-4.

HAYES, M.
Prisoner of the Congolese rebel army. *Nursing Mirror*, Dec. 3, 1965, p. 327-31.

HUMPHREYS, F. I.
SSAFA nursing service today. *Mother and Child*, May 1967, p. 12-13.

STEWART, A. C.
Ready to serve: a nurse recalls her experiences during the First World War. *American Journal of Nursing*, Sept. 1963, p. 85-7.

SUTHERLAND, D. J.
Nursing in the Peace Corps. *Nursing Outlook*, Dec. 1963, p. 888-90.

BIOGRAPHY

COLLECTIVE BIOGRAPHY

WILKINS, FRANCES
Six great nurses: Louise de Marillac, Florence Nightingale, Clara Barton, Dorothy Pattison, Edith Cavell, Elizabeth Kenny. Hamish Hamilton, 1962.

YOST, EDNA
American women of nursing. (3rd edn.) Philadelphia, Lippincott, 1965.

INDIVIDUAL BIOGRAPHY

ARMSTRONG, KATHARINE F.
Katharine F. Armstrong—nurse, teacher and writer, an appreciation. *Nursing Times*, Nov. 6, 1969, p. 1432.

BAGGALLAY, OLIVE
Olive Baggallay, MBE, LLB, SRN, SCM. 1894-1964. *The Nightingale Fellowship Journal*, Summer 1965, p. 16-17.

BEAMISH, RAHNO M.
Fifty years a Canadian nurse: devotion, opportunities and duty. New York, Vantage Press, 1970.

CAMERON, FLORA JEAN
Flora Jean Cameron—A tribute by Audrey Orbell. *The New Zealand Nursing Journal*, Feb. 1966, p. 5-6.

CARPENTER, MARY F.
Mary F. Carpenter by H.M.S. Director of Education, Royal College of Nursing. *Nightingale Fellowship Journal*, Jan. 1969, p. 46-47.

CARTER, MAYNARD LINDEN
Maynard Linden Carter, A.R.R.C. 1886-1962: a memoir, by Irene H. Charley. Reprinted from *International Journal of Nursing Studies*, July 1966, p. 161-7.

CAVELL, EDITH
Edith Cavell: pioneer and patriot, by A. E. Clark-Kennedy. Faber and Faber, 1965.

COCHRANE, MARY SMALLWOOD
League of Charing Cross Hospital Nurses. *The League News*, no. 27, Oct. 1965.

DOCK, LAVINIA LLOYD
Portrait of a leader: Lavinia Lloyd Dock, by T. E. Christy. *Nursing Outlook*, June 1969, p. 72-5.

FITZGERALD, ALICE
Nurse around the world: Alice Fitzgerald, by Iris Noble. New York, Julian Messner, 1964.

GEISTER, JANET M.
This I believe about my half-century in nursing. *Nursing Outlook*, Mar. 1964, p. 58-61.

GOOSTRAY, STELLA
Memoirs: half a century in nursing. Boston, Mass., University Mugar Memorial Library, Nursing Archive, 1969.

HEATHCOCK, RUTH
Sister Ruth, by Victor C. Hall. Spearman, 1968.

LEWIS, EDITH M.
Joy in the caring. (An autobiography.) Christchurch (N.Z.), N. M. Peryer, 1963.

LOCK, JOAN
Reluctant Nightingale. Dent, 1970.

MAASS, CLARA
Clara Maass, a nurse, a hospital, a spirit, by John T. Cunningham. Belleville, N.J., Rae Publishing Co. Inc., [1968?].

MALLON, MARY
Another look at Typhoid Mary. Mary Mallon, by M. L. Kretzer. *Nursing Science*, Dec. 1964, p. 487-91.

NEILL, GRACE
Grace Neill: the story of a noble woman, by J. O. C. Neill with a contribution by Flora J. Cameron. Christchurch, N.Z. Peryer, 1961.

NIGHTINGALE, FLORENCE
Florence Nightingale's influence on nursing to-day, by M. E. Baly. *Nursing Times*, Jan. 2, 1969, Occasional Papers, p. 1-4.

NIGHTINGALE, FLORENCE
Florence Nightingale: war nurse, by Anne Colver. Illinois, Garrard Publishing Co., 1961.
(This is a book for children.)

NIGHTINGALE, FLORENCE
As they saw her ... Florence Nightingale: the nurses with Florence Nightingale tell their stories, by Alan Delgardo. Harrap, 1970.

NIGHTINGALE, FLORENCE
Florence Nightingale, the legend that lives, by Myra E. Levine. *Nursing Forum*, vol. II, no. 4, 1963, p. 25-35.

NIGHTINGALE, FLORENCE
Florence Nightingale and the Goddess, by E. M. McInnes. *St. Thomas's Hospital Gazette*, Autumn 1963, p. 73-4.

NIGHTINGALE, FLORENCE
Florence Nightingale and State Registration, by E. W. Mills and J. Dale. *International Nursing Review*, vol. 11, no. 1, 1964, p. 31-6.

NIGHTINGALE, FLORENCE
Florence Nightingale curriculum vitae with information (sic) about Florence Nightingale and Kaiserswerth, by Anna Sticker. Düsseldorf-Kaiserswerth, Diakoniewerk, 1965.

NIGHTINGALE, FLORENCE
Florence Nightingale: rebel with a cause, by the Editors, the *RN Magazine*. Oradell, New Jersey, Medical Economics Book Division, 1970. Reprinted from *RN Magazine*, May 1970.

NIGHTINGALE, FLORENCE
The Nightingale Collection, part 1: a list of documentary and photographic material relating to Florence Nightingale deposited in the Greater London Record Office. The Office, 1969. [Typescript.]

NIGHTINGALE, FLORENCE
Florence Nightingale: nurse to the world, by Lee Wyndham. New York, World Publishing Company, 1969.

NUTTING, M. ADELAIDE
Portrait of a leader, M. Adelaide Nutting, by T. E. Christy. *Nursing Outlook*, Jan. 1969, p. 20-4.

OSBURN, LUCY
Lucy Osburn, c. 1836-1891: founder of the Nightingale System of Nursing at Sydney Hospital, by D. G. Bowd. Windsor, N.S.W., Hawkesbury Press, 1968.

OSBURN, LUCY
Miss Nightingale's young ladies: the story of Lucy Osburn and Sydney Hospital, by Freda MacDonnell. Angus & Robertson, 1970.

POWELL, MURIEL
Dame Muriel Powell, Chief Nursing Officer for Scotland. *British Hospital Journal and Social Service Review*, Sept. 12, 1969, p. 1686.

RISTORI, BRIDGET
Patients in my care: the autobiography of a nurse. Elek, 1967.

BIOGRAPHY

RUMSHEVICS, MARIA
Maria Rumshevics of Latvia, 1878-1962, by V. Bergman. *International Nursing Review*, vol. 10, no. 1, 1963, p. 10-11.

RUSSELL, EDITH KATHLEEN
A giant of nursing. *Canadian Nurse*, April 1964, p. 363-4.

RUSSELL, EDITH KATHLEEN
Edith Kathleen Russell—an appreciation, by D. C. Bridges. *Nursing Times*, June 26, 1964, p. 826.

RUSSELL, EDITH KATHLEEN,
Edith Kathleen Russell, by F. H. M. Emory. *International Nursing Review*, vol. 11, no. 2, 1964, p. 9-11.

SEACOLE, MARY
Mary Seacole: the Florence Nightingale of Jamaica, by M. Seivwright. *The Jamaican Nurse*, December 1961, p. 8.

SNELLMAN, VENNY
Venny Snellman—an appreciation by Marie Viitala. *International Nursing Review*, vol. 13, no. 2, 1966, p. 71-2.

STEWART, ISABEL MAITLAND
Portrait of a leader: Isabel Maitland Stewart, by T. E. Christy. *Nursing Outlook*, Oct. 1969, p. 44-8.

VINCENT DE PAUL
St. Vincent de Paul, by Leonard von Matt and Louis Cognet. Burns and Oates, 1960.

WALD, LILLIAN D.
Portrait of a leader: Lillian D. Wald, by T. E. Christy. *Nursing Outlook*, Mar. 1970, p. 50-4.

WILLIAMS, RACHEL
Florence Nightingale and the Goddess, by E. M. McInnes. *St. Thomas's Hospital Gazette*, Autumn 1963, p. 73-4.

NURSING AS A PROFESSION

GENERAL WORKS

ABDELLAH, F. G.
The nature of nursing science. *Nursing Research*, Sept.-Oct. 1969, p. 390-3.

ABEL-SMITH, B.
Crisis in nursing—The sociologist's view. *Nursing Times*, Sept. 29, 1961, p. 1262-3.

AICHLMAYR, R. H.
Creative nursing: a need to identify and develop the creative student. *Journal of Nursing Education*, Nov. 1969, p. 19-21 and 24-7.

AMERICAN MEDICAL ASSOCIATION
The AMA Committee on Nursing looks at nursing liaison activities in state medical societies, by F. M. Alexander. *Hospital Management*, April 1965, p. 110-2.

ANDERSON, A. M.
Concepts of leadership. *The New Zealand Nursing Journal*, March 1967, p. 7-10.

ANDERSON, ODIN W.
Towards an unambiguous profession? A review of nursing. Chicago, Center for Health Administration Studies, 1968. (Health Administration Perspectives, no. A6.)

ANELLO, M.
Responsibility for change and innovation in professional nursing. *International Nursing Review*, vol. 16, no. 3, 1969, p. 208-18.

ANSTICE, E.
Nursing. Miss Nightingale still has lots to answer for. *World Medicine*, July 2, 1968, p. 37-42.

ARWOLD, M. F.
Professionalism and changing concepts of administration. *The Journal of Nursing Education*, Jan. 1968, p. 5-14.

AYDELOTTE, MYRTLE K., *and* HUDSON, W. R.
Socio-engineering problem—the nursing profession. *Nursing Outlook*, Jan. 1962, p. 20-3.

BABICH, KAREN SUE
The perception of professionalism: Equality. *Nursing Forum*, vol. VII, no. 1, 1968, p. 14-20.

BANISTER, R. F. H.
Getting the best from others. *Nursing Times*, Dec. 18, 1969, Occasional Papers, p. 209-12.

BAZIAK, A. T.
Prospects for change in nursing. *Nursing Forum*, vol. VI, no. 2, 1967, p. 134-54.

BECK, F. S.
Professional responsibility and international relationships. *International Nursing Review*, vol. 9, no. 5, 1962, p. 45-50.

BELLINGER, A. C., *and* CLEVELAND, V. S.
A comparative analysis of Negro and Caucasian nurses on selected organismic and job-related variables. *Nursing Research*, Nov.-Dec. 1969, p. 534-8.

BENDALL, E. R. D.
Is nursing a backwater? *Nursing Times*, Nov. 19, 1970, p. 1498-9.

BENNETT, L. R.
This I believe... that nurses may become extinct. *Nursing Outlook*, Jan. 1970, p. 28-32.

BERGMAN, R. L.
Nursing and organised groups in society. *International Nursing Review*, vol. 12, no. 6, 1965, p. 28-31.

BERTHOLD, J. S.
Nurses and behavioral scientists: an alternate assessment. *Nursing Research*, Summer 1963, p. 153-6.

BRODT, D. E.
Excellence or obsolescence. *Nursing Forum*, vol. IX, no. 1, 1970, p. 19-26.

BROE, E.
The nurse—a world citizen. *Nursing Outlook*, Dec. 1963, p. 905-8.

BUDZYNA, A. H.
Cultural lag in the concepts of nursing. *Nursing Research*, Summer 1961, p. 132-40.

BUICK-CONSTABLE, B.
The professionalism spectre. *International Nursing Review*, vol. 16, no. 2, 1969, p. 133-44.

BUICK-CONSTABLE, B.
Technological change. Challenge to the professional nursing association. *New Zealand Nursing Journal*, Aug. 1969, p. 5-7.

BULLOUGH, BONNIE, *and* BULLOUGH, VERN, *editors*
Issues in nursing. New York, Springer, 1966.

CAMERON, F. J.
Quality nursing. *International Nursing Review*, vol. 10, no. 1, 1963, p. 21-7.

CAMPBELL, EMILY B.
Process of change. *American Journal of Nursing*, May 1967, p. 991-4.

CANADIAN NURSES ASSOCIATION
Course for the future, by Kasper D. Naegle. Ottawa, The Association, 1966.

CARR, A. J.
The problems and demands of change. *District Nursing*, Nov. 1968, p. 165-8.

CARVER, MARY
The nurse. Ward Lock, 1965.

CENTRAL OFFICE OF INFORMATION
Twenty questions about nursing in Scotland, prepared for the Scottish Home and Health Department by the Central Office of Information. Glasgow, H.M.S.O., 1963(?)

CHALK, D. N.
The decision making process in leadership. *American Association of Industrial Nurses Journal*, April, 1967, p. 10-12.

CHARBONNEAU, G.
Our professional obligations. *The Canadian Nurse*, Jan. 1966, p. 19-20.

CHERESCAVICH, G.
Shortage or misuse of professional nursing skills? *Nursing Forum*, vol. IX, no. 3, 1970, p. 224-33.

CHITTICK, R.
One nurse's utopia. *The Canadian Nurse*, June 1962, p. 507-15.

CHITTICK, R.
The troubled profession. *UNA Nursing Journal*, June 1968, p. 170-3.

CHOMLEY, P.
Some reflections and projections. Fourteenth Annual Oration—The New South Wales College of Nursing. *UNA Nursing Journal*, Mar. 1967, p. 75-81.

CHRISTMAN, L.
Knowledge, change and nursing care. *American Journal of Nursing*, Sept. 1966, p. 2027-9.

CHRISTMAN, L.
What the future holds for nursing. *Nursing Forum*, vol. IX, no. 1, 1970, p. 12-18.

NURSING AS A PROFESSION

CIARDI, J.
Nurses as writers. *American Journal of Nursing*, Dec. 1970, p. 2567-70.

CLARK, D. H.
Nurse and doctor. 1. Colleague or handmaiden? *Nursing Times*, Aug. 3, 1962, p. 978-80.

COLARDARCI, A. P.
What about that word profession? A new approach to deciding what nursing and its preparation should be, might clear up some of nursing's confusions. *American Journal of Nursing*, Oct. 1963, p. 116-8.

CONGALTON, ATHOL A.
The nurse and objective inquiry. *Australian Nurses' Journal*, Nov. 1962, p. 264-77.

CONGALTON, ATHOL A., *editor*
Nurses' evaluation of occupational status and other studies. Sydney, New South Wales College of Nursing, 1963.
(Research Reports in Nursing, no. 3).

CONGALTON, ATHOL A., *editor*
The public image of nursing. Sydney, New South Wales College of Nursing, 1962.
(Research Reports in Nursing, no. 1.)

CONGALTON, ATHOL A., *editor*
Young people look at nursing. Sydney, New South Wales College of Nursing, 1962.
(Research Reports in Nursing, no. 2.)

CORNELIUS, D. A.
The role of the nurse as a professional. *Jamaican Nurse*, Dec. 1968, p. 8-9 and 34.

CORWIN, R. G.
Role conception and career aspiration: a study of identity in nursing. *Sociology Quarterly*, April 1961, p. 69-86.

CORWIN, R. G., *and* MARVIN, J. T.
Some concomitants of bureaucratic and professional conceptions of the nurse role. *Nursing Research*, Fall 1962, p. 223.

CRANSTOUN, J.
The changing concept of nursing. *Canadian Hospital*, Dec. 1964, p. 40-3.

DAGSLAND, H.
Growing pains of professionalisation. *International Journal of Nursing Studies*, Dec. 1963, p. 45-50.

DAVID, OPAL D.
Anticipating the future for students and teachers in nursing: concepts about women are changing. *American Journal of Nursing*, Dec. 1962, p. 82-4.

DAVIS, FRED, *editor*
The nursing profession: five sociological essays. New York, John Wiley, 1966.

DE YOUNG, LILLIAN
The foundation of nursing as conceived, learned, and practiced in professional nursing. St. Louis, Mosby, 1966.

DILWORTH, A. S.
Goals for nursing. *Nursing Outlook*, May 1963, p. 336-40.

DONALDSON, F.
Is nursing a profession? *The Tasmanian Nurse*, July 1970, p. 6.

DREVES, K. D.
This I believe about nursing in a changing world. *Nursing Outlook*, Feb. 1964, p. 50-1.

DRYDEN, M. VIRGINIA
Nursing trends: a book of readings. Dubuque, Iowa, Brown, 1968.

DUCAS, DOROTHY
Modern nursing. New York, Henry Z. Walch, 1962.

DUNCANSON, M. B.
Who speaks for nurses and nursing? *The Canadian Nurse*, July 1963, p. 615-21.

DUNN, H. W.
Nursing service. *Hospitals*, April 1, 1964, p. 119-20 and 123-4.

DU PLESSIS, D. J.
The challenge to the nursing profession. Address given at the Congress of the South African Nurses Association, Durban, 1966. *South African Nursing Journal*, Dec. 1966, p. 30-4.

DURDIN, D. J.
Florence Nightingale oration. The future of others. *UNA Nursing Journal*, Nov. 1967, p. 341-9.

DUSTAN, LAURA C.
Is it the system? *Nursing Outlook*, May 1964, p. 58-61.

EDWARDS, MURIEL M.
Some nursing reports. *Nursing Times*, 1962.
(Originally published as articles in the *Nursing Times*, Mar., April and May 1962.)

ELLIS, ROSEMARY
The practitioner as theorist. *American Journal of Nursing*, July 1969, p. 1434-8.

ENSING, ELSIE C.
A new look at nursing. Pitman, 1966.

ETZIONI, AMITAI, *editor*
The semi-professions and their organization: teachers, nurses, social workers. New York, Free Press, 1969.

FAWKES, B. N.
Realistic nursing in a changing world. *Nursing Times*, Feb. 16, 1968, Occasional Papers, p. 25-8.

FAWKES, B. N.
Registration—passport to the world? *British Hospital and Social Service Journal*, Aug. 16, 1963, p. 986.

FAWKES, B. N.
European nursing. *Nursing Times*, May 5, 1967, p. 582-3.

FAWKES, B. N.
Towards a "European nurse". *Nursing Times*, Sept. 28, 1962, p. 1227.

FERLIC, A.
Existential approach in nursing. *Nursing Outlook*, Oct. 1968, p. 30-3.

FOLEY, J.
Wanted: a theory of nursing. *Royal Australian Nursing Federation Review*, Sept. 1970, p. 9-10; Oct. 1970, p. 6.

FOX, D., *and others*
Characteristics of basic nursing faculty. *Nursing Outlook*, Dec. 1964, p. 40-3.

FOX, RICHARD
Hostility towards doctors and nurses. 1. Public and profession. *Nursing Times*, July 20, 1962, p. 918-20.

FOX, RICHARD
Hostility towards doctors and nurses. 2. Face to face. *Nursing Times*, July 27, 1962, p. 956-8.

FRANK, SISTER CHARLES M.
Nursing needs more freedom. *American Journal of Nursing*, July 1962, p. 53-5.

FREEMAN, R. B.
The nurse as a writer. *Nursing Science*, Aug.-Sept. 1963, p. 156-61.

FRIEND, P. M.
Nursing in a technological age. *Nursing Mirror*, Nov. 11, 1966, p. 145-7.

GAINSBOROUGH, H.
The crisis in nursing—The physician's view. *Nursing Times*, Sept. 22, 1961, p. 1228-9.

GEORGOPOULOS, B. S.
 The hospital system and nursing: Some basic problems and issues. *Nursing Forum*, vol. V, no. 3, 1966, p. 8-35.

GILLAM, ROBERT
 Hierarchies in nursing. *International Nursing Review*, vol. 17, no. 4, 1970, p. 307-17.

GILLAM, ROBERT, *editor*
 Progress or retrogression? Realities in nursing; an edited account of a five-day workshop on facing reality in nursing, 1969, held at the New South Wales College of Nursing. Sydney, N.S.W. College of Nursing, 1969.

GINZBERG, E.
 What nurses need is a chance to grow. *The Modern Hospital*, April 1962, p. 103-6, 186 and 188.

GIRARD, A.
 A full partner in the health team. Address given at the Congress of the South African Nurses Association, Durban, 1966. *South African Nursing Journal*, Dec. 1966, p. 21-8.

GIRDWOOD, R. H.
 Some problems of nursing today. *British Medical Journal*, June 4, 1966, p. 1411-3.

GOODLAND, NORMAN L.
 Is nursing a "vocation"? *Nursing Mirror*, Jan. 20, 1967, p. 372-3.

GOODLAND, NORMAN L.
 The prestige of nursing. *Nursing Times*, Sept. 21, 1962, p. 1211-2.

GOODLAND, NORMAN L.
 The true state of nursing. *Quarterly Review*, Jan. 1965, p. 84-95.

GRAUHAN, A.
 A survey of the professional activities of former students of the School of Nursing, University of Heidelberg. *International Journal of Nursing Studies*, Aug. 1970, p. 125-33.

GRUNEAU RESEARCH LIMITED
 Study of attitudes of registered nurses in Ontario, conducted for the Registered Nurses Association of Ontario. Toronto, Gruneau Research, 1964.

HADLEY, B. J.
 Evolution of a conception of nursing. *Nursing Research*, Sept.-Oct. 1969, p. 400-5.

HALL, C. M.
 "Professional responsibility". *Nursing Times*, April 6, 1962, p. 451-2.

HANSEN, A. C., *and* THOMAS, D. B.
 Differences and changes in decision judgments within two role groups. *Nursing Researach*, July-Aug. 1969, p. 333-8.

HART, F.
 Crisis in nursing—The administrator's view. *Nursing Times*, Sept. 1, 1961, p. 1119.

HENDERSON, VIRGINIA
 Excellence in nursing. *American Journal of Nursing*, Oct. 1969, p. 2133-7.

HENDERSON, VIRGINIA
 The nature of nursing. *American Journal of Nursing*, Aug. 1964, p. 62-8.

HENDERSON, VIRGINIA
 The nature of nursing: a definition and its implications for practice, research and education. New York, Macmillan, 1966.

HOLLIDAY, J.
 The ideal characteristics of a professional nurse. *Nursing Research*, Fall 1961, p. 205-10.

HOSPITAL WORLD
 Are nurses professionals? *Hospital World*, Dec. 1970, p. 2.

INSTITUTE OF HOSPITAL MATRONS OF NEW SOUTH WALES AND AUSTRALIAN CAPITAL TERRITORY
 Report of the committee to consider all aspects of nursing. Part 1. The general nurse in the hospital environment. [Canberra], The Institute, 1967.

INTERNATIONAL COUNCIL OF NURSES
 Statement on nursing education, nursing practice and service and the social and economic welfare of nurses. Geneva, I.C.N., 1969.

ISRAEL. MINISTRY OF HEALTH. NURSING UNIT
 Nursing activities study: Israel—1966, [by M. Olga Weiss]. [Jerusalem], The Ministry, 1967.

JACOBS, D.
 The future of nursing, professionalization, profanation, prophecy. *International Nursing Review*, vol. 17, no. 1, 1970, p. 16-30.

JAHODA, MARIE
 Nursing as a profession. An address given at the 12th quadrennial meeting of I.C.N. *International Nursing Review*, May-June 1961, p. 11-18.

JAMESON, E. E., *and* MACKIE, E. J.
 Two departments of nursing. *Hospital Administration in Canada*, Oct. 1963, p. 36-9.

JENNINGS, M.
 On-the-job counseling ... a precious charge. *American Journal of Nursing*, Mar. 1961, p. 67-70.

JOHNSON, DOROTHY E.
 Today's action will determine tomorrow's nursing. *Nursing Outlook*, Sept. 1965, p. 38-41.

JOHNSON, R. L.
 Evaluating the effectiveness of an organization. *American Association of Industrial Nurses Journal*, April 1967, p. 15-19.

KAY, ELEANOR
 Nurses and what they do. New York, Franklin Watts, 1968.

KELBER, M.
 Accent on leadership. *International Nursing Review*, vol. 17, no. 1, 1970, p. 3-12.

KELLY, CORDELIA W.
 Dimensions of professional nursing. New York, Macmillan, 1962.
 2nd edn., 1968.

KING, I. M.
 A conceptual frame of reference for nursing. *Nursing Research*, Jan.-Feb. 1968, p. 27-31.

KRAMER, M.
 Collegiate graduate nurses in medical center hospitals: mutual challenge or duel. *Nursing Research*, May-June 1969, p. 196-210.

KRAMER, M.
 Comparative study of characteristics, attitudes and opinions of neophyte British and American nurses. *International Journal of Nursing Studies*, Dec. 1967, p. 281-93.

KRUSE, M.
 The next fifty years. *Irish Nurses' Journal*, Nov. 1969, p. 9-15.

KURTZ, R. A., *and* FLAMING, K. H.
 Professionalism. The case of nurses. *American Journal of Nursing*, Jan. 1963, p. 75-9.

LAMB, M. C. N.
 Current problems in nursing. *The Hospital*, June 1964, p. 350-3.

LAMBERTSEN, ELEANOR C.
 If nursing has changed, so have doctors and hospitals. *The Modern Hospital*, Nov. 1962, p. 124.

NURSING AS A PROFESSION

LAMBERTSEN, ELEANOR C.
Nurses must be teachers and must know these principles. *Modern Hospital*, Feb. 1968, p. 126.

LAMBERTSEN, ELEANOR C.
Why nurses should encourage change. *Modern Hospital*, Dec. 1968, p. 108.

LAMBERTSEN, ELEANOR C.
Reorganize nursing to re-emphasize care. *The Modern Hospital*, Jan. 1967, p. 68-72.

LANCASTER, A.
The reluctant profession. *International Nursing Review*, vol. 14, no. 6, 1967, p. 27-32.

LAWSON, M. G.
The Common Market—and its implications for nursing. *Nursing Mirror*, June 15, 1962, p. 198-200.

LEMINEN, A.
The theory of nursing. *International Nursing Review*, vol. 14, no. 6, 1967, p. 63-5 and 67-70.

LETHI, Y.
The conflict of generations in nursing. *International Nursing Review*, vol. 16, no. 2, 1969, p. 184-8.

LEVINE, M. E.
The four conservation principles of nursing. *Nursing Forum*, vol. VI, no. 1, 1967, p. 45-59.

LEVITT, E. E., *and others*
The student nurse, the college woman and the graduate nurse: a comparative study. *Nursing Research*, Spring 1962, p. 80-2.

LINDSEY, M.
Professional standards. Whose responsibility? *The American Journal of Nursing*, Nov. 1962, p. 84-7.

LORIG, K. R.
Consumer-controlled nursing. *Nursing Outlook*, Sept. 1969, p. 50-2.

LUKENS, L. G.
Personality patterns and choice of clinical nursing specialization. *Nursing Research*, Summer 1965, p. 210-21.

McGLOTHLIN, W. J.
The place of nursing among the professions. *Nursing Outlook*, April 1961, p. 214-6.

MACGREGOR, FRANCES C.
Nursing in transition: challenge for the future. [Geneva], W.H.O., 1967?

MACGREGOR, FRANCES C.
Nursing in transition. *International Nursing Review*, vol. 14, no. 6, 1967, p. 41-3.

MACGUIRE, J.
The development of identity with the role of the nurse. *International Journal of Nursing Studies*, Sept. 1966, p. 137-42.

McIVER, H.
What the community expects of nursing. *New Zealand Nursing Journal*, May 1970, p. 7-9.

McKAY, R.
Theories, models and systems for nursing. *Nursing Research*, Sept.-Oct. 1969, p. 393-9.

MACKENZIE, N.
The professional ethic. *International Nursing Review*, vol. 13, no. 4, 1966, p. 58-61.

MACLAGGAN, K.
The changing face of nursing. *The Canadian Nurse*, Nov. 1961, p. 1023-7.

MACLEOD, A. I.
The future role of nursing. *The Canadian Nurse*, Aug. 1965, p. 611-3.

MAJOR, D. M.
A profession . . . its growth and development. *Nursing Outlook*, Jan. 1963, p. 33-5.

MALKIN, S. A. S.
Crisis in nursing—The surgeon's view. *Nursing Times*, Sept. 8, 1961, p. 1150-1.

MALONE, M., *and others*
The paradox in nursing. *American Journal of Nursing*, Sept. 1961, p. 53.

MARRAM, G. D.
What is happening to nurses. *International Nursing Review*, vol. 16, no. 4, 1969, p. 320-6.

MARY PAULINA, SISTER
The heart of nursing [Nursing in Australia]. *South Australian Journal of Nursing*, Mar. 1969, p. 16 and 18-20.

MATHENEY, R. V.
The tragedy of the report of the Surgeon General's Consultant Group on Nursing. *Nursing Science*, April 1963, p. 4-10.

MATHIESON, J. B.
The Commonwealth level—a critical review of the nursing service. *International Nursing Review*, vol. 13, no. 4, 1966, p. 24-30.

MERENESS, D.
Freedom and responsibility for nursing students. *American Journal of Nursing*, Jan. 1967, p. 69-71.

MERENESS, D.
Recent trends in expanding roles of the nurse. *Nursing Outlook*, May 1970, p. 30-2.

MERTON, R. K.
Dilemmas of democracy in the voluntary associations. *American Journal of Nursing*, May 1966, p. 1055-61.

MERTON, R. K.
The nature of leadership. *International Nursing Review*, vol. 16, no. 4, 1969, p. 310-9.

MERTON, R. K.
The social nature of leadership. *American Journal of Nursing*, Dec. 1969, p. 2614-8.

MEYER, RALPH H.
Professional status of nursing. *Hospital Topics*, May 1964, p. 35-9.

MEYERS, MARY E., *editor*
Nursing fundamentals: a book of readings. Dubuque, Iowa, Brown, 1967.

MINISTRY OF HEALTH
The state of nursing. . . . from the Annual Report of the Chief Medical Officer of Health 1967. *Nursing Times*, Jan. 16, 1969, Occasional Papers, p. 9-12.

MOK, A. L.
Continuity and discontinuity in the nursing profession. *International Nursing Review*, vol. 16, no. 4, 1969, p. 296-307.

MORRIS, J. E.
Changing perspectives in nursing. *The Canadian Nurse*, Dec. 1962, p. 1079.

MOSBY, C. V. & Co.
Comprehensive review of nursing. 5th edn., New York, Mosby, 1961.
6th edn., 1965.
7th edn., 1969.

MURPHY, J. F.
Role expansion or role extension—some conceptual differences. *Nursing Forum*, vol. IX, no. 4, 1970, p. 380-90.

NAHM, H.
Nursing dimensions and realities. *American Journal of Nursing*, June 1965, p. 96-9; *International Nursing Review*, vol. 12, no. 6, p. 22-7.

NAHM, H.
Tribute to the past—prelude to the future. *International Nursing Review*, vol. 13, no. 4, 1966, p. 14-23.

NATIONAL LEAGUE FOR NURSING
Perspectives for nursing: report of the Committee on Perspectives. New York, The League, 1965.

NICOLAS, B.
British nurses and the Common Market. *Nursing Times*, Dec. 15, 1967, p. 1686-7.

NOBLE, M.
Social anthropology and nursing. *International Journal of Nursing Studies*, vol. 1, no. 3, 1964, p. 159-63.

NORRIS, C. M.
Towards a science of nursing—a method for developing unique content in nursing. *Nursing Forum*, vol. III, no. 3, 1964, p. 10-45.

NORTHERN IRELAND HOSPITALS AUTHORITY
Report of nursing committee. Sept. 1959. Belfast, N.I.H.A., 1960.

NURSING TIMES
Crisis in nursing—A nurse's view. *Nursing Times*, Oct. 13, 1961, p. 1324.

NURSING TIMES
Crisis in nursing—A nurse's view—2. Long-term policy. *Nursing Times*, Oct. 20, 1961, p. 1358.

NUSSBAUM, H.
Change and challenge. *The Canadian Nurse*, Sept. 1962, p. 798-801.

OGG, ELIZABETH
Your nursing services to-day and to-morrow. *Public Affairs Pamphlets*, 1961.

OLD INTERNATIONALS ASSOCIATION
Report of the Old Internationals Summer School, Aug. 1964. University of Edinburgh, 1964.

OLLERENSHAW, K.
The education service and the nursing profession. *Nursing Times*, June 14, 1963, p. 743-5.

PARKER, C.
The word nurse and its connotations. *Nursing Outlook*, Dec. 1962, p. 784-7.

PERKINS, E. W.
The registered nurse—a professional person? *American Journal of Nursing*, Feb. 1963, p. 90-2.

PETERSON, E.
The status of women today and its effect on nursing. *American Journal of Nursing*, Nov. 1963, p. 70-3.

PETROWSKI, DOROTHY D., *and*
PARTHEY ULLER, MARGARET T., *editors*
Forces affecting nursing practice. Washington, Catholic University of America Press, 1969.
(Nursing Education Workshop Proceedings.)

PLATOU, R. V., *and others*
Role of the nurse in medical education. New Orleans, Tulane University, 1964.

POTTER, T.
Are we too afraid of disturbing the "status quo" among our nurses? *Hospital Administration in Canada*, July 1970, p. 6 and 9.

POWELL, MURIEL B.
The fundamental problem in nursing. *Nursing Times*, Oct. 11, 1963, p. 1299-1300.

POWELL, MURIEL B.
Nursing—its contribution to society. Address given at the Annual General Meeting of the Association of Hospital Matrons, April 26, 1969. *Nursing Times*, July 17, 1969, Occasional Papers, p. 113-6; July 24, 1969, Occasional Papers, p. 117-20.

PRATT, HENRY
Doctor's view of the changing nurse-physician relationship. *Journal of Medical Education*, Aug. 1965, p. 767-71.

QUINN, S.
Keeping pace with the seventies. *Irish Nurses' Journal*, Nov. 1970, p. 11-13 and 19-20.

RAE, A. V.
Preparing the student nurse for responsibility. *Nursing Times*, Nov. 11, 1966, p. 1487-8.

RAVEN, K. A.
The future of the nursing profession. *Nursing Mirror*, May 26, 1961, p. 739-40; June 2, 1961, p. 843-5.

REINKEMEYER, AGNES M.
The myths by which we live. *International Nursing Review*, vol. 16, no. 1, 1969, p. 39-48.

REINKEMEYER, AGNES M.
Nursing's need: commitment to an ideology of change. *Nursing Forum*, vol. IX, no. 4, 1970, p. 340-55.

REVANS, R. W.
The student wants to learn—and live. *Nursing Times*, Feb. 11, 1966, p. 197-8.

ROBINSON, K.
Crisis in nursing—The politician's view. *Nursing Times*, Sept. 15, 1961, p. 1195.

ROGERS, MARTHA E.
An introduction to the theoretical basis of nursing. Philadelphia, Davis, 1970.

ROGERS, R., *and* BALLANTYNE, W.
Basic qualities of a good nurse. *Canadian Nurse*, Oct. 1963, p. 948-53.

ROREM, C. R.
The term "professional nurse" is just pious fiction. *Hospital Management*, Feb. 1967, p. 41-4.

ROY, SR. CALLISTA
Adaptation: a conceptual framework for nursing. *Nursing Outlook*, Mar. 1970, p. 42-5.

ROYAL COLLEGE OF NURSING AND NATIONAL COUNCIL OF NURSES OF THE UNITED KINGDOM
The duties and position of the nurse. Revised 1970.

ROYAL COLLEGE OF NURSING AND NATIONAL COUNCIL OF NURSES OF THE UNITED KINGDOM
The future of nursing in a changing society. Report of a conference held by the Rcn, at Porchester Hall, London, 29 June 1966. *Nursing Times*, July 8, 1966, p. 920-2.

RUBIN, R.
This I believe . . . about the structure of nursing in a changing society. *Nursing Outlook*, July 1966, p. 54-6.

SANNER, MARGARET C.
Trends and professional adjustments in nursing. Philadelphia, Saunders, 1962.

SCHLOTFELDT, ROZELLA M.
Towards new horizons of social responsibility. New York, American Nurses Association, 1966.

SCHLOTFELDT, ROZELLA M., *and* MACPHAIL, J.
An experiment in nursing. [Rationale and characteristics] [at the Case Western Reserve University Medical Centre, Cleveland, Ohio]. *American Journal of Nursing*, May 1969, p. 1018-23.

SCHLOTFELDT, ROZELLA M., *and* MACPHAIL, J.
An experiment in nursing: introducing planned change. *American Journal of Nursing*, June 1969, p. 1249-51.

SCHLOTFELDT, ROZELLA M., *and* MACPHAIL, J.
Experiment in nursing: implementing planned change. *American Journal of Nursing*, July 1969, p. 1475-80.

SCHMITT, M. H.
Role conflict in nursing. *American Journal of Nursing*, Nov. 1968, p. 2348-50.

NURSING AS A PROFESSION

SCHURR, M. C.
A comparative study of leadership in industry and the nursing profession, part I. *International Nursing Review*, vol. 16, no. 1, 1969, p. 16-29.

SCHURR, M. C.
A comparative study of leadership in industry and the nursing profession, part II. *International Nursing Review*, vol. 16, no. 2, 1969, p. 115-30.

SCOTFORD, H.
"The professional woman". *The Australian Nurses' Journal*, Dec. 1967, p. 245-8.

SEALE, J.
Crisis in nursing—The medical economist's view. *Nursing Times*, Oct. 6, 1961, p. 1286.

SEWARD, SR. JOAN MARIE
The role of the nurse: perceptions of nursing students and auxiliary nursing personnel. *Nursing Research*, Mar.-April 1969, p. 164-9.

SHEAHAN, J.
A stock-taking of British nursing—1. *Nursing Times*, Sept. 20, 1968, Occasional Papers, p. 145-8.

SHEAHAN, J.
A stock-taking of British nursing—2. *Nursing Times*, Sept. 27, 1968, Occasional Papers, p. 149-50.

SHEARS, L. W.
The characteristics of a profession. *UNA Nursing Journal*, Dec. 1964, p. 388-91.

SHELDON, E. B.
The use of behavioral sciences in nursing: an opinion. *Nursing Research*, Summer 1963, p. 150-2.

SIMMONS, L. W.
Past and potential images of the nurse. *Nursing Forum* Summer 1962, p. 16-33.

SKIPPER, J. K.
The nurse-role: an instrumental and/or expressive function? *The Canadian Nurse*, Feb. 1963, p. 139-42.

SMITH, D. W.
Change: how shall we respond to it? *Nursing Forum*, vol. IX, no. 4, 1970, p. 391-9.

SMITH, K. M.
Discrepancies in the role-specific values of head nurses and nursing education. *Nursing Research*, vol. 14, no. 3, 1965, p. 196-202.

SMOYAK, S. A.
Toward understanding nursing situations: a transaction paradigm. *Nursing Research*, Sept.-Oct. 1969, p. 405-10.

SOLOMON, L.
Resolving conflicts between education and service. *Nursing Outlook*, Feb. 1963, p. 102-4.

SPENCER FELTON, J.
Communicating in writing, part 1. *Occupational Health Nursing*, May 1970, p. 13-19.

STAUPERS, MABEL KEATON
No time for prejudice: a story of the integration of negroes in nursing in the United States. New York, Macmillan, 1961.

STEWART, W. H.
The challenge to nursing. *Public Health Reports*, Feb. 1967, p. 95-8.

STORLIE, F.
Nursing need never be defined. *International Nursing Review*, vol. 17, no. 3, 1970, p. 254-7.

TARLINTON, P.
The profession of nursing. . . . The importance of professional organization through a united association. *The Australian Nurses' Journal*, Mar. 1970, p. 56-62.

TAVES, MARVIN J., *and others*
Role conception and vocational success and satisfaction: a study of student and professional nurses, by Marvin J. Taves, Ronald G. Corwin, and J. Eugene Haas. Columbus, Ohio State University Bureau of Business Research, 1963.

THOMPSON, L. M.
The changing role of the nurse, part I. *The New Zealand Nursing Journal*, Mar. 1968, p. 19-20.

THOMPSON, L. M.
The changing role of the nurse, part II. *The New Zealand Nursing Journal*, April 1968, p. 7-8.

UPRICHARD, M.
Ferment in nursing. *International Nursing Review*, vol. 16, no. 3, 1969, p. 222-32.

WEDGERY, A.
The will to match our opportunity. *The Canadian Nurse* June 1966, p. 35-9.

WHITAKER, J. G.
The changing role of the professional nurse in the hospital. *American Journal of Nursing*, Feb. 1962, p. 65-9.

WHITAKER, J. G.
The nurse as a professional person. *Nursing Outlook*, April 1961, p. 217-9.

WHITAKER, J. G.
The professional nurse's dilemma: satisfying the conflicting demands of her clinical and managerial functions. *Hospitals*, Feb. 1962, p. 58-66 and 108.

WIEDENBACH, E.
The helping art of nursing. *American Journal of Nursing*, Nov. 1963, p. 54-7.

WIEDENBACH, E.
Nurses' wisdom in nursing theory. *American Journal of Nursing*, May 1970, p. 1057-62.

WILLIAMS, J. I.
Hospital nursing and the demand for change. *The Canadian Nurse*, July 1970, p. 38-41.

WILLIAMS, S.
Nursing in the Great Society. *Nursing Times*, Dec. 9, 1966, p. 1614-5.

WOLLOWICK, A.
Will the nursing profession become extinct? *Nursing Forum*, vol. IX, no. 4, 1970, p. 408-13.

WORLD HEALTH ORGANIZATION
Nurses. [Geneva] W.H.O., 1967.

WORLD HEALTH ORGANIZATION
Regional Office for the Eastern Mediterranean.
Report on the nursing seminar, Teheran, Iran, 9 November-19 November 1966. [The Organization], 1968.

WRIGHT, R. D.
New horizons for nursing. *Nigerian Nurse*, Feb. 1968, p. 23-4.

ZACHARIAH, A.
The public image of the nurse. *Nursing Journal of India*, Mar. 1969, p. 81 and 105.

MALE NURSES

ALDAG, J. C.
Occupational and nonoccupational interest characteristics of men nurses. *Nursing Research*, Nov.-Dec. 1970, p. 529-34.

BAGGOTT, E.
Male nurse administrators. *Nursing Times*, Mar. 26, 1965, p. 433.

BOORER, D. J.
Men nurses in Britain. *Nursing Outlook*, Nov. 1968, p. 24-6.

BROWN, R. G. S., *and* STONES, R. W. H.
Men who come into nursing. *Nursing Times*, Oct. 15, 1970, p. 153-5; Oct. 22, 1970, p. 157-9.

GREENE, J.
Male nurses in British psychiatric hospitals. *Nursing Outlook*, Sept. 1962, p. 607-8.

HARRIS, H. E.
21 years of male nursing in Western Australia. *Journal of the West Australian Nurses*, Nov. 1969, p. 15-17.

IRWIN, C.
Man nurses in New Zealand. *New Zealand Nursing Journal*, Sept. 1969, p. 33-4.

LLOYD, W. A.
The male nurse administrator. *Nursing Times*, Mar. 12, 1965, p. 363-4.

MANNINO, S. F.
The professional man nurse: why he chose nursing and other characteristics of men in nursing. *Nursing Research*, Summer 1963, p. 185-7.

PLANT, J.
Male nursing in Europe. *International Nursing Review*, vol. 13, no. 2, 1966, p. 36-47.

POPE, C.
Discrimination against male R.N's. grows more illogical as science increases the responsibilities of nursing staffs. *Hospital Administration in Canada*, Nov. 1962, p. 48.

SAINT PAUL, SISTER
Do our hospitals need male nurses? *Canadian Hospital*, Feb. 1963, p. 48-51.

SOCIETY OF REGISTERED MALE NURSES
Our society is founded, by G. Edwards. *Male Nurses Journal*, Oct. 1965, p. x-xii.

VYAS, R. W.
Why discrimination in nursing? [against male nurses]. *Nursing Journal of India*, Mar. 1969, p. 83 and 107.

WEDGERY, A. W.
The origins of a nursing stigma. *Canadian Hospital*, Nov. 1963, p. 63-6.

NURSING IN INDIVIDUAL COUNTRIES
GENERAL

BROADHURST, MARTHE JEANNE
Nurses from abroad: values in international exchange of persons. New York, American Nurses' Foundation, 1963.

LEE, C. M.
Be wise before the event. Preparation for nursing overseas. *Nursing Times*, May 3, 1968, p. 602-4.

MUMFORD, E.
The exchange nurse. Perspectives and prospects. *International Nursing Review*, vol. 16, no. 1, 1969, p. 49-55.

PRATT, R.
The challenge of nursing in developing countries. *International Nursing Review*, vol. 17, no. 2, 1970, p. 158-69.

AFRICA

BEAL, B.
Bantu nursing. *American Journal of Nursing*, Mar. 1970, p. 547-50.

SEARLE, C.
Professional advancement of the African nurse. *South African Nursing Journal*, Feb. 1961, p. 28.

CENTRAL AFRICA

MARAIS, J.
Nursing in Central Africa. *Nursing Mirror*, April 9, 1965, p. xii-xiii.

GHANA

KISSEIH, D. A. N.
Developments in nursing in Ghana. *International Journal of Nursing Studies*, Sept. 1968, p. 205-19.

KENYA

HOUGHTON, M.
Nursing in Kenya today. *Nursing Times*, Feb. 11, 1966, p. 186-8.

KOINANGE, M. W.
Communication with the local community in Kenya. *International Nursing Review*, vol. 12, no. 6, 1965, p. 32-4.

WERE, V.
The winds of change in Kenya. *The South African Journal of Nursing*, Dec. 1968, p. 4.

NIGERIA

JACOT, M.
Pioneer nurse, Niger. *World Health*, Sept.-Oct. 1969, p. 25-9.

MUIR, M.
Nursing in Nigeria. *Nursing Times*, April 21, 1967, p. 530-1.

WEST, T.
Rising above the difficulties. Wusasa Hospital, Zaria, Nigeria. *Nursing Times*, June 5, 1969, p. 716-9.

RHODESIA

O'CONNOR, A.
Nursing in Rhodesia—past, present and future. *Rhodesian Nurse*, Mar. 1969, p. 2-5.

SIERRA LEONE

NYLANDER, V. M.
The multi-purpose nurse of Sierra Leone. *International Journal of Nursing Studies*, Nov. 1969, p. 183-6.

SOUTH AFRICA

ROBERTS, E.
Nursing in Johannesburg. *Nursing Mirror*, Sept. 19, 1969, p. 39-41.

UGANDA

INTERNATIONAL COUNCIL OF NURSES
Nursing in a new member association—Uganda. *ICN Calling*, no. 10, Nov. 1969, p. [7-8].

MUSOKE, A. S. B.
Uganda's nurses and the hospitals they work in. *International Nursing Review*, vol. 15, no. 3, 1968, p. 254-68.

ZAMBIA

DOOLEY, J. W.
Community nursing in Zambia. *The Zambia Nurse*, Dec. 1968/Jan. 1969, p. 5 and 7-13.

RICHARDS, M.
Zambia and its health services. *Nursing Times*, Nov. 6, 1964, p. 1483-4.

ASIA
PAPUA

COGAN, E.
Nursing in Papua. *Journal of the West Australian Nurses*, Sept. 1968, p. 12-14.

HEARTFIELD, M.
Nursing in Papua. *The Tasmanian Nurse*, June 1970, p. 10-12.

THAILAND

AUDRIC, J.
Nurses and hospitals in Siam. *Nursing Mirror*, Oct. 27, 1967, p. ix-xi.

Foo Chong Ah
Solving nursing problems in the States of Malaya. *International Nursing Review*, vol. 13, no. 2, 1966, p. 13-16.

Kennedy, I. M.
A visit to Thailand, Malaysia and Singapore. *The South African Journal of Nursing*, Dec. 1968, p. 13-14.

VIETNAM

Williams, H.
Nursing programme in Vietnam. *Nursing Journal of India*, Sept. 1969, p. 320.

AUSTRALIA

Burchill, Elizabeth
Innamincka. Adelaide, Rigby, 1964.
[An account of the Australian Inland Mission.]

Forbes, D. N.
Nursing on aboriginal reserves. *South Australian Journal of Nursing*, Dec. 1969, p. 10-11.

Hollingsworth, E. B.
Tasmania—its hospitals and nurses. *Journal of the West Australian Nurses*, June 1969, p. 8 and 10-15.

Mathews, R. C.
Bush nursing in Marree. *South Australian Journal of Nursing*, Dec. 1969, p. 13-14.

Mead, B. P.
Nursing "down under". *Nursing Mirror*, Feb. 6, 1970, p. 39-41.

Paulina, Sr. Mary
Reflections on the future of nursing in Australia. *International Nursing Review*, vol. 16, no. 3, 1969, p. 258-66.

South Australian Journal of Nursing
Tasmania's hospitals and nurses. *South Australian Journal of Nursing*, Sept. 1969, p. 18.

BELGIUM

Ward, M. J., *and* Clampit, J.
A nursing experience in Belgium. *Nursing Times*, Dec. 17, 1970, p. 1614-6.

CANADA

Baldwin, J. T.
Nursing in a cold climate [North Canada]. *Nursing Mirror*, Dec. 25, 1970, p. 19-20 and 24.

Banfill, B. J.
Nurse of the islands. William Kimber, 1965.

Association of Canadian Hospital Administrators
Looking deeper into nursing. *Hospital Administration in Canada*, July 1964, p. 29-33.

Canadian Nurses' Association
Nursing Service Study. *Canadian Hospital*, Aug. 1963, p. 48.

Canadian Nurses' Association
A statement of nursing in Canada. *The Canadian Nurse*, June 1962, p. 533.

Copeland, Donalda M., *and* Myles, Eugenie Louise
Nurse among the Eskimos. Souvenir Press, 1964.

Diack, Lesley
Labrador nurse. Gollancz, 1963.

Fox, S.
Nursing in Vancouver. *Nursing Times*, Mar. 26, 1970, p. 414-5.

Gascoyne, R. A.
Nursing in Canada. *Nursing Mirror*, June 6, 1969, p. 26-8.

Gilbert, R. G.
The changing present and exciting future of nursing [in Canada]. *Hospital Administration in Canada*, Jan. 1970, p. 46 and 48-49.

King, M. P.
Nursing in the Canadian North. *Nursing Times*, Nov. 15, 1968, p. 1571-2.

Mussallem, H. K., *and* Lindabury, V. A.
Nursing in Canada. *Nursing Times*, Dec. 9, 1966, p. 1626-9.

Wilson, Amy V.
No man stands alone. Hodder & Stoughton, 1966.
[American edition entitled "A nurse in the Yukon", published by Dodd, Mead in New York.]

CARIBBEAN

Barbados Registered Nurses Association
Memorandum seeks better in-service conditions [Memorandum submitted to Ministry of Health by Barbados Registered Nurses Association]. *Barbados Nursing Journal*, April-May 1968, p. 16-20.

Barrow, N.
The role of the nurse in the changing Caribbean. *The Jamaican Nurse*, Sept. 1968, p. 6 and 25; *International Nursing Review*, vol. 16, no. 2, 1969, p. 167-71.

Bennett, B. A.
Journey to the West Indies. *Nursing Mirror*, Mar. 11, 1966, p. i-v; Mar. 18, 1966, p. x-xii; Mar. 25, 1966, p. i-iv; April 1, 1966, p. iv-vi, April 8, 1966, p. xii-xiii and xvi.

Caribbean Nurses' Organisation
Brochure on second biennial conference, St. Kitts-Nevis, 20th-26th August 1961. Antigua, the Organisation, 1961.

Caribbean Nurses' Organization
Sixth biennial conference report: the role of the nurse in the chang.ng Caribbean. Mary Seacole House, Kingston and University of West Indies, Kingston, 24th July-2nd August, 1968. Antigua, the Organisation, 1969.

Cowie, A. V.
The nursing services of Bermuda. *International Journal of Nursing Studies*, Aug. 1970, p. 159-63.

Jamaican Nurse
Main finding of the committee of enquiry and summary of Hart report on nursing. *The Jamaican Nurse*, April-May, 1967, p. 28-9.

Landauer, S.
Recent nursing developments in the English-speaking Caribbean. *International Nursing Review*, vol. 17, no. 2, 1970, p. 172-83.

Quinn, S.
The role of the professional nurses' association in the changing Caribbean. *The Jamaican Nurse*, Sept. 1968, p. 14-15 and 31.

Thompson, J.
The role of the nurse at present in the changing Caribbean. *The Jamaican Nurse*, Sept. 1968, p. 12 and 34.

DENMARK

White, D.
The structure of the hospital nursing service in Denmark. *Nursing Times*, Jan. 15, 1970, Occasional papers, p. 9-12.

EGYPT

Bull, M. R.
Nursing the fellahin in Egypt. *Nursing Mirror*, Dec. 13, 1963, p. viii-x.

FINLAND

Katajamaki, M.
Facts about nursing in Finland. *International Journal of Nursing Studies*, Nov. 1970, p. 249-52.

FRANCE

BADOUAILLE, MARIE-LOUISE
Present and future position of the nursing profession in France. *International Nursing Review*, vol. 17, no. 2, 1970, p. 146-55.

CARRUTHERS, B. M.
Nursing in France. *Rhodesian Nurse*, vol. 2, no. 3, 1969, p. 10-13.

GERMANY

GERMAN NURSES' FEDERATION
The German Nurses' Federation, 1948-1958. *Australian Nurses' Journal*, Feb. 1964, p. 36-40.

ICELAND

PETURSDOTTIR, M.
Nursing in Iceland. *International Journal of Nursing Studies*, vol. 3, no. 2, 1966, p. 81-7.

INDIA

ADRANVALA, T. K.
Nursing in India—1908-1968. *Nursing Journal of India*, Nov. 1968, p. 369-71.

KELLIE, G. A.
Expedition to Nepal. The Kozi Zonal Hospital, Biratuagar. *Nursing Times*, April 10, 1969, p. 480-1.

SYMONDS, S.
Healthier future for Nepal's children. *Nursing Mirror*, Oct. 16, 1970, p. 39-41; Oct. 23, 1970, p. 59-61.

IRELAND

SCANLAN, P.
Nursing education in Ireland. *International Nursing Review*, vol. 16, no. 2, 1969, p. 153-9.

ISRAEL

BERGMAN, R., *and* STRULOVICI, N.
Socio-demographic characteristics of Israeli student nurses. *International Journal of Nursing Studies*, June 1970, p. 67-78.

SKEET, M.
Israel. *Nursing Times*, April 17, 1969, Occasional Papers, p. 61-4.

WEISS, O.
Problems of peripatetic professionals. [Foreign nurses in Israel]. *International Nursing Review*, vol. 17, no. 1, 1970, p. 77-82.

JAPAN

CHINO, SHIZUKA
Nursing in Japan. *International Nursing Review*, vol. 11, no. 1, 1964, p. 19-22 and 24-6.

NAGANO, S.
Nursing in Japan. *Canadian Nurse*, June 1969, p. 35-6.

MAURITIUS

JUGOO, A. R.
Nursing in transition; Mauritius. *Nursing Times*, Oct. 29, 1970, p. 1406-7.

MIDDLE EAST

MOLONEY, SR. M. M.
Some impressions of nursing and nursing education in the Middle East. *Nursing Outlook*, Aug. 1970, p. 56-80.

RIFKA, G. E., *and* KHOURY, Y. G.
Nursing manpower in Lebanon. *International Nursing Review*, vol. 17, no. 3, 1970, p. 195-205.

WORLD HEALTH ORGANIZATION
Nursing in the Eastern Mediterranean Region. *W.H.O. Chronicle*, vol. 15, no. 4, April 1961.

PAKISTAN

JACOB, R. E.
The development of Pakistan nursing services. *International Nursing Review*, vol. 10, no. 4, 1963, p. 64-8.

OWEN, J. E.
Nursing in Pakistan. *Canadian Nurse*, June 1965, p. 449-50.

PORTUGAL

QUINN, S.
Nursing in Portugal. *International Nursing Review*, vol. 14, no. 3, 1967, p. 27-30.

SOUTH AMERICA

KINGSBURY, VIRGINIA
Nursing needs in Latin America. *Hospital Progress*, Dec. 1967, p. 43-7.

BOLIVIA

BECK, F. S.
Background to nursing in Bolivia. *International Nursing Review*, vol. 13, no. 2, 1966, p. 21-4.

BRAZIL

BRAZILIAN NURSING ASSOCIATION
Survey of needs and resources of nursing in Brazil. Rio de Janeiro, the Association, 1963.

DE ALCANTARA, GLETE
Obstacles in Brazilian society to the expansion of the nursing profession. *International Nursing Review*, vol. 11, no. 3, p. 12-14.

COLOMBIA

EASTON, R. E.
A study of the image of the graduate nurse in Colombia, South America. *International Nursing Review*, vol. 17, no. 1, 1970, p. 67-76.

RESTREPO, L. A., *and* DE GARZON, E. C.
Nursing in Colombia. *Canadian Nurse*, June 1969, p. 37-9.

PERU

DAVELUY, D.
Peruvian adventure. *Canadian Nurse*, Sept. 1969, p. 36-7.

KIBBLE, M. R.
From the Peruvian Andes. *Nursing Mirror*, April 10, 1970, p. 38-9.

MACKINTOSH, E. M.
Nursing in the Andes of Peru. *Nursing Mirror*, July 29, 1966, p. i-iv.

SPAIN

MANLY, R.
Nursing in Spain. *Nursing Mirror*, Mar. 15, 1963, p. x-xi.

SWEDEN

HOSPITAL WORLD
Nursing in Sweden. *Hospital World*, Aug. 1966, p. 5.

PECK, C.
Psychiatric nursing in Sweden. *Nursing Mirror*, Aug. 29, 1969, p. 27-30.

SWITZERLAND

BAECHTOLD, M.
Nursing in Switzerland. *International Nursing Review*, vol. 13, no. 6, 1966, p. 14-17.

TURKEY

TURER, A.
Turkey. Cradle of modern nursing. *International Nursing Review*, vol. 16, no. 1, 1969, p. 64-7.

NURSING AS A PROFESSION

UNION OF SOVIET SOCIALIST REPUBLICS

ERNSBERGER, R. G.
Nursing in Russia. *Nursing Outlook*, Dec. 1963, p. 883-7.

INGLES, T.
An American nurse visits the Soviet Union. *American Journal of Nursing*, April 1970, p. 754-62.

POWELL, A.
Nurse training in the USSR. *Nursing Times*, Dec. 2, 1966, p. 1600-1.

WORLD HEALTH ORGANIZATION
Report of the travelling seminar on nursing in the USSR. 6-28 October 1966. Geneva, W.H.O., 1967.

UNITED STATES OF AMERICA

HAYMAN, FRANCES
King country nurse. Angus & Robertson, 1965.

JONATHAN, M.
X-ray nurse in North America. *Nursing Mirror*, Dec. 5, 1969, p. 40-41.

JONES, P. E.
Foreign exchange visitor in the U.S.A. *Nursing Mirror*, Oct. 21, 1966, p. v-vii.

LEONE, L. P.
Nurses in the Federa Government. *Nursing Outlook*, April, 1961 p. 227.

STEWART, W. H.
The Surgeon General looks at nursing. *American Journal of Nursing*, Jan. 1967, p. 64-7.

WILLIAMS, E. M.
High rise nursing on Navajo Land. [Mexico]. *Occupational Health Nursing*, Sept. 1969, p. 9-13.

YATES, WILLIAM L.
Nursing in South Carolina, a statistical study of the quantity of nurses and the quality of their training. Columbia, South Carolina Hospital Association, 1963.

ASSOCIATIONS AND ORGANIZATIONS

GENERAL WORKS

BRIDGES, D. C.
The importance of professional organization—national and international. *International Nursing Review*, vol. 8, no. 1, 1961, p. 5-10.

BROWN, C.
Communication within and among nursing organizations. *International Nursing Review*, vol. 2, no. 5, 1965, p. 40-2.

CARPENA, E.
Better and stronger nurses' associations. *Jamaican Nurse*, Sept. 1968, p. 36 and 39.

GIRARD, A.
The professional Nursing Association—and You! *Australian Nurses' Journal*, June 1961, p. 135.

JARRETT, L.
The modern student nurse and her professional organization. *South Australian Journal of Nursing*, Mar. 1969, p. 22-4 and 26.

KERR, M. E.
Professional nurses' associations and good public relations. *The Canadian Nurse*, Nov. 1961, p. 1,056.

MERTON, R. K.
Organizational linkages in nursing. *Bedside Nurse*, Mar.-April 1969, p. 23-7.

AMERICAN NURSES' ASSOCIATION

AMERICAN NURSES' ASSOCIATION
Changing ANA to meet changing needs. Part I: Appraising the situation by F. L. A. Powell. *American Journal of Nursing*, Mar. 1964, p. 111-3.

AMERICAN NURSES' ASSOCIATION
Changing ANA to meet changing needs. Part II: Concern with practice, by F. L. A. Powell. *American Journal of Nursing*, April 1964, p. 113-6.

AMERICAN NURSES' ASSOCIATION
Changing ANA to meet changing needs. Part III: Resolving complex problems, by F. L. A. Powell. *American Journal of Nursing*, May 1964, p. 117-20.

AMERICAN NURSES' ASSOCIATION
Facts about nursing. New York, The Association, 1961-, in progress.

AMERICAN NURSES' ASSOCIATION
House of delegates sections reports 1964-1966. New York, The Association, [1966] and 1966-68. 1968.

AMERICAN NURSES' ASSOCIATION
House of delegates divisions on practice: proceedings. 46th convention, May 13-17, 1968, Dallas, Texas. New York, The Association, 1968.

AMERICAN NURSES' ASSOCIATION
Nurses, nursing and the ANA. *American Journal of Nursing*, April 1970, p. 808-15.

AMERICAN NURSES' ASSOCIATION
The profession prepares for its future. A report of the American Nurses' Association Convention, 1966. *American Journal of Nursing*, July 1966, p. 1548-67.

AMERICAN NURSES' ASSOCIATION
Report of a conference for State Boards of Nursing, April 6-7, 1961, Cleveland, Ohio. New York, the Association, 1961.

AMERICAN NURSES' ASSOCIATION
Study Committee on the functions of ANA: report. New York, the Association, 1962.

AMERICAN NURSES' ASSOCIATION
Putting our own house in order. What changes are needed in the American Nurses' Association, by M. B. Dolan. *American Journal of Nursing*, Dec. 1962, p. 76-9.

AMERICAN NURSES' ASSOCIATION
American Nurses' Foundation 1955-1970, by S. D. Taylor. *Nursing Research Report*, Dec. 1970, p. 1-6.

AMERICAN NURSES' ASSOCIATION *and* AMERICAN MEDICAL ASSOCIATION
Medical and nursing practice in a changing world; proceedings of first national conference for professional nurses and physicians, Feb. 13-15, 1964, Williamsburg, Va. New York, ANA/AMA, 1964.

ASSOCIATION OF HOSPITAL MATRONS

ASSOCIATION OF HOSPITAL MATRONS ANNUAL CONFERENCE 1963
Report of the meeting is given in—*Nursing Times*, May 31, 1963, p. 689.

ASSOCIATION OF HOSPITAL MATRONS
Report of 82nd General Meeting held at Middlesex Hospital Medical School, November 1964. *Nursing Mirror*, Nov. 13, 1964, p. 169-70.

ASSOCIATION OF HOSPITAL MATRONS
Annual General Meeting, Skegness, 1966. *British Hospital Journal and Social Service Review*, June 3, 1966, p. 1020.

ASSOCIATION OF HOSPITAL MATRONS
49th Annual General Meeting of the Association of Hospital Matrons is reported in—*Nursing Mirror*, May 24, 1968, p. 10-12.

ASSOCIATION OF HOSPITAL MATRONS
Anxiety and apprehension. [Report of a general meeting held in London, October 1969]. *Nursing Mirror*, Oct. 31, 1969, p. 14-16.

AUSTRALASIAN TRAINED NURSES' ASSOCIATION

AUSTRALASIAN TRAINED NURSES' ASSOCIATION
Extraordinary General Meeting of the Australasian Trained Nurses' Association held on 9th May 1970. [To discuss amalgamation with other nursing organisations]. *Australian Nursing Journal*, Aug. 1970, p. 173-4.

JARRETT, L.
Nursing organisation [in Australia]. *The Australian Nurses' Journal*, Dec. 1968, p. 264, 266-8 and 270.

BRITISH COMMONWEALTH NURSES' WAR MEMORIAL FUND

BRITISH COMMONWEALTH NURSES' WAR MEMORIAL FUND
Survey of the Fund through 21 years. [n.d.]

CANADIAN NURSES' ASSOCIATION

CANADIAN NURSES' ASSOCIATION
A call to action [Report of 35th biennial meeting, June 1970]. *Canadian Nurse*, Aug. 1970, p. 5-7 and 10-13.

CANADIAN NURSES' ASSOCIATION
Convention report [35th biennial meeting, June 1970]. *Canadian Nurse*, Aug. 1970, p. 24-9 and 34.

CANADIAN NURSES' ASSOCIATION
Countdown: Canadian nursing statistics. 1967-1968. Ottawa, The Association, 1969.

CANADIAN NURSES' ASSOCIATION
"Identity and destiny" [report of 34th general meeting of the Canadian Nurses Association]. *The Canadian Nurse*, Aug. 1968, p. 30-3.

CANADIAN NURSES' ASSOCIATION
The leaf and the lamp: the Canadian Nurses' Association and the influence which shaped its origins and outlook during the first sixty years. Ottawa, The Association, 1968.

CANADIAN NURSES' ASSOCIATION
Ad Hoc Committee
Special report on functions, relationships and fee structure. *The Canadian Nurse*, Mar. 1970, p. 35-8.

CARIBBEAN NURSES' ORGANIZATION

CARIBBEAN NURSES' ORGANIZATION
Brochure on second biennial conference, St. Kitts-Nevis, 20th-26th August 1961. Antigua, The Association, 1961.

CARIBBEAN NURSES' ORGANIZATION
Sixth biennial conference report: the role of the nurse in the changing Caribbean. Mary Seacole House, Kingston and University of West Indies, Kingston, 24th July-2nd August 1968. Antigua, The Organisation, 1969.

CENTRAL COUNCIL FOR DISTICT NURSING IN LONDON

CENTRAL COUNCIL FOR DISTRICT NURSING IN LONDON
History of the Central Council for District Nursing in London, 1914-1966. The Council, n.d.

CEYLON NURSES' ASSOCIATION

CEYLON NURSES' ASSOCIATION
Silver jubilee, 1943-1968. The Association, 1968.

COMMONWEALTH CARIBBAN NURSES

COMMONWEALTH CARIBBEAN NURSES
A regional nursing body for the Commonwealth Caribbean: report of the Commonwealth Caribbean nurses sponsored by the Commonwealth Foundation. Barbados, April 20-28, 1970.
[Canadian Nurses' Association for the Commonwealth Caribbean Nurses, 1970].

COMMUNITY OF THE NURSING SISTERS OF ST. JOHN THE DIVINE

COMMUNITY OF THE NURSING SISTERS OF ST. JOHN THE DIVINE
The story of the Community of the Nursing Sisters of Saint John the Divine, by F. Cartwright. [Hastings, The Community, 1968?].

FLORENCE NIGHTINGALE INTERNATIONAL FOUNDATION

FLORENCE NIGHTINGALE INTERNATIONAL FOUNDATION
The story of the Florence Nightingale International Foundation, by Marjorie Killby.
[Reprinted from International Nursing Review, vol. 10, no. 6, 1963, p. 25-36.]

GENERAL NURSING COUNCIL FOR ENGLAND AND WALES

GENERAL NURSING COUNCIL FOR ENGLAND AND WALES
The General Nursing Council for England and Wales, by Mary Henry. *Nursing Mirror*, Mar. 15, 1963, p. 522-4.

GENERAL NURSING COUNCIL FOR ENGLAND AND WALES
The General Nursing Council for England and Wales. 2. The training of nurses.
3. Examinations and assessments, by Mary Henry. *Nursing Mirror*, Mar. 22, 1963, p. 545-7 and 549.

GENERAL NURSING COUNCIL FOR ENGLAND AND WALES
The General Nursing Council for England and Wales. 4. Registration and enrolment, by Mary Henry. *Nursing Mirror*, Mar. 29, 1963, p. 561-2.

GENERAL NURSING COUNCIL FOR ENGLAND AND WALES
The General Nursing Council for England and Wales. 5. Miscellaneous duties, by Mary Henry. *Nursing Mirror*, April 5, 1963, p. 17-19.

GENERAL NURSING COUNCIL FOR ENGLAND AND WALES
A history of the General Nursing Council for England and Wales, 1919-1969, by Eve R. D. Bendall and Elizabeth Raybould. Lewis, 1969.

GENERAL NURSING COUNCIL FOR ENGLAND AND WALES
The next 50 years. *Nursing Times*, Jan. 30, 1969, p. 152-4.

GENERAL NURSING COUNCIL FOR ENGLAND AND WALES
Re-organisation of GNC for England and Wales, comments by the National Association of State Enrolled Nurses. *Nursing Mirror*, April 14, 1967, p. 30.

GENERAL NURSING COUNCIL FOR ENGLAND AND WALES
Report submitted to the Minister of Health [for years 1961—in progress].

GENERAL NURSING COUNCIL FOR ENGLAND AND WALES
Review of Constitution of Council and of the Mental Nurses and Enrolled Nurses Committees. *Nursing Times*, April, 21, 1967, p. 514-5.

GENERAL NURSING COUNCIL FOR ENGLAND AND WALES
Suggestions for the profession's consideration. *Nursing Times*, Oct. 21, 1966, p. 1397-8.

INTERNATIONAL COMMITTEE OF CATHOLIC NURSES
Eighth World Congress of catholic nurses: souvenir, Brighton, 2-12 June 1966. Brussels, The Committee, 1966.

INTERNATIONAL COMMITTEE OF CATHOLIC NURSES
Eighth World Congress of catholic nurses. The nurse and scientific progress. Paper given by C. Gagnon at the Congress held in Brighton, June 1966. *Nursing Times*, June 17, 1966, p. 818.

INTERNATIONAL COUNCIL OF NURSES

INTERNATIONAL COUNCIL OF NURSES
Do we need an International Council of Nurses? *Nursing Mirror*, Nov. 22, 1963, p. 185.

INTERNATIONAL COUNCIL OF NURSES
Focus on the future: proceedings of the 14th quadrennial Congress... Montreal (Canada), June 22-8, 1969. Basel, Karger, 1970.

NURSING AS A PROFESSION

INTERNATIONAL COUNCIL OF NURSES
A history of the International Council of Nurses, 1899-1964: the first sixty-five years, by D. C. Bridges. Pitman, 1967.

INTERNATIONAL COUNCIL OF NURSES
The International Council of Nurses (I.C.N.) from a historical viewpoint, by D. C. Bridges. *International Journal of Nursing Studies*, Dec. 1966, p. 191-6.

INTERNATIONAL COUNCIL OF NURSES
International Council of Nurses—its influence, by Helen Nussbaum. *International Journal of Nursing Studies*, Dec. 1963, p. 7-9.

INTERNATIONAL COUNCIL OF NURSES
International Council of Nurses. The immediate past, the urgent present and focus on the future, by S. Quinn. *International Nursing Review*, vol. 16, no. 3, 1969, p. 241-6.

INTERNATIONAL COUNCIL OF NURSES
ICN statement on nursing education, nursing practice and service and the social and economic welfare of nurses. *American Journal of Nursing*, Oct. 1969, p. 2177-9.

INTERNATIONAL COUNCIL OF NURSES
National reports of member associations, 1961. *The Council*, 1961.

INTERNATIONAL COUNCIL OF NURSES
National reports of member associations, 1965. *The Council*, 1965.

INTERNATIONAL COUNCIL OF NURSES
National reports of member associations, 1969: an international survey of Nursing. Basel, Karger, 1969.

INTERNATIONAL COUNCIL OF NURSES
Reports of standing committees 1961. The Council, 1961.

INTERNATIONAL COUNCIL OF NURSES
12th Quadrennial Congress: report of the President and General Secretary to the Grand Council, presented at Melbourne, Australia. April 1961, I.C.N. 1961.

INTERNATIONAL COUNCIL OF NURSES
12th Quadrennial Congress: some papers and reports presented at the I.C.N. 12th Quadrennial Congress, Melbourne, Australia, 17-22 April 1961. Geneva, W.H.O., 1961.

INTERNATIONAL COUNCIL OF NURSES
12th Quadrennial Congress, Melbourne, Australia, April 1961. Nursing as a profession by Marie Jahoda. *Nursing Mirror*, April 21, 1961, p. 237-9; April 28, 1961, p. 335-6 and 338.

INTERNATIONAL COUNCIL OF NURSES
12th Quadrennial Congress, Melbourne, Australia. April 1961. Interpreting nursing to the community, paper given by M. Mitchell. *Nursing Mirror* June 30, 1961, p. 1212; July 7, 1961, p. 1311.

INTERNATIONAL COUNCIL OF NURSES
13th Quadrennial Congress, Frankfurt, Germany, June 1965. Report of the Grand Council. *International Nursing Review*, vol. 12, no. 4, 1965, p. 3-16.

INTERNATIONAL COUNCIL OF NURSES
13th Quadrennial Congress, Frankfurt, Germany, June 1965. Report of the Grand Council. *American Journal of Nursing*, Aug. 1965, p. 88-97.

INTERNATIONAL COUNCIL OF NURSES
The 14th Quadrennial Congress, Montreal, 1969. The world of nursing meets in Montreal. *American Journal of Nursing*, Aug. 1969, p. 1685-99.

INTERNATIONAL COUNCIL OF NURSES
The 14th Quadrennial Congress, Montreal, June 1969, by A. M. C. Thompson. *International Nursing Review*, vol. 16, no. 4, 1969, p. 371-8.

INTERNATIONAL COUNCIL OF NURSES
14th Quadrennial Congress, Montreal, 1969. Congress report. *The Canadian Nurse*, Aug. 1969, p. 30-9.

INTERNATIONAL COUNCIL OF NURSES
TNAI and the ICN, by E. H. Paul. *Nursing Journal of India*, Oct. 1970, p. 326.

INTERNATIONAL COUNCIL OF NURSES. Basic Documents
Constitution and regulations, rules, procedure at meetings. I.C.N., 1966.

INTERNATIONAL COUNCIL OF NURSES
FLORENCE NIGHTINGALE INTERNATIONAL FOUNDATION
Report of the Conference [at the] Hellenic Red Cross School of Nursing, Athens, September 1967. The Foundation, 1967?

IRISH NURSES' ORGANISATION

IRISH NURSES' ORGANISATION
Summary of submissions by the Irish Nurses' Organisation to the Select Committee of the Oireachtas on the Health Services. *Irish Nurses Magazine*, Feb. 1963, p. 14-15.

NATIONAL ASSOCIATION OF STATE ENROLLED NURSES

NATIONAL ASSOCIATION OF STATE ENROLLED NURSES
NASEN considers its future. *Nursing Mirror*, Nov. 21, 1969, p. 25-6.

NATIONAL ASSOCIATION OF STATE ENROLLED NURSES
Professional associations and the unions—[document submitted to the Royal Commission on Trade Unions and Employers' Associations]. *Nursing Mirror*, Jan. 7, 1966, p. 439-40.

NATIONAL ASSOCIATION OF THEATRE NURSES

NATIONAL ASSOCIATION OF THEATRE NURSES
Theatre Nurses' first annual congress. [Held at Harrogate in October 1965]. *British Hospital Journal and Social Service Review*, Nov. 5, 1965, p. 2089-91.

NATIONAL ASSOCIATION OF THEATRE NURSES
A good start for NATN. Report of the National Association of Theatre Nurses First Annual Congress held 4-6 October 1965 in Harrogate. *Nursing Times*, Oct. 15, 1965, p. 1427-8.

NATIONAL ASSOCIATION OF THEATRE NURSES
Congress Report, Brighton, 1966. *NATNews*, Winter 1966, p. 19-21.

NATIONAL ASSOCIATION OF THEATRE NURSES
National Association of Theatre Nurses Report on the Association's second annual congress held at Brighton, Oct. 1966. *Nursing Mirror*, Nov. 4, 1966, p. 125-6.

NATIONAL ASSOCIATION OF THEATRE NURSES
Theatre nurses demand improved conditions of service. Report of the Third Annual Congress of the National Association of Theatre Nurses, held at Southport, 1967. *Nursing Mirror*, Oct. 27, 1967, p. 88-9.

NATIONAL ASSOCIATION OF THEATRE NURSES
NATN Congress at Southport, 1967. *Nursing Times*, Oct. 20, 1967, p. 1401-2.

NATIONAL ASSOCIATION OF THEATRE NURSES
NATN Congress Report Blackpool, October 1-4 1969. *NATNews*, Winter 1969, p. 18-20 and 23.

NATIONAL ASSOCIATION OF THEATRE NURSES
Theatre nurses meet in Blackpool [Report of NATN Congress]. *Nursing Mirror*, Oct. 17, 1969, p. 14.

NATIONAL LEAGUE FOR NURSING

NATIONAL LEAGUE FOR NURSING
Three score years and ten. 1893-1963. New York, The League, 1963.

NATIONAL LEAGUE FOR NURSING
6th Convention, Atlantic City, May 13-17, 1963. Report. *Nursing Outlook*, June 1963, p. 425-43.

NATIONAL LEAGUE FOR NURSING
Abstracts from selected papers given at the Sixth Biennial Convention of the National League for Nursing, held in Atlantic City, N.J., 13th-17th May 1963. *Hospital Topics*, July 1963, p. 31-8.

NEW ZEALAND REGISTERED NURSES' ASSOCIATION

BUICK-CONSTABLE, B.
Inside the RNA [New Zealand]. *The New Zealand Nursing Journal*, Mar. 1968, p. 5-17.

NEW ZEALAND REGISTERED NURSES' ASSOCIATION
Conference handbook, Wellington, April 2-4, 1968. [Wellington, The Association, 1968].

NEW ZEALAND REGISTERED NURSES' ASSOCIATION
Diamond Jubilee conference book, Wellington, April 15-17, 1969. [Wellington, The Association]. 1969.

NEW ZEALAND REGISTERED NURSES' ASSOCIATION
Reflections, messages and greetings. . . . The Diamond Jubilee of the New Zealand Registered Nurses' Association. *New Zealand Nursing Journal*, Sept. 1969, p. 5-24.

REGISTERED NURSES' ASSOCIATION OF NOVA SCOTIA

REGISTERED NURSES' ASSOCIATION OF NOVA SCOTIA
History of the nurses' official directory of the Registered Nurses' Association of Nova Scotia, Halifax Branch, by Anna Thorpe. Halifax, 1967.

ROYAL AUSTRALIAN NURSING FEDERATION

ROYAL AUSTRALIAN NURSING FEDERATION
Royal Australian Nursing Federation. First Biennial convention of the R.A.N.F. held at Sydney, September 1962. *The Australian Nurses' Journal*, Oct. 1962, p. 238-40.

ROYAL AUSTRALIAN NURSING FEDERATION
History of the Royal Australian Nursing Federation. *South Australian Journal of Nursing*, Sept. 1968, p. 11.

ROYAL COLLEGE OF NURSING AND NATIONAL COUNCIL OF NURSES OF THE UNITED KINGDOM

ROYAL COLLEGE OF NURSING AND NATIONAL COUNCIL OF NURSES OF THE UNITED KINGDOM
Charter and by-laws, 1963. The College, 1963.

ROYAL COLLEGE OF NURSING
Closing the gap between two worlds. An address given by Enoch Powell at the Royal College of Nursing Conference held in March 1963. *British Hospital Journal and Social Service Review*, Mar. 22, 1963, p. 334.

ROYAL COLLEGE OF NURSING AND NATIONAL COUNCIL OF NURSES OF THE UNITED KINGDOM
The College story. *Nursing Mirror*, April 5, 1963, p. 5-7.

ROYAL COLLEGE OF NURSING AND NATIONAL COUNCIL OF NURSES OF THE UNITED KINGDOM
The lamp and the book: the story of the Rcn 1916-1966, by Gerald Bowman. Queen Anne Press, 1967.

ROYAL COLLEGE OF NURSING AND NATIONAL COUNCIL OF NURSES OF THE UNITED KINGDOM
Past and present: a brief survey, by A. M. C. Thompson. The Library of Nursing, 1965.

ROYAL COLLEGE OF NURSING AND NATIONAL COUNCIL OF NURSES OF THE UNITED KINGDOM
Royal College of Nursing. Co-ordination within the Health Service—The Hospital Plan and its implications. *The Hospital*, April 1963, p. 221-4.

ROYAL COLLEGE OF NURSING AND NATIONAL COUNCIL OF NURSES OF THE UNITED KINGDOM
Fifty years of achievement. Golden Jubilee meetings: report and comment. *Nursing Mirror*, July 8, 1966, p. 335-40.

ROYAL COLLEGE OF NURSING AND NATIONAL COUNCIL OF NURSES OF THE UNITED KINGDOM
Rcn Golden Jubilee Supplement—This—is the college *Nursing Times*, June 24, 1966, p. 834-48.

ROYAL COLLEGE OF NURSING AND NATIONAL COUNCIL OF NURSES OF THE UNITED KINGDOM
The new voice of the Rcn. Report of first meeting of the Representative Body of the Rcn held in London, November 1967. *Nursing Mirror*, Nov. 10, 1967, p. 134-5.

ROYAL COLLEGE OF NURSING AND NATIONAL COUNCIL OF NURSES OF THE UNITED KINGDOM
Rcn Representative Body. Nurses look at the NHS. Report of a meeting held in London, 3rd and 4th November 1967. *Nursing Times*, Nov. 10, 1967, p. 1524-6.

ROYAL COLLEGE OF NURSING AND NATIONAL COUNCIL OF NURSES OF THE UNITED KINGDOM
Report of Annual General Meeting held in Harrogate, October 1969. Admission of SENs welcomed by Rcn. *Nursing Mirror*, Oct. 24, 1969, p. 9.

ROYAL COLLEGE OF NURSING AND NATIONAL COUNCIL OF NURSES OF THE UNITED KINGDOM
The story of the Royal College of Nursing Coat of Arms. *The Zambian Nurse*, Dec. 1966, p. 21-3.

ROYAL COLLEGE OF NURSING AND NATIONAL COUNCIL OF NURSES OF THE UNITED KINGDOM AND BRITISH MEDICAL ASSOCIATION
Responsibilities of nurses? *Nursing Times*, June 24, 1966, p. 823.

ROYAL COLLEGE OF NURSING AND NATIONAL COUNCIL OF NURSES OF THE UNITED KINGDOM
Words but not much action. Rcn Representative Body Meeting held in London, 16-17 October 1970. *Nursing Times*, Oct. 22, 1970, p. 1374-5.

SASKATCHEWAN REGISTERED NURSES' ASSOCIATION

SASKATCHEWAN REGISTERED NURSES' ASSOCIATION
Saskatchewan registered nurses' association: the first fifty years, by Marguerite E. Robinson. (Regina, Sask., The Association, 1967?).

SOUTH AFRICAN NURSES ASSOCIATION

SOUTH AFRICAN NURSING ASSOCIATION
Seventh biennial Congress, July 1970. *The Rhodesian Nurse*, Dec. 1970, p. 15-21.

SOUTH AFRICAN NURSING COUNCIL
The South African Nursing Council Silver Jubilee 1944-1969. *South African Nursing Journal*, Oct. 1969, p. 14-15.

TRAINED NURSES' ASSOCIATION OF INDIA

TRAINED NURSES ASSOCIATION OF INDIA
The TNAI and the nurse, by A. Surya Prakash Rao. *Nursing Journal of India*, Jan. 1970, p. 12.

NURSING JOURNALS

AMERICAN ASSOCIATION OF INDUSTRIAL NURSES JOURNAL
The history of the journal. *American Association of Industrial Nurses Journal*, Jan. 1966, p. 7-8.

NURSING MIRROR
Nursing Mirror through 75 years, by J. Elise Gordon. *Nursing Mirror*, Oct. 11, 1963, p. vi-viii and xiii.

Nursing Mirror through 75 years, by J. Elise Gordon. *Nursing Mirror*, Oct. 18, 1963, p. i-iii and x.

Nursing Mirror through 75 years, by J. Elise Gordon. *Nursing Mirror*, Oct. 25, 1963, p. v-vii.

Nursing Mirror through 75 years, by J. Elise Gordon. *Nursing Mirror*, Nov. 1, 1963, p. xi-xiii.

NURSING LEGISLATION

AMERICAN NURSES' ASSOCIATION
Bylaws, as amended May 1968. New York, The Association, 1968.

AMERICAN NURSES' ASSOCIATION
Conference on legislation, held in Washington, March 17-19, 1965; proceedings. New York, The Association, 1965.

AMERICAN NURSES' ASSOCIATION
Conference on legislation, held in Washington, March 15-17, 1967; proceedings. New York, The Association, 1967.

AMERICAN NURSES' ASSOCIATION
Legal aspects of nursing. New York, The Association, [1966?].
[A collection of reprints from *American Journal of Nursing* from Feb. 1962 to Nov. 1964.]

AMERICAN NURSES' ASSOCIATION
ECONOMIC SECURITY UNIT
Laws affecting nurses' economic security. New York, The Association, 1967.

BARBEE, G. C.
The legal basis of nursing. *Australian Nurses' Journal*, Dec. 1968, p. 279; Jan. 1969, p. 11-12.

BERNZWEIG, ELI P.
Liability for malpractice . . . its role in nursing education. *Journal of Nursing Education*, April 1969, p. 33-41.

BERNZWEIG, ELI P.
Nurse's liability for malpractice: a programmed course. New York, McGraw-Hill, 1969.

BOYLE, R.
Federal legislation: its impact on NLN's accrediting programs. *Nursing Outlook*, Mar. 1965, p. 34-9.

CHANDRA, J.
Medicolegal aspects of nursing care—nurse, patient and the law. *The Nursing Journal of India*, Oct. 1967, p. 253-6.

CREIGHTON, H.
The liability of the surgical nurse. Part 1. What is behind the increasing number of lawsuits? *Hospital Management*, Jan. 1965, p. 46-9, p. 46-9; Part 2, Feb. 1965. p. 70-3.

CROTIN, G. G.
Medicolegal problems *can* arise in the coronary care unit. *Canadian Nurse*, April 1969, p. 37-9.

DAS, D. M. H.
Legal implications in nursing. *Nursing Journal of India*, June 1970, p. 181-2 and 199.

DRISCOLL, J. R. M.
Medical legal responsibility of the nurse—1. *The Tasmanian Nurse*, Aug. 1969, p. 8-11.

DRISCOLL, J. R. M.
Medical legal responsibility of the nurse—2. *The Tasmanian Nurse*, Sept. 1969, p. 11 and 13-15.

EDE, L.
Legal relations in nursing. *Occupational Health Nursing*, Dec. 1969, p. 9-15.

GREAT BRITAIN. PARLIAMENT
Nurses' Act, 1964. H.M.S.O., 1964.

GREAT BRITAIN. PARLIAMENT
Nurses' Act, 1969. H.M.S.O., 1969.

GREAT BRITAIN. PARLIAMENT
Nurses' (Amendment) Act, 1961. H.M.S.O., 1961.

GREAT BRITAIN. PARLIAMENT
Teachers of Nursing Act, 1967. H.M.S.O., 1967.

GREAT BRITAIN. PARLIAMENT
Nurses and Midwives Act (Northern Ireland), 1970. Belfast. H.M.S.O., 1970.

HERSHEY, N.
Automation in patient care. The legal perspective. *American Journal of Nursing*, May 1967, p. 1037-9.

HERSHEY, N.
The law and the nurse. Medical records and the nurse—Part I. *American Journal of Nursing*, Feb. 1963, p. 110-2.

HERSHEY, N.
The law and the nurse. Medical records and the nurse—Part II. *American Journal of Nursing*, Mar. 1963, p. 94-7.

HERSHEY, N.
The law and the nurse. The surgeon was wrong. *American Journal of Nursing*, May 1970, p. 1063-4.

INTERNATIONAL COUNCIL OF NURSES
FLORENCE NIGHTINGALE INTERNATIONAL FOUNDATION
Principles of legislation for nursing education and practice: a guide to assist national nurses associations. Basel, Karger, 1969.

KUMAR, BISHNU
Legal aspects of nursing. *Nursing Journal of India*, Jan. 1970, p. 9-10 and 23.

THE LANCET
Should the nurse prescribe? *The Lancet*, April 6, 1963, p. 758-9.

LESNIK, MILTON J., *and* ANDERSON, BERNICE E.
Nursing practice and the law. 2nd. edn. Philadelphia, Lippincott, 1962.

NURSING MIRROR
The nurse's responsibilities in law. *Nursing Mirror*, Oct. 6, 1961, p. 5-6.

QUEEN'S INSTITUTE OF DISTRICT NURSING
SCOTTISH BRANCH
Scottish public health law: a digest for nurses, by H. E. Seiler and A. G. Mearns. Edinburgh, Livingstone, 1966.

ROYAL AUSTRALIAN NURSING FEDERATION *and*
NATIONAL FLORENCE NIGHTINGALE COMMITTEE OF AUSTRALIA
NATIONAL NURSING EDUCATION DIVISION
Teaching of the legal responsibility of the nurse. (Melbourne), The Federation, [1962].

SHAPIRO, F.
The LPN and the law. *Journal of Practical Nursing*, Oct. 1970, p. 24-5 and 52-4.

SPALDING, EUGENIA KENNEDY
Nursing legislation and education: a study of the role of national governments and voluntary nursing associations. Washington, Catholic University of America Press, 1963.

SPELLER, S. R.
Law notes for nurses . . . with supplement for Scotland by R. A. Bennett. 7th edn. Royal College of Nursing, 1970.

UNITED STATES PUBLIC HEALTH SERVICE
DIVISION OF NURSING
Nurse training act of 1964: program review report. Arlington, Virginia, U.S. Department of Health, Education and Welfare, 1967.
[Public health service publication, no. 1740.]

WATT, JAMES
Nurses and the law. Some comments on nurses' rights and responsibilities. *Nursing Times*, Feb. 13, 1969, p. 213-4.

ZARRAGA, M. G.
Medico-legal aspects of nursing practice. *The Philippine Journal of Nursing*, May-June 1964, p. 140-5.

SALARIES AND CONDITIONS OF WORK

ADAMSON, E. I. O.
Hours of duty and annual leave. *Nursing Times*, June 23, 1961, p. 814-5.

AMERICAN NURSES' ASSOCIATION
Collective bargaining: what is negotiable? *American Journal of Nursing*, Sept. 1969, p. 1891-5.

AMERICAN NURSES' ASSOCIATION
The role of the director of an organised nursing service in collective bargaining. *American Journal of Nursing*, Mar. 1970, p. 551-6.

AMERICAN NURSES' ASSOCIATION
RESEARCH AND STATISTICS UNIT
Survey of salaries and employment conditions in non-federal psychiatric hospitals, June 1965. New York, The Association, 1966.

AMERICAN NURSES' ASSOCIATION
RESEARCH AND STATISTICS UNIT
Survey of salaries and other employment conditions for teachers and administrators in nursing education programs, December 1965. New York, The Association, 1966.

AMERICAN NURSES' ASSOCIATION
RESEARCH AND STATISTICS UNIT
Survey of salaries and personnel practices in effect October 1960 for teachers and administrators in nursing educational programs. New York, The Association, 1961.

ASSOCIATION OF PROFESSIONAL NURSES OF THE PROVINCE OF QUEBEC
Who will bargain for Quebec's nurses? *Canadian Hospital*, Dec. 1964, p. 32-3.

AUSTRALIA. NEW SOUTH WALES
Public hospital nurses (state) award. *The Lamp*, Oct. 1967, p. 9-19.

CAMPBELL, N.
California nurses in revolt. *Hospital Topics*, Sept. 1966, p. 48-54.

CANADIAN HOSPITAL
Nursing salaries up 10 per cent in 1968 survey. *Canadian Hospital*, June 1969, p. 30-3.

CANADIAN NURSES' ASSOCIATION
Guidelines towards social and economic welfare. Ottawa, The Association, 1966.

CONLON, A. Y.
Bargaining rights for nurses. Convincing the legislature. *American Journal of Nursing*, Mar. 1966, p. 545-9.

COOK, F. P.
Background to negotiations. *Nursing Times*, May 24, 1968, Occasional papers, p. 81-4.

CORMICK, GERALD W.
The collective bargaining experience of Canadian registered nurses. Reprinted from *Labor Law Journal*, Oct. 1969, p. 667-82. Chicago, Commerce Clearing House, c. 1969.

CRISPO, J. H. G.
Collective bargaining and the professional. *Canadian Nurse*, Oct. 1963, p. 943-8.

DUNN, H. W.
Money and nursing. The nursing budget. *American Journal of Nursing*, Nov. 1963, p. M12-16.

EDWARDS, G.
Does the nursing profession need its own Members of Parliament? *Nursing Times*, Dec. 25, 1969, p. 1650-1.

ENG, E.
Better work schedules for nurses: four-week cycle raises morale, tightens supervision. *Hospitals*, Nov. 1, 1962, p. 64-7.

GINZBERG, E.
Money and nursing. The hospital and the nurse. *American Journal of Nursing*, Nov. 1963, p. M16-20.

HAWLEY, KAREN SUE
Economics of collective bargaining by nurses. Ames, Iowa, Industrial Relations Center, Iowa State University, 1967.

HENEMAN, H. G.
Collective bargaining. *American Journal of Nursing*, May 1968, p. 1039-42.

HILL, S. G.
Nurses and money. *Hospital and Social Service Journal*, Dec. 21, 1962, p. 1425.

INTERNATIONAL COUNCIL OF NURSES
Employment conditions of nurses in selected European countries 1964: report prepared by Mary E. Patten. The Council, 1965.

IU, SHEILA
Equal pay for equal work. [Hong Kong nurses campaign]. *The Hong Kong Nursing Journal*, Nov. 1970, p. 12-44.

JORDAN, C. H.
Where do nurse educators stand on the economic ladder? *American Journal of Nursing*, Aug. 1961, p. 70.

KELLY, DOROTHY N.
Equating the nurses' economic rewards with the service given. *American Journal of Nursing*, Aug. 1967, p. 1642-5.

KELLY, DOROTHY N.
Why economic security for nurses? New York, American Nurses' Association [1966].

KRUGER, D. H.
The changing roles of the hospital nurse and her economic status. *International Nursing Review*, vol. 10, no. 3, 1963, p. 44-8.

KRUSE, M.
A nurses' charter: halfway there. *International Nursing Review*, vol. 15, no. 3, 1968, p. 196-203.

KRUSE, M., and MUNCK, H.
Conditions of work of nurses in the northern European countries. *International Nursing Review*, vol. 12, no. 2, 1965, p. 50-4.

THE LANCET
Better use of nurses' time. *The Lancet*, Feb. 1, 1964, p. 257-8.

THE LANCET
The nurse's load. *The Lancet*, Aug. 28, 1965, p. 422.

LEWIS, E. P.
The New York City Hospital Story. An account of the disagreement between the New York City Council and the nursing staff of the City hospitals on their own working conditions and the welfare of patients. *American Journal of Nursing*, July 1966, p. 1526-35.

LEWIS, E. P.
The Bradenton story: a community crisis. Five nurses are fired in the course of a struggle for improved working conditions . . . and a sympathetic community is aroused to words and action. *American Journal of Nursing*, Oct. 1962, p. 58-63.

MAHONEY, A. B.
Bargaining rights for nurses. Convincing the membership. *American Journal of Nursing*, Mar. 1966, p. 544-8.

MEDICAL WORLD NEWSLETTER
Fair play for the nurses: a report on the pay dispute by the Medical Practitioners' Union. Medical Practitioners' Union, 1962.

MOSES, E. B.
Nursing's economic plight. *American Journal of Nursing*, Jan. 1965, p. 68-71.

NATIONAL ASSOCIATION OF STATE ENROLLED NURSES
Code of salaries, conditions of service, duties, responsibilities, ethical relationships, for State Enrolled Nurses employed in occupational health services. [The Association, 1969?]

NATIONAL BOARD FOR PRICES AND INCOMES
Pay of nurses and midwives in the National Health Service. H.M.S.O., 1968. [Report no. 60.]

NEW ZEALAND NURSING JOURNAL
Salaries and working conditions: nurses employed in public hospitals. *New Zealand Nursing Journal*, Jan. 1969, p. 5-18.

NURSING AS A PROFESSION

New Zealand Registered Nurses Association
R.N.A. makes momentous decision. *New Zealand Nursing Journal*, June 1964, p. 20-1.

New Zealand.
Special Committee of Cabinet
Report of the Lythgoe Committee. *New Zealand Nursing Journal*, Dec. 1964, p. 19-27.

Northern Nurses' Federation
Salary and employment conditions of nurses in the northern countries of Europe, July 1963. Oslo, The Federation, 1964.

Patten, M. K.
Better work schedules for nurses: shift rotation brings equality of working hours, more time off. *Hospitals*, Nov. 1 1962, p. 64, 74 and 77-8.

Pennsylvania Nurses' Association
Nurse employment conditions in Pennsylvania. The results of a survey made by the Pennsylvania Nurses' Association. *Pennsylvania Nurse*, Jan. 1967, p. 14-5.

Porter, E. K.
Money and nursing. Traditions and realities. *American Journal of Nursing*, Nov. 1963, p. M3-7.

Quinn, S. M.
Arbitration—its importance to the nursing profession. *Irish Nurse*, Aug. 1963, p. 5-10.

Quinn, S. M.
Raising the economic status of nurses: an international effort. *American Journal of Nursing*, Sept. 1966, p. 1990-4.

Registered Nurses Association of Ontario
Ontario nurses embrace collective bargaining. *Hospital Administration in Canada*, June 1964, p. 23-5.

Rogers, P. J.
Pay-as-you-eat. *Nursing Times*, Nov. 20, 1969, Occasional Papers, p. 193-6.

Rowsell, G.
Ups and downs of economic progress. *The Canadian Nurse*, Nov. 1967, p. 26-9.

Royal College of Nursing and National Council of Nurses of the United Kingdom
Comment by the Rcn Council on Report no. 60 of the National Board for Prices and Incomes. Rcn. 1968.

Ryan, J. R., *and* Boydston, G. D.
This flexible staffing plan puts nurses in right place at right time. *The Modern Hospital*, Sept. 1965, p. 114-7.

Seidman, J., *and others*
Professionals and economic security. *American Journal of Nursing*, Jan. 1965, p. 72-8.

Smith, F. E.
Internal night duty. *Nursing Times*, April 13, 1962, p. 464-5

Smith, P. M.
Influence of wage rates on nurse mobility. Chicago, Ill., Graduate program in hospital administration, University of Chicago, 1962.

Spencer, V.
The nurse and her employee labor relations. Part I. Unions are here to stay. *Hospital Management*, April 1964, p. 49-51; Part II. Problems that arise most frequently between the nurse and the union. May 1964, p. 44-8.

Sutherland, D.
Money and nursing. Money at the bedside. *American Journal of Nursing*, Nov. 1963, p. M7-12.

Trained Nurses' Association of India
First report of the economic welfare committee of the T.N.A.I., by G. P. Kapadia. *The Nursing Journal of India*, Jan. 1967, p. 11.

Trained Nurses' Association of India
Second report of the economic welfare committee of the T.N.A.I., by G. P. Kapadia. *The Nursing Journal of India*, Mar. 1967, p. 65-6.

Trained Nurses' Association of India
Third report of the economic welfare committee of the T.N.A.I., by G. P. Kapadia. *The Nursing Journal of India*, May 1967, p. 117-18.

Trained Nurses' Association of India
Fourth report of the economic welfare committee of the T.N.A.I., by G. P. Kapadia. *The Nursing Journal of India*, July 1967, p. 170-2.

Trained Nurses' Association of India
Fifth report of the economic welfare committee of the T.N.A.I., by G. P. Kapadia. *The Nursing Journal of India*, Sept. 1967, p. 227.

Trained Nurses' Association of India
Sixth report of the economic welfare committee of the T.N.A.I., by G. P. Kapadia. *The Nursing Journal of India*, Nov. 1967, p. 285.

United States
Bureau of Labour Statistics
How much nurses are paid. *American Journal of Nursing*, May 1961, p. 89-92.

Walmsley, P. Y.
Some comments on collective bargaining. *The Canadian Nurse*, Jan. 1966, p. 38-41.

Watkin, B.
Alternatives to Whitley. *Nursing Times*, July 10, 1969, Occasional Papers, p. 109-12.

Zimmerman, A.
Economic security in the decade ahead. *American Journal of Nursing*, Dec. 1962, p. 98-101.

HEALTH AND WELFARE

ACCOMMODATION

Carrington, M.
Living out and liking it. *Nursing Mirror*, Feb. 7, 1964, p. x-xii.

Great Britain. Ministry of Health
Accommodation for nursing staff. [H.M.S.O., 1961]. [Hospital Building Note no. 7.]

Great Britain. Ministry of Health
Accommodation for nursing staff. H.M.S.O., 1961. [Hospital Building Bulletin Series 2.]

Great Britain. Ministry of Health
Accommodation for nursing staff. H.M.S.O., 1963. [Hospital Equipment Note, no. 7.]

Great Britain. Ministry of Health
Residential accommodation for staff. H.M.S.O., 1964. [Hospital Building Note, no. 24.]

The Hospital
Design of nurses' homes. *The Hospital*, Sept. 1961, p. 559.

The Hospital
Torbay Hospital: a residential area for nursing staff. *The Hospital*, Jan. 1969, p. 22-4.

King Edward's Hospital Fund for London
Hospital Centre
Changing accommodation for non-resident staff. The Fund, [1965?].

London Hospital
Community life for nurses. A new concept for staff residence at The London Hospital, Whitechapel. *British Hospital and Social Service Journal*, Feb. 7, 1964, p. 176-7.

Malmi Hospital, Helsinki
Flats for nurses. *Nursing Mirror*, Jan. 4, 1963, p. v.

Marshall, D. G.
Building for nurses. [Nurses residences and a description of some Swiss examples]. *Nursing Times*, Aug. 14, 1969, p. 1035-7.

NETHER EDGE HOSPITAL, SHEFFIELD
Rented flats for nurses. *Nursing Mirror*, Oct. 13, 1967, p. 34-5.

NURSING TIMES
Students in residence. *Nursing Times*, Dec. 10, 1965, p. 1693

POSYNIAK, H.
Nursing residence at the Misericordia Hospital, Winnipeg. *Canadian Hospital*, Sept. 1963, p. 39-41.

ROYAL COLLEGE OF NURSING
WORKING PARTY ON SALARY STRUCTURE
Accommodation for nurses and midwives: a report of a study of accommodation provided for resident and non-resident nursing and midwifery staff in National Health Service hospitals in England, Scotland and Wales, 1959. The College, 1961.
[Studies in Nursing, no. 1.]

SICKNESS

BARR, A.
Absenteeism among hospital nursing staff. *The Hospital*, Jan. 1967, p. 9-12.

BARR, A.
Sickness absence among hospital nurses. Reprinted from *British Journal of Preventive and Social Medicine*, April 1960, p. 89-98. B.M.A., [1960].

BROWN, I. M.
Hospital staff health. *Occupational Health*, Jan./Feb. 1965, p. 4-9.

CHAI KEUM KIM
A study of health problems of student nurses. *The Korean Nurse*, vol. 5, no. 4, 1966, p. 44-6.

CHAMPAGNIE, L. E.
Nursing welfare—a review. *The Jamaican Nurse*, April/May 1969, p. 28.
[The activities of the Nursing Welfare Officer in the Ministry of Health in Jamaica.]

FLEWETT, T. H.
Virus diseases of the skin as occupational hazards to nurses. *Nursing Mirror*, Feb. 24, 1967, p. i-iii.

GARB, S.
Narcotic addiction in nurses and doctors. *Nursing Outlook*, Nov. 1965, p. 30-4.

GARLAND, T. O.
Care of hospital staff.
1. A neglected aspect of management.
Nursing Times, Feb. 16, 1968, p. 213-15.

GARLAND, T. O.
Care of hospital staff. A neglected aspect of management.
2. Student nurses.
Nursing Times, Feb. 23, 1968, p. 249-51.

GARLAND, T. O.
Care of hospital nursing staff. A neglected aspect of management.
3. Ward sisters.
Nursing Times, Mar. 1, 1968, p. 298-300.

GARLAND, T. O.
Care of hospital nursing staff. A neglected aspect of management.
4. Matrons and administrative sisters.
Nursing Times, Mar. 8, 1968, p. 328-9.

GINSBERG, F.
Where nurses err while handling radium. *The Modern Hospital*, Sept. 1962, p. 138.

GUNN, A. D. G.
Nurses' health. *Nursing Times*, Jan. 1, 1965, p. 7-8.

GUNN, A. D. G.
The sick nurse—so who cares? *Hospital World*, Nov. 1967, p. 1.

HAWARD, L. R. C.
Nursing and psychosis. *Nursing Mirror*, Feb. 24, 1961, p. 1903-4.

HEINEMANN, E., and OTHERS
Tuberculosis infection rates among nursing students. *Nursing Outlook*, Nov. 1962, p. 738-41.

HILLEBOE, H. E.
The mental and physical health of students of nursing. *Public Health Reports*, Sept. 1961, p. 737.

HOPKINS, T. D.
Sickness patterns of nursing staff. *Nursing Mirror*, April 16, 1965, p. 59-61.

MANOHARAN, A.
The health of nurses. *Berita Jururawat*, April 1967, p. 35-8.

MUNRO-ASHMAN, D.
Some aspects of dermatology. Contact dermatitis as a nursing hazard. *Nursing Times*, July 19, 1968, p. 974-6.

PORTER, I. A., and WILSON, J. S. P.
Staphylococcal infections treated with fusidic acid in nurses. *The Lancet*, Sept. 28, 1963, p. 658-9.

POUNDS, FRANCIS J.
The sick nurse: a ten-year review at King's College Hospital, London. The Hospital, 1964.
Part 11. A review of the years 1964-8, 1970.

ROSENTHAL, S. R., and others
BCG vaccination and tuberculosis in students of nursing. *American Journal of Nursing*, June 1963, p. 88-93.

THOMSON, W.
Some occupational hazards of nursing. *Nursing Times*, Nov. 26, 1970, p. 1526-8.

THURLOW, J.
Illness patterns in student nurses—a pilot project. Reprinted from the *Canadian Journal of Public Health*, Jan. 1967, p. 17-21.

TIMARU HOSPITAL, N.Z.
Smoking habits among student nurses at Timaru Public Hospital, 1962. *Nursing Gazette*, Mar. 1, 1963, p. 3.

TRICK, K.
Maintenance of nurse's mental health under stress. *Nursing Mirror*, Dec. 10, 1965, p. i-ii.

RECRUITMENT AND WASTAGE

ALLEN, V.
Getting and keeping nurses. *Nursing Mirror*, Dec. 8, 1961, p. v-vii.

ALLEN, V.
Getting and keeping nurses. *Nursing Mirror*, Dec. 15, 1961, p. iv-vi.

ALTSCHUL, A.
Tutors away. *Nursing Times*, Feb. 6, 1969, Occasional Papers, p. 21-4.

AMERICAN JOURNAL OF NURSING
Day care services help recruit nurses. *American Journal of Nursing*, Sept. 1963, p. 97-100.

AMERICAN NURSES' ASSOCIATION
Inventory of Professional Registered Nurses; Nation's Nurses. New York, The Association, 1965.

AMERICAN NURSES' ASSOCIATION
Statement on training for health occupations under the Manpower Development and Training Act of 1962. New York, the Association, 1962.

ANGUS, M. D.
Nursing shortage: a possible solution. Agencies should take steps to encourage the married nurse to return to the profession. *The Canadian Nurse*, June 1964, p. 563-5.

NURSING AS A PROFESSION

AULD, M. G.
An investigation into the recruitment and integration of part-time nursing staff in hospitals. *International Journal of Nursing Studies*, May 1967, p. 119-68.

AUSTRALASIAN NURSES' ASSOCIATION
Inquiry by the members of the Ward and Departmental Sisters' Group of Australasian Trained Nurses' Assn. into the difficulty of obtaining suitable sisters to work in hospital wards. *Australian Nurses' Journal*, Oct. 1969, p. 218-9.

AYDELOTTE, M. K., *and* HUDSON, W. R.
A socio-engineering problem—the nursing profession. The real measure of the "nursing shortage" is found in examining the length of time nurses devote to those activites which are in fact related to the patient's health and welfare. *Nursing Outlook*, Jan. 1962, p. 20-3.

BAIN, W.
Turnover of nursing and paramedical staff in 23 Ontario hospitals. *Canadian Hospital*, June 1969, p. 38-41.

BARKER, A. E., *and* STATON, E. E.
Inactive nurses. An untapped recruitment source. *Public Health Reports*, July 1965, p. 637-45.

BAYER, A. E.
Nurse supply: it's better than we thought. *The Modern Hospital*, July 1967, p. 75-9.

BENDALL, E. R. D.
Calculating wastage rates. *Nursing Times*, Sept. 29, 1967, p. 1300-1.

BENDALL, E. R. D.
A survey of wastage, sickness and allocation among student nurses, carried out by the School of Nursing, Hospital for Sick Children, Great Ormond Street, [1964].

BENDALL, E. R. D.
Wastage, sickness and allocation. A survey of student nurses. *Nursing Times*, June 4, 1965, p. 760-3.

BERNSTEIN, L., *and others*
Motivation for nursing. *Nursing Research*, Summer, 1965, p. 222-6.

BONHAM, A.
Day nursery for staff children. *British Hospital Journal and Social Service Review*, Aug. 16, 1968, p. 1508-9.

BOORER, D.
Nursery at Fulham Hospital. *Nursing Times*, Sept. 2, 1966, p. 1163-4.

BOORER, D.
Wanted—a rescue operation [shortages in nurses in special units could be overcome by Technical Nurse Flying Squads]. *Nursing Times*, May 7, 1970, p. 584-7.

BOURNE, M. W.
Recruitment of nursing staff at hospital level. *Nursing Times*, Jan. 14, 1966, p. 49-50.

BRITISH HOSPITAL JOURNAL AND SOCIAL SERVICE REVIEW
Attracting nurses. *British Hospital Journal and Social Service Review*, April 16, 1965, p. 689-91.

BRITISH HOSPITAL JOURNAL AND SOCIAL SERVICE REVIEW
Chertsey day nursery. *British Hospital Journal and Social Service Review*, April 3, 1970, p. 618-9.

BRUNCLIK, H. L., *and* THURSTON, J. R.
Nursing student attrition. *Nursing Outlook*, Nov. 1965, p. 57-9.

BURTON, R. A.
Nursing shortage: reality or illusion? *Hospital Topics*, Feb. 1967, p. 38-43.

CANADA. ROYAL COMMISSION ON HEALTH SERVICES
Sociological factors affecting recruitment into the nursing profession, by R. A. H. Robson. Ottawa, Queen's Printer, 1967.

CANADIAN HOSPITAL
Can hospitals curb high rate of nursing staff turnover? *Canadian Hospital*, Mar. 1970, p. 5.

CARPENTER, M. F.
Nursing—demands and supply. *International Nursing Review*, vol. 10, no. 2, 1963, p.29-32.

CARSON, RUTH
How we can get the nurses we need. New York, Public Affairs Committee, 1966.

CATANIA, J. J.
Why do nurses change jobs? *Hospital Management*, Aug. 1964, p. 93-4.

CHEW, D. C. E.
Wastage patterns in the nursing profession in Singapore: a study of manpower utilisation. *International Labour Review*, vol. 100, no. 6, 1969, p. 583-94.

CHEW, D. C. E.
Wastage patterns in the nursing profession in Singapore: a study of manpower utilisation. *International Nursing Review*, vol. 17, no. 4, 1970, p. 291-304 [reprint].

CLARK, B. F.
Solving the nurse shortage in Vermont. *JAMA*, Aug. 24, 1964, p. 643-4.

CLARK, D. F.
A survey of attitudes to nursing among comprehensive school pupils in Leicestershire. [The Author? 1967]
Note: Duplicated.

CLELAND, V., *and others*
Decision to reactivate nursing career. *Nursing Research*, Sept./Oct. 1970, p. 446-52.

CONGALTON, A. A., *and* SLOCUM, W. L.
Social characteristics of potential nurses. *Australian Nurses' Journal*, April, 1970, p. 70-5.

COOPER, S. S.
Activating the inactive nurse: a historical review. *Nursing Outlook*, Oct. 1967, p. 62-5.

COSTELLO, C. G.
Attitudes of nurses to nursing. *The Canadian Nurse*, June 1967, p. 42-4.

COULTER, P. P.
This I believe . . . about recruitment in an age of change. *Nursing Outlook*, April 1966, p. 31-3.

CROOKES, T. G., *and* FRENCH, J. G.
Intelligence and wastage of student mental nurses. *Occupational Psychology*, July 1961, p. 149.

CROSS, K. W.
Survey of student nurse wastage at 24 general nurse training schools [in the Birmingham region]. *International Journal of Nursing Studies*, Sept. 1968, p. 221-7.

CULLINAN, J.
Defining nursing shortage. *Nursing Times*, Aug. 12, 1966, p. 1059-60.

CULPAN, P.
Recruitment of the mature woman. *Nursing Times*, July 21, 1961, p. 926-7.

DALTON, B. M.
Withdrawal from training of RNMS student nurses. *Nursing Times*, Aug. 7, 1969, Occasional Papers, p. 125-8; *Nursing Times*, Aug. 14, 1969, Occasional Papers, p. 129-32.

DAN MASON NURSING RESEARCH COMMITTEE
Marriage and nursing: a survey of state registered and state enrolled nurses, by Gertrude A. Ramsden and Muriel H. Skeet. *The Committee*, 1967.

DARNELL, L. M.
Getting and keeping nurses. *Hospital and Social Service Journal*, Aug. 25, 1961, p. 1001-2.

DAVIES, R. P.
Selection for psychiatric nurse training. *Nursing Times,* June 21, 1968, Occasional Papers, p. 97-9.

DAVIS, A. E.
Hospital-operated nursery: project at Mount Sinai, Minneapolis, brings nurses back to work. *Hospital Topics,* Jan. 1966, p. 49-52, 57.

DAVIS, A. E.
Hospital-provided child care helps nurse-mothers return to work. *Hospital Topics,* Dec. 1965, p. 45-9.

DAVIS, ANNE J.
Self-concept, occupational role expectations, and occupational choice in nursing and social work. *Nursing Research,* Jan./Feb. 1969, p. 55-59.

DELORA, J. R., *and* MOSES, D. V.
Specialty preferences and characteristics of nursing students in baccalaureate programs. *Nursing Research,* Mar./April 1969, p. 137-44.

DOLAN, M. B.
More nurses, better nursing. *International Nursing Review,* vol. 17, no. 4, 1970, p. 337-45.

ELLIOTT, J. E.
ANA moves ahead to ease nurse shortage. *Empl. Serv. Rev.,* Nov. 1966, p. 13-43.

ENG, E.
A critical look at nursing service—why problems exist: how they can be solved. *Hospital Topics,* June 1963, p. 51-3.

FANNING, W. W.
Child-care nursery—one hospital's solution to nurse shortage. *Hospital Topics,* Dec. 1965, p. 51-3.

FERGUSON, V.
Come back to work! A review of what the nursing service administrator hopes the reactivated nurse will bring to the staff and patients. *Nursing Outlook,* Oct. 1970, p. 58-9.

FEYERHERM, A. M.
Nursing activity patterns: a guide to staffing. *Nursing Research,* Spring 1966, p. 124-33.

FINCHER, CAMERON
Nursing and paramedical personnel in Georgia: a survey of supply and demand. Atlanta, Georgia State College, 1962.

FLINT, R. T., *and* SPENSLEY, K. C.
Recent issues in nursing manpower: a review. *Nursing Research,* May/June 1969, p. 217-22.

FLITTER, HESSEL H.
Nursing in the South. Atlanta, Ga., Southern Regional Educational Board, 1968.

FORMAN, ALICE M.
Supply of nurses (in Turkey)
See
TAYLOR, CARL E., *and others.* Health manpower planning in Turkey, chapter 4. Baltimore, Johns Hopkins, 1968.

FULLER, D.
Bridging the gap. *Nursing Times,* June 25, 1965, p. 858-9.

GARVIN, M.
Why not a set of slides on nursing. *The Lamp,* Nov. 1969, p. 27-9.

GELMAN, S. J., *and* SMOLENS, J. B.
How to find nursing staff for 80,000 new beds. *The Modern Hospital,* June 1962, p. 96.

GENERAL NURSING COUNCIL FOR ENGLAND AND WALES
Student nurse wastage. *The Council,* 1966.

GINZBERG, E.
Nursing and manpower realities. *Nursing Outlook,* Nov. 1967, p. 26-9.

GISH, O.
Nursing and midwifery migration in Britain. *Nursing Times,* May 1, 1969, Occasional Papers, p. 69-72.

GOOD, S. R.
Considerations for nurse recruitment. *The Canadian Nurse,* Dec. 1967, p. 31-2.

GOODLAND, N. L.
Nurses from overseas. *Nursing Mirror,* June 4, 1965, p. 241-2.

GORDON, J. E.
Schoolgirl observers. A successful scheme for bridging the gap at Royal Cornwall Infirmary, Truro. *Nursing Mirror,* Aug. 28, 1964, p. vi-vii.

GRAYSON, G. A.
Small hospitals *can* attract and hold qualified nurses. *Hospitals,* April 16, 1969, p. 58-60.

GREAT BRITAIN. DEPARTMENT OF EMPLOYMENT AND PRODUCTIVITY
Guide to the regulations governing the entry of persons from overseas to training or employment in nursing and midwifery in Great Britain. The Department, 1970.

GREAT BRITAIN. MINISTRY OF LABOUR. NURSIN SERVICESG DIVISION
Training and employment of nurses from overseas. The Ministry, 1965.

GREAT BRITAIN. STUDENT NURSES' ASSOCIATION
Night duty during nurse training. *Nursing Times,* Aug. 14, 1964, p. 1058-9.

HALE, T.
Why the nursing shortage persists. *Hospital Topics,* Oct. 1964, p. 27-9.

HALL, J.
How not to obtain student nurses. *Nursing Times,* Oct. 1, 1970, Occasional Papers, p. 145-8; Oct. 8, 1970, Occasional Papers, p. 149-50; Oct. 29, 1970, Occasional Papers, p. 164.

HAMILTON, T. STEWART
Three ways to close the gap in nursing. *The Modern Hospital,* June 1961, p. 75.

HART, F.
Crisis in nursing. *British Hospital Journal and Social Service Review,* Oct. 31, 1969, p. 2030.

HEALEY, J. P.
Some causes of student nurse wastage. *Nursing Mirror,* Aug. 8, 1969, p. 10-11.

HILL, L. L., *and others*
Is there correlation between attrition in nursing schools and job turnover in professional nursing? *Nursing Outlook,* Sept. 1963, p. 666-9.

HILL, R. D.
Problems in providing nursing services. *International Nursing Review,* vol. 8, no. 6, 1961, p. 29-37.

HUME, B., *and* NORTH, N.
Welcoming married women back to nursing. *Nursing Times,* June 14, 1968, p. 786-8.

HUTTY, H. E.
Wastage. *Nursing Times,* May 8, 1964, p. 603-4.

ILLINOIS STUDY COMMISSION ON NURSING
Report of a 1966-1968 project to assess Illinois' nursing resources and needs, present and projected to 1980, and develop a program of action to meet the state's needs for nursing services, sponsored by the Illinois League for Nursing and the Illinois Nurses' Association [Chicago, Illinois League for Nursing], 1968.

JAMAICAN NURSE
What happens to Jamaica's trained nurses? *Jamaican Nurse,* Dec. 1964, p. 8-9.

JAMES, D.
Student nurse selection 1. *Nursing Times,* Aug. 4, 1967, p. 1023-6.

JAMES, D.
Student nurse selection. 2. Examinations and intelligence tests. *Nursing Times*, Aug. 11, 1967, p. 1070-1.

JAMES, D.
Student nurse selection. 3. Interviews and references. *Nursing Times*, Aug. 18, 1967, p. 1108-10.

JAMES, D.
Student nurse selection. 4. Selection in the future. *Nursing Times*, Aug. 25, 1967, p. 1131-2.

JAYAWARDENA, Y.
Launching of wastage survey. *Australian Nurses' Journal*, April 1969, p. 83-6.

JOINT COMMITTEE TO STUDY NURSING NEEDS AND RESOURCES IN ARIZONA
Interim report. Part 1. *Ariz. Nurse*, Nov./Dec. 1965, p. 23-38.

JOINT COMMITTEE TO STUDY NURSING NEEDS AND RESOURCES IN ARIZONA
Interim report. Part 2. *Ariz. Nurse*, May/June 1966, p. 14-22.

JONES, K.
Meeting the nursing shortage. Some practical answers. *International Nursing Review*, vol. 15, no. 3, 1968, p. 205-14.

JONES, R. E.
Personality, morale and rapid turnover among nurses. *Journal of Psychiatric Nursing*, July/Aug. 1970, p. 7-9.

KANSAS HEALTH FACILITIES INFORMATION SERVICE, INC.
Study of nursing needs and goals in Kansas through 1975. Topeka, Kans., The Service, 1965.

KEIDAN, O., and JONES, C.
Are married nurses dropouts? *Nursing Times*, May 21, 1970, Occasional Papers, p. 69-72.

KEMP, E., and PEITCHINIS, J.
Nurses' attitudes: fact or fallacy? *The Canadian Nurse*, Feb. 1968, p. 51-4.

KIBRICK, A. K.
Drop outs in schools of nursing: the effect of self and role perception. *Nursing Research*, Summer 1963, p. 140-9.

KING EDWARD'S HOSPITAL FUND FOR LONDON
Brochures for schools of nursing: report of an enquiry by the Hospital Centre. *The Fund*, 1965.

KING EDWARD'S HOSPITAL FUND FOR LONDON
HOSPITAL CENTRE
Nursing manpower. Report of a conference held at the Hospital Centre, June 1968. *British Hospital Journal and Social Service Review*, July 5, 1968, p. 1238-9.

KING EDWARD'S HOSPITAL FUND FOR LONDON
HOSPITAL CENTRE
Recruitment of student and pupil nurses. *Nursing Times*, June 14, 1968, Occasional Papers, p. 93-6.

KING EDWARD'S HOSPITAL FUND FOR LONDON and ROYAL COLLEGE OF NURSING AND NATIONAL COUNCIL OF NURSES OF THE UNITED KINGDOM
Factors affecting recruitment of nurse tutors: a survey carried out on behalf of the King's Fund and the Rcn by Ann Dutton. K.E.H.F., 1968.

KNIGHT, J. E.
Recruitment and wastage of nursing staff 1. *Nursing Times*, Nov. 5, 1965, p. 1502-3.

KNIGHT, J. E.
Recruitment and wastage of nursing staff 2. Who comes, stays or goes? *Nursing Times*, Nov. 12, 1965, p. 1540-2.

KNIGHT, J. E.
Recruitment and wastage of nursing staff 3. Summing up. *Nursing Times*, Nov. 19, 1965, p. 1572-4.

LAMBERTSEN, E. C.
Nurse staffing woes are only symptoms of a deeper problem. *Modern Hospital*, Nov. 1966, p. 146-8.

LAMBERTSEN, E. C.
Shortages of other specialists may be hidden in nurse shortage. *Modern Hospital*, Oct. 1969, p. 136.

THE LAMP
A rationalisation of student nurse intake. *The Lamp*, Jan. 1969, p. 13-4.

LAURIE, M.
The cost of error in student nurse recruitment. *Nursing Times*, Aug. 4, 1967, p. 1021-2.

LAWRENCE, J. G.
Attitudes to nursing among intelligent schoolgirls. [A survey made among schoolgirls in the West Riding of Yorks.] *British Medical Journal*, Oct. 17, 1964, p. 1001-3.

LAWSON, J. S.
Who will nurse in the seventies? A study of the nursing services in Victorian hospitals. *UNA Nursing Journal*, June 1969, p. 12-7, 20-2.

LAWTON, U.
Why nurses abandon the profession. *Nursing Times*, Aug. 6, 1970, p. 1022-3.

LESPARRE, MICHAEL
Retired nurses return to nursing. *Hospitals*, July 1, 1966, p. 46-50.

LEVINE, EUGENE
Some answers to the "nurse shortage". *Nursing Outlook*, March 1964, p. 30-4.

LEVINE, EUGENE
Nurse manpower: yesterday, today, and tomorrow. *American Journal of Nursing*, Feb. 1969, p. 290-6.

LUKENS, L. G.
Personality patterns and choice of clinical nursing specialization. *Nursing Research*, Summer 1965, p.210-21.

LYONS, T. F.
Reducing nursing turnover: social psychological research identifies factors affecting nursing turnover and suggests implications for administrators. *Hospitals*, Oct. 16, 1970, p. 74, 76-8.

LYONS, T. F.
Research shows lack of supervisor influence in nursing turnover patterns. *Hospitals*, Oct. 16, 1970, p. 78-80.

McCARRICK, H.
Minding the baby. *Nursing Times*, Oct. 13, 1967, p. 1365-7.

McEWAN, R.
An experience in selection—the person for the job.... *New Zealand Nursing Journal*, Nov. 1963, p. 8-9, 11-4.

McGREGOR, G.
The realities of staffing. *The American Journal of Nursing*, Nov. 1962, p. 56-63.

MACGUIRE, JILLIAN
Attrition from nursing training, 1 and 2. *International Nursing Review*, vol. 17, no. 1, 1970, p. 33-42; vol. 17, no. 2, 1970, p. 135-43.

MACGUIRE, JILLIAN
Research findings on recruitment and withdrawal. *Nursing Times*, Feb. 20, 1969, Occasional Papers, p. 29-31; Feb. 27, 1969, Occasional Papers, p. 33-6.

MACGUIRE, JILLIAN
Threshold to nursing: a review of the literature on recruitment to and withdrawal from nurse training programmes in the United Kingdom. Bell, 1969. (Occasional papers on social administration, no. 30.)

McKAY, J.
Selection of student nurses [Recruitment of nurses in Barbados]. *Barbados Nursing Journal*, April/May 1968, p. 12.

MALONE, M. F.
The dilemma of a professional in a bureaucracy. *Nursing Forum*, vol. III, no. 4, 1964, p. 36-60.

MARLOW, H. L.
Registered nurse and employee needs. *Nursing Outlook*, Nov. 1966, p. 62-5.

MARRAM, GWEN D.
An untapped source of registered nurses. [Foreign nurses in the U.S.] *Nursing Outlook*, July 1969, p. 48-9.

MARSH, DAVID C., *and* WILLCOCKS, ARTHUR J.
Focus on nurse recruitment: a snapshot from the provinces. Oxford University Press (for Nuffield Provincial Hospitals Trust), 1965.

MARSHALL, MELODY J., *and* BRUHN, J. G.
Refresher courses and the reactivation of nurses. *Nursing Outlook*, Jan. 1967, p. 59-61.

MAYES, N., *and others*
Commitment to nursing—how is it achieved? *Nursing Outlook*, July 1968, p. 29-31.

MELBIN, MURRAY, *and* TAUB, DORIS L.
High cost of replacing a nurse. *Hospitals*, Oct. 16, 1966, p. 112, 114, 117-8, 120, 122.

MEYER, MARY ARTHUR
Recruiting, selecting, retaining faculty. *Nursing Outlook*, Aug. 1962, p. 511-3.

MICHIGAN LEAGUE FOR NURSING AND MICHIGAN NURSES' ASSOCIATION
Nursing needs and resources in Michigan—to-day and tomorrow. Detroit, Mich., Cunningham Drug Company Foundation, 1966.

MINNESOTA BOARD OF NURSING
Nursing in Minnesota; a statistical review. St. Paul, Minn., The Board, 1967.

MITCHEL, MONROE
Recruiting nurses for long-term care. *Hospitals*, Nov. 1, 1965, p. 45-7.

MORGAN, B.
Bridge that gap. *Nursing Times*, April 14, 1967, p. 481-3.

NASH, MARY K.
Turnover of psychiatric staff nurses. *Nursing Outlook*, Aug. 1966, p. 29-30.

NATIONAL LEAGUE FOR NURSING
MEASUREMENT AND EVALUATION SERVICES
Let's examine attrition rates in schools of nursing. *Nursing Outlook*, Sept. 1970, p. 58.

NATIONAL UNION OF PUBLIC EMPLOYEES
Memorandum on nursing staff shortages. *The Union*, 1964.

NEW SOUTHGATE HOSPITAL MANAGEMENT COMMITTEE
Employment and wastage of nursing staff at a psychiatric hospital. *The Hospital*, Oct. 1965, p. 531-3.

NEW YORK STATE UNIVERSITY, STATE EDUCATION DEPARTMENT
Survey of registered professional nurses employed in hospitals in New York State. Albany, N.Y., State Education Department, 1965.

NORWOOD, R.
Sound advertising: the key to nurse recruitment. *Nursing Times*, Oct. 7, 1966, p. 1326-8.

OLLERENSHAW, K.
Changes in education: their effects on nurse recruitment. *Nursing Times*, Nov. 9, 1962, p. 1436-8.

PAYNE, G. O.
Need for re-appraisal in recruitment of student nurses. *Nigerian Nurse*, July 1970, p. 11-2.

PEIMER, S. C., *and others*
Experiment in retraining unemployed men for practical nursing careers. *Hospitals*, Oct. 16, 1966, p. 87-90, 164.

PLATOU, C. N., *and* PEDERSOM, W. D.
Can more part-time nurses be recruited? *Hospitals*, May 16, 1967, p. 77-8, and 82.

RAYNES, N. V.
Cadet courses as a means of recruitment to mental nursing. *Nursing Times*, Nov. 8, 1963, p. 1429-30.

REDMAN, B. K.
Nursing teacher perceptiveness of student attitudes. *Nursing Research*, Jan./Feb. 1968, p. 59-64.

REESE, DOROTHY E., *and others*
How many caps went on again? *Nursing Outlook*, Aug. 1962, p. 517-9.

REINKEMEYER, AGNES M.
It won't be hospital nursing! [Career plans of students taking university-associated nursing courses in Gt. Britain compared with the situation in the U.S.] *American Journal of Nursing*, Sept. 1968, p. 1936-40.

REVANS, R. W.
Hospital internal communications. Keeping the recruits. *British Hospital Journal and Social Service Review*, Aug. 28, 1965, p. 1583-4.

REVANS, R. W.
The measurement of supervisory attitudes. Manchester Statistical Society, 1961.

REVANS, R. W.
Standards for morale: cause and effect in hospitals. Oxford University Press (for Nuffield P.H.T.), 1964.

ROBSON, R. A. H.
Sociological factors affecting recruitment into the nursing profession. Ottawa, Queen's Printer, 1967. [Royal Commission on Health Services Study.]

ROTTKAMP, B. C.
Attrition rates in basic baccalaureate nursing programs. *Nursing Outlook*, June 1968, p. 44-7.

ROWE, H. R., *and* FLITTER, H. H.
Junior colleges hold their nursing students. *Nursing Outlook*, Feb. 1967, p. 35-7.

ROYAL AUSTRALIAN NURSING FEDERATION AND NATIONAL FLORENCE NIGHTINGALE COMMITTEE OF AUSTRALIA. NATIONAL NURSING EDUCATION DIVISION
Launching of wastage study report. *UNA Nursing Journal*, Feb. 1969, p. 2-6.

ROYAL AUSTRALIAN NURSING FEDERATION AND NATIONAL FLORENCE NIGHTINGALE COMMITTEE OF AUSTRALIA. NATIONAL NURSING EDUCATION DIVISION
Some information on the current wastage survey. *UNA Nursing Journal*, April/May 1964, p. 128-30.

ROYAL AUSTRALIAN NURSING FEDERATION AND NATIONAL FLORENCE NIGHTINGALE COMMITTEE OF AUSTRALIA. NATIONAL NURSING EDUCATION DIVISION
Survey report on the wastage of general trained nurses from nursing in Australia. Nov. 1960-Nov. 1967. Melbourne, Royal Australian Nursing Federation, 1969.

ROYAL COLLEGE OF NURSING AND NATIONAL COUNCIL OF NURSES OF THE UNITED KINGDOM. NURSE ADMINISTRATORS' SECTION
Day nurseries in hospitals for children of hospital staff. *The College* (1969?).

ROYAL COLLEGE OF NURSING AND NATIONAL COUNCIL OF NURSES OF THE UNITED KINGDOM. SCOTTISH BOARD, *et al.*
The problem of recruiting and retaining registered nurse tutors in the hospital service. Edinburgh, The College, 1965.

ROYAL MEDICO PSYCHOLOGICAL ASSOCIATION
Report of an investigation into recruitment and training of nursing staff of in-patient units for children and adolescents. The Association, 1970.

SALEH, S. D., *and others*
Why nurses leave their jobs: an analysis of female turnover. *Personnel Administration*, Jan./Feb. 1965, p. 25-8.

SCHLOTFELDT, R. M., *and* MCPHAIL, J.
An experiment in nursing: introducing planned change. *American Journal of Nursing*, June 1969, p. 1247-51.

SCHNEIDER, M.
Day nursery for staff's children helps New York City Hospital keep nurses. *The Modern Hospital*, Nov. 1964, p. 37-8.

SCHOENFELD, H.
"Hospitalers" relieve nursing shortage during critical periods. A New Jersey hospital solved its problem of personnel shortage in the nursing service department by establishing a new group of personnel... *Hospitals*, June 16, 1967, p. 54-6.

SCOTTISH HOME AND HEALTH DEPARTMENT
Student nurses in Scotland: characteristics of success and failure, by Margaret Scott Wright. Edinburgh, The Department, 1968. [Scottish Health Services Studies, no. 7.]

SEIVWRIGHT, M.
Project report on factors affecting mass migration of Jamaican nurses to the U.S. *The Jamaican Nurse*, Aug. 1965, p. 8-12.

SEN, AMYA
Problems of overseas students and nurses. National Foundation for Educational Research, 1970.

SIMPSON, H. M.
Satisfaction and dissatisfaction of student life. *International Nursing Review*, vol. 15, no. 4, October 1968, p. 329-36.

SPENCER, C. S., and MELE, F. M.
A community approach to nursing manpower. *Nursing Outlook*, Feb. 1969, p. 28-30.

STAHL, ADELE G.
Manpower development and training act; concerns for nursing. *American Journal of Nursing*, June 1964, p. 112-5.

STEVENS, B.
A new image for Florence Nightingale? *Industrial Society*, Oct. 1970, p. 12-4.

STEVENS, B. C., and FOSTER, JOANNA
Report on the selection and training of nurses at a hospital. Industrial Society [1969].

STREET, M. M
Staffing problems in nursing service. *The Canadian Nurse*, Feb. 1965, p. 91-3.

SYLVESTER, D. G. H.
A study of student nurse wastage. *Nursing Mirror*, Feb. 28, 1969, p. 37-8.

TABLER, M.
Welcome back to nursing. *Nursing Outlook*, Sept. 1965, p. 67-8.

TATE, BARBARA L.
Attrition rates in schools of nursing. *Nursing Research*, Spring 1961, p. 91-6.

TAYLOR, CALVIN W., and others
Selection and recruitment of nurses and nursing students: a review of research studies and practices by Calvin W. Taylor, Helen Nahm, Lorraine Loy, Mary Harms, Jeanne Berthold and John W. Wolfer. University of Utah Press, [1963].

TAYLOR, J. K., and RICHTER, F. S.
What motivates students into nursing? *Hospitals*, Jan. 1969, p. 59-61.

TEMPLETON, R. J.
Nurse recruitment. *Nursing Times*, Feb. 17, 1967, p. 209-10.

THURSTON, JOHN R., and others
Comprehensive manual for use with the Luther Hospital sentence completions, nursing sentence completions, nurse attitudes inventory, forms I and II, empathy inventory by John R. Thurston, Helen L. Brunclik and John F. Feldhusen. Eau Claire, Wisconsin, Nursing Research Associates, 1970.

THURSTON, JOHN R., and BRUNCLIK, HELEN L.
Luther Hospital sentence completions and nursing sentence completions. Wisconsin, Luther Hospital, 1965.

THURSTON, JOHN R., and BRUNCLIK, HELEN L.
Nurse attitudes inventory. Luther Hospital Research Project, Eau Claire, Wisconsin, 1965.

THURSTON, JOHN R. and others
The prediction of success in nursing education: a manual for the Luther Hospital Sentence Completions and the Nursing Sentence Completions. Phase I-II, 1959-67; Phase III, 1967-68, by John R. Thurston, Helen L. Brunclik and John F. Feldhusen. [Eau Claire, Wis., the Hospital, 1967-8.]

TIMS, N. S.
Competing for those eligible school-leavers. *The Hospital*, Sept. 1970, p. 301-3.

TOMPKINS, S.
A hard day's night [student nurse wastage]. *Industrial Society*, Oct. 1970, p. 15.

TORONTO. COMMITTEE FOR SURVEY OF HOSPITAL NEEDS IN METROPOLITAN TORONTO
Education and the provision of personnel: part sixteen of the study of the Committee. Toronto, The Committee, 1963.

TRINIDAD AND TOBAGO. MINISTRY OF HEALTH
Report on a quantitative and qualitative survey of nursing needs and resources. Trinidad, Government Printery, 1968.

UNITED KINGDOM COUNCIL FOR OVERSEAS STUDENT AFFAIRS
At home in London: report on a course for student nurses from overseas. The Council, [1970?].

U.S. NATIONAL CENTER FOR HEALTH STATISTICS
Employees in nursing and personal care homes, United States, May/June 1964. (Vital and Health Statistics, Series 12, no. 5) Washington, D.C., U.S. Government Printing Office, 1966.

U.S. PUBLIC HEALTH SERVICE
Health Manpower Source Book. Washington, D.C., U.S. Government Printing Office, 1963.

U.S. PUBLIC HEALTH SERVICE
Refresher programs for inactive professional nurses; a guide for developing courses for study. Washington, D.C., U.S. Government Printing Office, 1967.

U.S. PUBLIC HEALTH SERVICE, HEALTH MANPOWER BUREAU and THE AMERICAN HOSPITAL ASSOCIATION
Health Manpower Perspectives, 1967. Washington, D.C., U.S. Government Printing Office, 1967.

U.S. PUBLIC HEALTH SERVICE, HEALTH MANPOWER BUREAU and THE AMERICAN HOSPITAL ASSOCIATION
Manpower Resources in Hospitals, 1966. Chicago, Ill., American Hospital Association, 1966.

VAZ, D.
High school senior boys' attitudes toward nursing as a career. *Nursing Research*, Nov./Dec. 1968, p. 533-8.

WALLACE, M. B.
The nursing shortage. *Canadian Hospital*, Jan. 1964, p. 63-4, 78.

WALSH, S.
Finding prospective students. Realism seems the most effective approach in Gt. Britain. *The American Journal of Nursing*, May 1963, p. 123-4.

WARK, I. W.
Nurse wastage survey report. *Journal of the West Australian Nurses*, April 1969, p. 6-7.

WARK, I. W.
Survey report on the wastage of general trained nurses from nursing in Australia. *Queensland Nurses' Journal*, April 1969, p. 11, 13.

WEISS, O.
Motivation to enter nursing: eligible applicants to nursing schools in Israel—1968. *International Journal of Nursing Studies*, Aug. 1970, p. 135-49.

WELBROCK-SMITH, J.
Study days for trained nurses. An account of a successful experiment which is "bringing back the nurses" in the Oxford Region. *Nursing Mirror*, Dec. 22, 1961, p. xi-xii.

WHITE, J. H.
Some attitudes of South African nurses—a cross-cultural study. *Journal of Social Psychology*, vol. 69, 1966, p. 13-26.

WHITE, K. C.
Nurse training and recruitment. *The Hospital*, Oct. 1962, p. 677-9.

WHITTINGTON HOSPITAL
An analysis of the progress of student nurses entering training at Whittington Hospital since May 1960. *The Hospital* [1966?]

WIELAND, GEORGE F.
Studying and measuring nursing turnover. *International Journal of Nursing Studies*, July 1969, p. 61-9.

WILBUR, D. L.
Total manpower needs and resources—medicine and nursing. *Nursing Outlook*, Dec. 1969, p. 32-5.

WILBUR, MURIEL B., *and others*
Nursing needs and resources—a challenge to Rhode Island. *Rhode Island Medical Journal*, July 1965, p. 363.

WILSON, C. T., *and* HARRISON, S. E.
Recruitment, are we going about it the right way? *Nursing Times*, Aug. 27, 1970, Occasional Papers, p. 125-27.

WOLFE, H., *and* YOUNG, J. P.
Staffing the nursing unit.
Part 1. Controlled variable staffing.
Nursing Research, Summer, 1965, p. 236-43.
Part 2. Multiple assignment technique.
Nursing Research, Fall 1965, p. 299-303.

WRIGHT, MARGARET SCOTT
A study of the characteristics of successful and unsuccessful student nurses in Scotland up to the time of completing the Preliminary State examination of the General Nursing Council for Scotland. Edinburgh University, 1961. [Report of project as Boots Research Fellow in nursing.]

WURM, R.
The nursing crisis in hospitals. *Journal of the West Australian Nurses*, July 1970, p. 19-22.

YETT, DONALD E.
Nursing shortage and the nurse training act. *Hospital Topics*, June 1966, p. 28-31.

YETT, DONALD E.
The supply of nurses: an economist's view. Reprinted from *Hospital Progress*, Feb. 1965.

PART-TIME STAFF

ALLEN, V.
The successful use of part-time nurses. Staffing geriatric wards of a busy general hospital. *Nursing Mirror*, Sept. 15, 1961, p. 1557-9.

BENNETT, B. A.
Part-time nursing employment in Gt. Britain. *International Labour Review*, April 1962, p. 347-56.

CARR, A. J.
The part-time nurse's dilemma. *Nursing Times*, Nov. 25, 1966, p. 1544-6.

DE LA COURT, L. C.
The successful use of part-time nurses. Ten-year-old scheme at Queen Alexandra Hospital, Cosham. *Nursing Mirror*, Sept. 8, 1961, p. 1538-40.

HEWES, A.
Women part-time workers in the United States. *International Labour Review*, Nov. 1962, p. 443-52.

HODKINSON, M. A.
The successful use of part-time nurses. Pairing off part-timers (and full-time staff). *Nursing Mirror*, Aug. 25, 1961, p. 1488-90.

HOLLAND, S.
The successful use of part-time nurses. *Nursing Mirror*, Aug. 18, 1961, p. 1470-2.

HORSMAN, H. M.
Successful use of part-time nurses. *Nursing Mirror*, Jan. 19, 1962, p. 312-4.

HUGHES, W.
Successful use of part-time nurses. *Nursing Mirror*, Mar. 2, 1962, p. 433-4.

JACOBS, J.
Successful use of part-time nurses. *Nursing Mirror*, Jan. 26, 1962, p. 335-6.

JOHNSTON, M. D.
The part-time married nurse in hospital. *Nursing Times*, Sept. 8, 1967, p. 1215.

LIVESEY, A.
Successful use of part-time nurses. *Nursing Mirror*, Jan. 5, 1962, p. 257-9.

LYLE, M. R.
Successful use of part-time nurses. *Nursing Mirror*, Feb. 9, 1962, p. 371-4.

MCCALL, M. B.
Successful use of part-time nurses. *Nursing Mirror*, Feb. 2, 1962, p. 352-4.

MELVIN, J.
Part-time nursing. *Nursing Times*, June 24, 1966, p. 856.

PLATOU, C. N., *and* PEDERSON, W. D.
Can more part-time nurses be recruited? *Hospitals*, May 16, 1967, p. 77-81.

TAYLOR, M.
Successful use of part-time nurses. *Nursing Mirror*, Jan. 12, 1962, p. 283-5.

WALTON, A. M.
The successful use of part-time nurses. *Nursing Mirror*, Aug. 11, 1961, p. 1447-8.

WORMALD, E. G.
The successful use of part-time nurses. *Nursing Mirror*, Aug. 4, 1961, p. 1425-7.

APTITUDE AND PERSONALITY TESTS

BANNISTER, D., *and others*
The use of cognitive tests in nursing candidate selection. *Occupational Psychology*, Jan. and April, 1962, p. 75-8.

BENNETT, K., *and others*
Centralisation of applications for nurse training. *Nursing Times*, Sept. 4, 1969, Occasional Papers, p. 141-3; Sept. 11, 1969, Occasional Papers, p. 145-8.

CAMERON, F. J.
The selection of students for nursing. *The New Zealand Nursing Journal*, Aug. 1963, p. 4-5.

CORDINER, C. M.
Personality testing of Aberdeen student nurses. *Nursing Times*, Feb. 9, 1968, p. 178-80.

FRISBY, C. B.
The use of cognitive tests in nursing candidate selection: a comment. *Occupational Psychology*, Jan. and April 1962, p. 79-81.

GERSTEIN, A. I.
Development of a selection program for nursing candidates. *Nursing Research*, Summer 1965, p. 254-7.

GRUBER, EDWARD C.
Nursing school entrance examination. [4th edn.] New York, Arco Publishing Co., 1964 (reprinted 1965).

MCEWAN, R.
An experience in selection—the person for the job. *New Zealand Nursing Journal*, Nov. 1963, p. 8-9, 11-4.

MILLIOTT, H. L.
Selection of student nurses: a review of some studies relating to the selection of the general nursing student. Melbourne, Royal Australian Nursing Federation, 1963.

NATIONAL LEAGUE FOR NURSING
The use of tests in schools of nursing: the NLN achievement tests. 3rd edn. New York, The League, 1964.

PEARSON, P.
Selection at the pre-nursing stage. *Nursing Times*, Feb. 9, 1968, p. 188-9.

PSATHAS, G., and PLAPP, J.
Assessing the effects of a nursing program: a problem in design. *Nursing Research*, July/Aug. 1968, p. 336-42.

RYBACK, D.
A critical incident simulation technique for nurse selection. *International Journal of Nursing Studies*, May 1967, p. 81-9.

SMELTZER, C. H.
The interview in student nurse selection. New York, Putnam, 1968.

TATE, BARBARA L.
A method for rating the proficiency of the hospital staff nurse: manual of directions. New York, National League for Nursing, 1964.

THOMAS, M. J., and WEINSTEIN, A. S.
Comparisons of test scores in psychiatric nursing. *Nursing Outlook*, May 1965, p. 38-41.

EDUCATION AND TRAINING

BASIC TRAINING—GENERAL WORKS

ABRAMOVITZ, A. B., and BURNHAM, ELAINE
Self-understanding in professional education: a pilot project in schools of nursing in Wisconsin. Madison, Wisconsin State Board of Health [1965?].

AHAD, M. A.
Nursing education in India. *International Nursing Review*, vol. 17, no. 3, 1970, p. 224-37.

ALABAMA BOARD OF NURSING
Assessment of nursing education in Alabama, 1968. Margaret J. Koehler, study director. Montgomery, Ala., The Board [1968?].

ALBERTA NURSING EDUCATION SURVEY COMMITTEE
Report of nursing education survey committee province of Alberta 1961-63. Edmonton, Queen's Printer, 1963.

ALBERTA UNIVERSITY COMMITTEE ON NURSING EDUCATION
Survey of the schools of nursing in the province of Alberta. Edmonton, The University, 1963.

AMERICAN HOSPITAL ASSOCIATION
The nursing department's function in formalized educational programs. *Practical Approaches to Nursing Service Administration*, Summer 1969, p. 1-4.

AMERICAN JOURNAL OF NURSING COMPANY, EDUCATIONAL SERVICES DIVISION
The national survey of audiovisual materials for nursing 1968-1969. New York, The Company, 1970.

AMERICAN NURSES' ASSOCIATION
American Nurses' Association's first position on education for nursing. *American Journal of Nursing*, Dec. 1965, p. 106-11.

AMERICAN NURSES' ASSOCIATION
The continuing search for meaning. New York, The Association, 1964.

AMERICAN NURSES' ASSOCIATION
Educational preparation for nurse practitioners and assistants to nurses: a position paper. New York, The Association, 1965.

AMERICAN NURSES' ASSOCIATION
The knowledge explosion and its impact for health professions. New York, The Association, 1964.

AMERICAN NURSES' ASSOCIATION
Nurse! A guide for the establishment of refresher courses for registered nurses. New York, The Association, [1968].

AMERICAN NURSES' ASSOCIATION
Principles governing professional nursing education. *American Journal of Nursing*, April 1962, p. 56-8.

AMERICAN NURSES' ASSOCIATION. COUNCIL OF STATE BOARDS OF NURSING
Education for nursing practice, today and tomorrow: proceedings ANA educational conference for members and professional employees of State Boards of Nursing, Barbican Plaza Hotel, New York City, May 4-5, 1967. New York, The Association, 1967.

AMERICAN NURSES' ASSOCIATION. EDUCATION ADMINISTRATORS, CONSULTANTS AND TEACHERS SECTION
Guide for studying work load of teachers in education programs in nursing. New York, The Association, [1965].

ANDERSON, BERNICE E.
Nursing education in community junior colleges: a four-state, 5-year experience in the development of associate degree programs. Philadelphia, Lippincott, 1966.

BADGLEY, R. F.
The tragedy of nursing education. *Canadian Nurse*, Aug. 1963, p. 722-5.

BANU, A.
Suggestions supported by reasons for improvement of basic nursing education [in Pakistan]. *The Pakistan Nursing and Health Review*, July 1964, p. 13-6.

BERRY, C. E., and DRUMMON, E. J.
The place of the humanities in nursing education. *Nursing Outlook*, Sept. 1970, p. 30-1.

BESWETHERICK, MARGARET A.
Report on phasing out of nursing student service component in diploma schools of nursing in Nova Scotia. Halifax, Registered Nurses' Association of Nova Scotia, 1967.

BIGNOLD, V.
Training rural health nurses in Papua and New Guinea. *Nursing Mirror*, April 21, 1961, p. vii.

BISSONETTE, G.
The changing nature of nursing education. A sociological perspective. The Catherine R. Dempsey Lecture. *Occupational Health Nursing*, Sept. 1969, p. 19-20, 22-3, 26.

BLACK, C.
Nursing education: the *first* need is numbers. *Hospital Administration in Canada*, Dec. 1967, p. 29-31.

BLAIS, N., and BEAUDRY-JOHNSON, N.
Nursing education in Quebec—a new era. *The Canadian Nurse*, May 1968, p. 60-2.

BOMPAS, B. M.
Nurse education in Scandinavia. *Nursing Times*, July 14, 1967, p. 929-30.

BONE, A. I. C.
New development in nurse training in Ayr. *Nursing Mirror*, July 21, 1967, p. v-viii.

BONNET, P. D.
Hospital schools of nursing in 1984; two forecasts—part 1. Physician-administrator. *Hospitals*, Feb. 16, 1964, p. 62, 64-6.
Part II. *See* LAMBERTSEN, ELEANOR C.

BOYLE, R. E.
Critical issues in collegiate education in nursing—in relation to the qualifications and preparation of faculty, recruitment of students, advanced standing for graduate nurse students, achievement tests and the content of nursing. *Nursing Outlook*, Mar. 1962, p. 165-7.

BRENNAN, K.
Nurse training in Sweden. *Irish Nursing News*, May/June 1963, p. 6-7.

BRITISH COLUMBIA. DEPARTMENT OF HEALTH SERVICES AND HOSPITAL INSURANCE. MENTAL HEALTH SERVICES BRANCH
A combined course in psychiatric and general nursing. Final report of Mental Health Grant Project no. 609-5-136. Victoria, 1962. 2 vols. in 1.

BRODT, D. E.
Education today for nursing service tomorrow. *The Journal of Nursing Education*, Jan. 1966, p. 7-13.

BROWDER, J. J.
Assessing the value of student projects. *Nursing Outlook*, Aug. 1963, p. 588-9.

BROWN, RAY E.
Report of survey of nursing education in North Carolina. The North Carolina Board of Higher Education, and others, 1964.

BROWN, R. E., and BOOZER, H. R.
Recommendations for nursing education to relieve the nursing shortage in North Carolina. *Journal of Nursing Education*, Nov. 1965, p. 5-12.

BULL, MARY
Training nurses for Tunisia. *Nursing Mirror*, April 26, 1963, p. 76-8.

BUTLER, C. B., and GEITGEY, D. A.
A tool for evaluating teachers. *Nursing Outlook*, July 1970, p. 56-8.

CAMERON, F. J.
Pattern of basic nursing education in New Zealand. *Nursing Times*, April 7, 1961, p. 438-9.

CAMPBELL, K.
Training nurses in Natal. *Nursing Times*, Sept. 11, 1964, p. 1177-8.

CANADA. ROYAL COMMISSION ON HEALTH SERVICES
Nursing education in Canada, by Helen K. Mussallem. Ottawa, Queen's Printer, 1965.

CANADIAN NURSES' ASSOCIATION
A course for the future: a report based on the unfinished study of Kasper D. Naegele on the education of nurses in Canada. Ottawa, The Association, 1966.

CANADIAN NURSES' ASSOCIATION
Report on the Canadian Nurses' Association school improvement program. Ottawa, The Association, [1966].

CANADIAN NURSES' ASSOCIATION
Roles, functions, and educational preparation for the practice of nursing. Ottawa, The Association, 1967.

CARNEGIE, M. E.
Are Negro schools of nursing needed today. *Nursing Outlook*, Feb. 1964, p. 52-6.

CARPENTER, H. M.
Nursing education in Canada. *International Nursing Review*, vol. 13, no. 5, 1966, p. 29-35.

CATHCART, H. R.
Nursing education: an appraisal and a forecast. *Hospitals*, Aug. 16, 1968, p. 108-13.

CENTO
Cento conference on nursing education, held in Tehran, April 14-25, 1964. Ankara, Cento, n.d.

CHAMBERLAIN, EDITH M.
Orientation to nursing. New York, McGraw-Hill, 1962.

CHIONI, R. M., and SCHOEN, E.
Preparing tomorrow's nurse practitioner. *Nursing Outlook*, Oct. 1970, p. 50-3.

CHRISTIAN MEDICAL ASSOCIATION OF INDIA. NURSES' LEAGUE
A new text-book for nurses in India. 2nd edn. *Editor*: Ann Janama Zwemer. Vol. 1. The foundations of nursing. Madras, Christian Literature Society, 1968.

CHRISTIAN MEDICAL ASSOCIATION OF INDIA. NURSES' LEAGUE
A new text-book for nurses in India. Vol. 3. Nursing arts. Madras, Christian Literature Society, 1969.

CLARE MARIE, Sister
Survey of the schools of nursing in the province of Nova Scotia. Halifax, Registered Nurses' Association of Nova Scotia, 1966.

COE, C. R.
The relative importance of selected educational objectives in nursing. *Nursing Research*, Spring 1967, p. 141-5.

COLLEGE OF NURSING, AUSTRALIA
College of Nursing, Australia. Education policies adopted May 1969. *The Australian Nurses' Journal*, Nov. 1969, p. 233-4, and 236-40.

COLUMBIA UNIVERSITY. TEACHERS' COLLEGE. INSTITUTE OF RESEARCH AND SERVICE IN NURSING EDUCATION
Career decisions and professional expectations of nursing students, by David J. Fox, Lorraine K. Diamond and Nadia Jacobowsky. Columbia University, 1961.

CONANT, L. H.
Closing the practice-theory gap. *Nursing Outlook*, Nov. 1967, p. 37-9.

CONDER, P.
Tension: the needs of service and education. *Nursing Times*, Feb. 26, 1970, p. 274-6.

CONFERENCE OF CATHOLIC SCHOOLS OF NURSING
Nursing education and Catholic institutions: a report. Missouri, Conference of Catholic Schools of Nursing, 1963.

CONNOR, JOHN
Annapolis Valley nursing education study; a preliminary appraisal. Wolfville, N.S., Acadia University Institute, 1965.

COOKSON, J. S.
Nursing services of Iceland. *Nursing Mirror*, Aug. 18, 1961, p. v-vi.

COOPER, SIGNE S., and HORNBACK, MAY
Profile of the continuing learner in nursing. *Nursing Outlook*, Dec. 1966, p. 28-31.

COSTELLO, C. G.
The evaluation of a two-year experimental nursing program by C. G. Costello and T. Costonguay. Regina, Regina Grey Nuns' Hospital, School of Nursing, 1968.

COUNCIL OF EUROPE
European agreement on the instruction and education of nurses. [Strasbourg], The Council, 1967.
[Parallel text in English and French. European Treaty series, no. 59.]

CROOG S. H., and others
Career decisions of student nurses in Japan. *The Journal of Nursing Education*, Jan. 1966, p. 3-13.

DANAO, M. L.
Nursing scholarship in the Philippines. *Santo Tomas Nursing Journal*, Sept. 1965, p. 110-6.

DEAKIN, B. M.
Nursing education in relation to current social problems. *UNA Nursing Journal*, June 1967, p. 173-84

DEGARDIN, C.
Medical and nursing education in France. *World Hospitals*, April 1969 ,p. 81-6.

DENIS, M.
The training of African nurses then (1916) and now (1961). *South African Nursing Journal*, Nov. 1961, p. 25 and 33.

DRUMMOND, E. J.
The hospital school—as school. *Hospital Progress*, Feb. 1969, p. 45-8, 64.

DUSTAN, L. C.
Is it the system? Or is it the confusion in the interpretation of program purposes and objectives and lack of articulation between programs which characterizes the present 3-route approach to education for the practice of nursing? *Nursing Outlook*, May 1964, p. 58-61.

DUSTAN, L. C.
Needed: Articulation between nursing education programs and institutions of higher learning. *Nursing Outlook*, Dec. 1970, p. 34-7.

EICHHORN, S.
Trends in the professional education of doctors, nurses and other paramedical staff in the German Federal Republic. *World Hospitals*, April 1969, p. 77-80.

ELLIOTT, F. E., *and* MCGUINESS, A. F.
Experimental training in general and psychiatric nursing. *Nursing Mirror*, June 28, 1963, p. 275-8.

ERNE, Sister MARY J.
Implications of trends in nursing education. *Nursing Outlook*, Sept. 1968, p. 36-8.

ESPIRITU, T. M.
Problems of nursing education in the Philippines today. *Santo Tomas Nursing Journal*, Dec. 1965, p. 199-207.

FAHY, E.
Elements of comparative nursing education. *Nursing Science*, April 1965, p. 145-61.

FAWKES, B. N.
Budgeting and finance. *Nursing Times*, June 14, 1963, p. 731-2.

FAWKES, B. N.
General nurse training: a new concept. *Royal Society of Health Journal*, Nov./Dec. 1963, p. 295-9.

FAWKES, B. N.
Recent proposals for developments in nursing education in England and Wales. *International Nursing Review*, vol. 17, no. 3, 1970, p. 258-68.

FEIN, L. G.
Evidence of a curvilinear relationship between IPAT anxiety and achievement in nursing schools. *Journal of Clinical Psychology*, July 1963, p. 374-6.

FENSOME, J. E.
Community nurse training centre, Kaduna, Northern Nigeria. *International Nursing Review*, vol. 10, no. 5, 1963, p. 33-4.

FIELD, PEGGY ANNE
A follow-up survey of students graduating from the advanced practical obstetrics course, University of Alberta, Jan. 1960 to June 1965 (inclusive). Edmonton, School of Nursing, University of Alberta, 1966.

FIVARS, GRACE, *and* GOSWELL, DORIS
Nursing education: the problems and the process: the critical incident technique. New York, Macmillan, 1966.

FLETCHER, P. D.
Foresterhill College. A major development in nurse education. *The Hospital*, Aug. 1966, p. 376-9.

FOX, D. J., *and others*
Correlates of satisfaction and stress with selected clinical aspects of nursing school experience. *Nursing Research*, Spring 1963, p. 83-8; Summer 1963, p. 157-61.

FRANK, Sister CHARLES MARIE, *and* HEIDGERKEN, LORETTA E., *editors*
Perspectives in nursing education: educational patterns—their evolution and characteristics. Washington, Catholic University of America Press, 1963.

FUERST, ELINOR V., *and* WOLFF, LU VERNE
Fundamentals of nursing: the humanities and the sciences in nursing. 3rd edn. Philadelphia, Lippincott, 1964. 4th edn. 1969.

GAINSBOROUGH, H., *and* WATKIN, B.
Medical, nursing and paramedical education—recent thinking in Great Britain. *World Hospitals*, April 1969, p. 87-92.

GALLAGHER, ANNA HELEN
Educational administration in nursing. New York, Macmillan, 1965.

GAMMON, OLA M.
Texas plan. *Nursing Outlook*, May 1967, p. 58-9.

GEDDES, J. D. C.
Patient-centred teaching.
1. Facing the facts.
2. Change, choice or charybdis.
3. Telling isn't teaching and listening isn't learning.
4. Treat the cause not the symptoms.
5. Teaching with a purpose (i and ii).
Nursing Times, Dec. 27, 1968, p. 1756; Jan. 9, 1969, p. 43-4; Jan. 23, 1969, p. 116-7; Feb. 6, 1969, p. 176-7; Feb. 20, 1969, p. 239-41; Mar. 3, 1969, p. 305-7.

GEITGEY, D. A., *and* CROWLEY, D.
Preparing objectives. *American Journal of Nursing*, Jan. 1965, p. 95-8.

GENERAL NURSING COUNCIL FOR ENGLAND AND WALES
Record of practical instruction and experience for the certificate of general nursing. The Council, 1962.

GENERAL NURSING COUNCIL FOR ENGLAND AND WALES
Record of practical instruction and experience for the certificate of nursing of sick children. The Council, 1964.

GERCHBERG, LOUISE ROZARIO
An observational method for evaluating the performance of nursing students in clinical situations. New York, N.L.N., 1962.

GERSTEIN, A. I.
Development of a selection program for nursing candidates. *Nursing Research*, Summer 1965, p. 254-7.

GILLAM, R.
Through a veil, darkly: dilemmas in nursing education. *Australian Nurses' Journal*, Dec. 1969, p. 254-7.

GLASGOW ROYAL INFIRMARY
New Glasgow training scheme. *Nursing Times*, Aug. 9, 1963, p. 988-90.

GOODSON, M. R.
Professional education. *American Journal of Nursing*, April 1966, p. 798-801.

GOULD, M. E.
Area nurse training committees. *Nursing Times*, Nov. 8, 1963, p. 1420-1.

GREAT BRITAIN. FOREIGN AND COMMONWEALTH OFFICE
Nursing education. European agreement on the instruction and education of nurses (with recommendations). Strasbourg, Oct. 25, 1967. Treaty Series no. 92 (1970). H.M.S.O., 1970.
[This publication supersedes—Foreign Office Nursing education. European agreement . . . Cmnd. 3593.]

GRIFFEN, G. S., *and others*
New dimensions for the improvement of clinical nursing. *Nursing Research*, Fall 1966, p. 293-302.

GUINEE, KATHLEEN K.
The aims and methods of nursing education. New York, Macmillan, 1966.

GUMBLEY, C. N.
Projects. Their value in nurse education. *Nursing Times*, Feb. 5, 1965, p. 190-2.

HALE, T.
Divergent views of nurse education. *World Medical Journal*, July/Aug. 1967, p. 116-9.

HALL, B. L., and LITTLE, D. E.
Group project and learning outcomes. *Nursing Outlook*, June 1969, p. 82-3.

HAYNES, INEZ
Nursing education is not one program, it's four. *Modern Hospital*, Sept. 1963, p. 151-4.

HANGARTNER, C. A.
Re-examining the hospital's role in nursing education. *Hospital Progress*, Dec. 1969, p. 64-6, 70.

HARTY, M. B.
Trends in nursing education. *American Journal of Nursing*, April 1968, p. 767-72.

HASLAM, O.
Nurse training in Japan. *Nursing Mirror*, Feb. 19, 1965, p. 475-6.

HASSENPLUG, L. W.
The academician in nursing for tomorrow today. *Nursing Science*, Feb. 1964, p. 4-14.

HASSENPLUG, L. W.
Nursing education for a world of change. *The Canadian Nurse*, Sept. 1962, p. 802-8.

HECTOR, W. E.
How long? A review of the report on the Glasgow Experimental Scheme. *Nursing Times*, July 26, 1963, p. 937-8.

HECTOR, W. E.
Trends in nurse education. *Nursing Times*, Dec. 31, 1965, p. 1790-1.

HENDERSON, VIRGINIA
The nature of nursing: a definition and its implications for practice, research and education. New York, Macmillan, 1966.

HENRY, M.
Nurse training—future plans and aims. Paper given at the Twelfth Annual Conference of the Association of Hospital Management Committees, held at Scarborough, 1962. *Hospital and Social Service Journal*, June 22, 1962, p. 714-6.

HINES, PHYLLIS A.
Sweden. *The Lamp*, Mar. 1969, p. 13-5.

HONG KONG. NURSING BOARD
Report of the Nursing Board Working Party on Nursing Education and Training. [Hong Kong, The Board?], 1967. [Chairman: Sheila Iu.]

HOOPER, J.
Nurse training in Sweden, August 1968. *Nursing Times*, May 8, 1969, Occasional Papers, p. 73-6.

HOWARD, FRANCES M.
A study to determine the opinions of administrators and directors of nursing on five selected recommendations concerning nursing education included in the C.N.A. submission to the Royal Commission on Health Services. March 1962. Montreal, The Association, 1963.

HOWARD, M. I.
Professional status and educational standards. *Irish Nurse*, Oct. 1964, p. 43-8.

IAFOLLA, M. A. C.
Guidance in nursing education. *Journal of Nursing Education*, Jan. 1969, p. 15-21.

INNIS, MARY Q.
Nursing education in a changing society. Toronto, University of Toronto Press, 1970.

INTERNATIONAL COUNCIL OF NURSES
An enquiry into basic nursing education. *International Nursing Review*, vol. 12, no. 4, 1965, p. 27-39.

INTERNATIONAL COUNCIL OF NURSES
Report on nursing education from 12th Quadrennial Conference. *Nursing Mirror*, June 2, 1961, p. 839.

INTERNATIONAL DIGEST OF HEALTH LEGISLATION
Training of nurses, male nurses and children's nurses (Federal Republic of Germany). *International Digest of Health Legislation*, vol. 18, no. 1, 1967, p. 122-7.

INTERNATIONAL NURSING REVIEW
Nursing programmes in New Zealand. *International Nursing Review*, vol. 8, no. 2, 1961, p. 14-8.

THE INTERNATIONAL SCHOOL OF ADVANCED NURSING EDUCATION, LYON
The International School of Advanced Nursing Education, Lyon, France—after two years. *International Nursing Review*, vol. 14, no. 6, 1967, p. 11-6.

ISOLA-WILLIAMS, C. A.
Co-operation between nurse educators and nursing service personnel in the education of nurses. *Nigerian Nurse*, Jan. 1970, p. 52-4.

JACOBSON, M. D.
Effective and ineffective behavior of teachers of nursing as determined by their students. *Nursing Research*, Summer 1966, p. 218-24.

JAMAICAN NURSE
Nursing education. Proposed integration of general and psychiatric curriculum. *The Jamaican Nurse*, Dec. 1965, p. 28-9.

JAMES, A. R.
Technical education for nurses. *Nursing Times*, June 25, 1965, p. 877-8.

JAYACHANDRAN, V.
Nursing education in India today. *Nursing Journal of India*, Nov. 1963, p. 290-1.

JAYAWARDENA, Y. S.
The ICN and educational criteria for membership. *International Nursing Review*, vol. 9, no. 5, 1962, p. 55.

JONES, T. A.
The role of training in job participation. *Nursing Mirror*, Dec. 18, 1970, p. 33.

KAKOSH, MARGUERITE E.
Profile of the college graduate in basic nursing. *Nursing Outlook*, May 1967, p. 64-5.

KANEKO MITSU
A new aim of nursing education in Japan. *International Journal of Nursing Studies*, Sept. 1969, p. 141-8.

KEIM, D.
Practical nurse education in Alaska. *Nursing Outlook*, Aug. 1969, p. 32-5.

KERGIN, D.
Nurses and educational change. *Canadian Nurse*, Dec. 1969, p. 28-30.

KHAN, M. P.
Training of nurses in Pakistan. *The Pakistan Nursing and Health Review*, July 1967, p. 6-11.

KING, P. E.
Nursing education and cultural patterns in India. *International Journal of Nursing Studies*, April 1965, p. 33-8.

KINGSTON PUBLIC HOSPITAL, JAMAICA
Jamaica's first school of nursing. *The Jamaican Nurse*, Aug. 1965, p. 11.

KLAHN, J. E.
Self-concept and change-seeking need. *Journal of Nursing Education*, April 1969, p. 11-6.

KLONOFF, H., and MARCUS, A. M.
An innovation in nursing education. *The Canadian Nurse*, June 1965, p. 455-7.

KNOWLES, MALCOLM S.
The professional nurse looks at the learning climate. Washington, Leadership Resources, 1966. [Leadership in Nursing series, no. 14.]

NURSING AS A PROFESSION

KUHN, B. G.
Nursing education in Quebec, Canada. *Nursing Mirror*, Dec. 25, 1970, p. 21-4.

LAMB, M. C. N.
Modern trends in nursing education. *Irish Nurse*, Dec. 1963, p. 131-41.

LAMBERTSEN, ELEANOR C.
Changes in practice require changes in education. *American Journal of Nursing*, Aug. 1966, p. 1784-7.

LAMBERTSEN, ELEANOR C.
Hospital schools of nursing in 1984; two forecasts—part 2. Nurse-educator. *Hospitals*, Feb. 16, 1964, p. 63-4. Part 1, see BONNET, P. D.

LAMBERTSEN, ELEANOR C.
Would transfer of nurse education to campus improve patient care? *The Modern Hospital*, Feb. 1966, p. 128-30.

LAMONT, A. M.
Education for professional life. *S.A. Nursing Journal*, Nov. 1967, p. 8-9, 11-12 and 33.

LANGE, C. M.
A proposed approach to nursing education. *Nursing Outlook*, July 1966, p. 45-8.

LAPPING, A.
Training our nurses. *New Society*, Oct. 26, 1967, p. 589.

LEFKOWITZ, A. S., *and* HART, A. M.
Selection of laboratory facilities for collegiate nursing education. *Nursing Forum*, vol. IV, no. 1, 1965, p. 94-102.

LEIDERITZ, A. F.
New regulations for nurse training [in the Netherlands]. *World Hospitals*, April 1967, p. 151-2.

LEININGER, M.
Conference on the nature of science and nursing. *Nursing Research*, Nov./Dec. 1968, p. 484-507.

LEVINE, E., *and* HUDSON, H. H.
More nurses now have college degrees. *Nursing Outlook*, Oct. 1965, p. 31-3.

LEW, Y.
Trends in nursing education in Australia within the next decade. *Australian Nurses' Journal*, Oct. 1969, p. 202-8.

LEWIS, E. P.
The Fairview Story. *American Journal of Nursing*, Jan. 1966, p. 64-70.

LLEWELLYN-JONES, J. D.
Educated nurses. *The Australian Nurses' Journal*, Nov. 1968, p. 246-8.

LONG, L.
Changes in nursing education in Saskatchewan. *Canadian Nurse*, Oct. 1963, p. 935-41.

LONG, L.
Preparing the third-year student for responsibility. *The Canadian Nurse*, Aug. 1961, p. 750-4.

LONG, L.
Tomorrow's nursing education in Saskatchewan. *The Canadian Nurse*, April, 1967, p. 30-3.

LYMAN, KATHERINE
Basic nursing education programmes: a guide to their planning. Geneva, W.H.O., 1961. Public Health Papers, no. 7.

LYONS, B.
Educational trends overseas. *The Australian Nurses' Journal*, Nov. 1965, p. 272-5.

MCCLUSKEY, J. A.
Ladder education—why not? A challenge to nursing educators. *Journal of Practical Nursing*, May 1970, p. 24-5, 48, 50.

MACDONALD R.
London as a world centre for training nurses. *The Nursing Journal of India*, Nov. 1964, p. 323.

MCFARLANE, J.
Legacy for the seventies. [Future of nurse education.] *Nursing Times*, Jan. 15, 1970, p. 90-1; Jan. 22, 1970, p. 113-4.

MACGUIRE, J.
Nurses and graduates. An attempt to locate nurses with degrees. *Nursing Times*, April 2, 1970, Occasional Papers, p. 41-4; April 9, 1970, Occasional Papers, p. 45-8.

MACGUIRE, J., *and* POMERANZ, R.
Training for reality: the implications of demographic trends for the training of nurses. *Nursing Times*, July 26, 1968, Occasional Papers, p. 113-6; Aug. 2, 1968, Occasional Papers, p. 117-20.

MACGUIRE, J., *and* SPARKS, S.
The nurse/graduate in the United Kingdom: patterns and qualifications. *International Nursing Review*, v. 17, no. 4, 1970, p. 350-69.

MCINTOSH, D. M.
Educational background to nursing. 1—Education and human resources. *Nursing Mirror*, Nov. 16, 1962, p. 145-6 and 148.

MCINTOSH, D. M.
Educational background to nursing. 2—Educational objectives. *Nursing Mirror*, Nov. 23, 1962, p. 177-8 and 180.

MCINTOSH, D. M.
Educational background to nursing. 3—Beyond the school. *Nursing Mirror*, Nov. 30, 1962, p. 198-200.

MCINTOSH, D. M.
Educational background to nursing. 4—First principles. *Nursing Mirror*, Dec. 7, 1962, p. 217-8.

MCKAY, R.
A comparative approach to the development of nursing education. *Nursing Science*, April 1964, p. 125-37.

MCKENEMY, A.
An advanced standing diploma for LPNs. *Hospital Progress*, Sept. 1970, p. 77-80.

MCKENZIE, HEATHER
Report on overseas nursing education 1965-1966. [Sydney, New South Wales College of Nursing, 1967.]

MACLAGGAN, KATHERINE
Portrait of nursing: a plan for the education of nurses in the province of New Brunswick. Fredericton, the New Brunswick Association of Registered Nurses, 1965.

MCLAIN, Sister M. AMBROSE
A liberal approach to nursing education and nursing practice. *Nursing Outlook*, Oct. 1963, p. 732-5.

MCLEOD, I.
Symposium "The Future of Hospitals". Specialization for new nursing. *Canadian Hospital*, July 1965, p. 49-51.

MAJOR, DOROTHY M.
West Virginia plan 1965. *Nursing Outlook*, Dec. 1965, p. 22-5.

MAKHWADE, K. M. I.
Nursing education in Botswana: its role in the future development of nursing services—1 and 2. *International Journal of Nursing Studies*, Mar. 1970, p. 19-28; June 1970, p. 99-112.

MANCHESTER AREA NURSE TRAINING COMMITTEE
Report for the period 1st December 1961 to 30th September 1966. Manchester, The Committee, 1966.

MANDIN, J.
A new dimension in nursing education. *Hospital Progress*, Feb. 1968, p. 16 and 26.

MARKHAM, J.
Student nurse projects. *Nursing Times*, Dec. 8, 1961, p. 1600-2.

MARSHALL, MELODY J., *and* BRUHN, J. G.
Refresher courses and reactivation of nurses. *Nursing Outlook*, Jan. 1967, p. 59-61.

MARSON, S. N., *compiler*
Register of programmes for nurses. Revised edn. Sheffield. Programmed Instruction Centre for Industry, 1970.

MARTIN, J. R.
Correlation between pre-admission tests and graduation from nursing school. *Journal of Nursing Education*, Dec. 1962, p. 3-4, 23-5.

MATHENEY, R.
Can nursing live with open admissions? *American Journal of Nursing*, Dec. 1970, p. 2561-4.

MAXWELL, R. M.
Clinical nursing content in the graduate program. *Nursing Outlook*, Nov. 1962, p. 747-9.

MAXWELL, R. M.
The nursing service director as a graduate student. *Nursing Forum*, vol. II, no. 1, 1963, p. 9-13.

MERCADANTE, L.
Education for service—the challenge. *Nursing Forum*, vol. VIII, no. 2, 1969, p. 151-9.

MILLARD, R.
Liberal and professional nursing education. *Nursing Outlook*, July 1968, p. 22-5.

MILLER, J. M., *and others*
Needed: engineering courses in nursing education. *Hospital Topics*, Feb. 1966, p. 64-6.

MONAGHAN, J. R.
Nursing education in Malawi. *The Canadian Nurse*, June 1967, p. 35-7.

MONAGHAN, J R.
Student nurse training begins in Malawi. *Nursing Times*, April 21, 1967, p. 526-8.

MONTAG, M. L.
Technical education in nursing? *American Journal of Nursing*, May 1963, p. 100-3.

MORGAN, WINIFRED F.
An experiment in nurse training conducted in Glasgow Royal Infirmary 1956-1961. [Glasgow, Glasgow R.H.B., 1961.]

MOSER, D. H.
Changes in nursing education for the future—challenge or chagrin? *Journal American Association of Nurse Anesthetists*, June 1970, p. 203-8.

MULLANE, MARY K.
Care systems and nursing education. *Nursing Outlook*, Oct. 1963, p. 740-2.

MULLANE, MARY K.
Education in the hospital; changing responsibilities. *Hospital Topics*, Nov. 1965, p. 25-6.

MUSSALLEM, HELEN KATHLEEN
A path to equality: a plan for the development of nursing education programs within the general educational system of Canada. Ottawa, The Canadian Nurses' Association, 1964.

NAEGELE, KASPAR D.
Study of nursing education. Needed developments in the education of nurses in Canada: some general recommendations. *The Canadian Nurse*, Sept. 1964, p. 865-9.

NAEGELE, KASPAR D.
A course for the future; a report based on the unfinished study of Kaspar D. Naegele on the education of nurses in Canada. Ottawa, Canadian Nurses' Association, c. 1966.

NAGELE, M. F.
Faculty-student ratio in nursing. Part I. *Nursing Outlook*, Sept. 1962, p. 611-3.

NAGELE, M. F.
Faculty-student ratio in nursing. Part II—How to calculate enrollment to maintain a given ratio in a given program. *Nursing Outlook*, Oct. 1962, p. 683-6.

NAHM, H.
Nursing education—responsibility for preparation of leadership personnel. *International Journal of Nursing Studies*, vol. 2, no. 11, 1965, p. 95-103.

NATIONAL LEAGUE FOR NURSING
Extending the boundaries of nursing education: the preparation and the roles of the clinical specialist. Papers presented at the Third Conference of the Council of Baccalaureate and Higher Degree Programs held at Phoenix, Arizona, Nov. 13-15, 1968. New York, National League For Nursing, 1969.

NATIONAL LEAGUE FOR NURSING
The school improvement program of the National League for Nursing, 1951-1960. New York, The League, 1963.

NATIONAL LEAGUE FOR NURSING
Statement on nursing education. New York, The League, 1967.

NATIONAL LEAGUE FOR NURSING
Study on Cost of Nursing Education: Part I—Cost of Basic Diploma Programs. Part II—Cost of Basic Baccalaureate Programs and Associate Degree Programs, by H. R. Rowe and H. H. Flitter. New York, The League, 1964.

NATIONAL LEAGUE FOR NURSING
Teacher-practitioner: collaborators for the improvement of nursing care. New York, The League, 1965.

NATIONAL LEAGUE FOR NURSING. COMMITTEE ON CAREERS
Schools of professional nursing. New York, The League, 1964.

NATIONAL LEAGUE FOR NURSING. RESEARCH AND STUDIES SERVICE
Educational preparation for nursing, 1961. *Nursing Outlook*, Sept. 1962, p. 614-6.

NATIONAL LEAGUE FOR NURSING. RESEARCH AND STUDIES SERVICE
Educational preparation for nursing, 1962. *Nursing Outlook*, Sept. 1963, p. 674-6.

NATIONAL LEAGUE FOR NURSING. RESEARCH AND STUDIES SERVICE
Educational preparation for nursing, 1963. *Nursing Outlook*, Sept 1964, p. 60-2.

NATIONAL LEAGUE FOR NURSING. RESEARCH AND STUDIES SERVICE
Educational preparation for nursing, 1964. *Nursing Outlook*, Sept. 1965, p. 62-4.

NATIONAL LEAGUE FOR NURSING. RESEARCH AND STUDIES SERVICE
Educational preparation for nursing, 1965. *Nursing Outlook*, Sept. 1966, p. 58-61.

NATIONAL LEAGUE FOR NURSING. RESEARCH AND STUDIES SERVICE
Educatoinal preparation for nursing, 1966. *Nursing Outlook*, Sept. 1967, p. 64-8.

NATIONAL LEAGUE FOR NURSING. RESEARCH AND STUDIES SERVICE
Educational preparation for nursing, 1967. *Nursing Outlook*, Sept. 1968, p. 52-6.

NATIONAL LEAGUE FOR NURSING. RESEARCH AND STUDIES SERVICE
Educational preparation for nursing, 1968. *Nursing Outlook*, Sept. 1969, p. 76-9.

NURSING AS A PROFESSION

NATIONAL LEAGUE FOR NURSING. RESEARCH AND STUDIES SERVICE
Educational preparation for nursing, 1969. *Nursing Outlook*, Sept. 1970, p. 52-7.

NATIONAL LEAGUE FOR NURSING. RESEARCH AND STUDIES SERVICE
Nurse-faculty census 1966: various programs of nursing education, by Hessel H. Flitter. New York, The League, 1966.

NATIONAL LEAGUE FOR NURSING *and* UNITED STATES PUBLIC HEALTH SERVICE. JOINT COMMITTEE ON EDUCATIONAL FACILITIES FOR NURSING
Nursing education facilities: programming considerations and architectural guide: a report. Washington, U.S. Dept. Health, Education and Welfare, 1964.

NEW ENGLAND COUNCIL ON HIGHER EDUCATION FOR NURSING, REGIONAL NURSING PROGRAM
Proceedings of the 4th inter-university faculty, work conference: physical-biological basis for nursing care; implications for newer dimensions in generic nursing education, prepared by Winifred H. Griffin. Cape Cod, Mass., 1967. The Council [1967?].

NEW SOUTH WALES. HOSPITAL COMMISSION OF NEW SOUTH WALES
Commission of Inquiry to Study Education of Nurses in New South Wales. Interim report and recommendations. Sydney, The Commission, 1969.

NEW SOUTH WALES. HOSPITALS COMMISSION OF NEW SOUTH WALES
Committee of Inquiry to Study Education of Nurses in New South Wales. Report. New South Wales, Government Printer, 1970.

NEW YORK STATE NURSES' ASSOCIATION
Transition in nursing education. *American Journal of Nursing*, June 1967, p. 1211-4.

NICHOLS, G. A.
Clinical observations and actions of nursing students. *Journal of Nursing Education*, Nov. 1968, p. 15-22.

NICHOLLS, M. E.
The nursing home as a teaching laboratory. *Nursing Outlook*, April 1970, p. 35-7.

NORTHERN IRELAND HOSPITALS AUTHORITY
Nurse training in Northern Ireland. *Nursing Mirror*, July 7, 1967, p. 317.

NORTHERN IRELAND HOSPITALS AUTHORITY *and others*
Report by advisory committee on a pilot scheme for the exchange of nurse teachers. Belfast, The Authority, 1963.

NOTMAN, A. G.
Nurse education in Finland. *Nursing Times*, June 25, 1965, p. 862-3.

NURSING JOURNAL OF INDIA
Basic nursing education. *Nursing Journal of India*, July 1964, p. 199-201.

NURSING MIRROR
Soviet school for nurses. *Nursing Mirror*, Jan. 26, 1968, p. 24.

NURSING OUTLOOK
Characteristics of baccalaureate and graduate education in nursing. *Nursing Outlook*, July 1968, p. 36-7.

NURSING OUTLOOK
Turkey's new nursing schools. *Nursing Outlook*, Oct. 1965, p. 40-1.

NURSING RECRUITMENT SERVICE
Where should I train? *Nursing Times*, April 2, 1965, p. 448-9.

NURSING TIMES
A central admissions system to nurse training. *Nursing Times*, Oct. 9, 1969, p. 1305.

NURSING TIMES
Control of nurse training. *Nursing Times*, April 23, 1965, p. 545.

NURSING TIMES
Graduate to nurse.
St. Bartholomew's Hospital Undergraduates, by Winifred Hector.
The London Hospital Undergraduates, by Sheila Collins.
Nightingale School Graduates, by L. N. Jamieson.
Nursing Times, Feb. 27, 1969, p. 286-8.

NURSING TIMES
The schooling of 3,000 student nurses. *Nursing Times*, Feb. 14, 1964, p. 200-3.

NURSING TIMES
Training nurses in Moscow. *Nursing Times*, July 10, 1964, p. 888.

OGDEN, R. P.
Nursing education. *Hospitals*, April 1965, p. 129-33.

OXFORD AREA NURSE TRAINING COMMITTEE
From student to nurse: the induction period: a study of student nurses in the first six months of training in five schools of nursing. Headington, The Committee, 1961.

OXFORD AREA NURSE TRAINING COMMITTEE
From student to nurse, training and qualification: a study of student nurses in training in five schools of nursing [carried out by Jillian M. McGuire]. Headington, The Committee, 1966.

PALMER, MARY ELLEN
Self-evaluation of nursing performance based on clinical practice objectives. Boston University Press, 1962.

PAN-AMERICAN SANITARY BUREAU
Progress in nursing education in Latin America. *International Nursing Review*, vol. 14, no. 1, 1967, p. 64-6.

PAN-AMERICAN SANITARY BUREAU. REGIONAL OFFICE OF THE W.H.O.
Report of the survey of schools of nursing in the Caribbean area... March 1964 - August 1965. Washington, Pan-American Health Organization, 1966.

PATERSON, M. A.
Nurse training in 25 years' time. *Nursing Mirror*, July 29, 1966, p. 404-6.

PAULL, E. H.
Nursing programme of the Indian Red Cross Society. *International Journal of Nursing Studies*, Feb. 1967, p. 57-60.

PEART, MARGARET L.
Report of refresher programs in nursing pilot project for metropolitan Toronto 1968 co-sponsored by Ontario Hospital Association, Ontario Hospital Services Commission, and Registered Nurses' Association of Ontario. Toronto, 1970.

PELLEGRINO, E. D.
The communication crisis in nursing and medical education. *Nursing Forum*, vol. V, no. 1, 1966, p. 45-53.

PFNISTER, A. O.
The professions and education. *Nursing Outlook*, Jan. 1964, p. 29-32.

PIANA, B. M.
The Moscow School of Nursing. *Nursing Times*, Dec. 22, 1961, p. 1677.

PIEPGARAS, RUTH
Obsolescence of nursing skill. *American Journal of Nursing*, Sept. 1966, p. 1980-3.

PLAPP, J. M. *and others*
Intellective predictors and success in nursing school. *In* Proceedings of the 73rd Annual Convention of American Psychological Association, p. 307-8. Washington, D.C., American Psychological Association, 1965.

PONTE, M. L.
Observations on nursing education in Latin America. *International Journal of Nursing Studies*, Dec. 1964, p. 171-7.

PONTE, M. L.
Some Latin American attitudes—and how they affect nursing education. *International Journal of Nursing Studies*, May 1966, p. 21-5.

POST, S.
Nursing education and service cannot be separated. *Canadian Hospital*, Sept. 1969, p. 35-7.

POWELL, M. B.
The challenge of nursing education. The Ninth Nursing Mirror Lecture in Edinburgh, 1967. *Nursing Mirror*, Mar. 17, 1967, p. 551-4; Mar. 24, 1967, p. 581-4.

POWELL, M. B.
Nursing training and standards of care. *Nursing Times*, Aug. 30, 1963, p. 1081-2.

PRICE, ALICE L.
A handbook and charting manual for student nurses. 4th edn. St. Louis, Mosby, 1967.

PRINCESS MUNA COLLEGE OF NURSING, JORDAN
Princess Muna College of Nursing, Jordan. *Nursing Times*, Jan. 21, 1966, p. 93.

PUESCHEL, S. J.
A demographic analysis of the educational structure of American nursing. *Nursing Research*, May/June 1969, p. 211-6.

QUITTENTON, R. C.
Community colleges and nursing education in Ontario. Windsor, Ont., The St. Clair College of Applied Arts and Technology, 1968.

RALLA, E.
An Iranian assistant-nurse training school. *Nursing Mirror*, May 26, 1967, p. i-iii.

RAMSING, Sister BENEDICTE
Educational concepts in the basic programme in Denmark. *International Nursing Review*, vol. 10, no. 6, 1963, p. 47-54.

RASMUSSEN, E. H.
Preparation of faculty for schools of practical nursing. *Nursing Outlook*, Oct. 1965, p. 52-5.

REED, F. C.
Baccalaureate education and professional practice. *Nursing Outlook*, Jan. 1967, p. 50-2.

REGISTERED NURSES' ASSOCIATION OF BRITISH COLUMBIA
A proposed plan for the orderly development of nursing education in British Columbia. Part 1—Basic nursing education. Vancouver, 1967.

REINKEMEYER, Sister AGNES M.
New approaches to professional preparation. *Nursing Forum*, vol. IX, no. 1, 1970, p. 27-40.

RIAHI, A.
Nursing education in Iran. *International Journal of Nursing Studies*, Dec. 1968, p. 267-70.

RIDDELL, DOROTHY G.
Assessment report: nursing education in Lebanon, 20 April - 19 July 1968. [Geneva?] World Health Organization, Regional Office for the Eastern Mediterranean, 1968.

RINES, ALICE R.
Evaluating student progress in learning the practice of nursing. New York, Columbia University Teachers' College, Department of Nursing Education, 1963.

ROBB, K.
Study tour in Israel. *Nursing Times*, Feb. 19, 1965, p. 251-4.

ROBINSON, S. C.
A doctor looks at nursing education. *The Canadian Nurse*, July 1968, p. 38-40.

ROGERS, MARTHA E.
Educational revolution in nursing. New York, Macmillan, 1961.

ROGERS, MARTHA E.
Reveille in nursing. Philadelphia, F. A. Davis, 1964.

ROPER, N.
Making the most of ward experience. *Nursing Times*, Mar. 5, 1965, p. 335.

ROSE, Sister FRANCES
Basic nursing education in the "Land of the Midnight Sun". *Irish Nurse*, Sept. 1967, p. 252-6.

ROWSELL, GLENNA S.
Report on the Canadian Nurses' Association school improvement program. Ottawa, Canadian Nurses' Association, 1966.

ROYAL AUSTRALIAN NURSING FEDERATION *and* COLLEGE OF NURSING, AUSTRALIA
Submission on nursing education. The Federation, 1962.

ROYAL COLLEGE OF NURSING AND NATIONAL COUNCIL OF NURSES OF THE UNITED KINGDOM
The educational future of the Rcn. *Nursing Times*, Aug. 20, 1965, p. 1125.

ROYAL COLLEGE OF NURSING AND NATIONAL COUNCIL OF NURSES OF THE UNITED KINGDOM
A reform of nursing education: first report of a special committee on nurse education. The College, 1964. [*Chairman:* Sir Harry Platt.]

A reform of nursing education. Summary of the Platt Committee Report. *Nursing Times*, June 19, 1964, p. 813-4.

The Platt Report—a vital document, part I. *Nursing Mirror*, June 19, 1964, p. 271-3.

The Platt Report—a vital document, part II. *Nursing Mirror*, June 26, 1964, p. 287-9.

The Platt Report—a vital document, part III. *Nursing Mirror*, July 3, 1964, p. 307-9.

BALY, M.
The reform of nursing education—1. *Nursing Times*, June 25, 1965, p. 867-8.

BALY, M.
The reform of nursing education—2. *Nursing Times*, July 9, 1965, p. 955.

BALY, M.
The reform of nursing education—3. *Nursing Times*, July 16, 1965, p. 977-8.

BENDALL, E. R. D.
Implementing the Platt Report. A suggested training school programme for the Register. *Nursing Times*, July 10, 1964, p. 895-6.

CANADIAN NURSE
Review of the Platt Report. *The Canadian Nurse*, Sept. 1964, p. 880.

CHAVASSE, J.
The Platt Report. *Irish Nurse*, Oct. 1964, p. 49-52.

GENERAL NURSING COUNCIL FOR ENGLAND AND WALES
Platt report on a reform of nursing education: memorandum from the General Nursing Council for England and Wales. The Council, 1965.

GLASGOW ROYAL INFIRMARY *and* ASSOCIATED HOSPITALS BOARD OF MANAGEMENT
Report of a special committee to consider the Platt Report. *Nursing Mirror*, Oct. 22, 1965, p. 195-6.

GREENE, J.
Why a reform of nursing education is necessary. *Occupational Health*, Jan./Feb. 1965, p. 10-8.

MACIVER, A. A.
The Platt Report. Implications for Scotland. *Nursing Times*, Oct. 9, 1964, p. 1339-40.

NURSING AS A PROFESSION

MARTINA, P.
The Platt Report. *Santo Tomas Nursing Journal*, June 1965, p. 27-9.

SCOTTISH HOME AND HEALTH DEPT.
Group schools of nursing—an interim report on the Platt Report by a working party set up by the Scottish Home and Health Dept. *Nursing Mirror*, Oct. 11, 1968, p. 21-3.

SOUTH AFRICAN NURSING JOURNAL
A reform of nursing education. Summary of the Platt Report. *South African Nursing Journal*, Feb. 1965, p. 35-8.

ZAMBIA NURSE
The Platt Report. *Zambia Nurse*, Mar. 1966, p. 8-11.

ROYAL WOMEN'S HOSPITAL, MELBOURNE
Centenary of nurse training in Australia, 1862-1962. Melbourne, The Royal Women's Hospital, 1962.

ST. THOMAS'S HOSPITAL, NIGHTINGALE SCHOOL
Graduate to nurse. *Nursing Times*, Feb. 1, 1963, p. 123 and 152.

SALMIN, D.
Accreditation: A challenge to nursing education. *The Philippine Journal of Nursing*, Jan./Mar. 1968, p. 47.

SALMON, E. B.
Education for nursing. *The New Zealand Nursing Journal*, Sept. 1968, p. 5-8.

SASKATCHEWAN. BOARD OF NURSING EDUCATION
Evaluation of the state of nursing education in the province of Saskatchewan. Regina, 1969.

SASKATCHEWAN. DEPARTMENT OF PUBLIC HEALTH.
Ad hoc Committee on Nursing Education.
Report. Regina, Queen's Printer, 1966.

SASKATCHEWAN REGISTERED NURSES' ASSOCIATION
A brief presented to the *ad hoc* committee on nursing education to the Minister of Public Health, Government of Saskatchewan. Regina, the Association, 1965.

SCHLOTFELDT, ROZELLA M., and MONTAG, MILDRED L.
Preparation of nurses for faculty positions. *Nursing Outlook*, Jan. 1967, p. 26-31.

SCHMIDT, M. D.
Implications of current trends in nursing education upon industrial nursing. *American Association of Industrial Nurses' Journal*, July 1964, p. 10-2.

SCHWEER, JEAN E.
Creative teaching in clinical nursing. St. Louis, Mosby, 1968.

SCOTTISH HOME AND HEALTH DEPARTMENT
Experimental nurse training at Glasgow Royal Infirmary: final report of the assessment committee appointed by the Secretary of State for Scotland and the Nuffield Provincial Hospitals Trust. Edinburgh, H.M.S.O., 1963.

SEARLE, CHARLOTTE
Developments in nursing education at South African universities. *International Journal of Nursing Studies*, July 1969, p. 107-12.

SEARLE, CHARLOTTE
Overview of nursing education in South Africa, 1914-1964. *South African Nursing Journal*, Sept. 1964, p.52-6, 61-85.

SHANKS, M. D.
Evaluation of faculty. *Nursing Outlook*, Oct. 1965, p. 63-4.

SHARPE, MOLLY E.
A revolution in nurse training, 1952-64, at Gt. Ormond Street. *Nursing Times*, June 5, 1964, p. 714-6.

SHETLAND, M. L.
The responsibility of the professional school for preparing nurses for ethical, moral, and humanistic practice. *Nursing Forum*, vol. VIII, no. 1, 1969, p. 17-27.

SIME, E., *and others*
Faculty-supervisor: a dual position. *Nursing Outlook*, Mar. 1970, p. 39-41.

SIMPSON, M. JUNE
The "walk-around" laboratory practical examination in evaluating clinical nursing skills. *Journal of Nursing Education*, Nov. 1967, p. 23-6.

SKAGGS, K. G.
Mobility in nursing careers. *Bedside Nurse*, Nov./Dec. 1968, p. 21-3.

SLATER, P. V.
Comprehensive training. *UNA Nursing Journal*, June 1963, p. 202-10.

SLATER, P. V.
The education of the nurse. Florence Nightingale Oration. *UNA Nursing Journal*, Oct. 1963, p. 344-53.

SLATER, P. V.
What's new for nurses. *Australian Nurses' Journal*, May 1963, p. 134-7.

SMELTZER, C. H.
Psychological evaluation in nursing education. Collier-Macmillan, 1965.

SMITH, D. M.
Nursing education and nursing service. *Journal of Psychiatric Nursing*, May/June 1965, p. 220-7.

SMITH, J. P.
Basic nursing education in Scandinavia. *Nursing Mirror*, Jan. 10, 1969, p. 22-4.

SNEDDEN, B. M.
The establishment of the committee on overseas professional qualifications. *The Australian Nurses' Journal*, May 1969, p. 109-10.

SOUTH AFRICAN NURSING ASSOCIATION
Report on nursing education in the Republic of South Africa, submitted by the Board of the South African Nursing Association to the biennial congress of the S.A.N.A., October, 1966.
[Pretoria, The Association, 1966.]

SPOHN, ROBERTA R.
The future of education for professional practice: a guide for the study of ANA's proposed goal on nursing education and principles of nursing education. New York, A.N.A., 1962.

STEIN, R. F., and GREEN, E. J.
The graduate record examination as a predictive potential in the nursing major. *Nursing Research*, Jan./Feb. 1970, p. 42-7.

STEINDLER, FRANCES M., *editor*
Changing patterns in health and in professional education: a nursing symposium. Rutgers, The State University, College of Nursing, 1966.

STEPHENSON, E.
Studying nursing, midwifery and health visiting at university. *Midwife and Health Visitor*, July 1965, p. 90-1.

STOKES, O. J. J.
Records of practical instruction. *Nursing Times*, Mar. 26, 1965, p. 417.

STOOPS, MICHAEL
Comparison of student nurse profiles. Berkeley, Calif. Program in Hospital Administration, University of California, 1966.

STRYKER, RUTH P.
Refresher course—a series of surprises. *Nursing Outlook*, April, 1962, p. 232-5.

SWANSBURG, R. C.
Blueprint for a refresher course. *Nursing Outlook*, Feb. 1966, p. 54-5.

TATE, BARBARA L.
Rate of graduation in schools of nursing. *International Nursing Review*, vol. 15, no. 4, 1968, p. 339-46.

TATE, BARBARA L., *and* KNOPF, LUCILLE
Nurse career-pattern study. Part 1—Practical nursing programs. New York, National League for Nursing, 1968.

TATTERSALL, E. R.
School of Nursing, Lagos University Teaching Hospital. *Nigerian Nurse*, Feb. 1968, p. 14-9.

THOMPSON, V. D.
Sensitivity training and nursing education: a process study. *Nursing Research*, Spring 1965, p. 132-7.

THURSTON, J. R., *and* BRUNCLIK, H. L.
The relationship of personality to achievement in nursing education. *Nursing Research*, Summer 1965, p. 203-9.

TIMMINS, N. G.
Nursing against the odds (Nigeria). *Nursing Times*, Dec. 24, 1965, p. 1763-4.

TORONTO. COMMITTEE FOR SURVEY OF HOSPITAL NEEDS IN METROPOLITAN TORONTO
Education and the provision of personnel: part sixteen of the study by the Committee. Toronto, The Committee, 1963.

TORONTO. UNIVERSITY SCHOOL OF NURSING
Continuing education for nurses; a study of the need for continuing education for registered nurses in Ontario by . . . and Division of University Extension. Toronto, 1968.

TORRANCE, P. N.
Does nursing education reduce creativity? *Nursing Outlook*, July 1964, p. 27-30.

TOSIELLO, F.
A liberal education for nursing. *Nursing Outlook*, Mar. 1965, p. 64-6.

TRAINED NURSES' ASSOCIATION OF INDIA
Nurses' inquiry commission recommends improvement in hospitals and nursing schools. *Nursing Journal of India*, May 1969, p. 157-8.

TROUTEN, F.
Are changes in nursing education removing students from operating room experience? *Hospital Administration in Canada*, Aug. 1968, p. 64-6.

TSCHUDIN, M. S.
Educational preparation needed by the nurse in the future. *Nursing Outlook*, April 1964, p. 32-5.

TURNER, W. K.
Must the patient pay for nursing education? *Hospitals*, Dec. 16, 1961, p. 53-5 and 104.

UDDOH, C.
Report of the first symposium of the Nigerian Association of Nurse Tutors. *Nigerian Nurse*, Jan. 1970, p. 87-9.

UNITED STATES. PUBLIC HEALTH SERVICE
Refresher programs for inactive professional nurses; a guide for developing courses for study. Washington, D.C., U.S. Government Printing Office, 1967. (Publication no. 1611.)

UNITED STATES. PUBLIC HEALTH SERVICE, DIVISION OF NURSING
Nurse training act of 1964. Rev. edn. Washington, The Department, 1965.
[Public Health Service Publication 1154.]

UNITED STATES. PUBLIC HEALTH SERVICE, DIVISION OF NURSING
Nurse training act of 1964: program review report. Arlington, Virginia, U.S. Department of Health, Education and Welfare, 1967.
[Public Health Service Publication no. 1740.]

VAILLOT, M. C.
Nursing theory, levels of nursing, and curriculum development. *Nursing Forum*, vol. IX, no. 3, 1970, p. 234-49.

VAUGHAN-RICHARDS, G. A.
A review of nursing education in Nigeria. *Nigerian Nurse*, Feb. 1968, p. 25-7.

WALLACE, M. B.
Hospitals should retain their schools of nursing. *The Canadian Nurse*, Feb. 1966, p. 27-8.

WATKIN, BRIAN
Bedside teaching. Macmillan, 1962.

WATKIN, BRIAN
Self-help and higher education. *Nursing Mirror*, July 3, 1970, p. 11-2.

WATKIN, BRIAN, *and* TAYLOR, MARK
An experiment in management education for nurses.
In
MCLACHLAN, GORDON, *editor*
Problems and progress in medical care. 4th series, 1970. Chapter 6. Oxford U.P. (for Nuffield P.H.T.)

WATSON, MARION
Development programme. [Changes in nursing education in hospitals in N.S.W.] *The Lamp*, Mar. 1969, p. 17-20.

WESTERN COUNCIL ON HIGHER EDUCATION FOR NURSING
Today and tomorrow in western nursing. Boulder, Colorado, Western Interstate Commission for Higher Education, 1966.

WESTERN COUNCIL ON HIGHER EDUCATION FOR NURSES
Toward more effective teaching in WCHEN schools: the report of a short-term course in improving instruction through the use of selected teaching tools and techniques under the direction of Jo Eleanor Elliott. Colorado, Western Interstate Commission for Higher Education, 1964.

WHITE, DOROTHY T.
Abilities needed by teachers of nursing in community colleges. New York, N.L.N., 1961.

WHITE, DOROTHY T.
Have our values in nursing really changed—or were we sidetracked? *Nursing Science*, April 1963, p. 48-57.

WILKINSON, MAY G.
Refresher practice. *American Journal of Nursing*, Feb. 1965, p. 108-9.

WILLIAMS, HEATHER M.
The integrated nurse/health visitor course: a report of the first five years of the experimental course organized by the University of Southampton and the Nightingale School, St. Thomas' Hospital. [Southampton University], 1962.

WILSON, K. J. W.
The common-sense of nursing science. *International Journal of Nursing Studies*, no. 3, 1964, p. 119-24.

WILSON, W. L., *and* POIRIER, W. A.
Nursing education in New Hampshire. *Nursing Outlook*, Dec. 1961, p. 739-41.

WOOD, VIVIAN
Accreditation and the Canadian school of nursing diploma program. London, Ontario, 1961 (no publisher).

ZDERAD, LORETTA, *and* BELCHER, HELEN C.
Developing behavioral concepts in nursing: report of the Regional project in teaching psychiatric nursing in baccalaureate programs. Atlanta, Ga., Southern Regional Education Board, 1968.

ZINBERG, N. E., *and others*
Some vicissitudes of nursing education. *Nursing Outlook*, Dec. 1962, p. 795-8.

ZODIACAL, C. P.
Philosophy and aims of clinical instruction. *Santo Tomas Nursing Journal*, Dec. 1965, p. 211-3.

Associate Degree Programmes

ANDERSON, K. C.
An associate degree nursing program in a medical center. *The Journal of Nursing Education*, Feb./Mar. 1963, p. 17-8.

CAFFERTY, KATHRYN W.
Faculty orientation and in-service education in one associate degree program. *Journal of Nursing Education*, April 1964, p. 19-23.

CHATER, S. S.
Selection of content for associate degree programs. *Nursing Outlook*, July 1970, p. 50-2.

DECHOW, G. H.
Accreditation of associate degree nursing programs. *Journal of Nursing Education*, Aug. 1965, p. 27-32.

DUNLAP, MARJORIE S.
Preparation of nurse faculty for associate degree nursing program. *Nursing Science*, June 1964, p. 223-34.

GEITGEY, DORIS A.
Teacher in associate degree programs. *Nursing Outlook*, Feb. 1967, p. 30-2.

LEWIS, E. P.
The associate degree program. *American Journal of Nursing*, May 1964, p. 78-81.

LOGAN, W. W.
Overview of the Associate Degree in Nursing in the U.S.A.: Possible applications to nursing education in the United Kingdom. *International Journal of Nursing Studies*, Aug. 1967, p. 245-53.

MARTIN, A. B.
Associate degree nursing ... are changes needed in the practice field for new graduates? *Journal of Nursing Education*, Aug. 1969, p. 7-12.

MONTAG, MILDRED L.
Nurse faculty in associate degree programs. *Nursing Outlook*, July 1964, p. 40-2.

MONTAG, MILDRED L.
Utilization of graduates of associate degree nursing programs. *Journal of Nursing Education*, April 1966, p. 5-9.

NATIONAL LEAGUE FOR NURSING. DEPARTMENT OF DIPLOMA AND ASSOCIATE DEGREE PROGRAMS
Criteria for the evaluation of educational programs in nursing leading to a diploma. Rev. edn. New York, N.L.N., 1962.

NATIONAL LEAGUE FOR NURSING. DEPARTMENT OF DIPLOMA AND ASSOCIATE DEGREE PROGRAMS
Report on associate degree programs in nursing. New York, N.L.N., 1961.

NATIONAL LEAGUE FOR NURSING. DEPARTMENT OF DIPLOMA AND ASSOCIATE DEGREE PROGRAMS.
Trends in continuing education; a report of the 1960 regional meetings. New York, N.L.N., 1961.

NATIONAL LEAGUE FOR NURSING. DEPARTMENT OF DIPLOMA AND ASSOCIATE DEGREE PROGRAMS
Utilization of faculty in associate degree programs in nursing: report of a Conference held in St. Louis, Missouri, April 3-4, 1964. New York, The League, 1964.

NEW YORK STATE UNIVERSITY, STATE EDUCATION DEPARTMENT
New York State Associate Degree Nursing Project, 1959-1964. Final report to the W. K. Kellogg Foundation. Albany, N.Y. State Education Department, 1964.

PARSE, ROSEMARIE R.
Advantages of the associate degree nursing program. *Journal of Nursing Education*, Aug. 1967, p. 15-21, and 24-5.

SCHMIDT, MILDRED S.
Factors affecting the establishment of associate degree programs in nursing in community junior colleges. New York, National League for Nursing, Department of Associate Degree Programs, 1966.

SCHMIDT, MILDRED S.
Obtaining and keeping faculty in an associate degree nursing program. Atlanta, Ga., Southern Regional Education Board, 1965.

WALKER, C. N.
The associate degree nurse. *Hospital Management*, Aug. 1967, p. 70-2.

ZEITZ, ANN N., *and others*
Associate degree nursing: a guide to programs and curriculum development. St. Louis, C. V. Mosby, 1969.

ZIMMERMAN, ESTHER D.
Associate degree program graduate in nursing service. *Journal of Nursing Education*, April 1966, p. 11-3, 15-6, and 39-41.

Bibliographies

CUMULATIVE INDEX TO NURSING LITERATURE
1956 to 1960, vols. 1-5, edited by Ella J. Crandall and Fumiko Oiye. Glendale, Calif., Seventh-Day Adventist Hospital Association, 1961 [in progress].
Cover title: Nursing literature index.

INTERNATIONAL NURSING INDEX
New York, American Journal of Nursing Co. and National Library of Medicine, cumulative vols. Vol. 1, 1966 [in progress].

NURSING STUDIES INDEX
An annotated guide to reported studies, research methods, and historical and biographical materials in periodicals, books and pamphlets published in English. Prepared by Yale University School of Nursing Index Staff, under the direction of Virginia Henderson. Philadelphia, Lippincott.
Vol. II, 1930-49 (1970).
Vol. III, 1950-6 (1966).
Vol. IV, 1957-9 (1963).

THOMPSON, ALICE M. C., *editor*
A bibliography of nursing literature, 1859-1960, with an historical introduction. Library Association, for the Royal College of Nursing and National Council of Nurses of the United Kingdom in association with King Edward's Hospital Fund for London, 1968.

Careers in Nursing

ALEXANDER, FLORENCE M.
Education for a career in nursing. *JAMA*, Feb. 14, 1966, p. 591-3.

BENJAMIN, NANCY, *and* CICATIELLO, PATRICIA
Needed: career counseling for nursing students. *Nursing Outlook*, Oct. 1964, p. 56-7.

CARB, GENEVIEVE R.
Tutoring project is gateway to nursing careers for underprivileged girls. *Hospitals*, Sept. 1, 1967, p. 59-61, and 154.

CENTRAL YOUTH EMPLOYMENT EXECUTIVE
Nursing and midwifery. 3rd edn. H.M.S.O., 1965.
4th edn., 1968. [Choice of careers, no. 82].

CENTRAL YOUTH EMPLOYMENT EXECUTIVE
Nursing for men. 2nd edn. H.M.S.O., 1962.
3rd edn., 1967. [Choice of careers, no. 89.]

DARNELL, LILIAN M.
Nursing. 3rd edn. Hale, 1965.

DAVIS, FRED, *and* OLESEN, VIRGINIA L.
Career outlook of professionally educated women; the case of collegiate student nurses. *Psychiatry*, Nov. 1965, p. 334-45.

EDWARDS, C. N., *and* GRIBBLE, G.
Nursing as a career. How students perceive it. *American Journal of Nursing*, June 1969, p. 1223-5.

FRACKLETON, DOROTHY L., *and* FAVILLE, KATHERINE
Opportunities in nursing for disadvantaged youth. *Nursing Outlook*, April 1966, p. 26-8.

BIBLIOGRAPHY OF NURSING

GILLAM, ROBERT
Schoolgirls' interest in nursing as a career. School of Hospital Administration, University of New South Wales, 1968.
[Australian studies in health service administration—3.]

GORDON, J. E.
Nursing as a second career. *British Hospital Journal and Social Service Review*, Sept. 24, 1965, p. 1818-9.

GRAVELIUS, E. M.
Shall I take up nursing? *Nursing Times*, May 7, 1965, p. 639.

HEIDGERKEN, L. E.
Nursing as a career: is it relevant? *American Journal of Nursing*, June 1969, p. 1217-22.

HEIDGERKEN, L. E.
Work values and career preferences of nurses for teaching and clinical nursing practice. *Nursing Research*, May/June 1970, p. 219-30.

INDEX OF OPPORTUNITY IN THE NURSING PROFESSION
A directory of career opportunities for registered nurses with hospitals, nursing homes, sanitariums and other medical, health and welfare institutions. Princeton, Resource Publications, Inc., 1969.

KATZELL, M. E.
Upward mobility in nursing: helping students up the career ladder in nursing. *Nursing Outlook*, Sept. 1970, p. 36-9.

KING, CHRISTINE
Your career in... nursing and physiotherapy. Cornmarket: *Daily Express*, 1970.

KNUDSON, E. G.
Deterrents to developing interest in occupational advancement among nurses. *The Journal of Nursing Education*, Jan. 1968, p. 27-30.

KNUDSON, E. G.
Nurses and occupational advancement. *Nursing Outlook*, Aug. 1969, p. 29-31.

LANDE, S.
Nursing career perceptions among high school students. *Nursing Research*, Fall 1966, p. 337-42.

LEONETTI, ANN N.
Status of guidance services for potential nurse candidates in selected senior high schools. *Journal of Nursing Education*, Aug. 1965, p. 9-13.

MAJOR, DOROTHY M.
Career planning of high-ranking senior students. *Nursing Research*, Spring 1961, p. 68-74.

NURSING JOURNAL OF INDIA
Trends in health services and implications for nursing. *Nursing Journal of India*, July 1964, p. 197-9.

PANKRATZ, L. D., and PANKRATZ, D. M.
Determinants in choosing a nursing career. *Nursing Research*, Spring 1967, p. 169-72.

POWERS, ELEANORE FRANCIS
Attitudes toward professionalization and career plans: a study of nursing students in sectarian and non-sectarian baccalaureate degree program. *Journal of Nursing Education*, Aug. 1964, p. 17-23.

RAMPHAL, M.
Needed: a career ladder. *American Journal of Nursing*, June 1968, p. 1234-7.

RAYNER, CLAIRE
Shall I be a nurse? Exeter, Wheaton, 1967.

ROSS, AILEEN D.
Becoming a nurse. Toronto, Macmillan, 1961.

SHETLAND, M. L.
This I believe... about career ladders, new careers and nursing education. *Nursing Outlook*, Sept. 1970, p. 32-5.

WEISS, M. OLGA
Opportunities in nursing careers. New York, Universal Publishing and Distributing Corporation, 1964.

Collegiate Schools

BULLOUGH, B., and BULLOUGH, V.
Collegiate nursing in the United States. An historical review. *International Nursing Review*, vol. 10, no. 1, 1963, p. 41-7.

COLUMBIA UNIVERSITY. TEACHERS' COLLEGE
Development of general education to collegiate nursing programs: role of the administrator, by Mary Kohl Pillepich. Bureau of Publications, Teachers' College, Columbia University, 1962.
[Nursing Education Monographs, no. 2.]

COULTER, PEARL PARVIN
The winds of change: a progress report of regional co-operation in collegiate nursing education in the West 1956-1961. Colorado, Western Interstate Commission for Higher Education, 1963.

COULTER, PEARL PARVIN, and LEINO, AMELIA
Validation of the collegiate nursing curriculum through use of the critical incident: report of a study by a committee of the Baccalaureate Seminar of the Western Council on Higher Education for Nursing, Western Interstate Commission for Higher Education. Boulder, Colo., the Council, 1965.

DINEEN, M. A.
Current trends in collegiate nursing education. *Nursing Outlook*, Aug. 1969, p. 22-6.

DREVES, K. D.
University of Minnesota School of Nursing. An account of the first American collegiate nursing programme. *Nursing Outlook*, Jan. 1961, p. 14-8.

MACDONALD, GWENDOLINE
Development of standards and accreditation in collegiate nursing education. New York, Teachers' College, Columbia University, 1965.

NATIONAL LEAGUE FOR NURSING. DEPARTMENT OF BACCALAUREATE AND HIGHER DEGREE PROGRAMS
Excellence in education: the role of accreditation in collegiate nursing education: a report of a Conference held... in co-operation with the National Commission on Accrediting, St. Louis, Missouri, Nov. 10-1, 1960. New York, N.L.N., 1961.

Curricula and Syllabus

BANKS, I.
Designing the training programme for student nurses. [By computer.] *Nursing Times*, Nov. 29, 1968, Occasional Papers, p. 186-8.

COKER, N.
Implications of the 1969 General Nursing Council. Syllabus of the nursing services. *Nursing Times*, Oct. 8, 1970, Occasional Papers, p. 151-2.

CORONA, D. F.
A continuous progress curriculum in nursing. *Nursing Outlook*, Jan. 1970, p. 46-8.

DICKOFF, J., and JAMES, P.
Beliefs and values: bases for curriculum design. *Nursing Research*, Sept./Oct. 1970, p. 415-27.

GENERAL NURSING COUNCIL FOR ENGLAND AND WALES
Syllabus of subjects for examination and record of practical instruction and experience for the certificate of nursing of the mentally subnormal. The Council, 1970.

GENERAL NURSING COUNCIL FOR ENGLAND AND WALES
Syllabus of subjects for examination and record of practical instruction and experience for the certificate of general nursing. The Council, 1969.

GENERAL NURSING COUNCIL FOR ENGLAND AND WALES
Guide to the syllabus of subjects for examination for the certificate of nursing of sick children. The Council, 1964.

NURSING AS A PROFESSION

GENERAL NURSING COUNCIL FOR ENGLAND AND WALES
Guide to the syllabus of subjects for examination for the certificate of general nursing. The Council, 1962.

HARMS, M. T., *and* MCDONALD, F. J.
A new curriculum design. *Nursing Outlook*, Sept. 1966, p. 50-3.

HOLDSWORTH, J. N.
A creative approach to curriculum development. *Journal of Nursing Education*, April 1969, p. 3-5.

JORDON, M.
Vision and revision: report of a curriculum revision project in a practical nursing program. New York, National League for Nursing, Dept. of Practical Nursing Programs, 1966.

LUM, J. L. J., *and* KIM, H. T.
A faculty undertakes a major curriculum revision [at School of Nursing in the College of Applied Sciences, University of Hawaii]. *The Journal of Nursing Education*, Aug. 1967, p. 19-23.

MCDONALD, F. J., *and* HARMS, M. T.
A theoretical model for an experimental curriculum. *Nursing Outlook*, Aug. 1966, p. 48-51.

Dictionaries, Glossaries, Year Books, Directories

AMERICAN PSYCHIATRIC ASSOCIATION. COMMITTEE ON PUBLIC INFORMATION
A psychiatric glossary: the meaning of words most frequently used in psychiatry. 2nd edn. Washington, The Association, 1964.

AUSTRALASIAN hospital directory and nurses' year book, 1963; compiled and annotated by A. L. Hart. Sydney, New South Wales Nurses' Association, 1963 [in progress].

CARTER, GLADYS B., *and others*
A dictionary of midwifery and public health, by G. B. Carter, Gladys H. Dodds, and P. J. Cunningham. 2nd edn. Faber, 1963.

DAVIES, PAUL M.
Medical terminology in hospital practice: a guide for all those engaged in professions allied to medicine. Heinemann, 1969.

FITCH, GRACE E., *and* DUBINY, MARY JANE, *editors*
The Macmillan dictionary for practical and vocational nurses. New York, Macmillan, 1966.

FRENAY, Sister MARY AGNES CLARE
Understanding medical terminology. 3rd edn. St. Louis, Missouri, Catholic Hospital Association, 1966.

MORTEN, HONNOR
The nurses' dictionary of medical terms and nursing treatment, compiled for the use of nurses ... 25th edn. Faber, 1962.

OAKES, LOIS, *and* DAVIE, THOMAS B.
A new dictionary for nurses. 11th edn. Edinburgh, Livingstone, 1961.
12th edn., 1966.
13th edn., 1969. [All edited by Nancy Roper.]

OAKES, LOIS, *and* DAVIE, THOMAS B.
A pocket medical dictionary. 9th edn., comp. by Nancy Roper. Edinburgh, Livingstone, 1961.
10th edn., 1966.

SCHMIDT, J. E.
Practical nurses' medical dictionary: a cyclopedic medical dictionary for practical nurses, vocational nurses and nurses' aides. Springfield, Ill., Thomas, 1968.

STEDMAN'S MEDICAL DICTIONARY
A vocabulary of medicine and its allied sciences, with pronunciations and derivations. 21st edn. Edinburgh, Livingstone, 1966.

STRAND, HELEN R.
An illustrated guide to medical terminology. Baltimore, Williams & Wilkins, 1968.

THOMAS, D., *and* THOMAS, J.
English for nurses. Edward Arnold, 1969.

Diploma Schools

CANADIAN NURSES' ASSOCIATION
Criteria for the evaluation of diploma programms in nursing. Ottawa, The Association, 1966.
[French and English text.]

DRUMMOND, E. J.
The future of the diploma school in nursing education. *Hospitals*, Aug. 1, 1965, p. 59-62.

ERICKSON, E. H.
Why nurses need a college education. *Modern Hospital*, Feb. 1963, p. 89-90 and 146.

HARVEY, E. L.
Financing diploma schools of nursing. *Hospital Management*, Dec. 1961, p. 26.

LAMBERTSEN, E. C.
How diploma nursing schools view accreditation—report of a survey. *Hospitals*, May 1, 1962, p. 54.

NATIONAL LEAGUE FOR NURSING
Education for nursing—the diploma way: information about NLN-accredited diploma programs in nursing. New York, The League, 1968.

NATIONAL LEAGUE FOR NURSING. DEPARTMENT OF DIPLOMA AND ASSOCIATE DEGREE PROGRAMS
Nursing education in community colleges. Proceedings of the Conference on Nursing Education in Community Colleges held on Nov. 1, 1962, at Newton Junior College, Newtonville, Massachusetts. New York, The League, 1964.
[League Exchange no. 68.]

NATIONAL LEAGUE FOR NURSING. DEPARTMENT OF DIPLOMA AND ASSOCIATE DEGREE PROGRAMS
To-day's diploma schools of nursing, prepared by Elizabeth V. Cunningham. New York, National League for Nursing, 1963.

PETERSON, F. K.
The new diploma schools. *American Journal of Nursing*, May, 1964, p. 68-72.

PSATHAS, GEORGE
The student nurse in the diploma school of nursing. New York, Springer, 1968.

ROWE, HAROLD R., *and* FLITTER, HESSEL H.
Study on cost of nursing education. Part 1—Cost of basic diploma programs. New York, National League for Nursing, 1964.

STEED, M. E.
Trends in diploma nursing education. *The Canadian Nurse*, Feb. 1968, p. 40-1.

Examinations

ALLEN, C.
Sitting examinations. *Nursing Times*, Mar. 29, 1963, p. 386-8.

ANDERSON, D.
The gentle art of the examiner. *The Australian Nurses' Journal*, Nov. 1965, p. 266-8.

BEVAN, JAMES
State final questions and answers for nurses. Faber, 1962.
2nd edn., 1964.
3rd edn., 1966.
4th edn., 1968.

BRIGGS, M. R., *and* MACGUIRE, J. M.
Towards a ward-based final practical examination: an assessment of a pilot scheme in four general hospitals. *Nursing Times*, July 19, 1968, Occasional Papers, p. 109-11.

BROWN, M. H.
How much do tests and grades motivate learning? *Nursing Outlook*, Oct. 1968, p. 60-2.

CONGALTON, A. A.
To test or trap? *Nursing Times*, Jan. 8, 1965, p. 62-3.

GENERAL NURSING COUNCIL FOR ENGLAND AND WALES
Changes in State Final Examinations for the general part of the register. *Nursing Times*, Sept. 8, 1961, p. 1145.

GENERAL NURSING COUNCIL FOR ENGLAND AND WALES
GNC Intermediate Examination changes. *Nursing Mirror*, Nov. 7, 1969, p. 17.

GENERAL NURSING COUNCIL FOR ENGLAND AND WALES
Revised general training syllabus, *Nursing Mirror*, May 25, 1962, p. 151.

GENERAL NURSING COUNCIL FOR ENGLAND AND WALES
Revised training regulations of the General Nursing Council for England and Wales. *Nursing Mirror*, Mar. 11, 1966, p. 675.

GRUNHUT, I.
How to pass—the art of taking an examination. *Nursing Times*, Oct. 1, 1970, p. 1274-5.

JAMES, D. E.
Answering examination questions. *Nursing Times*, Mar. 18, 1966, p. 385-6.

JAMES, D. E.
Aspects of examinations—1. Examinations in perspective. *Nursing Times*, Sept. 16, 1966, p. 1216-7.

JAMES, D. E.
Aspects of examinations—2. Form and function in examinations. *Nursing Times*, Sept. 23, 1966, p. 1261-3.

JAMES, D. E.
Aspects of examinations—3. Setting and marking examinations. *Nursing Times*, Sept. 30, 1966, p. 1290-1.

JAMES, D. E.
Aspects of examinations—4. Effects of examinations on nursing education. *Nursing Times*, Oct. 7, 1966, p. 1333-4.

JAMES, D. E.
Revising for examinations. *Nursing Times*, Mar. 11, 1966, p. 346-8.

KIRWIN, W. B.
The art of examining. *Nursing Mirror*, June 26, 1970, p. 25-7.

NATIONAL LEAGUE FOR NURSING
Let's examine ... Development of a National League for Nursing standardized achievement test. *Nursing Outlook*, Mar. 1966, p. 65.

NATIONAL LEAGUE FOR NURSING
Let's examine—differences in test scores of students in diploma and degree programs. *Nursing Outlook*, Sept. 1962, p. 617.

NATIONAL LEAGUE FOR NURSING
Let's examine—grids for teacher-made tests. *Nursing Outlook*, May 1962, p. 339.

NOTMAN, A. G.
Is it a success? The 1962 syllabus. *Nursing Times*, April 1, 1966, p. 454-5.

OWEN, S. V., *and* FELDHUSEN, J. F.
Effectiveness of three models of multivariate prediction of academic success in nursing education. *Nursing Research*, Nov./Dec. 1970, p. 517-25.

RAJABALLY, J.
Is the GNC system of examining obsolete? *Nursing Mirror*, Dec. 18, 1970, p. 10-1.

ROBERTS, T.
How practical is the practical final examination for psychiatric student nurses? *Nursing Mirror*, June 16, 1967, p. 252-4.

ROYAL COLLEGE OF NURSING, SCOTLAND
Clinical instructors' course—students' evaluation. *Nursing Times*, Aug. 25, 1961, p. 1102-4.

SCOTT, W. A.
Art and practice of examining—1 and 2. *Nursing Times*, Sept. 7, 1962, p. 1133-4; Sept. 14, 1962, p. 1160-2.

UNIVERSITY OF ARIZONA COLLEGE OF NURSING
Curriculum subcommittee on rating scales. Let's examine: a method of developing performance rating scales. *Nursing Outlook*, Oct. 1970, p. 57.

WHYTE, B. BRYSSON
Practical examinations in the ward. *Nursing Times*, Nov. 26, 1970, Occasional Papers, p. 179-80.

WHYTE, B. BRYSSON, *and* DAVIS, A.
Multiple choice questions. *Nursing Times*, Feb. 9, 1968, p. 190-3.

In-Service Education

ANDERSON, P. S. B.
A familiar process in a new dress. *The Canadian Nurse*, May 1962, p. 415-7.

BIRCH, N. M.
In-service training for sisters. *Nursing Times*, May 31, 1963, p. 692.

CALLIN, M. E.
In-service education. *The Canadian Nurse*, Aug. 1967, p. 32-4.

DAS, D. M. H.
In-service education—"A tool for Health Care". *The Nursing Journal of India*, July 1969, p. 233, and 237.

DAUK, C. S.
In-service education: its application. *The Canadian Nurse*, May 1962, p. 419-20.

DEOCAMPO, MARIE ANNE DE JESUS
The in-service education for nursing service personnel. *Santo Tomas Nursing Journal*, Mar. 1965, p. 296-303.

FOGT, J. R.
In-service concerns everyone. *American Journal of Nursing*, Nov. 1963, p. 83-5.

FOSTER, R.
Here's how in-service education works. *Modern Hospital*, Oct. 1970, p. 95-96 and 134.

GAUTHIER, L., *and others*
Unit-based in-service education. *The Canadian Nurse*, Aug. 1967, p. 39-42.

GERMAINE, A.
Nursing administration. In-service programs face challenge. *Hospital Administration in Canada*, July 1969, p. 42-3.

KANE, M.
An in-service program for professional nurses. *Nursing Outlook*, May 1964, p. 38-9.

LEVA, I.
In-service education for nursing personnel in the Children's Hospital in Helsinki. *International Journal of Nursing Studies*, Dec. 1967, p. 319-22.

LINDEMAN, C. A., *and* VAN AERNAM, A. B.
Staff develops in-service programs to teach itself. *Modern Hospital*, Oct. 1970, p. 98-100.

LOCHORE, M. S.
In-service education [report of Inter-country Workshop held in Bangkok, 1967]. *The New Zealand Nursing Journal*, Aug. 1968, p. 26-7.

MCPHETRIDGE, M.
In-service nursing education. *Hospital Management*, May 1963, p. 54, 56, 58, 60 and 61.

MILLER, M. A.
In-service education—conceptual handicaps, parts I and II. *Nursing Outlook*, Oct. 1962, p. 691; Nov. 1962, p. 753.

MILLER, M. A.
In-service education—are orientation and skill training true in-service education? *Nursing Outlook*, Dec. 1962, p. 787.

MILLER, M. A.
In-service education—what, why, where, how, when? *Nursing Outlook*, Aug. 1962, p. 541-3.

MILLER, M. A.
Sources for assistance in in-service education. New York, National League for Nursing, 1962.

MUHS, E. J.
In-service education: an investment in nursing. *Nursing Outlook*, Feb. 1969, p. 50-1.

NELSON, E. M.
Teaching students at night. *The American Journal of Nursing*, June 1962, p. 105.

OSCAR, M., *and* GARRETSON, A. M.
"Tomispstare": a formula for planning and carrying out meaningful, practical in-service education programs for nursing service personnel. *Nursing Outlook*, Oct. 1970, p. 38-41.

PALK, M. L.
In the Victorian Order of Nurses. In in-service education there is no room for complacency. *The Canadian Nurse*, May 1962, p. 424.

PETTUS, M. A.
Staff nurses plan their own in-service program. *American Journal of Nursing*, June 1963, p. 82-4.

PIRNIE, F. A.
Why, what, and how of in-service education. *Nursing Outlook*, Jan. 1964, p. 47-51.

POST, S.
In-service for teachers too? *Canadian Nurse*, Sept. 1969, p. 29-30.

SEWELL, E. M.
An over-view of in-service education. A statement of the general principles underlying a staff education program. *The Canadian Nurse*, May 1962, p. 413-4.

SWANSBURG, RUSSELL C.
A design for an in-service education program. *Nursing Outlook*, March 1965, p. 40-2.

SWANSBURG, RUSSELL C.
In-service education. New York, Putman, 1968.

TOSIELLO, F.
University-oriented in-service education. *Nursing Outlook*, April 1964, p. 40-2.

VETERANS' ADMINISTRATION. DEPARTMENT OF MEDICINE AND SURGERY
In-service education activities in nursing service. Washington, The Administration, 1963.

WHITEFORD, L. J.
In the health service for Indians and Eskimos. Orientation, like all learning, is continuous and does not end at the completion of two weeks. It is all part of in-service education which leads to good nursing care. *The Canadian Nurse*, May 1962, p. 427.

WORLD HEALTH ORGANIZATION
Guide for in-service education of nursing personnel, prepared by Ingrid Hamelin. Geneva, W.H.O., 1967.

YUN-O, LU
In-service education programmes. *International Nursing Review*, vol. 10, no. 1, 1963, p. 24-30.

Integrated Courses

ALTSCHUL, A.
Conflict. A basic training for general and psychiatric nursing. *Nursing Times*, Dec. 17, 1965, p. 1712-3.

BENDALL, E. R. D.
A change in pattern of nurse training. The integrated scheme at the Hospital for Sick Children, Gt. Ormond Street, London. *Nursing Mirror*, Aug. 7, 1964, p. x-xiii.

BRYDEN, E. G. M.
Integrated course of nurse education: a study of an experiment ... conducted by Hammersmith Hospital and Royal Post-Graduate Medical School, Battersea College of Technology (now University of Surrey), Queen's Institute of District Nursing. The Institute, 1969.

CHITTICK, R.
The integration of general and psychiatric nursing in the curriculum. *The Jamaican Nurse*, Dec. 1966, p. 10-1.

DEAN, D. J.
Basic training for general and psychiatric nursing? *Nursing Mirror*, June 24, 1966, p. 275-6.

GODDEN, G. M.
Obstetric secondment. A pilot scheme at Hammersmith Hospital. *Nursing Times*, Feb. 23, 1962, p. 239-42.

HALE, R.
An integrated course of nurse education. *Nursing Mirror*, June 14, 1963, p. v-vi.

ILLING, M.
Integrated course. King's College Hospital, Royal College of Nursing. *District Nursing*, Nov. 1965, p. 208-9.

KENNETH, H. Y.
Medical and nursing students learn together. *Nursing Outlook*, Nov. 1969, p. 46-9.

LLEWELLYN, E. M.
Integrated course. Hillingdon and West Middlesex Hospitals. Chiswick Polytechnic. *District Nursing*, Nov. 1965, p. 209.

MORTON, P.
Diploma in community nursing course. Manchester University, Crumpsall Hospital, Queen's Institute of District Nursing. *District Nursing*, Nov. 1965, p. 206-8.

ST. GEORGE'S HOSPITAL, LONDON
An experiment in integrated training by G. V. Marsh. *The Hospital*, Oct. 1965, p. 528-31.

SOUTHAMPTON UNIVERSITY/ST. THOMAS' HOSPITAL, LONDON
Students' eye view of integrated training scheme for health visitors at University of Southampton and St. Thomas' Hospital, London. *Nursing Mirror*, Jan. 5, 1962, p. v-vii.

Pre-Nursing Courses

BRISTOW, A.
Hospital cadet courses in transition. *Nursing Times*, Jan. 31, 1964, p. 154-5.

CHAMBERS, V.
Cadet schemes, recruitment and wastage. *Nursing Times*, Jan. 20, 1961, p. 89-90.

CLARKE, V. H.
Education for pre-nursing cadets. [An experiment in block release education for pre-nursing cadets undertaken by the Sheffield Regional Hospital Board.] *Nursing Mirror*, Dec. 6, 1968, p. 15.

DRUMMOND, E. J.
The hospital school—as school. [Hospitals schools of nursing seen in relation to other branches of higher education.] *Hospital Progress*, Feb. 1969, p. 45-8 and 64.

ERITH TECHNICAL COLLEGE, WOOLWICH
New gateway to nursing for school-leavers. *Nursing Times*, Feb. 8, 1963, p. 165-6 and 175.

GRANT, R.
Sheffield's pre-nursing innovation. *Nursing Mirror*, July 26, 1968, p. 18-21.

OXFORD REGIONAL HOSPITAL BOARD
Nursing cadet schemes: analysis of replies relating to 471 cadets. Oxford, The Board, 1970.

REVANS, R. W.
Hospital cadet schemes—a study in the Manchester region. *International Journal of Nursing Studies*, May 1964, p. 65-74.

SAWKINS, E. M.
Pre-nursing studies and colleges of further education. *Nursing Times*, May 29, 1969, p. 697-8.

SCOTTISH EDUCATION DEPARTMENT
Report of a study group on the future pattern of pre-nursing courses in Scotland. Edinburgh, Scottish Education Department, 1963.
[*Chairman:* W. S. Gray.]

WARCABA, B.
Project for nursing cadets. *Nursing Times*, Aug. 25, 1967, p. 1146-7.

Student Status

ADAMS, J.
Considerations in assessing changes in personality characteristics of nursing students. *Journal of Psychiatric Nursing*, Nov./Dec. 1970, p. 12-6.

BAILEY, J. T., *and* CLAUS, K. E.
Comparative analysis of the personality structure of nursing students. *Nursing Research*, July/Aug. 1969, p. 320-6.

BASHFORD, A. J.
Nursing and the universities. A student's view. *Nursing Times*, Oct. 15, 1970, p. 1340-1.

BENDALL, E. R. D.
Human problems of student nurses. *Mental Health*, April 1965, p. 69-71.

BERZON, F. C.
Use of extended care facility for beginning students. *Nursing Outlook*, Nov. 1970, p. 44-6.

CASWELL, G.
Keeping the balance: some aspects of student nurse allocation and training. *Nursing Times*, Sept. 6, 1968, Occasional Papers, p. 137-40.

DEVANESON, BERYL A.
Counselling. *Nursing Journal of India*, Dec. 1968, p. 390-1 and 397.

DUSTAN, LAURA C.
Characteristics of students in three types of nursing education programs. *Nursing Research*, Spring 1964, p. 159-66.

FOX, D. J., *and others*
The nursing student in the hospital setting. *Hospitals*, July 1, 1963, p. 50-4 and 56.

FREDERICKS, M. A., *and others*
A model for teaching student nurses social concepts. *Hospital Progress*, Dec. 1969, p. 37-40.

GENERAL NURSING COUNCIL FOR ENGLAND AND WALES
Minimum age of entry to nurse training. *Nursing Times*, May 7, 1970, Occasional Papers, p. 61-3.

GUNTER, L. M.
The developing nursing student. Part I—A study of self-actualizing values. *Nursing Research*, Jan./Feb. 1969, p. 60-4.

GUNTER, L. M.
The developing nursing student. Part II—Attitudes toward nursing as a career. *Nursing Research*, Mar./April 1969, p. 131-6.

GUNTER, L. M.
The developing nursing student. Part III—A study of self-appraisals and concerns reported during the sophomore year. *Nursing Research*, May/June 1969, p. 237-43.

GUNTER, L. M.
The effects of segregation on nursing students. *Nursing Outlook*, Feb. 1961, p. 74-6.

HARVEY, L. H.
Educational problems in minority group nurses. *Nursing Outlook*, Sept. 1970, p. 48-50.

JOHNSTON, M. E.
The mature student. *Nursing Times*, Nov. 2, 1962, p. 1390.

KAUFMAN, E. S., *and* BLAYLOCK, E.
Individual programming for students. *Nursing Outlook*, June 1970, p. 41-3.

KELLER, M. J.
The student program: participation, not observation. *Occupational Health Nursing*, Nov. 1970, p. 17-9.

KING, H. M.
Ward reports: an effort to be fair. *Nursing Times*, Feb. 9, 1968, Occasional Papers, p. 21-4.

KING EDWARD'S HOSPITAL FUND FOR LONDON. HOSPITAL CENTRE
A study of student nurses' progress reports; interim report. The Hospital Centre, [1966].

MCKNEW, DONALD HARRISON, *and* EASTERLY, JUDITH
Psychosocial seminars for nursing students. *Nursing Outlook*, July 1969, p. 44-6.

NURSING FORUM
Introduction to views on student protest. [College of Nursing, Rutgers, New Jersey.] *Nursing Forum*, vol. VIII, no. 2, 1969, p. 118-43.

OGSTON, D. G., *and* OGSTON, K. M.
Counseling students in a hospital school of nursing. *Canadian Nurse*, April 1970, p. 52-3.

OSTLUND, L. A.
An adjustment program for nursing students. *Hospital Topics*, July, 1965, p. 58-61.

PENNY, M.
Excerpts from a study on student nurses. *New Zealand Nursing Journal*, Mar. 1970, p. 7-9; April 1970, p. 16-7.

QUINT, J. C.
Role models and the professional nurse identity. *The Journal of Nursing Education*, April, 1967, p. 11-5.

RYBACK, D.
The student nurse. *Journal of Psychiatric Nursing*, July/Aug. 1968, p. 219-23.

SANFORD, N.
Students and studies. *American Journal of Nursing*, April 1968, p. 805-6.

SMITH, G. M.
The role of personality in nursing education. A comparison of successful and unsuccessful nursing students. *Nursing Research*, Winter 1965, p. 54-8.

STEIN, R. F.
The student nurse. A study of needs, roles and conflicts. Part I. *Nursing Research*, July/Aug. 1969, p. 308-15.

STEIN, R. F.
The student nurse. A study of needs, roles and conflicts. Part II. *Nursing Research*, Sept./Oct. 1969, p. 433-40.

STOOPS, MICHAEL
Comparison of student nurse profiles. Berkeley, California, Program in Hospital Administration, University of California, 1966.

TATE, B., and KNOPF, L.
Nursing students—who are they? A long range study of the characteristics of students initiated in 1962 by the National League for Nursing. *American Journal of Nursing*, Sept. 1965, p. 99-102.

THURSTON, J. R., and BRUNCLIK, H. L.
The relationship of personality to achievement in nursing education. *Nursing Research*, Summer 1965, p. 203-9.

TREECE, E. M.
Students' opinions concerning patient selection for clinical practice. *Journal of Nursing Education*, April 1969, p. 17-22.

WILSON, C.
The effects of cloisterization on students of nursing. *American Journal of Nursing*, Aug. 1970, p. 1726-9.

WOOD, V.
Examining student nurses' problems by the case method. *The Canadian Nurse*, Feb. 1970, p. 31-5.

ZACCARIA, J. S., and REYNOLDS, GENEVIEVE H.
Nursing students' attitudes toward their careers: challenge for nursing education. *Journal of Nursing Education*, Aug. 1966, p. 31-4.

Evaluation of Students

ALLEN, M. G.
A course in practical assessment. *Nursing Times*, May 14, 1970, p. 634-5.

ARANETA, N. C., and MILLER, C. L.
Philosophical systems of weighting clinical performance in nursing. *International Journal of Nursing Studies*, Nov. 1970, p. 235-41.

ARMIGER, B.
Evaluation of student nurses. *Hospital Progress*, Jan. 1962, p. 70-4.

BRESTER, M., and others
Evaluating nursing students. *The American Journal of Nursing*, May 1962, p. 117-9.

BARE, CAROLE E.
Behavioral change through effective evaluation. *Journal of Nursing Education*, Nov. 1967, p. 7-9.

BROOME, W. E.
Nursing standards [student assessment]. *Nursing Mirror*, Aug. 28, 1970, p. 14-5.

CLISSOLD, G. K., and METZ, E. A.
Evaluation—a tangible process. *Nursing Outlook*, Mar. 1966, p. 41-5.

DIAMENT, M. L., and GOLDSMITH, R.
A method of keeping student records and its application to the evaluation of examinations. *British Journal of Medical Education*, June 1970, p. 138-44.

FLANAGAN, J. C., and others
Evaluating student performance. *American Journal of Nursing*, Nov. 1963, p. 96-9.

FRASER, J. R.
Some aspects of trainee nurses' evaluation of their term of operating theatre nursing duties. *Australian Nurses' Journal*, Jan. 1969, p. 16-21.

GILLIES, DEE ANN, and ALYN, IRENE BARRETT
Saunders tests for self-evaluation of nursing competence. Philadelphia, Saunders, 1968.

HESLIN, P.
Evaluating clinical performance. *Nursing Outlook*, May 1963, p. 344-5.

JESCHKE, D. B.
Exceptional students in nursing. *Nursing Outlook*, Oct. 1962, p. 689.

JOURARD, S. M.
The servo theory. A suggested method in evaluation of nursing students. *The Canadian Nurse*, Jan. 1965, p. 40-2.

LOGAN, W. W., and GROSVENOR, P. A.
Students' reactions to an educational programme—1. *Nursing Times*, Feb. 26, 1970, Occasional Papers, p. 33-5.

LOGAN, W. W., and GROSVENOR, P. A.
Students' reactions to an educational programme—2. *Nursing Times*, Mar. 5, 1970, Occasional Papers, p. 37-9.

MALASPINA, H.
How to evaluate nurses' work. *The Modern Hospital*, Aug. 1961, p. 70-4.

MATHENEY, RUTH V.
Pre- and post-conferences for students. *American Journal of Nursing*, Feb. 1969, p. 286-9.

MIMS, F. H.
Students evaluate faculty. *Nursing Outlook*, July 1970, p. 53-5.

MOORE, M. A.
A point of view on evaluation. *Nursing Outlook*, July 1968, p. 54-7.

MORITZ, D. A., and SEXTON, D. L.
Evaluation: a suggested method for appraising quality. *Journal of Nursing Education*, Jan. 1970, p. 17-21, 24-5, 27, 29, and 31-4.

MORMAN, R. R., and others
Predictions of academic achievement of nursing students. *Nursing Research*, Summer 1965, p. 227-30.

MUNDAY, L., and HOYT, D. P.
Predicting academic success for nursing students. *Nursing Research*, Fall 1965, p. 341-4.

NANCE, J. L.
On the delegation of responsibility. [An experiment in self-evaluation with students.] *The Canadian Nurse*, Nov. 1969, p. 29-30.

ROBERTS, T.
Assessing nursing performance. *Nursing Mirror*, July 3, 1970, p. 14-5.

ROSEN, A., and ABRAHAM, G. E.
Evaluation of a procedure for assessing the performance of staff nurses. *Nursing Research*, Spring 1963, p. 78-81.

TATE, B. L.
Evaluating the nurse's clinical performance. *Nursing Outlook*, Jan. 1962, p. 35-7.

THURSTON, J. R., and others
A method for evaluating the attitudes of prospective nursing students. *The Journal of Nursing Education*, May/June, 1963, p. 3-7 and 23-6.

VILLEGAS, E. L.
Evaluation in nursing education. *The Philippine Journal of Nursing*, July/Aug. 1967, p. 200-6.

WORLD HEALTH ORGANIZATION. REGIONAL OFFICE FOR EUROPE
The evaluation of nursing education: report of a working party, Copenhagen, Dec. 1968. Copenhagen, Regional Office for Europe, 1969.

Teaching and Learning

ADEBAJO, S. O.
The role of the ward sister in the teaching team of the hospital. *The Australian Nurses' Journal*, June 1970, p. 116-20.

ANDREWS, J.
Ward tests for students and pupils. *Nursing Times*, Feb. 27, 1969, p. 280-2.

ASBURY, G.
Basic principles underlying ward teaching. *Nursing Mirror*, Nov. 22, 1968, p. 33-5.

BARNES, M.
Some thoughts and experiences of clinical teaching. *Nursing Mirror*, Dec. 31, 1965, p. 415.

BERGGREN, H. J., and ZAGORNIK, A. D.
Teaching nursing process to beginning students. *Nursing Outlook*, July 1968, p. 32-5.

BERITA JURURAWAT
The clinical instructor. *Berita Jururawat*, April 1967, p. 45-7.

BIGGIN, K. M.
Learning nursing—1. *Nursing Times*, Jan. 18, 1963, p. 85.

BIGGIN, K. M.
Learning nursing—2. *Nursing Times*, Jan. 25, 1963, p. 118-9.

BUMBALO, J., and STEELE, S.
Independent study: an expreience for senior students. *Nursing Outlook*, Jan. 1970, p. 40-3.

BURTON, G.
The instructor-counselor. *Journal of Nursing Education*, Dec. 1962, p. 5-6 and 8-10.

CLISSOLD, GRACE K.
How to function effectively as a teacher in the clinical area: a resource unit. New York, Springer, 1962.

COLLINS, S. M.
Learning to nurse at the London Hospital—1. *Nursing Times*, Mar. 15, 1963, p. 321-3.

COLLINS, S. M.
Learning to nurse at the London Hospital—2. *Nursing Times*, Mar. 22, 1963, p. 363-6.

DEEGAN, M.
The tutorial concept permits acceleration in nursing. *Journal of Nursing Education*, April 1970, p. 23-7.

DENMAN, K. M.
Clinical investigations as a basis for teaching. *Nursing Times*, Sept. 28, 1962, p. 1240-1.

DUNBAR, V. M.
The instructor of history of nursing. *Nursing Outlook*, May 1962, p. 307-10.

EASTWOOD, C. G.
The tactics of teaching. *Nursing Mirror*, Jan. 6, 1961, p. 1237.

EMENS, A. E.
The clinical instructor in the psychiatric hospital. *Nursing Times*, April 28, 1967, p. 556-8.

FOSHAY, A. W.
Beware, your future students are learning to think. *Nursing Outlook*, Oct. 1965, p. 47-9.

FRANK, E. D.
Teaching without learning? *Nursing Forum*, vol. IX, no. 2, 1970, p. 130-45.

FRERICHS, M.
Generalizations in nursing instruction. *Journal of Nursing Education*, Jan. 1970, p. 35-8.

FUERST, ELINOR V., and WOLFF, LU VERNE
Teaching fundamentals of nursing: method content and evaluation. 4th edn. Philadelphia, Lippincott, 1963.

FULLER, E. D., and DISMUKES, L. M.
An open-chest preparation in the laboratory for teaching coronary care. *Nursing Forum*, vol. VIII, no. 3, 1969, p. 302-10.

GOWELL, E. C.
Helping student nurses to become involved. *International Journal of Nursing Studies*, Nov. 1970, p. 225-33.

GRIFFIN, G. J., and others
Clincial nursing instruction and closed circuit TV. *Nursing Research*, Summer 1964, p. 196-204.

HARMS, M. T., and MCDONALD, F. J.
The teaching process. *Nursing Outlook*, Oct. 1966, p. 54-7.

HASSENPLUG, L. W.
The good teacher. *Nursing Outlook*, Oct. 1965, p. 24-7.

HASTINGS, B.
Clinical instruction in the mental hospital. *Nursing Times*, Aug. 2, 1963, p. 958-60.

HAWKINS, R. B.
The how and why of teachers' speech. *Journal of the American Association of Nurse Anesthetists*, Dec. 1969, p. 441-9.

HECTOR, W. E.
Buying equipment for the school of nursing. *Nursing Times*, June 14, 1963, p. 746-8.

HOSPITAL MANAGEMENT
Issue devoted to hospital training, including nurse training with descriptions of individual centres. *Hospital Management* Sept./Oct. 1969, p. 409-51.

HUNT, V.
Tutors in the wards. *Nursing Times*, Aug. 16, 1963, p. 1021-3.

HYMOVICH, D. P.
Coordinated student learning [by working in teams with flexibility of roles]. *Nursing Outlook*, July 1970, p. 62-4.

JARVIS, J. M.
Simple psychology—1, 2, 3, 4. *Nursing Times*, Mar. 11, 1966, p. 335-7; Mar. 18, 1966, p. 370-2; Mar. 25, 1966, p. 408-9; April 1, 1966, p. 436-8.

JOURARD, S.
How do people learn? *Canadian Nurse*, April 1964, p. 347-50.

KELLER, N. S.
Teaching by concepts. *Nursing Outlook*, Jan. 1969, p. 32-4.

KOVACS, M.
The new approach to instruction in nursing education. *The Journal of Nursing Education*, Feb./Mar. 1963, p. 3-4 and 20-21.

LAMBERTSEN, E. C.
No school can prepare nurses for all the hospital situations. *The Modern Hospital*, Feb. 1967, p. 127.

LAYTON, Sister MARY MICHELE
How instructors' attitudes affect students. *Nursing Outlook*, Jan. 1969, p. 27-9.

LISTER, D. W.
Clinical exploration of nursing theory. *Nursing Outlook*, Nov. 1967, p. 58-62.

MCCAFFERY, M.
What is the student learning in the clinical laboratory? *The Journal of Nursing Education*, Nov. 1968, p. 3-9.

MAJOR, D. M.
Keys to a philosophy of teaching. *Nursing Outlook*, Aug. 1962, p. 506-10.

MOORE, L., and WHITE, G. D.
Comparison of teaching methods in maternal and infant care. *Nursing Outlook*, May 1965, p. 74-6.

MULLER, T. G.
The head nurse as a teacher. *Nursing Outlook*, Jan. 1963, p. 46-8.

NAYLOR, P. N.
Methods of teaching the art of nursing. *Nursing Mirror*, Sept. 27, 1963, p. 549-51.

NEEDHAM, R. C.
The staff nurse as a clinical instructor. *Nursing Mirror*, Dec. 14, 1962, p. 231.

POHL, MARGARET L.
Teaching activities of the nursing practitioner. *Nursing Research*, Winter 1965, p. 4-11.

POHL, MARGARET L.
Teaching function of the nursing practitioner. Dubuque, Iowa, Brown, 1968.

PORTER, D. L.
Modern teaching techniques. *Nursing Mirror*, April 30, 1965, p. xiv-xvi.

REID, F.
Ward and classroom: correlating training. *Nursing Times*, Feb. 9, 1968, p. 181.

SAMSON, E. G.
Clinical instruction. *Santo Tomas Nursing Journal*, Dec. 1965, p. 208-10.

SCHMIDT, M. S.
The Hospital: a laboratory for the teaching of nursing. *Journal of Nursing Education*, April 1966, p. 17-22.

SHETLAND, M. L.
Teaching and learning in nursing. *American Journal of Nursing*, Sept. 1965, p. 112-6.

SHOLTIS, LILLIAN A., *and* BRAGDON, JANE SHERBURN
The art of clinical instruction: medical and surgical nursing. Philadelphia, Lippincott, 1961. [Originally published as "Teaching medical and surgical nursing". 1955.]

SIMONDS, A.
Two methods of teaching in the OR. *Nursing Outlook*, Feb. 1970, p. 29-31.

SKINNER, J. E.
Methods of teaching and learning. *Nursing Times*, April 3, 1964, p. 451-2.

SORIANO-CABRERA, V.
Ethics in clinical instruction. *Santo Tomas Nursing Journal*, Dec. 1965, p. 219-24.

SOUTH WEST METROPOLITAN AREA NURSE-TRAINING COMMITTEE
Report on pilot investigation into methods of teaching in nurse-training schools, by A. Catnach and M. Houghton. The Committee, 1961.

SPALDING, E. K.
What is a teacher? *International Nursing Review*, vol. 11, no. 3, 1964, p. 49-59.

TRIBOU, M.
The incident process in teaching. *Nursing Outlook*, Jan. 1965, p. 36-9.

WHITE, M. A.
Teaching the superior nursing student. *Journal of Nursing Education*, April 1965, p. 9-13.

WHYTE, B. BRYSSON
Teaching nursing. *Nursing Mirror*, Feb. 4, 1966, p. ix and xvi.

WIEDENBACH, ERNESTINE
Meeting the realities in clinical teaching. New York, Springer, 1969.

WILLIAMS, M. M.
Role-playing: a teaching method for increasing professional skills. *Nursing Times*, Feb. 23, 1968, Occasional Papers, p. 32.

WOLFORD, H. G.
Dialogue as a method of teaching. *Journal of Nursing Education*, Aug. 1965, p. 21-5.

WOLFORD, H. G.
Let the teacher be the patient. *Journal of Nursing Education*, May/June 1963, p. 17-20.

WOOD, V.
Measurement and evaluation in nursing education. *The Canadian Nurse*, April 1966, p. 54-8.

WOOLLEY, A. S.
The effect of organic factors and attitudes on learning in schools of nursing. *Journal of Nursing Education*, Aug. 1966, p. 13-9.

Teaching Machines and Programmed Learning

BITZER, MARYANN D.
Clinical nursing instruction via the PLATO simulated laboratory. *Nursing Research*, Sept. 1966, p. 144-50.

BITZER, MARYANN D., *and* BOUDREAUX, M. C.
Using a computer to teach nursing. *Nursing Forum*, vol. VIII, no. 3, 1969, p. 234-54.

BUCKBY, E., *and others*
Programme writing. *Nursing Times*, Mar. 11, 1966, p. 326-8.

CALIANDRO, G.
Programmed instruction and its use in nursing education: a review of the literature. *Nursing Research*, Sept./Oct. 1968, p. 450-4.

CLEINO, B.
Teaching machines and programmed learning. *Journal of Nursing Education*, Jan. 1964, p. 13-5 and 28.

COYE, DOROTHY H.
Programmed instruction for staff education. *American Journal of Nursing*, Feb. 1969, p. 325-7.

CRAYTOR, J. K., *and* LYSAUGHT, J. P.
Programmed instruction in nursing education: a trial use. *Nursing Research*, Fall 1964, p. 323-6.

FELDMAN, HERMAN
Learning transfer from programmed instruction to clinical performance. *Nursing Research*, Jan./Feb. 1969, p. 51-4.

GEIS, G. L., *and* ANDERSON, M. C.
Programmed instruction in nursing education. Part I—Some basic principles of the technique and essential features. *Nursing Outlook*, Aug. 1963, p. 592-4.

GEIS, G. L., *and* ANDERSON, M. C.
Programmed instruction in nursing education. Part II—Applying principles of the technique in producing materials. *Nursing Outlook*, Sept. 1963, p. 662-5.

HECTOR, WINIFRED E.
For and against programmed learning. *Nursing Times*, Jan. 17, 1964, p. 85-7.

HECTOR, WINIFRED E.
Making a programme—1. *Nursing Times*, June 5, 1964, p. 738.

HECTOR, WINIFRED E.
Making a programme—2. *Nursing Times*, June 12, 1964, p. 777.

HECTOR, WINIFRED E.
Making a programme—3. *Nursing Times*, June 19, 1964, p. 809-10.

HECTOR, WINIFRED E.
Making a programme—4. *Nursing Times*, June 26, 1964, p. 844.

HECTOR, WINIFRED E.
Programmed learning. *Nursing Times*, Sept. 13, 1963, p. 1146-7.

HECTOR, WINIFRED E.
Programmed learning in hospitals. *British Hospital and Social Service Journal*, Oct. 18, 1963, p. 1268-9.

HECTOR, WINIFRED E.
Tape recorder in clinical teaching. *Nursing Times*, April 6, 1962, p. 439-40.

HULL, E. J., *and* ISAACS, B. J.
Programming on the job in a nurse training school. *Nursing Times*, Sept. 11, 1969, p. 1166-8.

Hull, E. J., and Isaacs, B. J.
Two years' experience of programmed teaching. Part 1—Linear programmes. *Nursing Times*, Mar. 11, 1966, p. 333-4.

Hull, E. J., and Isaacs, B. J.
Two years' experience of programmed teaching. Part 2—Branching programmes. *Nursing Times*, Mar. 18, 1966, p. 373-4.

Hutchins, N.
Mediated self-instruction in nursing education. *The Journal of Nursing Education*, April 1968, p. 3-6.

Kidd, D. E.
Milk kitchen technique—teaching by programmed learning. *Nursing Mirror*, June 27, 1969, p. 29-31.

King Edward's Hospital Fund for London. Hospital Centre
Teaching aids: assessment of needs in pupil nurse training schools. A survey... by Heinemann Training Services Ltd. The Fund, 1968.

Klaiman, R. R.
Programmed instruction—can we use it? *The Canadian Nurse*, July 1967, p. 44-7.

Koehler, M. L.
Programmed instruction—potential uses in nursing. *Hospital Topics*, Aug. 1963, p. 48-50.

Krueger, Elizabeth A.
The hypodermic injection: a programmed unit. [New York] Columbia University, Teachers' College, 1966.

Linden, K.
The multimedia approach to teaching nursing. *Nursing Outlook*, May 1969, p. 36-40.

Mackenzie, F.
Audiovisual aids. *Nursing Times*, Sept. 18, 1969, p. 1205-6.

Marson, S.
Progress in programmed instruction. *Nursing Times*, Oct. 30, 1969, Occasional Papers, p. 181-4.

Mechner, F.
Learning by doing through programmed instruction. *American Journal of Nursing*, May 1965, p. 98-104.

Nursing education through multi-sensory approaches. University Center, Mich., Delta College, 1966.

Porter, P.
Programmed instruction—a challenge for nursing. *Nursing Forum*, vol. V, no. 4, 1966, p. 40-9.

Raine, N. L.
An experiment in programmed learning. A progress report: 1—First stages in planning. *Nursing Times*, June 3, 1966, p. 733-5.

Raine, N. L.
An experiment in programmed learning. A progress report: 2—Preparing to write a programme. *Nursing Times*, June 10, 1966, p. 764-6.

Redman, B. K., and Harlow, S. J.
Instructional qualities of television visuals for fundamentals of nursing. *Journal of Nursing Education*, Nov. 1969, p. 35-41.

Seedor, Marie M.
Can nursing be taught with teaching machines? *American Journal of Nursing*, May 1963, p. 117-20.

Seedor, Marie M.
Programmed instruction for a unit on asepsis. *Hospital Topics*, Aug. 1963, p. 50-5.

Seedor, Marie M.
Programmed instruction for nursing in the community college. Columbia University, Teachers' College, 1963.

Seedor, Marie M.
Programmed learning adds new dimensions to nursing curriculum. *Hospitals*, Sept. 1, 1966, p. 71, 74 and 76.

Smith, Genevieve Love, and Davis, Phyllis E.
Medical terminology: a programmed text. New York, John Wiley, 1963.
2nd edn., 1967.

Watson, M. W.
Programmed learning. *Irish Nurse*, Dec. 1964, p. 79-84.

Whyte, B. Brysson
The teaching machine in nurse training. *Nursing Times*, Nov. 16, 1962, p. 1471-2.

Whyte, B. Brysson
Teaching machines in schools of nursing. *Nursing Times*, Oct. 11, 1963, p. 1277-8.

Visual Aids

Anderson, L. D.
Telecourse in nursing. *American Journal of Nursing*, July 1964, p. 79-82.

Anderson, L. D.
Use of television in nursing education. *International Journal of Nursing Studies*, Mar. 1970, p. 31-5.

Bassett, R. L.
Medical teaching by film. *Nursing Mirror*, Nov. 10, 1967, p. xii-xiii.

Dixon, N.
Visual aids in teaching. *Nursing Times*, Aug. 3, 1962, p. 987.

Graves, J.
Audiovisual techniques in the USA. *Nursing Mirror*, Jan. 16, 1970, p. 28-31; Jan. 23, 1970, p. 39-43.

Griffin, Gerald J., and others
Clinical nursing instruction and closed circuit T.V. *Nursing Research*, Summer 1964, p. 196-204.

Griffin, Gerald J., and others
Clinical nursing instruction by television: a report on a two-year experiment using closed-circuit television to teach clinical nursing, by Gerald J. Griffin, Robert E. Kinsinger and Avis J. Pitman. New York, Columbia University Teachers' College, Dept. of Nursing Association, 1965.

Harty, M. B.
Role playing as a teaching technique. *Nursing Outlook*, Sept. 1961, p. 563-4.

Hector, Winifred E.
Closed-circuit television for schools of nursing. *Nursing Times*, Jan. 29, 1970, p. 136-8.

Hector, Winifred E.
Uses of the tape-recorder in teaching student nurses. *Nursing Times*, Jan. 4, 1693, p. 26.

Hilton, A.
Visual aids: their use and abuse. *District Nursing*, Oct. 1966, p. 165-7.

Huff, M., and Langhoff, H.
An overview of audiovisual modes of instruction. *AORN Journal*, Oct. 1969, p. 50-3.

Keveren, R. H.
Educational television. *Nursing Times*, Feb. 10, 1967, p. 173-5.

Kinsella, C.
Educational television for a hospital system. *American Journal of Nursing*, Jan. 1964, p. 72-5.

Lester, B. A.
Use of visual aids in education. *Nursing Mirror*, July 19, 1963, p. 341-2.

NURSING AS A PROFESSION

McKenzie, F. L.
Use of the overhead projector in schools of nursing. *Nursing Times*, Mar. 13, 1969, p. 336-7.

Remillet, J. G.
The 8 mm film in student and patient education. *The Journal of Nursing Education*, April 1968, p. 27-34.

Roeschlaub, E. L.
Audio-visual self-teaching aids can bolster in-service program. *Hospital Topics*, Oct. 1969, p. 38-42.

Royle, G. C.
Closed-circuit television as a teaching aid. *Nursing Times*, Sept. 1, 1967, p. 1178-9.

Schofield, H.
The overhead projector as a blackboard. *Nursing Mirror*, July 10, 1970, p. 40-1.

Sommer, R.
Say it with tape. *The American Journal of Nursing*, Jan. 1962, p. 71.

Tornyay, R. de
Instructional technology and nursing education. *Journal of Nursing Education*, April 1970, p. 3-8 and 34-5.

Weddige, D.
New York City's experiment with educational television in nursing. *Nursing Outlook*, April 1963, p. 254-5.

Westley, B. H., *and* Hornback, M.
An experimental study of the use of television in teaching basic nursing skills. *Nursing Research*, Summer 1964, p. 205-9.

Whyte, B. Brysson
Visual aids—a practical approach. *Nursing Times*, June 14, 1963, p. 737-8.

Wilcox, J.
Closed circuit television: a tool for nursing research. *Nursing Research*, Summer 1964, p. 210-6.

Wood, J. J.
Make your own films. *Nursing Times*, Sept. 6, 1963, p. 1120-1.

Worledge, C. B.
Teaching nursing by television. *Journal of Nursing Education*, April 1966, p. 33-7.

University Courses

Abbott, M.
The nurse and the university. *International Journal of Nursing Studies*, Mar. 1969, p. 17-24.

Alexander, M. E. F.
First university course for non-European nurses in South Africa. *International Nursing Review*, vol. 10, no. 2, 1963, p. 23-6.

Barbus, A. J., *and* Carbol, K. L.
Experiences in problem-solving for the baccalaureate student in nursing. *The Journal of Nursing Education*, Sept. 1963, p. 11-4, 16-7 and 19-20.

Batey, M. V.
The two normative worlds of the university nursing faculty. *Nursing Forum*, vol. VIII, no. 1, 1969, p. 4-16.

Brockington, Fraser
A university course in nursing: a report on the first four years of the University of Manchester experimental course in nurse education. Manchester, Crumpsall Hospital School of Nursing, 1964.

Canadian Nurse
University schools of nursing in Canada. *Canadian Nurse*, Dec. 1966, p. 34-43.

Canadian Nurse
University schools of nursing in Canada. *Canadian Nurse*, April 1970, p. 41-51.

Chittick, R.
Post-basic nursing in the University of Ghana. *International Journal of Nursing Studies*, April 1965, p. 39-42.

Chittick, R.
University education for nurses. *Australian Nurses' Journal*, Oct. 1969, p. 213-5; *New Zealand Nursing Journal*, Oct. 1969, p. 5-7.

Christy, Teresa E.
Cornerstone for nursing education: a history of the Division of Nursing Education at Teachers' College, Columbia University, 1899-1947. New York, Columbia University, Teachers' College Press, 1969.

Cooper, S. S.
The contributions of the university to the continuing education of nurses [with particular reference to the University of Wisconsin]. *International Journal of Nursing Studies*, Dec. 1968, p. 273-8.

Gowan, M. Olivia
Influence of graduate nurses on the formative years of a university school of nursing [Catholic University of America School of Nursing]. *Nursing Research*, Summer 1967, p. 261-6.

Grauhan, A.
Practical nurse training at Heidelberg University. *Nursing Mirror*, May 12, 1961, p. 545.

Gupta, A.
The development of university education for nurses in India. *Nursing Journal of India*, July 1964, p. 206-7.

Hassenplug, L. W.
This I believe... about university nursing education. *Nursing Outlook*, May 1970, p. 38-40.

Hornback, M. S.
University sponsored staff education in nursing via a telephone/radio network. *International Journal of Nursing Studies*, Nov. 1969, p. 217-23.

Hubert, Sister Mary
British nursing and the universities.
See
Reinkemeyer, Agnes.

Lee, Eleanor
Neighbours 1892-1967: a history of the Department of Nursing, Faculty of Medicine, Columbia University 1937-1967 and its predecessor the School of Nursing of the Presbyterian Hospital, New York, 1892-1937. [New York?] Columbia University-Presbyterian Hospital School of Nursing, Alumnae Association, 1967.

Manchester University/Crumpsall Hospital
University diploma in community nursing. Description of integrated course. *Nursing Mirror*, Oct. 6, 1961, p. i-iv.

Marsh, N., *and* Morton, P.
Towards a university degree in nursing. At the University of Manchester.
1. The course programme: organization and assessment.
2. Opinions on the course and follow-up of students.
Nursing Times, Jan. 1, 1970, Occasional Papers, p. 1-3; Jan. 8, 1970, Occasional Papers, p. 5-6.

Graduate nurses. (A criticism of the University of Manchester/Crumpsall Hospital scheme of nurse training.) *The Hospital*, Mar. 1964, p. 129-30.

Montag, M. L.
The logic of associate degree programs in nursing. *Nursing Science*, June 1964, p. 188-98.

New York State University, State Education Department
New York State Associate degree nursing project, 1959-1964. Final report to the W. K. Kellogg Foundation. Albany, N.Y. State Education Department, 1964.

New Zealand Nurses' Association
University education programme for nurses. *The New Zealand Nursing Journal*, May 1965, p. 20.

NURSING TIMES
University/basic nursing courses. *Nursing Times*, Dec. 17, 1965, p. 1735.

O'CONNELL, P. E.
University education and the future nurse. *International Journal of Nursing Studies*, Dec. 1963, p. 1-6.

PALMER, I. S.
The responsibility of the university faculty in nursing. *Nursing Forum*, vol. IX, no. 2, 1970, p. 120-9.

PELLEGRINO, E. P.
Rationale for nursing education in the university. *American Journal of Nursing*, May 1968, p. 1006-9.

POLLACK, H. P.
Training for nurses at university level [in South Africa]. *The Rhodesian Nurse*, Dec. 1970, p. 45-54.

REID, A.
The place of nursing in the university. *The New Zealand Nursing Journal*, Sept. 1965, p. 5-9; *The Nursing Gazette*, Nov. 1965, p. 1-5.

REINKEMEYER, AGNES
British nursing and the Universities—an American view. 1. Four basic university courses. *Nursing Times*, Oct. 6, 1967, p. 1335-7.

REINKEMEYER, AGNES
British nursing and the universities—an American view. 2. University attitude; a fundamental measure of fit. *Nursing Times*, Oct. 13, 1967, p. 1375-6.

REINKEMEYER, AGNES
British nursing and the universities—an American view. 3. Structural and functional relationships. *Nursing Times*, Oct. 20, 1967, p. 1415-7.

REINKEMEYER, AGNES
British nursing and the universities—an American view. 4. The faculty and students of nursing within the university. *Nursing Times*, Oct. 27, 1967, p. 1453-5.

REINKEMEYER, AGNES
British nursing and the universities—an American view. 5. The nursing course: the weakest university link. *Nursing Times*, Nov. 3, 1967, p. 1485-7.

REINKEMEYER, AGNES
British nursing and the universities—an American view. 6. Pause on the university threshold. *Nursing Times*, Nov. 10, 1967, p. 1519-20.

REINKEMEYER, AGNES
British nursing and the universities—an American view. 7. The future. *Nursing Times*, Nov. 17, 1967, p. 1553-4.

REINKEMEYER, AGNES
A nursing paradox. *Nursing Research*, Jan./Feb. 1968, p. 4-9.

REINKEMEYER, AGNES
The limited impact of basic university programs in nursing: a British case study; dissertation submitted in partial satisfaction of the requirements for the degree of Doctor of Philosophy in Education in the graduate division of the University of Berkeley. Berkeley, Calif., The author, 1966.

ROWSELL, G. S.
University nursing education—facts and trends. [Nursing education in Canada.] *The Canadian Nurse*, Dec. 1966, p. 31-3.

SCHMITT, L. M.
University education for nurses. *The Australian Nurses' Journal*, July 1968, p. 144-8.

SHEATH, H. C.
University nurse training scheme is off to a good start in New South Wales. *The Lamp*, Mar. 1969, p. 29-31.

SHETLAND, M. L.
Research—a function of baccalaureate education? *Nursing Science*, Oct. 1964, p. 381-90.

SMITH, D. W.
Some problems of baccalaurate programs. *American Journal of Nursing*, Jan. 1970, p. 120-3.

THOMAS, L., *and* JOHNSON, M. M.
Research in the associate in arts degree program in nursing. *Journal of Nursing Education*, Aug. 1964, p. 31-5.

TUNIS, BARBARA LOGAN
In caps and gowns: the story of the school for graduate nurses, McGill University 1920-1964. Montreal, McGill University Press, 1966.

WILLIAMS, R. M.
Professional training and the universities. *New Zealand Nursing Journal*, June 1970, p. 9-11.

WILSON, K. J.
British nursing and the universities: a Scottish view. *Nursing Times*, Feb. 9, 1968, p. 175-7.

LIBRARIES

ABRAMSON, G. K.
Nursing's place in a library. *Nursing Outlook*, Dec. 1967, p. 62.

AMERICAN NURSES' ASSOCIATION
Using and improving the keys to knowledge; papers presented at . . . biennial convention . . . New Jersey, June 18, 1964. New York, The Association, 1964.

ANGUS, M. D.
Project X completed! Books are, apart from the work and influence of the teacher, the chief instruments in education. *Canadian Nurse*, April 1964, p. 353-4.

ANNAN, G. L.
The Library—a force for better nursing care. *Nursing Outlook*, April 1964, p. 56-8.

BENNETT, C.
Some nursing books are for keeps. *Nursing Outlook*, Dec. 1969, p. 53-5.

BOORER, D.
Libraries for nurses. 1—Mansfield General Hospital. *Nursing Times*, Dec. 10, 1965, p. 1688-90.

BOORER, D.
Libraries for nurses. 2—Lincoln County Hospital. *Nursing Times*, April 15, 1966, p. 505-7.

BOORER, D.
Libraries for nurses. 3—Changes at Southampton. *Nursing Times*, June 26, 1969, p. 816-7.

BOORER, D.
Nurses' libraries, time to come in from the cold . . . *Nursing Times*, Sept. 10, 1970, p. 1171.

BOORER, D.
Nurses who do not read. *Nursing Times*, July 31, 1969, p. 984-5.

BRITISH HOSPITAL AND SOCIAL SERVICE JOURNAL
Hospital and nursing libraries. *British Hospital and Social Service Journal*, April 3, 1964, p. 440.

BROWN, M. C.
The library and nursing education. *Canadian Nurse*, April 1964, p. 350-2.

BUNCH, ANTONIA J., *and* CUMMING, EILEEN E.
Libraries in hospitals; a review of services in Scotland Scottish Hospital Centre, 1969.

CONCORDIA, MARY
Library procedure manual, Queen of Angels School of Nursing. California, The School, 1963.

DUANA, INES
Selected library references in Spanish for basic nursing programs in Latin-America. New York, The Rockefeller Foundation, 1966.

NURSING AS A PROFESSION

EATON, E. S., *and* KNOWLES, L. N.
The library as a classroom. *Nursing Outlook*, April 1964, p. 62-3.

FENN, L. J. S.
Building up a library. *Nursing Times*, April 26, 1968, p. 562.

FLANDORF, V. S.
A library for students and staff. *Nursing Outlook*, May 1961, p. 288-9.

FLANDORF, V. S.
Combining medical and nursing libraries. *Hospital Progress*, Sept. 1969, p. 42, 48, 50 and 54.

FULCHER, J. M.
Learning how to "do it yourself" in the library. *Nursing Outlook*, April 1964, p. 59-61.

GALL, G.
Psychiatric hospital libraries and internal news service. *Nursing Mirror*, Oct. 11, 1968, p. 47-8.

GILES, G.
Suggested books and journals for hospital libraries. *Canadian Hospital*, Feb. 1967, p. 51-7.

HENDERSON, V.
Library resources in nursing—their development and use. *International Nursing Review*, vol. 15, no. 2, 1968, p. 164-74; vol. 15, no. 3, 1968, p. 236-46; vol. 15, no. 4, 1968, p. 348-53.

HOLDSWORTH, J. N.
Vicarious experience of reading a book in changing nursing students' attitudes. *Nursing Research*, Mar./April 1968, p. 135-9.

HUTTON, J. M.
Library provision for the modern nurse. *Nursing Times*, Dec. 1, 1967, p. 1614-6.

INTERAGENCY COUNCIL ON LIBRARY TOOLS FOR NURSING
Reference tools for nursing. *Nursing Outlook*, May 1966, p. 67-72.

INTERAGENCY COUNCIL ON LIBRARY TOOLS FOR NURSING
References for nursing. *Nursing Outlook*, April 1970, p. 47-52.

INTERNATIONAL NURSING INDEX
The International Nursing Index. *American Journal of Nursing*, April 1966, p. 783-6.

IRWIN, J. E.
Widen your horizons. A list of suggested reading to help a nurse broaden her outlook and become a generalist as well as a specialist. *The Canadian Nurse*, July 1968, p. 41-2.

KING EDWARD'S HOSPITAL FUND FOR LONDON. HOSPITAL CENTRE
Hospital libraries. Report of a conference held on 9th February 1966. *British Hospital Journal and Social Service Review*, Feb. 25, 1966, p. 362-3.

KING EDWARD'S HOSPITAL FUND FOR LONDON. THE HOSPITAL CENTRE AND THE LIBRARY ASSOCIATION
Libraries in hospitals. Conference at the Hospital Centre. *Nursing Times*, Feb. 18, 1966, p. 230-1.

KONA, W.
The library and the nurse. *International Nursing Review*, vol. 11, no. 6, 1964, p. 33-5.

KONA, W.
Nursing school libraries in Metropolitan Chicago. *International Nursing Review*, vol. 11, no. 6, 1964, p. 35-9.

KUCHINSKY, S.
The hospital's medical and nursing libraries. *Hospital Topics*, April 1963, p. 35-7 and 47.

LIBRARY ASSOCIATION
Hospital libraries: recommended standards for libraries in hospitals. The Association, 1965.

LOUGHLIN, T. M., *and others*
A comparative study of supervised and unsupervised library periods for student nurses in psychiatric nursing. *Journal of Psychiatric Nursing*, July/Aug. 1964, p. 345-9.

MCCABE, Sister MARY CONCEPTA
A suggested annotated bibliography for a reference collection in nursing education. *Hospital Progress*, May 1966, p. 46-9.

MANCHESTER REGIONAL HOSPITAL BOARD
The use of books in nurse training. *Nursing Mirror*, April 28, 1961, p. 333; *Nursing Times*, April 28, 1961, p. 519.

MANSFIELD GENERAL HOSPITAL
Libraries for nurses. Mansfield General Hospital. *Nursing Times*, Dec. 10, 1965, p. 1688-90.

MILE END HOSPITAL, LONDON
Libraries for nurses. *Nursing Times*, July 22, 1966, p. 967.

MINK, G.
Publication explosion—control or chaos? *American Journal of Nursing*, May 1964, p. 104-6.

MONAGHAN, MARGARET A.
The library committee in a school of nursing. *Hospital Progress*, Feb. 1961, p. 104 and 106.

MORPURGO, J. E.
Book and journal services for doctors and nurses: an interim report on a National Book League investigation. Nuffield Provincial Hospitals Trust, 1966.

MORTON, K.
The hospital centre library and information service. *The Hospital*, April 1967, p. 135-6.

MORTON, L. T.
The library in medical communication. *World Medical Journal*, July/Aug. 1968, p. 94-5.

MORTON, L. T.
Research and the library. *Physiotherapy*, April 1966, p. 119-20.

MUNSON, A. H.
Make friends with your library. *Nursing Outlook*, April 1963, p. 261-2.

NATIONAL LEAGUE FOR NURSING
Library service in the health service: papers presented at the program meeting of the Interagency Council on Library Tools for Nursing at the 1967 Convention of the National League for Nursing. New York, The League, 1967.

NATIONAL LEAGUE FOR NURSING. DEPARTMENT OF DIPLOMA AND ASSOCIATE DEGREE PROGRAMS
The Bellevue classification system for nursing school libraries. New York, The League, 1965.

NATIONAL LEAGUE FOR NURSING. DIVISION OF NURSING EDUCATION
The library—a force for better nursing care. New York, The League, 1964.

NILES, A. McK.
Nursing dial access. A taped library for professional nurses. *Nursing Forum*, vol. VIII, no. 3, 1969, p. 328-36.

NURSING OUTLOOK
What happens to the libraries of nursing schools in transition? *Nursing Outlook*, April 1969, p. 40-1.

NURSING RESEARCH
Nursing libraries—today and tomorrow. *Nursing Research*, Fall 1965, p. 291.

NURSING TIMES
Textbooks and stationery. *Nursing Times*, May 26, 1967, p. 681.

PARKIN, M. L.
Library service and the nursing profession in Canada. *International Nursing Review*, vol. 16, no. 1, 1969, p. 58-61.

PARKIN, M. L.
Our new library. *The Canadian Nurse*, March 1966, p. 32-3.

PARKIN, M. L.
Resources and use of CNA library. *Canadian Nurse*, Mar. 1969, p. 32-4.

PEMBURY HOSPITAL
Libraries for nurses: Pembury Hospital. *Nursing Times*, Sept. 16, 1966, p. 1229.

PIEHLER, P.
Literature's place in the nursing curriculum. *Nursing Outlook*, May 1963, p. 346-8.

PINGS, VERN M.
Nursing libraries in historical perspective. *American Journal of Nursing*, Nov. 1965, p. 115-20.

PINGS, VERN M.
A plan for indexing the periodical literature of nursing: report of a study for bibliographic control of the scholarly record of nursing. New York, American Nurses' Foundation, 1966.

PINGS, VERN M.
Study of a plan for an index of nursing periodical literature, working paper no. 2: nursing libraries, a review of the literature, 1900-1963. New York, American Nurses' Foundation, 1964.

RAYBOULD, E.
Building a nursing school library. *Nursing Times*, June 5, 1964, p. 724-6.

RODIL-MARTIRES, C., and GOCHOCO, V. S.
Reading abilities of nursing student applicants for Cebu City Nursing Schools. *The Philippine Journal of Nursing*, Mar./April 1967, p. 103-6.

ROYAL COLLEGE OF NURSING. LIBRARY OF NURSING
A library guide for schools of nursing [by A. M. C. Thompson]. Royal College of Nursing, 1962. 2nd edn., 1967.

SHAVER, MARY C.
The library's contribution to nursing education. *Canadian Nurse*, June 1961, p. 553-5.

STEARNS, N. S., and others
The hospital library—part 1. *Hospitals*, Mar. 1, 1970, p. 55-9.

STEARNS, N. S., and others
The hospital library—part 2. *Hospitals*, Mar. 16, 1970, p. 88-90.

STEARNS, N., and others
A core nursing library for practitioners. *American Journal of Nursing*, April 1970, p. 818-23.

SULLIVAN, J. J.
The value of books and libraries to the nurse. Part 2—Reading for personal reasons. *Nursing Mirror*, June 23, 1961, p. 1133-4 and 1139.

TABOR, R. B.
Library services in hospitals and the medical profession. From: Report of the Library Association London and Home Counties Branch annual weekend conference, 18th - 20th April, 1969, Canterbury, Kent.

THOMPSON, A. M. C.
Libraries in nursing schools—1 and 2. *Nursing Times*, Aug. 24, 1962, p. 1090-1; Aug. 31, 1962, p. 1116-7.

THOMPSON, A. M. C.
A sense of values. A library is vital to any educational establishment. It is also a professional necessity for a trained staff. *Nursing Times*, June 14, 1963, p. 735-6.

THOMPSON, G.
The value of books and libraries to the nurse. Part 1—Reading for professional reasons. *Nursing Mirror*, June 16, 1961, p. 1029-30.
[For Part 2 see SULLIVAN, J. J.]

WILKINSON, P.
Getting nurses to use the library. *Nursing Times*, Feb. 10, 1967, p. 187-8.

WILLIAMS, E. V.
The Janet Geister Memorial Library. *American Association of Industrial Nurses' Journal*, June 1968, p. 7-9.

POST BASIC EDUCATION

AGNES KARLL NURSES' ASSOCIATION
Post-certificate training in Germany. *Nursing Mirror*, Jan. 10, 1964, p. i.

ALTSCHUL, A., and others
How nurse tutors use their time: an investigation. *Nursing Times*, June 5, 1964, p. 744-5.

AMERICAN NURSES' ASSOCIATION
Avenues for continued learning. New York, The Association, 1967.

BARRITT, E., and OHLIGER, J. F.
Continuing education. *American Journal of Nursing*, Oct. 1969, p. 2170-1.

BATLEY, NORMA
Further education and the nurse. *Nursing Times*, June 28, 1968, Occasional Papers, p. 101-4.

BERGERON, Sister RITA MARIE
The nursing departmental chairman in the liberal arts college: a comparative study of the role of the liberal arts and the nursing departmental chairman in nineteen private liberal arts colleges. Washington, Catholic University of America Press, 1963.

BERGMAN, R.
Operation action: from philosophy to practice. [Two post-basic nursing programs in Israel]. *Journal of Nursing Education*, Aug. 1968, p. 21-6.

BOYD, E., and SALMON, G. B.
Post-basic nursing education in New Zealand. *International Nursing Review*, vol. 17, no. 1, 1970, p. 43-51.

BRAND, V. R.
Graduates of a basic baccalaureate program and of a baccalaureate program for registered nurses compared. *Nursing Research*, Fall 1967, p. 347-51.

BRANDT, EDNA MAE, and others
Comparison of on the job performance of graduates with school of nursing objectives. *Nursing Research*, Winter 1967, p. 50-60.

BROWDER, J. J.
Advanced nursing for senior students. *Nursing Outlook*, Dec. 1962, p. 810-1.

BUDGE, U. V.
A tutor's lot is not a happy one. *Nursing Times*, Aug. 9, 1963, p. 1011.

CAMPBELL, JEAN
Current trends in the admission of registered nurses to baccalaureate programs. In Modern Dialogue: Nursing in the Community. [Brochure no. 4.] Albany, N.Y., New York State League for Nursing, 1964, p. 33-46.

CAMPBELL, JEAN
Masters' education in nursing: report of a study conducted in Spring 1963. New York, National League for Nursing, 1964.

CARROLL, M. C.
Teacher preparation must improve. *American Journal of Nursing*, Dec. 1962, p. 86-8.

CHATER, S. S.
Differential characteristics of graduate students in nursing. *Nursing Research*, Spring 1967, p. 146-53.

CHERIAN, A.
Post basic nursing education in India. *The Nursing Journal of India*, July 1964, p. 202.

NURSING AS A PROFESSION

COOPER, S. S.
Continuing education: an imperative for nurses. *Nursing Forum*, vol. VII, no. 3, 1968, p. 289-97.

DAVIS, FRED, *and* OLESEN, VIRGINIA L.
Baccalaureate students' images of nursing; a study of change, consensus, and consonance in the first year. *Nursing Research*, Winter 1964, p. 8-15.

DUNLAP, MARJORIE S.
Preparation of nurse faculty for associate degree nursing program. *Nursing Science*, June 1964, p. 223-34.

FIELD, W. E., JR.
Differentiating between graduate and baccalaureate nursing education. *The Journal of Nursing Education*, Aug. 1966, p. 9-11.

FRITZ, EDNA
Baccalaureate nursing education; what is its job? *American Journal of Nursing*, June 1966, p. 1312-6.

GARNER, G. S., *and* LOWE, A.
Group dynamics in graduate education of nurses. *Nursing Research*, Spring 1965, p. 146-50.

GENERAL NURSING COUNCIL FOR ENGLAND AND WALES
An experimental course for the preparation of nurse tutors. *Nursing Times*, May 14, 1965, p. 657.

GOOD, S.
Post-basic baccalaureate education for nurses in Canada. *International Nursing Review*, vol. 16, no. 2, 1969, p. 147-51.

GORTNER, S. R.
Nursing majors in twelve western universities: a comparison of registered nurse students and basic senior students. *Nursing Research*, Mar./April 1968, p. 121-9.

GOYAL, K.
Post-basic B.Sc. nursing programme, College of Nursing, Chandigarh. *Nursing Journal of India*, May 1967, p. 116-8.

GRAHAM, L. E.
Are we motivating students to go on for graduate education? *Nursing Outlook*, Aug. 1968, p. 48-50.

GRAHAM, L. E.
A faculty research development project in a baccalaureate program in nursing [in the department of nursing in Columbia Union College, Takoma Park, Maryland]. *Nursing Research*, July/Aug. 1968, p. 321-6.

GREAT BRITAIN. DEPARTMENT OF HEALTH AND SOCIAL SECURITY
Report of the nurse tutor working party. The Department, 1970.

HAYTER, J.
A follow-up study of graduates of the baccalaureate degree program in nursing. *Nursing Research*, Winter 1963, p. 45-7.

HECTOR, W. E.
Some problems of the tutor. *Nursing Times*, Feb. 9, 1968, p. 172-4.

HEDRICKS, J. A.
Practices of granting college credit by examination. *Nursing Research*, Summer 1961, p. 160-5.

HEIDGERKEN, L. E.
Preference for a teaching or clinical nursing practice career: influence of significant others. *Nursing Research*, July/Aug. 1970, p. 292-302.

INDIANA UNIVERSITY. BULLETIN OF THE SCHOOL OF EDUCATION
The persistence of registered nurses in supplementing the school of nursing diploma with study toward the baccalaureate degree in general nursing on Indiana university regional campuses, by Lucy Perry. Bloomington, Indiana, Bureau of Educational Studies and Testing, 1964. [Bulletin of the School of Education, Indiana University, vol. 40, no. 6, Nov. 1964.]

JOHNSON, D. E.
Nursing and higher education. *International Journal of Nursing Studies*, Dec. 1964, p. 219-25.

JOHNSON, D. E.
Post-masters' education. *Nursing Outlook*, Jan. 1964, p. 33-5.

KENDALL, K. K.
$ and sense of baccalaureate degrees. *American Association of Industrial Nurses' Journal*, Oct. 1966, p. 7-11.

LOGAN, W. M.
Recruiting and retaining tutors. *Nursing Times*, Oct. 8, 1965, p. 1367-71.

LOGAN, W. M.
The shortage of nurse educators—report of a research project carried out in Scotland. *International Journal of Nursing Studies*, Feb. 1966, p. 283/92.

MACDONALD, G.
Baccalaureate education for graduates of diploma and associate degree programs. *Nursing Outlook*, June 1964, p. 52-6.

McWEE, AGNES C.
Preparing for the future: a study of secondment among tutor and administrative students in Scotland—part 1 and part II. *International Journal of Nursing Studies*, June 1968, p. 135-55; Sept. 1968, p. 231-48.

MAXWELL, R. M.
The preparation of teachers of nursing. *Nursing Forum*, vol. VII, no. 4, 1968, p. 365-74.

MENTAL HEALTH TUTORS' ASSOCIATION
Shortage of nurse tutors in the mental health field. The Association, 1961.

MILLER, D. M.
Characteristics of graduate students in four clinical nursing specialties. *Nursing Research*, Spring 1965, p. 106-13.

MONTAG, M.
Preparation of nurses for faculty positions. *Nursing Outlook*, Jan. 1967, p. 27 and 29-31.

NAHM, H.
Changing attitudes and approaches to nursing care through continuing education. *Journal of Nursing Education*, Aug. 1969, p. 31-6.

NAHM, H.
Expectations of students in graduate education. *Nursing Forum*, Fall 1962, p. 19-27.

NAHM, H.
The registered nurse and baccalaureate education. *Nursing Forum*, vol. VI, no. 1, 1967, p. 28-44.

NAHM, H., *and others*
Doctoral preparation for nurses. *Nursing Forum*, vol. V, no. 3, 1966, p. 36-63.

NATIONAL LEAGUE FOR NURSING
Some statistics on baccalaureate and higher degree programs in nursing—1969. New York, The League, 1970.

NATIONAL LEAGUE FOR NURSING. DEPARTMENT OF BACCALAUREATE AND HIGHER DEGREE PROGRAMS
Baccalaureate education for the registered nurse student. New York, The League, 1966.

NATIONAL LEAGUE FOR NURSING. DEPARTMENT OF BACCALAUREATE AND HIGHER DEGREE PROGRAMS
Policies and procedures of accreditation of the department of baccalaureate and higher degree programs of the National League for Nursing. New York, The League, 1963.

NATIONAL LEAGUE FOR NURSING, DEPARTMENT OF BACCALAUREATE AND HIGHER DEGREE PROGRAMS, COUNCIL OF MEMBER AGENCIES
Statement of beliefs and recommendations regarding baccalaureate nursing programs admitting registered nurse students. *Nursing Outlook*, June 1964, p. 57.

NATIONAL LEAGUE FOR NURSING. RESEARCH AND STUDIES SERVICE
Faculty study, 1964. New York, The League, 1964.

PAPE, R. H.
Higher education for the nurse practitioner. *Nursing Outlook*, Feb. 1967, p. 48-52.

PENTZ, M.
The Open University: an opening for nurses. *Nursing Times*, June 11, 1970, p. 754-6.

PETERS, L.
Post-basic nursing education at Trivandrum, Kerala. *The Nursing Journal of India*, July 1964, p. 207.

PONTE, M. L.
A rapid glance at Brazilian post-graduate nursing education. *International Journal of Nursing Studies*, Feb. 1967, p. 37-45.

POPIEL, ELDA S.
The director of continuing education in perspective. *Nursing Forum*, vol. VIII, no. 1, 1969, p. 86-93.

POPIEL, ELDA S.
The many facets of continuing education in nursing. *Journal of Nursing Education*, Jan. 1969, p. 3-13.

PRICE, ELMINA MARY
Learning needs of registered nurses. New York, Teachers' College Press, Columbia University, 1967.

REED, FAY C.
Baccalaureate education and professional practice. *Nursing Outlook*, Jan. 1967, p. 50-2.

REESE, D. E., and others
How many caps went on again? A follow-up study of the work patterns of nurses completing a refresher course. *Nursing Outlook*, Aug. 1962, p. 517-9.

SALMON, B.
New Zealand post-graduate school for nurses. *New Zealand Nursing Journal*, Sept. 1969, p. 25-6.

SASKATCHEWAN REGISTERED NURSES' ASSOCIATION
A guide for refresher courses for inactive nurses. Regina, The Association, 1966.

SAVAGE, W. W.
Prescription for a professional degree. *Nursing Outlook*, Aug. 1962, p. 530-2.

SCHLOTFELDT, R. M.
Preparation of nurses for faculty positions. *Nursing Outlook*, Jan. 1967, p. 26, and 28-9.

STRYKER, RUTH PERIN
Back to nursing. Philadelphia, Saunders, 1966.

UNITED STATES. PUBLIC HEALTH SERVICE. DEPARTMENT OF HEALTH, EDUCATION AND WELFARE
Nurses for leadership: the professional nurse traineeship program. Washington, The Department, 1963.

WATKIN, B.
The Lyons International School of Advanced Nursing Education. *Nurse*, vol. 5, no. 12, 1966, p. 1-4.

WEDGERY, A. W.
Post-basic courses . . . a major nursing need. *Canadian Hospital*, Jan. 1968, p. 45-6.

WELTER, MARY L.
The art of scholarship and the essence of sustained education for faculty in schools of nursing. *Journal of Nursing Education*, April 1964, p. 5-6 and 25-6.

TRAINING SCHOOLS

AMERICAN NURSES' ASSOCIATION
Commercial schools of nursing. New York, The Association, 1966.

BONNET, P. D.
Hospital schools of nursing in 1984: two forecasts. *Hospitals*, Feb. 16, 1964, p. 62-6.

BRISTOL. UNITED BRISTOL HOSPITALS
Schools of nursing operational policies. Bristol, Royal Infirmary, [1967?].

BUTLER, R.
Birth of a training school. Queen Elizabeth II Hospital, Welwyn Garden City. *Nursing Times*, April 12, 1968, p. 495-7.

CABOT, R.
Suggestions for the improvement of training schools for nurses. *Nursing Forum*, vol. V, no. 1, 1966, p. 55-9.

CHARING CROSS GROUP OF HOSPITALS
School of nursing. The Group [1970].

DUNDEE COLLEGE OF NURSING
Dundee College of Nursing. *Nursing Mirror*, July 18, 1969, p. 20-1.

FLORENCE NIGHTINGALE COLLEGE OF NURSING, TURKEY
Faculty organization. Istanbul, Ministry of Health and Social Welfare, 1961.

FULHAM HOSPITAL
"Seven-weeks" teaching department. *Nursing Times*, Jan. 31, 1964, p. 151.

GOUGH, M. A.
Planning and budgeting for a new pupil nurse training school. *Nursing Times*, Mar. 20, 1964, p. 374 and 390.

HALE, T.
The hospital school of nursing. *Hospital Management*, Nov. 1966, p. 72-6.

HOLDER, S.
"Any mistakes are mine" [The planning of the School of Nursing, St. Mary's Hospital, Paddington]. *Nursing Mirror*, Oct. 3, 1969, p. 9-12.

IPSWICH AND DISTRICT ENROLLED NURSE TRAINING SCHOOL
Ipswich and District Enrolled Nurse Training School. *Nursing Times*, Mar. 20, 1964, p. 378-90.

KAUNDA, B.
Planning a school of nursing for Zambia. *The Zambia Nurse*, Aug./Sept. 1968, p. 3-9.

LIVERPOOL ROYAL INFIRMARY
Nurses' training school, 1862-1962. Liverpool, The Infirmary, 1962.

MCCARRICK, H.
Foresterhill College, Aberdeen. *Nursing Times*, June 23, 1967, p. 828-30.

MCLEAN, CATHERINE D.
A report on the establishment of the Quo Vadis school of nursing and the selection of the first class of students. Toronto, The School, 1964.

NATIONAL LEAGUE FOR NURSING. RESEARCH AND STUDIES SERVICE
State-approved schools of practical and vocational nursing, meeting minimum requirements set by law and board rules in the various jurisdictions. New York, The League, 1965. [In progress.]

NATIONAL LEAGUE FOR NURSING. RESEARCH AND STUDIES SERVICE
State-approved schools of professional nursing, meeting minimum requirements set by law and board rules in the various jurisdictions. New York, The League, 1965.

UNITED STATES PUBLIC HEALTH SERVICE. DIVISION OF NURSING
A guide for projecting space needs for schools of nursing. Washington, U.S. Government Printing Office, [1966].

WEST, NOEL
A new school for new nurses. School of Nursing Medical Centre, University of Malaysia. *World Health*, Nov. 1970, p. 18-20.

WOLFSON SCHOOL OF NURSING, WESTMINSTER HOSPITAL
The Wolfson School of Nursing. *Hospital and Social Service Journal*, April 7, 1961, p. 395.

WOLFSON SCHOOL OF NURSING, WESTMINSTER HOSPITAL
Wolfson School of Nursing, Westminster Hospital. *Hospital Management Planning and Equipment*, April 1966, p. 208-9.

NURSING RESEARCH

ABDELLAH, F. G.
Criterion measures in nursing for experimental research.
See
WALTER REED ARMY INSTITUTE OF RESEARCH
Report on nursing research conference, 1959. 1961.

ABDELLAH, F. G.
Frontiers in nursing research. *Nursing Forum*, vol. V, no. 1, 1966, p. 28-38.

ABDELLAH, F. G.
Overview of nursing research 1955-1968, part 1. *Nursing Research*, Jan./Feb. 1970, p. 6-17.

ABDELLAH, F. G.
Overview of nursing research 1955-1968, part 2. *Nursing Research*, Mar./April 1970, p. 151-62.

ABDELLAH, F. G.
Overview of nursing research 1955-1968, part 3. *Nursing Research*, May/June 1970, p. 239-52.

ABDELLAH, F. G., *and* LEVINE, E.
The aims of nursing research. *Nursing Research*, Winter 1965, p. 27-32.

ABDELLAH, F. G. *and* LEVINE, E.
Better patient care through nursing research. Collier-Macmillan, 1965.

ABDELLAH, F. G., *and* LEVINE, E.
Better patient care through nursing research. *International Journal of Nursing Studies*, April 1965, p. 1-12.

ABDELLAH, F. G., *and* LEVINE, E.
Future directions of research in nursing. *American Journal of Nursing*, Jan. 1966, p. 112-6.

ABRAHAM, G. E.
Promoting nursing research in an organized nursing service. *American Journal of Nursing*, April 1968, p. 818-21.

AMERICAN NURSES' ASSOCIATION
An expanding concern with research. *The American Journal of Nursing*, Aug. 1962, p. 45.

AMERICAN NURSES' ASSOCIATION
The nurse in research. *American Journal of Nursing*, July 1968, p. 1504-7.

AMERICAN NURSES' ASSOCIATION
The nurse in research. ANA guidelines on ethical values. *Nursing Research*, Mar./April 1968, p. 104-7.

AMERICAN NURSES' ASSOCIATION
[First] nursing research conference 1965, New York. New York, The Association, 1965.

AMERICAN NURSES' ASSOCIATION
[Second] nursing research conference, 1966, Phoenix, Arizona. New York, The Association, 1966.

AMERICAN NURSES' ASSOCIATION
[Third] nursing research conference, 1967, Seattle, Washington. New York, The Association, 1967.

AMERICAN NURSES' ASSOCIATION
[Fourth] nursing research conference, New York City. New York, The Association, 1968.

AMERICAN NURSES' ASSOCIATION. COMMITTEE ON RESEARCH AND STUDIES
ANA blueprint for research in nursing. *The American Journal of Nursing*, Aug. 1962, p. 69-71.

AMERICAN NURSES' FOUNDATION
Effects of different nursing approaches on psychological and physiological responses. *Nursing Research Report*, Mar. 1970, p. 1, and 5-7.

BATEY, M. V.
Some methodological issues in research. *Nursing Research*, Nov./Dec. 1970, p. 511-6.

BATTLE, A. O.
Quasi-experimental research designs in nursing. *Nursing Outlook*, Oct. 1964, p. 30-2.

BECK, F. S.
Some reflections on research in nursing. *International Nursing Review*, vol. 14, no. 2, 1967, p. 59-62.

BENDALL, E.
Nurses and research. *Nursing Times*, Dec. 3, 1970, Occasional Papers, p. 181-4.

BENDER, J.
The nurse in medical research. *RN Magazine*, May 1970, p. 62-5 and 101-2.

BENNE, K. D., *and* BENNIS, W.
What is real nursing? Role confusion and conflict in nursing. *Canadian Nurse*, Feb. 1961, p. 122-7.

BERTHOLD, JEANNE S.
Advancement of science and technology while maintaining human rights and values. *Nursing Research*, Nov./Dec. 1969, p. 514-22.

BERTHOLD, JEANNE S., *and others*
Symposium on theory development in nursing. *Nursing Research*, May/June 1968, p. 196-227.

BEST, L. A.
Nursing research in the National Health Service. *Irish Nurse*, April 1968, p. 10-3; May 1968, p. 10-1 and 13.

BHATIA, B. D.
Selecting a research problem. *Nursing Journal of India*, Oct. 1963, p. 261 and 265.

BOYLE, RENA E.
Administrative planning for project initiation and completion.
See
WALTER REED ARMY INSTITUTE OF RESEARCH
Report on nursing research conference, 1959. 1961.

BOYLE, RENA E.
Methods of data collection.
See
WALTER REED ARMY INSTITUTE OF RESEARCH
Report on nursing research conference, 1959. 1961.

BROWN, M. I.
Research in the development of nursing theory. *Nursing Research*, Spring 1964, p. 109-112.

BROWN, M. I.
Symposium on theory development in nursing. Social theory in geriatric nursing research. *Nursing Research*, May/June 1968, p. 213-7.

BUDZYNA, A. H.
Cultural lag in the concepts of nursing. *Nursing Research*, Summer 1961, p. 132.

BUEKER, K.
Reactions to a questionnaire survey. *Journal of Psychiatric Nursing and Mental Health Services*, Sept./Oct. 1969, p. 215-7 and 220-1.

BUNGE, H. L.
The first decade of nursing research. *Nursing Research*, Summer 1962, p. 133-7.

BYERLEY, E. L.
The nurse researcher as participant-observer in a nursing setting. *Nursing Research*, May/June 1969, p. 230-6.

CAMPBELL, M. A.
Identifying nursing problems. *The Canadian Nurse*, Feb. 1965, p. 96-9.

CANADIAN NURSES' ASSOCIATION
Index of Canadian nursing studies, 1969. Ottawa, The Association, 1969.

BIBLIOGRAPHY OF NURSING

CANADIAN NURSES' ASSOCIATION
List of studies on nursing in Canada. Ottawa, The Association, 1964.

CARNEVALI, D. S., *and* LITTLE, D. E.
Effects of a clinical nursing research study on a hospital. *Hospitals*, Sept. 1, 1965, p. 70-4.

COHEN, H.
The survey: a tool for appraisal. *Nursing Outlook*, Jan. 1961, p. 24-6.

CONANT, L. H.
On becoming a nurse researcher. *Nursing Research*, Jan./Feb. 1968, p. 68-71.

COYLE, M., *and others*
Research in nursing. An account of an introductory course in nursing research held at the New Zealand Postgraduate School for Nurses. *New Zealand Nursing Journal*, Dec. 1966, p. 19.

CRAMP, B.
Role of the nurse in metabolic research. *Nursing Mirror*, Sept. 20, 1968, p. 10-3.

CULLINAN, J.
Nursing research findings and their implementation. [Report of a conference held at The Hospital Centre, 26-27 February, 1969.] *Nursing Times*, April 3, 1969, Occasional Papers, p. 53-6.

DAVIES, J. O. F.
Reflections on the reasons for and the implications of nursing research.
See
MCLACHLAN, GORDON, *editor*.
Problems and progress in medical care... Oxford U.P. (for Nuffield P.H.T.), 1964.

DICKOFF, J., *and* JAMES, P.
Symposium on theory development in nursing. A theory of theories: a position paper. Researching research's role in theory development. *Nursing Research*, May/June 1968, p. 197-206.

DICKOFF, J., *and others*
Theory in a practice discipline. *Nursing Research*, Nov./Dec. 1968, p. 545-54.

DIERS, D.
Faculty research development at Yale. *Nursing Research*, Jan./Feb. 1970, p. 64-71.

DIERS, D.
This I believe... about nursing research. *Nursing Outlook*, Nov. 1970, p. 50-4.

DIERS, D., *and* LEONARD, R. C.
Interaction analysis in nursing research. *Nursing Research*, Summer 1966, p. 225-8.

DILWORTH, AVA S.
Problem formulation and resume of research processes.
See
WALTER REED ARMY INSTITUTE OF RESEARCH
Report on nursing research conference, 1959. 1961.

DIPIETRO, M. H.
An undergraduate course in nursing research. *Nursing Outlook*, May 1967, p. 52-3.

DOWNS, F. S.
Ethical inquiry in nursing research. *Nursing Forum*, vol. VI, no. 1, 1967, p. 12-20.

DOWNS, F. S.
Some critical issues in nursing research. *Nursing Forum*, vol. VIII, no. 4, 1969, p. 393-404.

DWYER, J. M.
The nurse and medical research. *Nursing Outlook*, May 1965, p. 51-3.

DUNSTON, B. N.
Nursing research: its challenges and its opportunities. *Nursing Science*, Oct. 1964, p. 368-76.

ELLIOTT, J. E.
Research in nursing: its contribution to present and future improvement of health care. *The Lamp*, Dec. 1968, p. 24-6; Jan. 1969, p. 9-11 and *The Tasmanian Nurse*, Feb. 1969, p. 9-11.

ELLIS, R.
Symposium on theory development in nursing. Characteristics of significant theories. *Nursing Research*, May/June 1968, p. 217-22.

FAWKES, B. N.
Why research in public health nursing? European nursing: The General Nursing Council for England and Wales and Registration. *International Journal of Nursing Studies*, Dec. 1967, p. 341-6.

FERGUSON, M., *and* WRIGHT, M. SCOTT
Scientific group on research in nursing: background paper. Geneva, W.H.O., 1963.

FIVARS, GRACE, *and* GOSNELL, DORIS
Nursing evaluation: the problems and the process: the critical incident technique. New York, Macmillan, 1966.

FOLTA, J. R., *and* SCHATZMAN, L.
Education in research for nurses. *The Journal of Nursing Education*, Nov. 1965, p. 29-35.

FOX, DAVID J.
Fundamentals of research in nursing. New York, Appleton-Century-Crofts, 1966.
2nd edn., 1970.

FOX, DAVID J.
A proposed model for identifying research areas in nursing. *Nursing Research*, Winter 1964, p. 29-36.

FOX, DAVID J., *and others*
Factors and practices project: the potential for satisfaction and stress of selected aspects of nursing school experience, by David J. Fox, Lorraine K. Diamond and Ruth C. Walsh. New York, Columbia University, Teachers' College, Institute of Research and Services in Nursing Education, 1962.

FOX, DAVID J., *and* KELLY, RUTH LUNDT
The research process in nursing. New York, Appleton-Century-Crofts, 1967.

FRANCES PAYNE BOLTON SCHOOL OF NURSING
Research—how will nursing define it? Papers presented at a symposium held May 4, 1966:
1. Quint, J. C. The case for theories generated from empirical data.
2. Conant, L. H. A search for resolution of existing problems in nursing.
3. Cleland, V. S. The use of existing theories.
4. Kolthoff, N. J. The use of the laboratory.
Nursing Research, Spring 1967, p. 108-29.

GARCIA, P. J.
Research opportunities in nursing. *Santo Tomas Nursing Journal*, Mar. 1965, p. 285-91.

GEITGEY, D. A., *and* METZ, E. A.
A brief guide to designing research proposals. *Nursing Research*, July/Aug. 1969, p. 339-44.

GREENBERG, BERNARD G.
The philosophy and methods of research.
See
WALTER REED ARMY INSTITUTE OF RESEARCH
Report on nursing research conference, 1959. 1961.

GREENFIELD, RUTH L.
Research tools for the nurse practitioner.
See
WALTER REED ARMY INSTITUTE OF RESEARCH
Report on nursing research conference, 1959. 1961.

GULABANI, L.
Abstracts of studies on Indian nursing problems. *The Nursing Journal of India*, April 1966, p. 106.

NURSING AS A PROFESSION

GUNTER, L. M.
Notes on a theoretical framework for nursing research. *Nursing Research*, Fall 1962, p. 219-22.

GUNTER, L. M.
Notes on teaching nursing research. *Journal of Nursing Education*, Aug. 1964, p. 13-6.

GUNTER, L. M.
Research techniques applied to nursing. *Nursing Research*, Summer 1964, p. 230-2.

HALSEY, FRANCIS Y.
Specific guides for writing research reports.
See
WALTER REED ARMY INSTITUTE OF RESEARCH
Report on nursing research conference, 1959. 1961.

HASSENPLUG, L. W.
Report of the Surgeon General's Consultant Group on Nursing. Significance and implications for research in nursing. *Nursing Research*, Spring 1963, p. 68 and 70.

HAWARD, L. R.
The nurse as a research associate. *International Journal of Nursing Studies*, Dec. 1964, p. 211-7.

HAWLEY, J.
Reconciling nursing with research. *Nursing Outlook*, June 1968, p. 34-5.

HEIDGERKEN, LORETTA E.
Nursing research—its role in research activities in nursing. *Nursing Research*, Summer 1962, p. 140-3.

HEIDGERKEN, LORETTA E.
Evaluation of reported research in nursing.
See
WALTER REED ARMY INSTITUTE OF RESEARCH
Report on nursing research conference, 1959. 1961.

HESS, IRENE, and others
Probability sampling of hospitals and patients, by Irene Hess, Donald C. Riedel and Thomas B. Fitzpatrick. Ann Arbor, University of Michigan, 1961.

HILBERT, H.
A trial plan for abstracting reports of studies in nursing. *Nursing Research*, Summer 1962, p. 173-5.

HOCKEY, L.
The place of research in district nursing. *Nursing Mirror*, Mar. 18, 1966, p. 685-6.

HOLLIDAY, J.
Clinical research training and subjective reactions of nursing service staff to the study process. *Nursing Research*, Summer 1967, p. 219-27.

HUBERT, Sister MARY
An inherited pathology.
See
REINKEMEYER, AGNES

HUGHES, P. E.
Research and problem solving in nursing. *New Zealand Nursing Journal*, Feb. 1969, p. 6-7 and 9.

HULICKA, I. M., and HULICKA, K.
To design experimental research. *The American Journal of Nursing*, Feb. 1962, p. 100-3.

JAHODA, M.
What is research? *Nursing Mirror*, Mar. 10, 1961, p. 2097-8; Mar. 17, 1961, p. 2199-200.

JENKINSON, V. M.
The ward sister in relation to administration and research. *International Journal of Nursing Studies*, April 1965, p. 105-13.

JOHNSON, D. E.
Symposium on theory development in nursing. Theory in nursing: borrowed and unique. *Nursing Research*, May/June 1968, p. 206-9.

JOHNSON, J. E., and others
Research projects for teaching methodology. *Nursing Outlook*, Nov. 1968, p. 27-9.

KEMPF, F. C.
What is research? *American Association of Industrial Nurses' Journal*, April 1964, p. 11 and 31.

LA FLAIR, EDNA I.
The public health nurse in research. *Canadian Nurse*, July 1961, p. 658-60.

LAMBERTSEN, ELEANOR C.
Identification of problems in nursing.
See
WALTER REED ARMY INSTITUTE OF RESEARCH
Report on nursing research conference, 1959. 1961.

LEE, A. S.
Search or research? An experience with a faculty research development project. *Nursing Outlook*, May 1965, p. 73.

LEININGER, M. M.
The research critique. *Nursing Research*, Sept./Oct. 1968, p. 444-9.

LENTZ, E. M., and MICHEALS, R. G.
Personality contrasts among medical and surgical nurses. *Nursing Research*, Winter 1965, p. 43-8.

LEONARD, R. C.
Developing research in a practice-oriented discipline. *American Journal of Nursing*, July 1967, p. 1472-5.

LINDEMAN, C. A., and VAN AERNAM, A. B.
Research program for nurses. *Hospitals*, June 1, 1970, p. 89-91.

LOWE, M. L., and FREEMAN, R. B.
Search and research. *Nursing Outlook*, May 1961, p. 313-5.

MACGREGOR, F. C.
Research potential in collegiate nursing students. *Nursing Research*, Summer 1964, p. 259-64.

MCMANUS, R. LOUISE
The place of research in nursing: past, present and future.
See
WALTER REED ARMY INSTITUTE OF RESEARCH
Report on nursing research conference, 1959. 1961.

MCMANUS, R. LOUISE
Nursing research—its evolution. *American Journal of Nursing*, April 1961, p. 76-9.

MCMANUS, R. LOUISE
Today and tomorrow in nursing research. *American Journal of Nursing*, May 1961, p. 68-71.

MAJOR, D. M., and CONN, V. S.
Research and the undergraduate student. *Journal of Nursing Education*, Aug. 1964, p. 9-12.

MALONE, M.
From practitioner to researcher. *The American Journal of Nursing*, Aug. 1962, p. 65-8.

MALONE, M. F., and BERKOWITZ, N. H.
Development of research skills in graduate nursing students. *Journal of Nursing Education*, Aug. 1964, p. 5-14.

MATHEWS, B. P.
Measurement of psychological aspects of the nurse-patient relationship. *Nursing Research*, Summer 1962, p. 154-62.

MERENESS, D.
Preparing the nurse researcher. *American Journal of Nursing*, Sept. 1964, p. 78-80.

MEYER, BURTON, and HEIDGERKEN, LORETTA E.
Introduction to research in nursing. Philadelphia, Lippincott, 1962.

MINCKLEY, BARBARA B.
O.R. nursing research. *AORN Journal*, Nov. 1969, p. 65-6.

MINCKLEY, BARBARA B.
O.R. nursing research. *AORN Journal*, Dec. 1969, p. 47-9.

MORRIS, M.
A new field for nursing research: preventive nursing. *Nursing Research*, Sept./Oct. 1969, p. 441-3.

MURRAY, V. P.
The role of the research sister. *New Zealand Nursing Journal*, Mar. 1970, p. 5-6.

MUSSALLEM, HELEN K.
Trends in research in nursing (Canada and the USA) [Geneva], W.H.O., 1963.

NEWTON, M. E.
As nursing research comes of age. *The American Journal of Nursing*, Aug. 1962, p. 46.

NEWTON, M. E.
The case for historical research. *Nursing Research*, Winter 1965, p. 20-6.

NORTHERN NURSES' FEDERATION
A seminar on research methods applied to nursing, 5th to 17th December, 1966. Stockholm, The Federation, [1967].

NORTON, D.
Nursing research—and how it can help. *British Hospital and Social Service Journal*, Jan. 22, 1965, p. 147 and 149.

NORTON, D.
Research for progress. *Nursing Mirror*, Jan. 22, 1965, p. 390-3.

NOTTER, L.
Nursing research is every nurse's business. *Nursing Outlook*, Jan. 1963, p. 49-51.

NURSING OUTLOOK
The research attitude in nursing. *Nursing Outlook*, May 1965, p. 33.

NURSING OUTLOOK
Search or research? Translation: from rough ideas to project plans. *Nursing Outlook*, Oct. 1964, p. 39.

ORAM, P. G., and ROUTHIER, W. R.
Research as in-service education. *Nursing Outlook*, Sept. 1968, p. 20-2.

PAIR, N.
Problems encountered in the conduct of nursing resources survey. *Journal of Nursing Education*, Aug. 1964, p. 27-9.

PEARSALL, M.
Participant observation as role and method in behavioral research. *Nursing Research*, Winter 1965, p. 37-42.

PUNSHON, P. M.
Perceptions of a research interviewer. *Nursing Outlook*, May 1965, p. 62-4.

QUINT, J. C.
Search or research? Some problems in applying the findings of research. *Nursing Outlook*, Aug. 1965, p. 53.

REINKEMEYER, AGNES
An inherited pathology. *Nursing Outlook*, Nov. 1967, p. 51-3.

REUELL, V. M.
Running a research ward. *American Journal of Nursing*, Dec. 1961, p. 80-2.

ROYAL COLLEGE OF NURSING
Nursing research at the College. *Nursing Times*, Mar. 1, 1963, *Royal College of Nursing Supplement*, p. 5-6.

ROYAL COLLEGE OF NURSING and NATIONAL COUNCIL OF NURSES OF THE UNITED KINGDOM
Nursing research. Report of conference held at Bournemouth, March 1965. *Nursing Times*, May 14, 1965 (*Rcn Supplement*, p. 19-20.)

ROYAL COLLEGE OF NURSING and NATIONAL COUNCIL OF NURSES OF THE UNITED KINGDOM
Nursing research. Report of a conference held at Bournemouth, March 1965. *Nursing Times*, June 11, 1965. (*Rcn Supplement*, p. 23-4).

ROYAL COLLEGE OF NURSING and NATIONAL COUNCIL OF NURSES OF THE UNITED KINGDOM
Nursing research. Report on conference held at Bournemouth, March 1965. *Nursing Times*, July 9, 1965 (*Rcn Supplement*, p. 27-8).

ROYAL COLLEGE OF NURSING and NATIONAL COUNCIL OF NURSES OF THE UNITED KINGDOM
Nursing research. Report of a conference held at Bournemouth, March 1965. *Nursing Times*, Aug. 13, 1965 (*Rcn Supplement*, p. 30-1).

ROYAL COLLEGE OF NURSING and NATIONAL COUNCIL OF NURSES OF THE UNITED KINGDOM
Nursing research. Report of the Conference held at Bournemouth, March 1965. *Nursing Times*, Sept. 10, 1965 (*Rcn Supplement*, p. 36).

ROYAL COLLEGE OF NURSING and NATIONAL COUNCIL OF NURSES OF THE UNITED KINGDOM
Nursing research. Report of a conference held at Bournemouth in March 1965. *Nursing Times*, Oct. 8, 1965 (*Rcn Supplement*, p. 39-41).

ROYAL COLLEGE OF NURSING and NATIONAL COUNCIL OF NURSES OF THE UNITED KINGDOM
Nursing research—a reappraisal. *Nursing Times*, June 2, 1967, p. 731.

SCHLOTFELDT, R. M.
Report of the Surgeon General's Consultant Group on Nursing. Significance and implications for research in nursing. *Nursing Research*, Spring 1963, p. 69 and 71.

SCHMITT, L. M.
Research in nursing. *The Australian Nurses' Journal*, Sept. 1968, p. 194-8.

SCHWARTZ, D. R.
The value of small local nursing studies. *American Journal of Nursing*, June 1966, p. 1327-9.

SCOTTISH HOSPITAL CENTRE
The nurse and research. Meeting at the Scottish Hospital Centre on Friday, 6th November, 1970. Edinburgh, The Centre, [1971].

SEIVWRIGHT, M. J.
Nursing research and you. *The Jamaican Nurse*, June 1961, p. 19.

SEIVWRIGHT, M. J.
Nursing research: a progress report. *The Jamaican Nurse*, Dec. 1961, p. 35.

SEYFFER, C.
Research and development in nursing. *International Nursing Review*, vol. 14, no. 2, 1967, p. 39-42.

SHARP, L. J.
The behavioral scientist in nursing research. *Nursing Research*, Fall 1964, p. 327-32.

SHARP, L. J., and TSCHUDIN, M. S.
Nursing faculty research development: report of an experience. *Nursing Research*, Spring 1967, p. 161-6.

SHELDON, ELEANOR B.
A report on an experimental program in nursing research. *Nursing Research*, Winter 1964, p. 16-9.

SHELDON, ELEANOR B., *and others*
A progress note: an experimental program in nursing research. *Nursing Research*, Spring 1961, p. 105-7.

SIMMONS, LEO W., and HENDERSON, VIRGINIA
Nursing research, a survey and assessment. New York, Appleton-Century-Crofts, 1964.

SIMPSON, H. M.
Nursing research. Report of the Special Interest Session held at the ICN Quadrennial Congress, Montreal, 1969. *International Nursing Review*, vol. 17, no. 2, 1970, p. 110-32 bibliogs., p. 119-22; history of research projects, p. 125-32).

SIMPSON, H. M.
Research for improvement of nursing service. [Geneva], W.H.O., 1967?

SIMPSON, H. M.
[Guest editorial.] Research in nursing in the United Kingdom. *International Nursing Review*, vol. 17, no. 2, 1970, p. 99-100.

SIMPSON, H. M.
Research into nursing. *Occupational Health*, Sept./Oct. 1966, p. 246-50.

SPRATT, I. H., *and others*
Some practical outcomes of a research study. *Nursing Outlook*, June 1969, p. 66-7.

STEELE, R.
Methodology of a study in hospital utilization. *Canadian Hospital*, Nov. 1961, p. 34.

STEPHENSON, E.
Fields of research in nursing. *Nursing Mirror*, Mar. 24, 1961, p. 2299-300.

STEPHENSON, E.
The need for nursing research. *International Journal of Nursing Studies*, Feb. 1966, p. 279-82.

STRYKER, R. P.
Precepts for a method study. *Nursing Outlook*, May 1965, p. 65-7.

TAO-CHEN YU
Teaching research concepts in the basic nursing programme. *International Nursing Review*, vol. 11, no. 5, 1964, p. 20-4.

THIGPEN, LORNA W.
Guidelines for research in clinical nursing. New York, National League for Nursing, 1967. [League exchanges, no. 81.]

THIGPEN, LORNA W., *and* DRANE, J. W.
The Venn diagram: a tool for conceptualization in nursing. *Nursing Research*, Summer 1967, p. 252-60.

TOBIN, M. J.
Applied research for the nurse administrators.
See
MCLACHLAN, GORDON, *editor*
Problems and progress in medical care ... Oxford U.P. (for Nuffield P.H.T.), 1964, p. 99.

UNITED STATES. PUBLIC HEALTH SERVICE. DIVISION OF NURSING
Current nursing research grants, supported by the Division of Nursing. January 1968, 1969. Washington, Government Printing Office, 1968-9.

UNITED STATES. PUBLIC HEALTH SERVICE. DIVISION OF NURSING
Current research project grants. Revised edn. Washington, U.S. Dept. of Health, 1970.

UNITED STATES. PUBLIC HEALTH SERVICE. DIVISION OF NURSING
Research in nursing 1955-1968. Research grants: projects supported with funds administered by the Division of Nursing. Bethesda, Maryland, U.S. Dept. of Health, 1969.

VERHONICK, PHYLLIS J.
Note taking and organizing materials for writing.
See
WALTER REED ARMY INSTITUTE OF RESEARCH
Report on nursing research conference, 1959. 1961.

WALLER, M. V.
Nurse interviewers on a health research team. *Nursing Outlook*, May 1965, p. 60-2.

WALTER REED ARMY INSTITUTE OF RESEARCH
Report on nursing research conference, 24th February - 7th March, 1959, edited by Harriet H. Werley. Washington, Walter Reed Army Medical Center, 1961.

WANDELT, MABEL A.
Guide for the beginning researcher. New York, Appleton-Century-Crofts, 1970.

WAX, J.
Attitudes of nursing students toward research. *Nursing Outlook*, April 1966, p. 70-2.

WESTERN COUNCIL ON HIGHER EDUCATION FOR NURSING
Communicating nursing research: the research critique, edited by Marjorie V. Batey. Boulder, Co., The Council, 1968.

WESTERN COUNCIL ON HIGHER EDUCATION FOR NURSING
Newly initiated and completed research in the field of nursing by faculty of WCHEN schools of nursing. Boulder, Colorado, The Council, 1964.

WESTERN COUNCIL ON HIGHER EDUCATION FOR NURSING
Newly initiated and completed research in the field of nursing by faculty of WCHEN schools of nursing. Boulder, Colorado, The Council, 1965.

WHALEY, P. J.
Nursing research: limbo or liberty. *American Journal of Nursing*, Aug. 1967, p. 1675-7.

WHITING, L., *and* J. F.
Finding the core of hospital nursing. *The American Journal of Nursing*, Aug. 1962, p. 80-3.

WILLIAMS, M. M.
Research and its uses. *Nursing Times*, Dec. 8, 1961, p. 1609.

OPERATIONAL RESEARCH

JEFFRIES, I. J.
Operational research and the ward sister. *New Zealand Nursing Journal*, Oct. 1963, p. 14-5.

KING EDWARD'S HOSPITAL FUND FOR LONDON *and* MINISTRY OF HEALTH
Operational research in nursing. *Nursing Times*, Sept. 10, 1965, p. 1248-9.

LOWE, S.
The contribution of operational research to contemporary nursing service. *New Zealand Nursing Journal*, Feb. 1963, p. 15-17.

THE PATIENT—RESEARCH

BARTON, R., ELKES, A., *and* GLEN, F.
Unrestricted visiting in a mental hospital. An inquiry into its effects and nursing-staff attitudes. *The Lancet*, June 3, 1961, p. 1220-2.

LAMBERTSEN, E. C.
Nursing research: the process begins with the patient in the hospital setting. *The Modern Hospital*, May 1967, p. 142.

LETOURNEAU, C. U.
Patient environment—a new area for research. *Hospital Management*, April 1964, p. 43-5.

THE WORK OF THE NURSE

BRINCKLOW, P., *and* SMELLIE, H.
Cut flowers and antiseptics. In one ward it was estimated that 14 nurse-hours a week were being spent "doing the flowers". This article describes how this time could be reduced. *Nursing Times*, Oct. 25, 1963, p. 1348-50.

CHARLOTTE, SR. M., *and* HOPKINS, V. L.
A study of the professional and personal characteristics of full and part-time nurses at Mercy Hospital, Pittsburgh. *Hospital Progress*, July 1967, p. 100-4.

JAYAWARDENA, Y.
Research in operating theatre nursing. *International Nursing Review*, vol. 10, no. 4, 1963, p. 25-33.

Mason, R., and Major, K.
Health visitors with a medical research unit. *Nursing Times*, Aug. 24, 1962, p. 1081-3.

Pearson, E.
Research into nursing equipment at Manor Park Hospital, Bristol. *Nursing Times*, May 6, 1966, p. 604-6.

Petrowski, D. D.
How do public health nurses use the telephone? *Nursing Outlook*, Jan. 1965, p. 42-4.

NURSING ETHICS

American Nurses' Association
Code for nurses. *American Journal of Nursing*, Dec. 1968, p. 2581-5.

American Nurses' Association
Ethics, the code, and the nurse. New York, The Association, 1964.

American Nurses' Association
The nurse in research: ANA guidelines on ethical values. [New York] The Association, [1968?]

American Nurses' Association. Committee on Ethical, Legal and Professional Standards
Code for nurses with interpretive statements. [Rev. edn.] New York, The Association, 1968.

Berthold, J. S.
Advancement of science and technology while maintaining human rights and values. *Nursing Research*, Nov./Dec. 1969, p. 514-22.

Cross, Y.
The nurse and the nursing press. *District Nursing*, Nov. 1963, p. 174.

Dent, M. J. W.
Should nurses diagnose death? *Nursing Mirror*, Dec. 5, 1969, p. 20-3.

Drage, E., and Lange, B.
Ethical considerations in the use of patients for demonstration [of group therapy]. *American Journal of Nursing*, Oct. 1969, p. 2161-5.

General Nursing Council for England and Wales
The profession's good name. *Nursing Times*, Aug. 23, 1963, p. 1061-2.

Guild of St. Barnabus for Anglican Nurses
Amended constitution . . . 1964. *The Guild*, n.d.

Guild of St. Barnabus for Anglican Nurses
Manual. *The Guild*, n.d.

Guild of St. Barnabas for Anglican Nurses
To the Anglican nurse. Rev. edn. Church Information Office, 1969.

Gunter, L. M.
The effects of segregation on nursing students. *Nursing Outlook*, Feb. 1961, p. 74-6.

Hayes, Edward J., and others
Moral principles of nursing, by Edward J. Hayes, Paul J. Hayes and Dorothy Ellen Kelly. New York, Macmillan, 1964.

International Committee of the Red Cross
Rights and duties of nurses, military and civilian medical personnel under the Geneva Conventions of August 12, 1949. Red Cross Principles. Geneva, The Committee, 1969.

Komorita, N. I.
Nursing diagnosis. *American Journal of Nursing*, Dec. 1963, p. 83-6.

Lippitt, Gordon L.
The professional nurse looks at ethics. Washington, Leadership Resources, 1966.
[Leadership in Nursing Series, no. 13.]

McDevitt, B. A.
Ethics and the nurse—1. *Nursing Times*, April 15, 1966, p. 503-4.

McDevitt, B. A.
Ethics and the nurse. 2—Responsibilities of the nurse to her patient. *Nursing Times*, April 22, 1966, p. 542-3.

National Federation of Licensed Practical Nurses
Code of ethics for the licensed practical nurse. *Bedside Nurse*, Mar./April 1968, p. 6.

Pole, K. F. M.
Handbook for the catholic nurse. Robert Hale, 1964.

Rothberg, J. S.
Why nursing diagnosis? *American Journal of Nursing*, May 1967, p. 1040-2.

Shield, B.
Ethics in the basic nursing programme. *UNA Nursing Journal*, Nov. 1966, p. 325-8.

Speller, S. R.
Professional confidence. *Nursing Mirror*, Jan. 12, 1968, p. 352-4; Jan. 19, 1968, p. 381-2.

Stock, W.
Planning a syllabus for teaching ethics to student nurses. *UNA Nursing Journal*, Nov. 1966, p. 319-23.

NURSE-PATIENT RELATIONSHIP

Aasterud, M.
Defenses against anxiety in the nurse-patient relationship. *Nursing Forum*, Summer 1962, p. 35-59.

Aguilera, D. C.
Relationship between physical contact and verbal interaction between nurses and patients. *Journal of Psychiatric Nursing*, Jan./Feb. 1967, p. 5-21.

American Nurses' Association
Innovations in nurse-patient relationships: automatic or reasoned nurse actions. N.Y., A.N.A., 1962.
[ANA Convention, 1962, clinical monographs no. 6.]

American Nurses' Association
Innovations in nurse-patient relationships: nursing the patient with problems of response. N.Y., A.N.A., 1962.
[ANA Convention, 1962, clinical monographs no. 7.]

American Nurses' Association
The nurse and groups of patients or clients. N.Y., A.N.A., 1962.
[ANA Convention, 1962, clinical monographs no. 10.]

American Nurses' Association
The nurse-patient-doctor triadic relationships: effects on nursing care of the patient. N.Y., A.N.A., 1962.
[ANA Convention, 1962, clinical monographs no. 21.]

Boorer, David
A question of attitudes: an account of a series of meetings held at The Hospital Centre from October 1968 to January 1970 during which nurses explored their attitudes to their patients. King's Fund Hospital Centre, 1970.

Bray, R. E., and Bird, T. E.
The art of listening. *Nursing Mirror*, Jan. 1, 1965, p. 307-8.

Brown, J. A., and Goldstein, L. S.
Nurse-patient interaction before and after the substitution of street clothes for uniforms. *The International Journal of Social Psychiatry*, Winter 1967-8, p. 32-43.

Burke, J. L., and Lafave, H. G.
A structured group programme for patient-staff communication. *International Journal of Social Psychiatry*, Spring 1964, p. 142-8.

Burton, Genevieve
Nurse and patient: the influence of human relationships. Tavistock, 1965.

NURSING AS A PROFESSION

BYE, W. G., *and* BERNALL, M. E.
The effects of two patient behaviors upon psychiatric nurses' ratings of the patient. *Nursing Research*, May/June 1968, p. 251-5.

CARNEVALI, D., *and* LITTLE, D.
Tuberculosis patients and nurse specialists. *Nursing Outlook*, May 1965, p. 78-80.

CONANT, L. H.
Use of Bales' interaction process analysis to study nurse-patient interaction. *Nursing Research*, Fall 1965, p. 304-9.

COOPER, J.
Morale in the ward. *Nursing Times*, July 12, 1963, p. 875-7.

CUTHBERT, B. L.
Switch off, tune in, turn on. [Nurses' attitudes to patients.] *American Journal of Nursing*, June 1969, p. 1206-11.

ECKELBERRY, G.
The nurse as a patient. *Nursing Outlook*, Dec. 1964, p. 20-3.

HAGERMAN, Z. J.
Teaching beginners to cope with extreme behavior. *American Journal of Nursing*, Sept. 1968, p. 1927-9.

HALE, S. L.
Terminating the nurse-patient relationship. *American Journal of Nursing*, Sept. 1963, p. 116-9.

HALL, B. L.
Human relations in the hospital setting. *Nursing Outlook*, Mar. 1968, p. 43-5.

HAY, SHEILA
Human relations in hospital. *International Journal of Nursing Studies*, May 1964, p. 99-112.

HAYES, WAYLAND J., *and* GAZAWAY, RENA
Human relations in nursing. 3rd edn. Philadelphia, Saunders, 1964.

HAYS, J. S.
Analysis of nurse-patient communications. *Nursing Outlook*, Sept. 1966, p. 32-5.

INGLES, T.
Understanding the nurse-patient relationship. *Nursing Outlook*, Nov. 1961, p. 698-700.

KING, J. M.
A nurse's communication patterns and a patient's use of denial. *Nursing Research*, Spring 1967, p. 137-40.

KIRKPATRICK, W. J.
The nurse as a patient-counsellor. *Nursing Times*, Oct. 22, 1965, p. 1461-2.

LAMBERTSEN, E. C.
Patient service will improve if nurse-doctor communications do. *The Modern Hospital*, Dec. 1965, p. 108.

LEWIS, G. K.
Communication: a factor in meeting emotional crises. *Nursing Outlook*, Aug. 1965, p. 36-9.

LEWIS, G. K.
Nurse-patient communication. Dubuque, Iowa, 1969.

LOS ANGELES COUNTY GENERAL HOSPITAL. CORONARY CARE UNIT
Protocol for patient care. *American Journal of Nursing*, Nov. 1967, p. 2314-7.

LUM, J. L. J.
Interaction patterns of nursing personnel. *Nursing Research*, July/Aug. 1970, p. 324-30.

MCQUEEN, RONALD J.
Introducing ... the liaison nurse. *Hospital Administration in Canada*, May 1964, p. 41-2.

MADLAND, L.
Nurse-patient relationships. *The Canadian Nurse*, Aug. 1964, p. 762-5.

MALLORY, E.
Patient care needs as seen by a nurse. *Pennsylvania Nurse*, May 1969, p. 10-4.

MANASER, JANICE CLACK, *and* WERNER, ANITA MARIE
Instruments for study of nurse-patient interaction. New York, Macmillan, 1964.

MARCUS, A. M.
The nurse and the sociopathic personality. *Canadian Nurse*, Oct. 1969, p. 49-50.

MARY ELENA OF THE CROSS
Improving nurse-patient relationship. *Santo Thomas Nursing Journal*, Sept. 1965, p. 102-9.

METHVEN, D., *and* SCHLOTFELDT, R. M.
The social interaction inventory. *Nursing Research*, Spring 1962, p. 83-8.

MILLER, A.
The patient's right to know the truth. *The Canadian Nurse*, Jan. 1962, p. 25-9.

MULLER, H. M.
The role of sociology in nursing education. *Journal of Nursing Education*, Jan. 1964, p. 21-3.

NEHREN, J. G., *and* BATEY, M. V.
The process recording [a method of teaching interpersonal relationship skills]. *Nursing Forum*, vol. II, no. 2, 1963, p. 65-73.

NEW ZEALAND. DEPARTMENT OF HEALTH. OPERATIONAL RESEARCH UNIT
Patient-nurse dependency: exploratory study, by I. J. Jeffery and Shirley M. Lowe. Wellington, The Department, 1963.

NEW ZEALAND. DEPARTMENT OF HEALTH. RESEARCH AND PLANNING UNIT
Patient-nurse dependency: general survey data: an analysis of survey data from three public hospitals in Christchurch 1962. Wellington, Owen, 1965.

NORRIS, C. M.
Direct access to the patient. [The doctor as a barrier to the nurse-patient relationship.] *American Journal of Nursing*, May 1970, p. 1006-10.

NURSING CLINICS OF NORTH AMERICA
Symposium on compassion and communication in nursing. *Nursing Clinics of North America*, Dec. 1969, p. 651-729.

O'CONNOR, D., *and* HAGAN, F.
Liaison nurse. *American Journal of Nursing*, June 1964, p. 101-3.

ORLANDO, IDA JEAN
The dynamic nurse-patient relationship; function, process and principles. New York, Putnam, 1961.

PRANGE, ARTHUR J., *and* MARTIN, HARRY W.
Aids to understanding patients. *American Journal of Nursing*, July 1962, p. 98-100.

ROCH, S.
The care of the dying. *Nursing Times*, Oct. 11, 1968, Occasional Papers, p. 157-60.

SHEPS, C. G., *and* BACHAR, M. E.
Changing patterns of practice—nursing and medical. *Journal of Psychiatric Nursing*, Mar./April 1965, p. 151-9.

SHORTHOUSE, M. A.
Patients' questions and nurses' answers. *Nursing Times*, Aug. 2, 1963, p. 952-4.

SKIPPER, J. K. *and* LEONARD, R. C.
Communication and patient care. *The Canadian Nurse*, July 1965, p. 562-5.

SMITH, D. M.
Myth and method in nursing practice. *American Journal of Nursing*, Feb. 1964, p. 68-72.

STEIN, R. F.
Sociological foresight and hindsight in nursing. *International Journal of Nursing Studies*, Dec. 1967, p. 311-6.

STEVENS, L. F.
Nurse-patient discussion groups. *American Journal of Nursing*, Dec. 1963, p. 67-9.

UJHELY, G. B.
What is realistic emotional support? *The American Journal of Nursing*, April 1968, p. 758-62.

WESSLER, R. L.
Patient opinions: what do they really mean? *Hospital Progress*, July 1968, p. 50-3.

WINTERS, M. C., and GILMER, L.
The nurse's judgment and the patient's understanding. *American Journal of Nursing*, Dec. 1961, p. 50-4.

PROFESSIONAL STAFF RELATIONSHIPS

BATES, B., and CHAMBERLIN, R. W.
Physician leadership as perceived by nurses. *Nursing Research*, Nov./Dec. 1970, p. 534-9.

BERKOWITZ, NORMAN H., and MALONE, MARY F.
Intra-professional conflict. *Nursing Forum*, vol. VII, no. 1, 1968, p. 50-71.

BEYTELL, J. H.
The need for hospital counsellors. *South African Nursing Journal*, Sept. 1963, p. 29-30.

BRIDGES, D. E.
What the nurse expects of the doctor. *World Medical Journal*, Sept. 1961, p. 328-9.

BUSH, CHRISTINE H.
Personal and vocational relationships for practical nurses. Philadelphia, Saunders, 1961.
2nd edn., 1966.

CHASE, P. H.
FEL—a process for teaching interpersonal relationships. *American Journal of Nursing*, Mar. 1970, p. 524-8.

CHRISTMAN, L. P.
Nurse-physician communications in the hospital. *International Nursing Review*, vol. 12, no. 4, 1966, p. 49-57.

CLARKE, D. H.
Nurse and doctor—1. Colleague or hand-maiden. *Nursing Times*, Aug. 3, 1962, p. 978-80.

CLARK, L.
Individualizing hospital staff orientation. *American Journal of Nursing*, Oct. 1962, p. 102.

DAKE, MARCIA A.
What's wrong with the nurse-physician relationship in today's hospitals? A nurse's views. *Hospitals*, Dec. 16, 1966, p. 70-4 and 122.

DREWERY, J., and KEAR-COLWELL, J. J.
An evaluation of nursing attitudes—a preliminary communication. *Nursing Times*, Nov. 27, 1969, Occasional Papers, p. 197-200.

ELLIS, G.
Nurse and doctor—2. Mothers and fathers. *Nursing Times*, Aug. 10, 1962, p. 1022-3.

GALBRAITH, J. M.
What the physician expects of the nurse. *World Medical Journal*, Sept. 1961, p. 325-7.

GILDNER, JOHN L.
Pilot study of the meaning of words between physicians and nurses in hospital communications as measured by the Semantic differential. Minnesota, University of Minnesota School of Public Health, 1964.

GOZZI, E. K., and others
Gaps in doctor-patient communication. Implications for nursing practice. *American Journal of Nursing*, Mar. 1969, p. 529-33.

GRAULOU, R.
Integration of young nurses in hospital life. *International Nursing Review*, vol. 9, no. 2, 1963, p. 39-41.

HEFFNER, W. W.
Medical staff counsellors aid nursing students. *Hospital Topics*, Feb. 1967, p. 44-6.

JENKINSON, V.
Nurse and doctor—3. Doctor in the ward. *Nursing Times*, Aug. 17, 1962, p. 1041-3.

KING, E. S., and FASSO, T. E.
How nursing and social work dovetail. *American Journal of Nursing*, April 1962, p. 89-90.

KRAMER, M.
Role conceptions of bacalaureate nurses and success in hospital nursing. *Nursing Research*, Sept.-Oct. 1970, p. 428-39.

LETOURNEAU, C. U.
The changing pattern of the nurse-physician relationships. *Hospital Management*, July 1964, p. 55-6 and 58.

MARTIN, J.
What the nurse thinks of the doctor. *World Medical Journal*, Sept. 1961, p. 330-1.

MARY BLAISE
Who is a practical nurse? Relations between registered nurses and licensed practical nurses. *American Journal of Nursing*, Oct. 1962, p. 76-8.

MATTHIAS, A. N.
Nurse and doctor—4. Surgeon in the theatre. *Nursing Times*, Aug. 24, 1962, p. 1078-80.

MENZIES, ISABEL E. P.
The functioning of social systems as a defence against anxiety: a report on a study of the nursing service of a general hospital. Tavistock Publications, 1961.
Re-issued 1967.

MERTON, R. K.
Relations between registered nurses and licensed practical nurses. Status-orientations in nursing. *American Journal of Nursing*, Oct. 1962, p. 70-3.

MESOLELLA, D. W.
Teachers—you are trespassing! [hostility between nurse educators and ward staff]. *The Canadian Nurse*, July 1970, p. 21.

MITCHELL, H. E., and others
Nursing students look at their problems across three years of training. *Nursing Research*, Winter 1962, p. 21-5.

NEHREN, J., and KILLEN, B.
Preventive counselling for nursing students. *Nursing Outlook*, Jan. 1967, p. 37-9.

OLESEN, VIRGINIA L., and WHITAKER, ELVI W.
The silent dialogue: a study in the social psychology of professional socialization. San Francisco, Jossey-Bass, 1968.

OLIVER, S.
Problems of the newly appointed ward staff. *British Hospital Journal and Social Service Review*, Oct. 17, 1970, p. 2055-6.

OSTLUND, L. A.
An adjustment program for nursing students. *Hospital Topics*, July 1965, p. 58-61.

PELLEGRINO, E. D.
What's wrong with the nurse-physician relationship in today's hospitals? A physician's view. *Hospitals*, Dec. 16, 1966, p. 70, 77-8 and 80.

POWELL, M.
The eternal triangle [regulations between doctors, nurses and administrators]. *British Medical Journal*, May 16, 1970, p. 416-8.

PRATT, HENRY
Doctor's view of the changing nurse-physician relationship. *Journal of Medical Education*, Aug. 1965, p. 767-71.

PRICE, G.
The adviser to students and her advice. *American Journal of Nursing*, April 1964, p. 130-2.

RASMUSSEN, E. H.
Changing organizational relations. Relations between registered nurses and licensed practical nurses. *American Journal of Nursing*, Oct. 1962, p. 73-6.

RAYNER, C.
Doctor-nurse relationships in a hospital environment. *The Lancet*, Dec. 30, 1961, p. 1448-50.

ROSE, P.
Using the student diary to identify stress-satisfactions. *American Journal of Nursing*, Aug. 1962, p. 94-6.

ROSS, CARMEN
Personal and vocational relationships in practical nursing. Philadelphia, Lippincott, 1961.

SCHLOTFELDT, ROZELLA M.
Nurse's view of the changing nurse-physician relationship. *Journal of Medical Education*, Aug. 1965, p. 772-7.

SPALDING, EUGENIA KENNEDY *and* NOTTER, LUCILLE E.
Professional nursing . . . 7th edn. Philadelphia, Lippincott, 1965.
[Earlier edition of this work published under the title: Professional adjustments in nursing . . .]
8th edn., 1970.

STEVENS, MARION KEITH
Personal and vocational relationships of the practical nurse. Philadelphia, Saunders, 1967.

VAILL, PETER B.
The professional nurse looks at staff-line relations. Washington, Leadership Resources, 1966.
[Leadership in Nursing series, no. 12.]

VAILLOT, MADELEINE CLEMENCE
Commitment to nursing: a philosophic investigation. Philadelphia, Lippincott, 1962.

WHELDON, M.
Anxiety in ward sisters. *Nursing Mirror*, July 27, 1962, p. 323-4.

YOUNG, E. H.
Inter-personal relationships in nursing. *The Journal of Nursing Education*, Sept. 1963, p. 7-10 and 44-5.

WORK OF THE NURSE

GENERAL WORKS

AHAD, M. A.
Approach to clinical nursing. *Nursing Journal of India*, Dec. 1968, p. 394, and 408.

AMERICAN NURSES' ASSOCIATION
ANA clinical sessions. . . . 1966 San Francisco. New York, Appleton-Century-Crofts, 1967.

AMERICAN NURSES' ASSOCIATION
Culture, atmosphere and social organization: effects on nursing care of the patient. N.Y., A.N.A., 1962. [ANA Convention 1962, clinical monographs no. 18.]

AMERICAN NURSES' ASSOCIATION
Emergency intervention by the nurse. N.Y., A.N.A., 1962. [ANA Convention 1962, clinical monographs no. 1].

AMERICAN NURSES' ASSOCIATION
Exploring progress in medical-surgical nursing practice. New York, the Association, 1966.

AMERICAN NURSES' ASSOCIATION
Exploring progress in nursing practice. New York, the Association, 1966.

AMERICAN NURSES' ASSOCIATION
Improvement of nursing practice: speeches presented at the Section Regional Conference for Professional Nurses. New York, A.N.A., 1961.

AMERICAN NURSES' ASSOCIATION
Nursing and the patient's motivations. N.Y., A.N.A., 1962. [ANA Convention 1962, clinical monographs no. 19.]

AMERICAN NURSES' ASSOCIATION
Nursing approaches to denial of illness. N.Y., A.N.A., 1962. [ANA Convention 1962, clinical monographs no. 12.]

AMERICAN NURSES' ASSOCIATION
Phases in human development: relevance in nursing. N.Y., A.N.A., 1962. [ANA Convention 1962, clinical monographs no. 14.]

AMERICAN NURSES' ASSOCIATION
Phases in human development: relevance in nursing. N.Y., A.N.A., 1962. [ANA Convention 1962, clinical monographs no. 15.]

AMERICAN NURSES' ASSOCIATION
Phases in human development: relevance in nursing. N.Y., A.N.A., 1962. (ANA Convention 1962, clinical monographs no. 16.]

AMERICAN NURSES' ASSOCIATION
Technical innovations in health care: nursing implications. N.Y., A.N.A., 1962. (ANA Convention 1962, clinical monographs, no. 5.)

AMERICAN NURSES' ASSOCIATION
Technical innovations in health care: nursing implications. N.Y., A.N.A., 1962. [ANA Convention, 1962, clinical monographs no. 3.]

AMERICAN NURSES' ASSOCIATION
Technical innovations in health care: nursing implications. N.Y., A.N.A., 1962. [ANA Convention 1962, clinical monographs no. 4.]

ANDERSON, MAJA C.
Basic nursing techniques: a programed introduction to nursing fundamentals. Philadelphia, Saunders, 1968.

ASK, R.
Are attitudes important in nursing? *The Nursing Journal of India*, July 1969, p. 227, and 230.

BAIN, B.
The therapeutic role of the staff nurse. *Nursing Forum*, vol. II, no. 2, 1963, p. 90-7.

BARBATA, JEAN C., *and others*
A workbook of medical-surgical nursing. New York, Putnam, 1961.

BARBATA, JEAN C., *and others*
A textbook of medical-surgical nursing by Jean C. Barbata, Deborah M. Jensen and William G. Patterson. New York, Putnam, 1964.

BELAND, IRENE L.
Clinical nursing: pathophysiological and psychosocial approaches. New York, Macmillan, 1965.
2nd edn., 1970.

BENDALL, EVE R. D.
Nursing in a technological age. From a paper given at Royal College of Nursing Golden Jubilee Conference. *Nursing Times*, July 15, 1966, p. 951-2.

BENDALL, EVE R. D., *and* RAYBOULD, ELIZABETH
Basic nursing. H. K. Lewis, 1963.
2nd edn., 1965.
3rd edn., 1970.

BENDALL, EVE R. D., *and* RAYBOULD, ELIZABETH
A guide to medical and surgical nursing. H. K. Lewis, 1965.
2nd edn., 1970.

BERGERSEN, BETTY S., *and others, editors*
Current concepts in clinical nursing. St. Louis, Mosby, 1967. vol. 2, 1969.

BERMOSK, LORETTA SUE, *and* MORDAN, MARY JANE
Interviewing in nursing. New York, Macmillan, 1964.

BERNARD, JESSIE, *and* JENSEN, DEBORAH MACLURG
Sociology. 6th edn. St. Louis, Mosby, 1962.
7th edn., 1966.
8th edn., 1970.

BERNSTEIN, LEWIS, *and* DANA, RICHARD H.
Interviewing and the health professions. New York, Appleton-Century-Crofts, 1970.

BONNEY, VIRGINIA, *and* ROTHBERG, JUNE
Nursing diagnosis and therapy: an instrument for evaluation and measurement. New York, National League for Nursing, 1963.

BOWDEN, E. A. F.
Nurses' attitudes toward hospital nursing services. *Nursing Research*, Summer 1967, p. 246-51.

BRANDT, EDNA MAE, *and others*
Comparison of on-the-job performance of graduates with school of nursing objectives. *Nursing Research*, Winter 1967, p. 50-60.

BRITTEN, JESSIE D.
Practical notes on nursing procedures. 4th edn. Edinburgh, Livingstone, 1963.
5th edn., 1966.

BROWN, ELIZABETH A., *and* KRAMER, JEANNETTE R.
Clinical experience in a nursing home. *Nursing Outlook*, Dec. 1968, p. 52-3.

BRODT, D. E.
A synergistic theory of nursing. *American Journal of Nursing*, Aug. 1969, p. 1674-5.

BROWN, ESTHER LUCILE
Nursing reconsidered: a study of change. Philadelphia, Lippincott, 1970.
Part 1. The professional role in institutional nursing.

BRUNNER, LILIAN SHOLTIS, *and others*
Textbook of medical-surgical nursing, by Lillian Sholtis Brunner, Charles Phillips Emerson, Jr., L. Kraeer Ferguson and Doris Smith Suddarth. Philadelphia, Lippincott, 1964.
2nd edn., 1970.

CARLSON, CAROLYN E., *editor*
Behavioral concepts and nursing intervention. Philadelphia, Lippincott, 1970.

CARNEVALI, D., *and* BREUCKNER, S.
Immobilization—reassessment of a concept. *American Journal of Nursing*, July 1970, p. 1502-7.

CHERESCAVICH, G.
The expanding role of the professional nurse in a hospital. *Nursing Forum*, vol. III, no. 4, 1964, p. 9-20.

CHRISTMAN, LUTHER
Specialism and generalism in clinical nursing. *Hospitals*, Jan. 1, 1967, p. 83-6.

COOMBS, R. P.
Active-care hospital nurse expands her role. *Canadian Nurse*, Oct. 1970, p. 23-9.

COOPER, SIGNE SKOTT
Contemporary nursing practice: a guide for the returning nurse. New York, McGraw-Hill, 1970.

CULVER, VIVIAN M.
Modern bedside nursing. 7th edn. Philadelphia, W. B. Saunders, 1969.

CUNNINGHAM, LYDA SUE
Advanced medical-surgical nursing. Dubuque, Iowa, Brown, 1966.

DAHLSTEDT, J. M.
Rearrangements to enrich bedside nursing. *American Journal of Nursing*, June 1969, p. 1254-7.

DARWIN, JOAN, *and others*
Bedside nursing: an introduction, by Joan Darwin, Joan Markham and Brysson Whyte. Heinemann, 1964.
2nd edn., 1967.

DAVISON, T.
Labour-saving methods in nursing. *Nursing Mirror*, Feb. 7, 1969, p. 44-5; Feb. 14, 1969, p. 44-5.

DICKOFF, J., *and others*
Theory in a practice discipline. Part 1. Practice oriented theory. *Nursing Research*, Sept./Oct. 1968, p. 415-35.

DICKOFF, J., *and others*
Theory in a practice discipline. Part 2. Research. *Nursing Research*, Nov./Dec. 1968, p. 545-54.

DISON, NORMA GREENLER
An atlas of nursing techniques. St. Louis, Mosby, 1967.

DODGE, J. S.
Factors related to patients' perceptions of their cognitive needs. *Nursing Research*, Nov./Dec. 1969, p. 502-13.

DUGAN, A. B.
Nursing autonomy: key to quality nurturance. *Hospital Progress*, April 1970, p. 47-9, and 60.

DUNN, J. B.
Where the action is—RMP [Regional Medical Programs]. *Nursing Outlook*, Feb. 1969, p. 31-2.

ELLIS, GERALDINE L.
A patient-centered study guide in medical-surgical nursing. New York, Macmillan, 1962.

FIELO, SANDRA B., *and* EDGE, SYLVIA C.
Technical nursing of the adult: medical, surgical and psychiatric approaches. Macmillan, 1970.

FINCH, J.
Systems analysis: a logical approach to professional nursing care. *Nursing Forum*, vol. VIII, no. 2, 1969, p. 176-90.

FRANK, C. M.
Satisfactions in nursing practice. *Nursing Outlook*, May 1962, p. 302-4.

GOLDIN, P., *and* RUSSELL, B.
Therapeutic communication. *American Journal of Nursing*, Sept. 1969, p. 1928-30.

GOODLAND, N. L.
The male nurse in a general hospital. *Nursing Mirror*, Mar. 19, 1965, p. 577-8.

GORHAM, W. A.
Staff nursing behaviors contributing to patient care and improvement. *Nursing Research*, Spring 1962, p. 68-79.

GRAFFAM, S. R.
Nurse response to the patient in distress—development of an instrument. *Nursing Research*, July/Aug. 1970, p. 331-6.

GRIFFIN, G. S., *and others*
New Dimensions for the improvement of clinical nursing. *Nursing Research*, Fall 1966, p. 293-302.

HALSTEAD, HELEN H., *and others*
Contemporary studies in medical-surgical nursing. Philadelphia, Davis, 1967.

HART, G. S.
Success and shortcomings of modern nursing practice. *Nursing Mirror*, Dec. 1, 1961, p. 167.

HECTOR, WINIFRED
Modern nursing: theory and practice. 2nd edn. Heinemann 1962.
3rd edn., 1965.
4th edn., 1968.
5th edn., 1970.

NURSING AS A PROFESSION

HECTOR, WINIFRED
Practical techniques for nurses in training. British Broadcasting Corporation, 1970.
[Prepared for use in conjunction with a series of 10 BBC television programmes, Spring 1971].

HOLDSWORTH, VIVIAN E.
Fundamentals of bedside nursing. New York, Macmillan, 1968.

HOLMES, MARGUERITE C., *and* LEVINE, HARRIET, *editors*
Medical-surgical nursing: 1,500 multiple choice questions and referenced answers. 2nd edn. New York, Medical Examination Publishing Co., 1967.
[Nursing examination review book, vol. 1.]

HOUGHTON, MARJORIE, *and* PARNELL, J. E.
Practical procedures for nurses. Bailliere, Tindall and Cassell, 1969.
[Formerly entitled "Tray and trolley setting".]

HOUGHTON, MARJORIE, *and* WHITTOW, MARY
Aids to medical nursing. 6th edn. Bailliere, 1962.
[Originally published as "Aids to medical nursing" by Margaret Hitch.]
7th edn., 1967.

HOUGHTON, MARJORIE *and* WHITTOW, MARY
Aids to practical nursing. 10th edn. Bailliere, Tindall & Cox, 1965.

HULL, E. J., *and* ISAACS, B. J.
Do-it-yourself revision for nurses, vols. 1 & 2. Bailliere, 1970.

INGLES, T.
A concept of nursing practice. *International Nursing Review*, vol. 12, no. 2, 1966, p.7-12.

JACOX, A. K.
Who defines and controls nursing practice? *American Journal of Nursing*, May 1969, p. 977-82.

JENNY, M. R.
A development for nursing [Regional Medical Programs]. *Nursing Outlook*, Feb. 1969, p. 35-6.

JOEL, ALMA L., *and others*
Workbook and study guide for medical-surgical nursing: a patient-centered approach. 2nd edn. Saint Louis, C. V. Mosby, 1969.

JOHNSON, MAE M., *and others*
Problem-solving in nursing practice, by Mae M. Johnson, Mary Lou C. Davis and Mary Jo Bilitch. Iowa, Wm. C. Brown, 1970.

KEANE, CLAIRE BRACKMAN
Essentials of nursing, a medical-surgical text for practical nurses. Philadelphia, W. B. Saunders, 1964.
2nd edn., 1969.

KOCH, HARRIETT B., *and others*
Workbook and study guide for medical-surgical nursing: a patient-centered approach, by Harriett B. Koch, Barbara Puras, Mary Ann Pugh, Lois S. Carter, Alma L. Joel, Dorothy Savich and Marjorie Beyers. St. Louis, C. V. Mosby, 1965.

LAMBERTSEN. ELEANOR C.
How nursing rounds become professional. *Modern Hospital*, Feb. 1969, p. 128.

LAMBERTSEN, ELEANOR C.
Nurses have been trained to nurse people, not machines. (Modern Nursing Practice Department.) *Modern Hospital*, Oct. 1965, p. 144.

LEE, RUTH M.
Workbook for nursing in emotional and physical problems. New York, McGraw-Hill, 1967.

LEININGER, M.
The culture concept and its relevance to nursing. *The Journal of Nursing Education*, April 1967, p. 27-33 and 35-7.

LEONE, LUCILE P.
Attack on heart disease, cancer, and stroke; is nursing ready? *American Journal of Nursing*, May 1965, p. 68-72.

LEVINE, MYRA E.
The pursuit of wholeness. *American Journal of Nursing*, Jan. 1969, p. 93-8.

LONG, S. E.
Labour-saving methods in nursing. *Nursing Mirror*, Jan. 24, 1969, p. 22-3.

MCBRIDE, M. A., *and others*
Nurse-researcher: the crucial hyphen. *American Journal of Nursing*, June 1970, p. 1256-60.

MCCAIN, R. F.
Nursing by assessment—not intuition. *American Journal of Nursing*, April 1965, p. 82-4.

MCCUTCHEON, MAUREEN
Care of the patient with common medical-surgical disorders: a textbook for nurses. New York, McGraw-Hill, 1970.

MCLEAN, M. D.
Improvement of nursing practice. *The Canadian Nurse*, Oct. 1964, p. 955-60.

MANGAN, H. M.
Care, coordination and communication in the Life Island setting. *Nursing Outlook*, Jan. 1969, p. 40-4.

MANTHEY, M., *and others*
Primary nursing. *Nursing Forum*, vol. IX, no. 1, 1970, p. 65-83.

MANTHEY, M., *and* KRAMER, M.
A dialogue on primary nursing. *Nursing Forum*, vol. IX, no. 4, 1970, p. 356-79.

MARKHAM, JOAN
"To relieve sometimes . . ." *Nursing Times*, July 6, 1962, p. 858.

MARKHAM, JOAN
". . . to comfort always." *Nursing Times*, July 13, 1962, p. 894.

MATHENEY, RUTH V.
Technical nursing practice. New York, National League for Nursing, [1967].

MATHENEY, RUTH V.
The technical practice of nursing. *Pennsylvania Nurse*, Jan. 1970, p. 12-4.

MAUKSCH, H. O.
Organizational context of nursing practice.
In
DAVIS, FRED, *editor*
Nursing profession; five sociological essays. New York, Wiley, 1966, p. 109-37.

MILES, B.
Basic bedside nursing—still important. *Nursing Times*, May 19, 1967, p. 665-6.

MOORE, M. A.
The professional practice of nursing: the knowledge and how it is used. *Nursing Forum*, vol. VIII, no. 4, 1969, p. 361-73.

MUMFORD, EMILY, *and* SKIPPER, JAMES K.
Sociology in hospital care. New York, Harper & Row, 1967.

MURRAY, J. B.
Self-knowledge and the nursing interview. *Nursing Forum*, vol. II, no. 1, 1963, p. 69-78.

NATIONAL LEAGUE FOR NURSING. COMMITTEE ON QUALITY OF ORGANIZED NURSING SERVICE IN HOSPITAL
A self-evaluation guide for nursing services in hospitals and related institutions. New York, The League, 1967.

NATIONAL LEAGUE FOR NURSING.
DEPT. OF HOSPITAL NURSING
Blueprint for progress in hospital nursing. Proceedings of the 1962 regional conferences sponsored by the Department of Hospital Nursing and the Regional Councils of State Leagues for Nursing. New York, The League, 1963.

NEWLAND, R. A.
Goodbye to sheets and blankets? *Nursing Mirror*, Aug. 14, 1970, p. 22-4.

NORDMARK, MADELYN TITUS, *and* ROHWEDER, ANNE W.
Scientific foundations of nursing. 2nd edn. Pitman Medical Publishing Co., 1967.
[For previous edition, *see* Science principles applied to nursing, by the same authors.]

NORRIS, CATHERINE M., *editor*
Proceedings: second Nursing Theory Conference, University of Kansas Medical Center, Department of Nursing Education, October 9-10, 1969. Kansas, University of Kansas Medical Center, Department of Nursing Education, [1969].

NORRIS, CATHERINE M., *editor*
Proceedings: third Nursing Theory Conference, University of Kansas Medical Center, Department of Nursing Education, Jan. 29-30, 1970. Kansas, University of Kansas Medical Center, Department of Nursing Education, [1970].

NURSING MIRROR
Casebook for 1963. Iliffe Technical Publications (for *Nursing Mirror*), 1963.

NURSING TIMES
The art of the case study. Macmillan, 1962.

O'MALLEY, C. D.
Nursing in a space-age hospital. *American Journal of Nursing*, Dec. 1962, p. 54.

OSBORNE, O. H.
Anthropology and nursing: some common traditions and interests. *Nursing Research*, May-June 1969, p. 251-5.

OXFORD REGIONAL HOSPITAL BOARD.
OPERATIONAL RESEARCH UNIT
Chance or choice in nursing. Oxford, the Board, 1963.

PEARCE, EVELYN CLARE
A general textbook of nursing: a comprehensive guide to the final state examinations. 16th edn. Faber, 1963.
17th edn., 1967.

PRICE, ALICE L.
The art, science and spirit of nursing. 3rd edn. Philadelphia, Saunders, 1965.

PUGH, W. T. GORDON
Practical nursing, including hygiene and dietetics. 19th edn. Edinburgh, Blackwood, 1962.
20th edn., 1965.
21st edn., 1969.

RAINS, A. J. HARDING, *and others*
Urgencies and emergencies for nurses, by A. J. Harding Rains, Valerie Hunt and Margaret D. Mackenzie. English Universities Press, 1965.

RAMPHAL, M. M.
Values of routines in nursing. *Nursing Forum*, vol. VI, no. 3, 1967, p. 337-40.

RATNER, MURIEL
Study guide to medical and surgical nursing. 2nd edn. Philadelphia, Davis, 1961.

REVANS, R. W.
The adjustment of nurse and patient in hospital life. *Journal of Chronic Diseases*, vol. 15, 1962, p. 857-65.

ROPER, NANCY
Principles of nursing. Edinburgh, Livingstone, 1967.

ROSS, JANET S., *and* WILSON, KATHLEEN J. W.
Foundations of nursing. 3rd edn. Edinburgh, Livingstone, 1963.
4th edn. Foundations of nursing and first aid, 1965.

RUBIN, R.
Symposium on theory development in nursing. A theory of clinical nursing. *Nursing Research*, May/June 1968, p. 210-2.

ST. JOHN AMBULANCE ASSOCIATION *and others*
Nursing; the authorised manual of the St. John Ambulance Associations of the Order of St. John, the St. Andrew's Ambulance Association and the British Red Cross Society. 2nd edn. Publ. jointly by the Societies, 1964.
3rd edn., 1969.

SCHMAHL, J. Z.
Ritualism in nursing practice. *Nursing Forum*, vol. III, no. 4, 1964, p. 74-84.

SCHMIEDING, N. J.
Relationship of nursing to the process of chronicity. *Nursing Outlook*, Feb. 1970, p. 58-62.

SECOR, JANE
Patient studies in medical-surgical nursing. Philadelphia, Lippincott, 1967.

SELLEW, GLADYS, *and* FURFEY, PAUL HANLY
Sociology and its use in nursing service. 5th edn. Philadelphia, Saunders, 1962.
[Formerly entitled "Sociology and social problems in nursing service".]

SHAFER, KATHLEEN NEWTON, *and others*
Medical-surgical nursing. 2nd edn. St. Louis, Mosby, 1961.
3rd edn., 1964.
4th edn., 1967.

SKINNER, G.
What do practicing nurses want to know? *American Journal of Nursing*, Aug. 1969, p. 1662-3.

SMITH, S.
The psychology of illness. *Nursing Forum*, vol. III, no. 1, 1964, p. 35-47.

SMOYAK, S.
Cultural incongruence: the effect on nurses' perceptions. *Nursing Forum*, vol. VII, no. 3, 1968, p. 234-7.

SNELLMAN, V.
Nurses in the publishing business. *The American Journal of Nursing*, Aug. 1962, p. 90-1.

SOUTH WESTERN REGIONAL HOSPITAL BOARD
The green book: nursing procedures taught to pupil nurses at Notton House Training School, Lacock, Wiltshire. Bristol, the Board, 1966.

STOCKWELL, M. L., *and* NISHIKAWA, H. A.
The third hand: a theory of support. *Journal of Psychiatric Nursing and Mental Health Services*, May/June 1970, p. 7-10.

SUTTON, AUDREY LATSHAW
Bedside nursing techniques in medicine and surgery. Philadelphia, Saunders, 1964.
2nd edn., 1969.

THOMPSON, ELLA M., *and* MURPHY, CONSTANCE
Textbook of basic nursing. 8th edn. Philadelphia, Lippincott, 1966.
[Previous edns. called "Simplified nursing", by Florence Dakin, *et al.*]

TRAVELBEE, JOYCE
Interpersonal aspects of nursing. Philadelphia, Davis, 1966.

TURK, HERMAN, *and* INGLES, THELMA
Clinic nursing: explorations in role innovation. Philadelphia, Davis, 1963.

VLOK, MARIE E., *and* RYKHEER, GLOUDINA M.
Manual for general nurses: a comprehensive textbook for the South African general nurse. Johannesburg, Radford Adlington (printers), 1962.
3rd edn., 1969.

WALD, F. S., *and* LEONARD, R. C.
Towards development of nursing practice theory. *Nursing Research*, Fall 1964, p. 309-13.

WEISS, JAMES M. A., editor
Nurses, patients, and social systems: the effects of skilled nursing intervention upon institutionalized patients. Columbia, Miss., University of Missouri Press, 1968.

WEST, N. C.
A handbook for nurses: common medical and surgical conditions. English Universities Press, 1967.

WHITESIDE, J. E.
Medical nursing. Sydney, Angus and Robertson, 1970.

WIEDENBACH, ERNESTINE
Clinical nursing: a helping art. New York, Springer, 1964.

WILL, HILDA E.
Practice of nursing in a nursing home. *Journal of Practical Nursing*, Aug. 1970, p. 22-3, and 38-9.

WILLCOCK, H. D.
Nursing methods in a general hospital: a comparative study of two medical units in a general hospital, in each of which a different method of nursing was practised. An inquiry carried out by Government Social Survey for the Department of Health for Scotland, between September 1957, and January, 1958. Government Social Survey, 1961.

WINSOR, T.
Clinical thermography. *Nursing Mirror*, June 3, 1966, p. iv-v.

WOOLDRIDGE, POWHATAN, and others
Behavioral science, social practice and the nursing profession. Cleveland, Ohio, Western Reserve University, 1968.

ADMINISTRATION
General Works

AMERICAN HOSPITAL ASSOCIATION
The nursing department's function in hospital studies. *Practical Approaches to Nursing Service Administration*, Spring 1969, [p. 1-4].

AMERICAN HOSPITAL ASSOCIATION
Philosophy and objectives of the Department of Nursing. *Practical Approaches to Nursing Service Administration*, Summer 1970, p. [4].

ANDERSON, R. M.
Activity preferences and leadership behavior of head nurses: Part I. *Nursing Research*, Summer 1964, p. 239-43.

ANDERSON, R. M.
Activity preferences and leadership behavior of head nurses: Part 2. *Nursing Research*, Fall 1964, p. 333-7.

AYDELOTTE, MYRTLE K.
Issues of professional nursing: the need for clinical excellence. *Nursing Forum*, vol. VII, no. 1, 1968, p. 72-86.

BARABAS, MARY HELEN
Contemporary head nursing. New York, Macmillan, 1962.

BARRETT, JEAN
The head nurse. New York, Appleton-Century-Crofts, 1962.
2nd edn., 1968, entitled "The Head Nurse—her changing role."

BARRETT, JEAN
The head nurse's changing role. *Nursing Outlook*, Nov. 1963, p. 800-4.

BECKHARD, RICHARD
The professional nurse looks at the consultative process. Washington, Leadership Resources, 1966.
[Leadership in Nursing series, no. 10.]

BENDALL, E. R. D.
The position of the staff nurse. *Nursing Times*, May 3, 1963, p. 561-2.

BENNETT, THOMAS R.
The professional nurse looks at planning for change. Washington, Leadership Resources, 1966.
[Leadership in Nursing series, no. 6.]

BHATTACHARYA, A.
Functional leadership in nursing. *Nursing Times*, Aug. 6, 1970, p. 1001-3; Aug. 13, 1970, p. 1033-4.

BLACK, M.
The changing role of the nurse. *Nursing Times*, Jan. 19, 1968, Occasional papers, p. 12.

BOORER, D.
The road to the top. Administrative opportunities for men. *Nursing Times*, Mar. 12, 1965, p. 357-60.

BRODT, DAGMAR E.
Service manager, innovation for nursing and health organization. *Hospital Progress*, Sept. 1966, p. 69-70 & 74.

BROWN, DAVID S.
The professional nurse looks at decision making. Washington, Leadership Resources, 1966.
[Leadership in Nursing series, no. 4.]

BROWN, DAVID S.
The professional nurse looks at authority and hierarchy. Washington, Leadership Resources, 1966.
[Leadership in Nursing series, no. 8.]

BROWN, E. L.
Preparation for nursing. *American Journal of Nursing*, September 1965, p. 70-3.

BRUNEL UNIVERSITY HOSPITAL ORGANIZATION. RESEARCH UNIT
Ward housekeeping—1. Sapiential authority and secondment: the organization of housekeeping staff in the ward. 2. The ward housekeeper: a proposal based on organizational analysis. *Nursing Times*, Dec. 4, 1969, Occasional Papers, p. 201-3; Dec. 11, 1969, Occasional papers, p. 205-7.

BUCHANAN, PAUL C.
The professional nurse looks at individual motivation. Washington, Leadership Resources, 1966.
[Leadership in Nursing series, no. 5.]

CALENDER, TINY M.
Unit administration. New York, Saunders, 1962.

CAMPBELL, E. B.
The process of change. *American Journal of Nursing*, May 1967, p. 991-4.

CAMPBELL, M., and BARKER, B. L.
Nursing: management education. *Hospitals*, Dec. 1, 1970, p. 100, 102, and 104.

CHRISTMAN, L. B.
Nursing and leadership. Style and substance. *American Journal of Nursing*, Oct. 1967, p. 2091-3.

CHRISTMAN, L. B.
The role of systems engineering in meeting the nursing challenge. *International Nursing Review*, vol. 17, no. 4, 1970, p. 320-5.

CHRISTMAN, L. B.
The role of nursing in organizational effectiveness. *International Nursing Review*, vol. 16, no. 3, 1969, p. 248-55.

CLARK, M. A., and JONES, M.
Social psychiatry and the senior nurse. *Nursing Mirror*, April 9, 1965, p. 45-7; April 16, 1965, p. 64-6.

COOPER, R.
Aspects of effective leadership. *Nursing Mirror*, Mar. 11, 1966, p. xiii-xvi.

CRAWFORD, M .P.
Role-confusion among matrons and tutors. *International Journal of Nursing Studies*, Dec. 1966, p. 161-7.

CRICHTON, ANNE, and CRAWFORD, MARION P.
"The legacy of Nightingale"? A consideration of some of the problems of nursing staff in Welsh hospitals today. [Cardiff], Welsh Hospital Board, 1966.

DAVIDSON, LOUISE COLIN
Students' perception of leadership in nursing care. *Nursing Outlook*, Dec. 1968, p. 30-1.

DELLER, H. J., *and others*
Who wants to be a manager? *Nursing Times*, Jan. 9, 1969, Occasional Papers, p. 5-8.

DE MONTFORT, SR. M.
Aspects of management in nursing. *New Zealand Nursing Journal*, July 1969, p. 20-1.

DESMOND, Sr. M.
Personnel function in the hospital: viewpoint of a nursing director. *Canadian Hospital*, June 1970, p. 35-9.

DIETRICH, B. J., *and* MILLER, D. I.
Nursing leadership—a theoretical framework. *Nursing Outlook*, Aug. 1966, p. 52-5.

DUGAN, A. B.
Problems in leader initiated change studies. *Journal of Psychiatric Nursing and Mental Health Services*, May/June 1970, p. 17-20.

DUNN, H.
Facing realities in nursing administration today. *American Journal of Nursing*, May 1968, p. 1013-8.

EDWARDS, M. M.
Committees. 1. General. *Nursing Times*, June 7, 1963, p. 713-4.

EDWARDS, M. M.
Committees. 2. Nurse education committees. *Nursing Times*, June 14, 1963, p. 749-51.

EDWARDS, M. M.
Committees. 3. Members, secretary, chairman. *Nursing Times*, June 21, 1963, p. 780-2.

EXCHAQUET, N. F.
The role of the head nurse in the management of the ward. *International Nursing Review*, vol. 14, no. 5, 1967, p. 29-37.

FERNANDEZ, C. G.
Ward administration in Singapore. *Berita Jururawat*, April 1967, p. 17-20.

FITZGIBBON, M.
A changing night administration. *Nursing Times*, Oct. 29, 1970, Occasional Papers, p. 161-3.

FOSTER, V. L.
The night nurse is very special. *Nursing Outlook*, Dec. 1961, p. 765-6.

FREEMAN, R. B.
Organization for a purpose in an organization with a purpose. *Nursing Outlook*, Aug. 1966, p. 35-7.

GEITGEY, DORIS A.
A handbook for head nurses. Philadelphia, Davis, 1961.

GEORGIA INSTITUTE OF TECHNOLOGY. SCHOOL OF INDUSTRIAL ENGINEERING *and* MEDICAL COLLEGE OF GEORGIA
An objective basis for in-patient nursing unit design: an interim research report by [John R. Freeman and Harold E. Smalley]. Atlanta, Georgia, The Authors, 1968.
[Program in hospital and medical systems. Program bulletin no. 2.]

GERMAIN, L. D.
Needed: changes in hospitals to utilize the new practitioner in nursing. *Journal of Nursing Education*, Aug. 1969, p. 25-9.

GERMAINE, A.
Are we facing professional suicide? [can nursing cope with change?] *Hospital Administration in Canada*, Feb. 1969, p. 54-5.

GERMAINE, A.
Hospital design has dramatic effect on nursing efficiency. *Hospital Administration in Canada*, July 1970, p. 64-5.

GODDARD, H. A.
Joint consultation. *Nursing Mirror*, Mar. 1, 1968, p. 43-4.

GODDARD, H. A.
The art of interviewing—1 *and* 2. *Nursing Mirror*, Feb. 16, 1968, p. 45-50; Feb. 23, 1968, p. 39-40.

GODDARD, H. A.
Personnel management. *Nursing Mirror*, Feb. 2, 1968, p. 18 and 31.

GODDARD, H. A.
Personnel policy. *Nursing Mirror*, Feb. 9, 1968, p. 45-7.

GOURLAY, D.
Middle management for nurses. [School of Business Management Studies, Robert Gordon's Institute of Technology, Aberdeen]. *British Hospital Journal and Social Service Review*, Apr. 24, 1970, p. 759.

GRANT, J. V.
Women in management. *Nursing Times*, Aug. 4, 1967, p. 1036-7.

GREAT BRITAIN. DEPARTMENT OF HEALTH AND SOCIAL SECURITY. NATIONAL NURSING STAFF COMMITTEE
A report... on management development of senior nursing staff in the hospital service. [The Department], 1968.

GREAT BRITAIN MINISTRY OF HEALTH *and* SCOTTISH HOME AND HEALTH DEPARTMENT
Report of the committee on senior nursing staff structure. H.M.S.O., 1966.
[*Chairman:* Brian Salmon.]

ALLGOOD, J.
Salmon in a psychiatric hospital group. 3. A ward sister's view of the Salmon structure. *Nursing Mirror*, Nov. 13, 1970, p. 32-3.

ASSOCIATION OF HOSPITAL MATRONS
Assessment of the Salmon Committee Report. Report of a meeting of the Association of Hospital Matrons held at Skegness, May 1966. *Nursing Times*, May 27, 1966, p. 721-2.

ASSOCIATION OF HOSPITAL MATRONS
A further assessment of the Salmon Report. Report of Annual General Meeting of the Association of Hospital Matrons. *Nursing Mirror*, Nov. 11, 1966, p. 134.

BENDALL, EVE
The Salmon Report—A Tutor's View. *Nursing Times*, May 27, 1966, p. 718-9.

BRITISH HOSPITAL JOURNAL AND SOCIAL SERVICE REVIEW
Salmon Report. *British Hospital Journal and Social Service Review*, May 13, 1966, p. 853-855.

BROMLEY, R.
Implementing a Salmon Pilot Scheme. *Nursing Times*, May 31, 1968, p. 87-8.

CHISHOLM, M. K.
A public health look at the Salmon Report. *Nursing Mirror*, Dec. 15, 1967, p. xiii and xvi.

COLLINS, SHEILA M.
Implications for the Rcn and the education of nurses. *Nursing Times*, June 17, 1966, p. 816-7.

CONFEDERATION OF HEALTH SERVICE EMPLOYEES
Comments on the report of the Salmon Committee. *Health Services Journal*, Oct. 1966, p. 2-3.

DODWELL, B. I. R.
Senior nursing staff structure. *British Hospital Journal and Social Service Review*, Oct. 17, 1969, p. 1942-3.

FRANKS, G. L.
A nursing officer's view of Salmon. *British Hospital Journal and Social Service Review*, July 17, 1970, p. 1391-2.

FRANKS, G. L.
Salmon in a psychiatric hospital group. 1. The Salmon Unit. *Nursing Mirror*, Oct. 30, 1970, p. 23-5.

FRIEND, PHYLLIS M.
A matron looks at Salmon. *Nursing Times*, Sept. 23, 1966, p. 1269-70.

GENERAL NURSING COUNCIL FOR ENGLAND AND WALES
Comments on senior nursing staff structure (Salmon Report). *Nursing Times*, April 7, 1967, p. 459-61.

GETTINGS, B.
Implementing Salmon in Berkshire. *Nursing Mirror*, Nov. 7, 1969, p. 23-5.

GREAT BRITAIN. DEPARTMENT OF HEALTH AND SOCIAL SECURITY
National Health Service: appointment of senior nursing staff: an introduction to Salmon management structures. (H.M. 69, 33). Dept. of Health, April, 1969.

GREAT BRITAIN. DEPARTMENT OF HEALTH AND SOCIAL SECURITY NATIONAL NURSING STAFF COMMITTEE
National Health Service: an interim report ... on assimilation of existing staff introduction of Salmon management structures. Dept. of Health, Dec. 1968.

GREAT BRITAIN. DEPARTMENT OF HEALTH AND SOCIAL SECURITY *and* WELSH OFFICE
The senior nursing organization in hospitals: an introduction to the report of the Salmon Committee. Dept. of Health, 1969.

GREAT BRITAIN. MINISTRY OF HEALTH
The Salmon Teaching Division: three viewpoints. GNC's views, by Barbara Fawkes; Rcn's views, by Christine Brown; DOHSS's views, by Sheila A. G. Garrett; An RHB Pilot, by Ethel Hodgkinson; A Teaching Hospital Pilot, by Betty Hoare. *Nursing Times*, Feb. 27, 1969, p. 269-78.

GROVES, M. D.
Salmon in a psychiatric hospital group. 6. The group Secretary's view of Salmon and the future. *Nursing Mirror*, Dec. 25, 1970, p. 34-5.

HAMILTON, D.
Salmon versus Tutors. *Nursing Times*, Feb. 26, 1970, p. 268-70.

HARDY, G. F. R.
Salmon as seen by a treasurer. *The Hospital*, Dec. 1969, p. 414-6.

HAYWOOD, S. C., *and others*
What do nurses think of the Salmon report? *Nursing Times*, May 14, 1970, Occasional papers, p. 65-6.

HILL, S. G.
Comment [on Salmon Committee Report]. A group secretary's views. *Nursing Times*, July 15, 1966, p. 931-2.

THE HOSPITAL
Nursing administration reshaped. *The Hospital*, June 1966, p. 253-6.

HOSPITAL MANAGEMENT PLANNING AND EQUIPMENT
Comment [on Salmon Committee Report]. Management, matrons and make-believe. *Hospital Management Planning and Equipment*, June 1966, p. 353.

INSTITUTE OF HOSPITAL ADMINISTRATORS
The Salmon Report. Comments of the Institute of Hospital Administrators. *The Hospital*, Dec. 1966, p. 589-91.

LANCET
The nursing hierarchy: the Salmon Committee Report. *The Lancet*, May 14, 1966, p. 1085-6.

LLOYD, W. A.
Salmon—and the problems of administration. *Nursing Times*, Mar. 10, 1967, p. 313.

LLOYD, W. A.
Salmon in a psychiatric hospital group. 5. The chief nursing officer's view of the Salmon Structure. *Nursing Mirror*, Dec. 18, 1970, p. 36-7, and 39.

LOCKE, J. T.
The Salmon Report. *International Journal of Nursing Studies*, May 1967, p. 105-10.

MACHIN, DOROTHY
More thoughts about Salmon. *Nursing Times*, Dec. 16, 1966, p. 1669-70.

MIDWIVES CHRONICLE AND NURSING NOTES
The Salmon Report. *Midwives Chronicle and Nursing Notes*, July 1966, p. 256-7.

MIDWIVES CHRONICLE AND NURSING NOTES
Salmon and the midwives. *Midwives Chronicle and Nursing Notes*, June 1969, p. 191-2.

MILLWARD, R. C.
Salmon structure in relation to administrative organization. *Hospital*, Jan. 1969, p. 7-9.

MOSS, H. J. L.
The Salmon Report. Comment. *District Nursing*, Aug. 1966, p. 124.

NATIONAL ASSOCIATION OF HOSPITAL MANAGEMENT COMMITTEE GROUP SECRETARIES
Comments on the report of the committee on senior nursing staff structure—the Salmon Report. The Association, 1966.

NURSE TEACHERS' ASSOCIATION
Comments on the report of the committee on senior nursing staff structure 1966. Epsom, The Association, 1966.

NURSE TEACHERS' ASSOCIATION
Nurse education in the context of Salmon. Report of a conference held by the Nurse Teachers' Association at Wakefield, in September 1967. *Nursing Times*, Oct. 20, 1967, p. 1417.

NURSING MIRROR
Salmon Committee Report on senior nursing staff structure. *Nursing Mirror*, May 13, 1966, p. 145-8.

NURSING MIRROR
Salmon Committee report on senior nursing staff structure. *Nursing Mirror*, May 27, 1966, p. 185-8.

NURSING MIRROR
Implications of the Salmon Report. Open Forum Session at the 51st Nursing Mirror Conference. *Nursing Mirror*, Feb. 24, 1967, p. 483-7 and 492.

NURSING TIMES
Structure according to Salmon. *Nursing Times*, May 13, 1966, p. i-viii.

NURSING TIMES
Junior view of Salmon. Comments by students and pupil nurses. *Nursing Times*, Sept. 9, 1966, p. 1188-9.

PEERS, R. E.
The King's Fund and Salmon. *Nursing Times*, Aug. 19, 1966, p. 1089.

REVANS, R. W.
The Salmon Report. No longer the clinical long-stop. *Nursing Times*, June 24, 1966, p. 855.

RICHARDSON, B.
Salmon in a psychiatric hospital group. 4. The Salmon unit in subnormality. *Nursing Mirror*, Dec. 11, 1970, p. 23-4.

ROYAL COLLEGE OF NURSING *and*
NATIONAL COUNCIL OF NURSES OF THE UNITED KINGDOM
Comment on Salmon. The College, 1966.

ROYAL COLLEGE OF NURSING *and*
NATIONAL COUNCIL OF NURSES OF THE UNITED KINGDOM
Report of Rcn Conference on the Salmon Report, held at Church House, London, September 1966. *Nursing Mirror*, Oct. 7, 1969, p. 5-9.

ROYAL COLLEGE OF NURSING *and*
NATIONAL COUNCIL OF THE UNITED KINGDOM
N. IRELAND BOARD
Salmon Conference. Rcn Northern Ireland Board. *Nursing Times*, Mar. 24, 1967, p. 397.

ROYAL COLLEGE OF NURSING *and*
NATIONAL COUNCIL OF NURSES OF THE UNITED KINGDOM
SCOTTISH BOARD
The Salmon Report debated in Edinburgh . . . Report of Rcn Scottish Conference held 15th October 1966 in Edinburgh. *Nursing Times*, Oct. 28, 1966, p. 1417-8.

ROYAL COLLEGE OF NURSING *and*
NATIONAL COUNCIL OF NURSES OF THE UNITED KINGDOM
WELSH BOARD
Welsh thinking on Salmon. Report of Rcn Welsh Board Conference held in Cardiff on 24th September 1966. *Nursing Times*, Sept. 30, 1966, p. 1298-9.

TAYLOR, D.
Salmon in a psychiatric hospital group. 2. From assistant matron to nursing unit officers. *Nursing Mirror*, Nov. 6, 1970, p. 23.

WEBSTER, LIAM
A critical look at Salmon. 1. Salmon and the Ward Sister/Staff Nurse. 2. Is Salmon for nurse tutors. 3. Salmon and the managers. *Nursing Times*, Aug. 4, 1967, p. 1039; Aug. 11, 1967, p. 1079; Aug. 18, 1967, p. 1105.

WHITEHEAD, J.
Salmon: its objectives and achievements as seen from the centre. *Nursing Times*, Dec. 17, 1970, p. 1626-7 and 1632.

WLOCH, N.
Salmon in the Isle of Wight. *Nursing Times*, Oct. 9, 1969, Occasional Papers, p. 161-4.

GREEN, M. D.
First-line management. *Nursing Times*, Feb. 3, 1967, p. 150-1.

GRUN, J.
Management training for nurses. *Nursing Times*, April 19, 1968, Occasional papers, p. 64.

HAGEN, ELIZABETH, *and* WOLFF, LUVERNE
Nursing leadership behavior in general hospitals. New York, Columbia University, 1961.

HALL, M. F.
Social science and decision making. *Nursing Mirror*, May 17, 1968, p. 35-7.

HALL, O.
Problems affecting the nurse's status. *The Canadian Nurse*, July 1964, p. 655-62.

HAMIL, E. M.
The changing director of nurses. *Nursing Outlook*, Dec. 1969, p. 64-5.

HANHAM, H. J.
The nurse and social administration. *Nursing Mirror*, Sept. 3, 1965, p. 553-5.

HARDMAN, ELIZABETH
An introduction to ward management. Oxford, Blackwell, 1970.

HAUGLAND, B.
Preparing the nurse for the leadership role. *Jamaican Nurse*, Dec. 1968, p. 14-5.

HAYWOOD, S., *and* TURNER, F. W.
A first-line management course. *Nursing Times*, Aug. 4, 1967, p. 1038-9.

HENDERSON, CYNTHIA
Freeing the nurse to nurse. *American Journal of Nursing*, Mar. 1964, p. 72-7.

HENDERSON, J. E.
Unit manager system helps to redefine role of head nurse. *Hospital Administration in Canada*, June 1970, p. 52-7.

HILL, MURIEL
Regional nursing officers. *International Journal of Nursing Studies*, May 1964, pp. 93-7.

HOSPITAL ADMINISTRATION IN CANADA
Blind spots in nursing leadership. *Hospital Administration in Canada*, Sept. 1963, p. 4.

HUGHES, D. M.
Management training in nursing 1. *Nursing Times*, Aug. 13, 1965, p. 1120.

HUGHES, D. M.
Management training in nursing 2. *Nursing Times*, Aug. 20, 1965, p. 1149-50.

HYDE, L.
A philosophy of change in reorganization. *Nursing Outlook*, Aug. 1966, p. 38-9.

INGRAM, J. T.
Journey among women. (1) Leadership in nursing. (2) Responsibility at the top. *Nursing Times*, May 28, 1970, Occasional Papers, p. 73-6; June 4, 1970, Occasional Papers, p. 79-80.

IRVINE, M.
Principles of management applied to nursing services, 1 *and* 2. *Nursing Times*, June 19, 1969, Occasional Papers, p. 97-100; June 26, 1969, Occasional Papers, p. 101-4.

ISHIYAMA, T., *and others*
Resolving a nursing leadership crisis. *American Journal of Nursing*, Mar. 1965, p. 106-8.

JOHNSON, D. E.
Today's action will determine tomorrow's nursing. *Nursing Outlook*, Sept. 1965, p. 38-41.

KELBER, M.
Communication or conflict. Paper given at the 13th Quadrennial Congress of the International Council of Nurses held at Frankfurt, 1965. *Australian Nurses' Journal*, July 1965, p. 159-65.

KEMBLE, E. L.
The Dean—born or made? *Nursing Outlook*, Oct. 1963, p. 737-40.

KILLAM, L.
The nursing director as group facilitator. *American Journal of Nursing*, Aug. 1970, p. 1686-90.

KING EDWARD'S HOSPITAL FUND FOR LONDON
The King's Fund and its part in management training for nurses. *Nursing Times*, Oct. 13, 1967, p. 1360.

KNOWLES, MALCOLM S.
The professional nurse looks at self-development. Washington, Leadership Resources, 1966. [Leadership in Nursing series, no. 11.]

KRIEGEL, JULIA
The head nurse: thoughts and decisions. New York, Macmillan, 1968.

KUCHA, D. H.
The human relations approach to nursing administration. *Nursing Forum*, vol. IX, no. 2, 1970, p. 162-8.

LAMB, M.
The role of the nurse in the future. *Jamaican Nurse*, Sept. 1968, p. 16-7 and 40.

LAMBERTSEN, ELEANOR C.
Expertness in administration is essential for director of nursing. *Modern Hospital*, April 1964, p. 136.

LAMBERTSEN, ELEANOR C.
The implications of new techniques in ward management as they affect nursing. *International Nursing Review*, vol. 16, no. 1, 1969, p. 4-13.

NURSING AS A PROFESSION

LAMBERTSEN, ELEANOR C.
We're not using the nurses we have to best advantage. *Modern Hospital*, May 1968, p. 146.

LAMBERTSEN, ELEANOR C.
Why can't nurses manage to manage? *The Modern Hospital*, July 1962, p. 85.

LAMBERTSEN, ELEANOR C.
Why head nurse often favors doctor over administrator. *The Modern Hospital*, April 1968, p. 134.

LARSON, L. G.
The role of the nurse in regional medical programs. *Cardio-Vascular Nursing*, May/June 1969, p. 9-14.

LEMIN, B.
Middle management course. *Nursing Times*, June 4, 1970, Occasional Papers, p. 77-8.

LEMIN, B.
An introduction to management and its principles—I. *District Nursing*, Sept. 1970, p. 112-3.

LEMIN, B.
An introduction to management and its principles—II. *District Nursing*, Oct. 1970, p. 137-8.

LETOURNEAU, C. U.
Unit managers—one solution to the nursing shortage. *Hospital Management*, Dec. 1967, p. 31-2.

LINSKY, A. S.
Why evaluate work conferences? *Nursing Outlook*, Sept. 1963, p. 656-9.

LINVILLE, C. H., and HUDSON, W. R.
We taught our nurses how to become managers. *The Modern Hospital*, April 1963, p. 96-7, 150 and 152.

LIPPITT, GORDON L., and SEASHORE, EDITH
The professional nurse looks at group effectiveness. Washington, Leadership Resources, 1966. [Leadership in Nursing series, no. 2.]

LITTLE, DOLORES E., and CARNEVALI, DORIS L.
Nursing care planning. Philadelphia, Lippincott, 1969.

LUCK, G. M.
The sister's role in ward management. *Nursing Times*, Dec. 6, 1968, p. 1654-6.

MCLAUGHLIN, H.
What shape is best for nursing units. *The Modern Hospital*, Dec. 1964, p. 84-9.

MCLEMORE, S. DALE, and HILL, RICHARD J.
Management-training effectiveness: a study of nurse managers. Austin, University of Texas, Bureau of Business Research, 1965.

MCNAIR, E.
The influence of ward organization on patient care and nursing education. *UNA Nursing Journal*, May 1966, p. 123-4.

MCNICHOLAS, E. L.
International nurse-practitioner committees. *International Nursing Review*, vol. 16, no. 3, 1969, p. 279-85.

MACHEN, W. V.
Nursing rounds—their purpose and value. *Nursing Outlook*, Oct. 1969, p. 52-4.

MACHEY, D.
Management, training and nurses: cause for concern? *Nursing Times*, Sept. 17, 1970, p. 1206-7.

MALASPINA, H.
How to evaluate nurses' work. *The Modern Hospital*, Aug. 1961, p. 70.

MARCHESINI, E. H.
From head nurse to supervisor. *Nursing Outlook*, June 1963, p. 421-4.

MARLOW, H. L.
Registered nurse and employee needs. *Nursing Outlook*, Nov. 1966, p. 62-5.

MARY DONALD, SR., and MARY SUZANNE, SR.
Nursing? Administration? or Both?... This is The Head Nurse's dilemma. *Hospital Progress*, April 1965, p. 76-9.

MATHEW, G.
What causes frustration among nurses. Need for socio-psychological study. *The Nursing Journal of India*, Oct. 1968, p. 321-2.

MAUKSCH, H. O.
Organizational context of nursing practice.
In
DAVIS, FRED, *editor*
Nursing profession; five sociological essays. New York, Wiley 1966 p. 109-37.

MEILICKE, C. A.
Administration and the changing role of the nurse. *The Canadian Nurse*, Nov. 1961, p. 1051-5.

MEYER, G. R., and HOFFMAN, M. J.
Nurses' inner values and their behavior at work. *Nursing Research*, Summer 1964, p. 244-9.

MICHAELSON, M.
Ward clerks at St. Joseph's [General Hospital, Port Arthur, Ontario] free head nurse of 50% clerical burden. *Hospital Administration in Canada*, June 1967, p. 34-6.

MOOTH, ADELMA E., and RITVO, MIRIAM M.
Developing the supervisory skills of the nurse: a behavioral science approach. Collier-Macmillan, 1966.

MUSSALLEM, H. K.
The changing role of the nurse. *Canadian Nurse*, Nov. 1968, p. 35-7; *American Journal of Nursing*, Mar. 1969, p. 514-7.

NORRIS, C. M.
Administration for creative nursing. *Nursing Forum*, Summer 1962, p. 88-105.

NORTH-EASTERN REGIONAL HOSPITAL BOARD
WORK STUDY DEPARTMENT
Nurses' work in hospitals in the North-Eastern region: report of a research project. ... Edinburgh, Scottish Home and Health Department, 1967. [Scottish Health Service Studies, 3.]

NURSING CLINICS OF NORTH AMERICA
Symposium on administration on the patients' behalf. *Nursing Clinics of North America*, June 1970, p. 277-357.

NURSING MIRROR
Training for leadership. Report of refresher course arranged by Gloucester City and County, April 1966. *Nursing Mirror*, April 29, 1966, p. 97-8.

NURSING OUTLOOK
An internship for leadership in nursing—a symposium. A combined education-service program, by V. M. Ross. Education—the primary purpose, by C. E. Bradshaw. Benefits to nursing service, by B. A. Gentry. An intern's experience, by B. Leventhal. *Nursing Outlook*, Feb. 1966, p. 40-5.

O'MALLEY, C. D.
Application of systems engineering in nursing. *American Journal of Nursing*, Oct. 1969, p. 2155-60.

ORBELL, A.
Nursing to-day and to-morrow. *The New Zealand Nursing Journal*, Aug. 1964, p. 15-6.

PALMER, H.
Nurses for nursing. *Canadian Nurse*, May 1969, p. 36-9.

PANTALL, J., and COND, R.
Nursing managers—what should they read? *Nursing Times*, Aug. 6, 1970, Occasional Papers, p. 113-6; Aug. 13 1970, Occasional Papers, p. 117-8.

PELLEGRINO, E. D.
The changing role of the professional nurse in the hospital. *Hospitals*, Dec. 16, 1961, p. 56, 59-60 and 62.

PERRY, ELLEN L.
Ward administration and teaching: the work of the ward sister. Bailliere, Tindall & Cassell, 1968.

PETERSON, G. C.
Do nursing administrators need advanced clinical preparation? *American Journal of Nursing*, Feb. 1970, p. 297-303.

PICTON, L. V.
Management responsibility. *South African Nursing Journal*, Aug. 1967, p. 17-20.

PLESSIS, D. J. DU
Nursing in this scientific age. An address given at the Third Biennial Conference of the South African Nursing Association. *South African Nursing Journal*, Nov. 1962, p. 35.

POWELL, M. B.
The image of the matron. *Nursing Times*, May 17, 1963, p. 617-8.

RAMOS, PAZ GOMEZ, *and others*
A study of graduates of vocational nursing programs in California: conducted by Paz Gomez Ramos, reported by Jeanne M. Tague, project director, Melvin L. Barlow. Los Angeles, University of California, 1961.
[Sponsored by the Bureau of Industrial Education, California State Department of Education.]

REDMAN, P.
The nurse as manager. *Nursing Times*, Mar. 8, 1968, p. 330-1.

REED, D. A.
Relieving the nursing shortage . . . what administration can do. *Hospital Progress*, April 1966, p. 96-100.

REVANS, R. W.
The measurement of supervisory attitudes. Manchester Statistical Society, 1961.

RIMMER, T.
Ward management. Report from the I.H.F. Congress, Chicago, 1967. *British Hospital Journal and Social Service Review*, Oct. 6, 1967, p. 1877-81.

ROSEN, A., *and* ABRAHAM, G. E.
Attitudes of nurses toward a performance appraisal system. *Nursing Research*, Fall 1966, p. 317-22.

ROSS, C. F., *and* HAIDUCK, A.
Seminars improve rapport between Registered Nurses and Licensed Practical Nurses. *Hospitals*, Nov. 1964, p. 64 and 68.

ROYAL COLLEGE OF NURSING *and*
NATIONAL COUNCIL OF NURSES OF THE UNITED KINGDOM
Plans for the health and welfare services. Report of conference, December 1963. *Nursing Times*, Dec. 13, 1963, p. 1567-8.

RUDGE, P. F.
The executive role of the ward sister. *The Australian Nurses' Journal*, Oct. 1967, p. 197-8.

RUTHERFORD, R.
What bothers staff nurses. *American Journal of Nursing*, Feb. 1967, p. 315-8.

RUTHERFORD, W. L.
Can evening and night nursing supervisors meet their administrative demands? *Hospital Topics*, Nov. 1963, p. 33-5.

SCHMIDT, WARREN H.
The administrative nurse looks at her leadership responsibilities. Washington, Leadership Resources, 1966.
[Leadership in Nursing series, no. 1.]

SCHURR MARGARET C.
Management training or education for leadership? *Nursing Times*, Mar. 8, 1968, p. 314-5.

SCHURR MARGARET C.
Leadership and the nurse: an introduction to the principles of management. English Universities Press, 1968.

SCHURR, MARGARET C.
A comparative study of leadership in industry and the nursing profession. *International Nursing Review*, vol. 16, no. 1, 1969, p. 16-29; vol. 16, no. 2, 1969, p. 115-30.

SCHWIER, M. E., *and* GARDELLA, F. A.
Planning, orienting and preparing for a new kind of nurse leadership. *Nursing Outlook*, May 1970, p. 42-6.

SCOTTISH HOME AND HEALTH DEPARTMENT
SCOTTISH NURSING STAFFS COMMITTEE
Selection and appointments procedures assessment reporting system. Edinburgh, The Department, 1970.
Scottish Hospital Memorandum no. 69/1970.

SEARLE, CHARLOTTE
The place of the nurse in building a healthy nation. *South African Nursing Journal*, Nov. 1968, p. 14-7, and 13.

SEWARD, J. F.
Professional practice in a bureaucratic structure. *Nursing Outlook*, Dec. 1969, p. 58-61.

SEYFFER, C.
The social sciences and nursing. Tomorrow's nurse in a changing world. *International Nursing Review*, vol. 12, no. 4, 1965, p. 66-72.

SHEAFOR, M. M.
The case method at work: graduate students in nursing administration must learn group dynamics. *Nursing Outlook*, Sept. 1970, p. 40-1.

SJOBERG, K.
Unit assignment—a new concept. *The Canadian Nurse*, July 1969, p. 29-31.

SKERRY, W. J.
The function of the nurse in the hospital of the future. *AORN Journal*, July 1969, p. 45-9.

SLACK, M.
The art of interviewing—1. *Nursing Times*, Jan. 21, 1966, p. 83-4.

SLACK, M.
The art of interviewing—2. Assessment of casework from the student's angle. *Nursing Times*, Jan. 28, 1966, p. 117-8.

SLACK, M.
The art of interviewing—3. Evaluation of casework from the supervisor's angle. *Nursing Times*, Feb. 4, 1966, p. 157-8.

SMITH, C. A.
Job satisfaction in hospital nursing. *The Canadian Nurse*, Feb. 1963, p. 147-55.

STINSON, S. M.
The future begins now for nursing in the year 2000. *Hospital Administration in Canada*, Sept. 1968, p. 86-91.

TAYLOR, CAROLE
How unit manager system works for us. *The Modern Hospital*, Aug. 1962, p. 69.

TAYLOR, CAROLE
In horizontal orbit: hospitals and the cult of efficiency. New York, Rinehart and Winston, 1970.

THOMAS, L. A.
Action for change. A rationale for nursing administration. *American Journal of Nursing*, April 1969, p. 774-6.

TORONTO GENERAL HOSPITAL
Orientation directs the new nurse. *Hospital Administration in Canada*, Nov. 1962, p. 24-7.

TORRIE, P. J.
The nature of management. *Nursing Times*, April 19, 1968, Occasional papers, p. 61-3.

NURSING AS A PROFESSION

UNITED STATES SURGEON-GENERAL
Action for critical nursing problems proposed. A digest of the complete report of the Consultant Group on Nursing. *American Journal of Nursing*, Mar. 1963, p. 69-74.

WATKIN, B.
Nurses and hospital management. *Nursing Mirror*, Sept. 2, 1966, p. 527-9.

WESCHLER, IRVING R.
The professional nurse looks at creativity. Washington, Leadership Resources, 1966.
[Leadership Resources Series, no. 9.]

WHITE, R.
Delegation and control. *Nursing Mirror*, May 31, 1968, p. 19-21.

WHITE, R.
Principles of management. *Nursing Mirror*, May 9, 1969, p. 48-50.

WIENS, A. N., *and others*
Interview interaction behavior of supervisors, head nurses and staff nurses. *Nursing Research*, Fall, 1965, p. 322-9.

WILLIAMS, DEREK
Administrative contribution of the nursing sister. Royal Institute of Public Administration, 1969.

WILLIAMS, DEREK, *and* MESSAGE, M. C.
Management courses for senior nursing staff. *International Nursing Review*, vol. 16, no. 4, 1969, p. 329-37.

WRIGHT, M. SCOTT
Implementation of change in nursing. *Nursing Times*, Feb. 13, 1969, Occasional Papers, p. 25-7.

YOUNG, L. S.
The modern nurse administrator. *Journal of Nursing Education*, Aug. 1969, p. 13-7 and 20-4.

Automation

ALEXANDER, FLORENCE M., *and* ZIX, LORRAINE G.
Streamlining nurses' reports: tape recordings. *Hospitals*, Jan. 1, 1963, p. 48-9.

BAILEY, A.
Electronics in nursing. *Nursing Mirror*, April 2, 1965, p. i-iii.

BANKS, ALICE W., *and others*
Tape-recorded nurses' notes. *Nursing Outlook*, Oct. 1966, p. 42-4.

BARTEL, G. J., *and* FAHEY, J. J.
Nursing station is home base for phone-printer system. *Modern Hospital*, Nov. 1969, p. 85-8.

CLARK, N.
Automation as it affects the general nurse and her patients. *Journal of the West Australian Nurses*, Oct. 1968, p. 8-10.

COULTER, PEARL P.
Programing for nursing service. *Nursing Outlook*, Sept. 1967, p. 33-8.

DAVIS, M., *and* SAUNDERS, R.
Allocating student nurses by computer. *Nursing Times*, April 8, 1966, p. 467-9.

DAVIS, M., *and* SAUNDERS, R.
Scheduling of student nurses with the aid of a computer. *The Hospital*, Sept. 1966, p. 423-7.

DEMARCO, J. P.
Automating nursing's paper work. *American Journal of Nursing*, Sept. 1965, p. 74-7.

DEMARCO, J. P., *and* SNAVELY, SHIRLEY A.
Nurse staffing with a data processing system. *American Journal of Nursing*, Oct. 1963, p. 122-5.

EDELSTEIN, R. R.
Automation: its effect on the nurse. *American Journal of Nursing*, Oct. 1966, p. 2194-8.

GALBRAITH, G.
Medical electronics: an established aid which makes new demands of nursing staff. *Hospital Administration in Canada*, Aug. 1968, p. 46-8.

GILLAM, R.
The use of computers in nursing. *International Nursing Review*, vol. 15, no. 4, Oct. 1968, p. 308-25.

GIVEN, C. W., *and* GIVEN, B.
Automation and technology: A key to professionalized care. *Nursing Forum*, vol. VIII, no. 1, 1969, p. 74-81.

GREAT BRITAIN. MINISTRY OF HEALTH
Patient/nurse call systems. H.M.S.O., 1966.
[Hospital Technical Memorandum no. 15.]

GREENBERG, R. C.
This technological age: are nurses in it? Mechanical aids. *Nursing Times*, Dec. 3, 1970, p. 1558-60.

ISBERG, R. A.
Someday the kidney will talk to the nurse. Rapid development of electronic technology may eliminate I.C.U.s, automate physical exams., and let computers analyze diagnostic test results. *The Modern Hospital*, July 1967, p. 81.

MCLEAN, M. D.
Automation and the nurse. *The Canadian Nurse*, May 1965, p. 363-4.

OLSSON, D. E.
Automating nurses' notes—first step in a computerized record system. *Hospitals*, June 16, 1967, p. 64, 69-70, 74, 76 and 78.

ONTARIO REGISTERED NURSES' ASSOCIATION
Are nurses ready for automation in patient care? *Hospital Administration in Canada*, June 1967, p. 48-9.

PAYNE, L. C.
Computers and patient management. *Nursing Times*, Oct. 1, 1965, p. 1339-41.

PAYNE, L. C.
Medical automation: a professional necessity. *Nursing Mirror*, May 14, 1965, pp. v-vii.

PRICE, E.
Data processing [computers]. *American Journal of Nursing*, Dec. 1967, p. 2558-64.

RICHMAN, A.
Nursing; knobs; and know-how. The impact of hospital automation. *International Journal of Nursing Studies*, July 1965, p. 145-7.

ROSENBERG, M., *and others*
Attitudes of nursing students toward computers. *Nursing Outlook*, July 1967, p. 44-6.

ROWAN, R. L.
Automation. Its effect on the hospital. *American Journal of Nursing*, Oct. 1966, p. 2199.

SALMON, B.
Nursing in the age of automation. *New Zealand Nursing Journal*, Dec. 1969, p. 20-1.

SHERMAN, ROGER
Computer system clears up errors, lets nurses get back to nursing. *Hospital Topics*, Oct. 1965, p. 44-6.

SMITH, A.
The application of computers to health and medical care. *International Journal of Nursing Studies*, Dec. 1968, p. 281-90.

SMITH, B.
Computer in the ward [King's College Hospital]. *Nursing Times*, Nov. 5, 1970, p. 1426-9.

SMITH, J. L.
The computer: its impact on the physician, the nurse and the administrator. *Hospitals*, Sept. 16, 1969, p. 61-5.

Speed, Eunice L., and Young, Nancy A.
SCAN: data processed printouts of a patient's basic care needs. *American Journal of Nursing*, Jan. 1969, p. 108-10.

Tarrant, B. J.
Automation. Its effect on the patient. *American Journal of Nursing*, Oct. 1966, p. 2190-4.

Thomas, F. A., and others
A new automated psychiatric nursing report. *Perspective in Psychiatric Care*, Sept./Oct. 1970, p. 222-9.

United States. National Institute of General Medical Sciences
Advances in micro-electronics. *Nursing Mirror*, Aug. 25, 1967, p. vii-x.

Weil, T. P., and Weil, J. W.
The use of computer systems in patient care. *Nursing Forum*, vol. VI, no. 2, 1967, p. 207-17.

Communication

American Nurses' Association
Communicating—keystone of administration, by Helen W. Dunn. New York, The Association, 1964.

Armstrong, E.
Nursing and public relations. *The Lamp*, Feb. 1969, p. 13-21.

Awon-Khan, V.
Means of communication within the nursing profession and with other professions and occupational groups. *International Nursing Review*, vol. 8, no. 3, 1961, p. 92-8.

Brigden, Raymond J.
A matter of public relations. *Nursing Times*, Sept. 16, 1966, p. 1218-20.

Carstairs, Vera
Channels of communication: report on an enquiry carried out in hospitals in Scotland for the Working Party on Suggestions and Complaints in Hospitals. Edinburgh, Scottish Home and Health Department, 1970. [Scottish Health Service Studies, no. 11.]

Central Health Services Council
Communication between doctors, nurses and patients . . . [a summary]. *Nursing Times*, July 12, 1963, p. 859.

Central Health Services Council,
Joint sub-committee of the Standing Medical and Standing Nursing Advisory Committees
Communication between doctors, nurses and patients: an aspect of human relations in the hospital service. H.M.S.O. 1963.

Clark, J. A. P.
Fundamentals of communication. *Canadian Nurse*, Jan. 1961, p. 19-23.

Davis, A. J.
The skills of communication. *American Journal of Nursing*, Jan. 1963, p. 66-70.

Dean, D. J.
Internal communications in a psychiatric hospital. *Nursing Times*, Mar. 15, 1968, Occasional Papers, p. 43-8.

Dunn, H. W.
Good communication/Good administration. *Nursing Outlook*, Nov. 1961, p. 670-2.

Eng, E.
An effective communication plan for the nursing service. *Hospitals*, Sept. 1, 1964, p. 103-4, 106, 108 and 110, 113-4.

Hawthorne Experiment
Hospital internal communications. The Hawthorne Experiments. *Nursing Times*, Sept. 3, 1965, p. 1213-4.

Horton Hospital, Epsom
Who does what? (Liaison and communication difficulties between nurses and occupational therapists). *Nursing Mirror*, May 15/June 5, 1970, p. 17-9.

Jessee, R.
Educating nurses for communication. *International Nursing Review*, July/Aug. 1965, p. 43-5.

Kelber, M.
Communication or conflict. *International Nursing Review*, vol. 12, no. 3, 1965, p. 29-36.

Kron, Thora
Communication in nursing. Philadelphia, Saunders, 1967.

Lockerby, Florence K.
Communications for nurse. 2nd edn. St Louis, Mosby, 1963.

McGinty, P.
One solution to the problem of communications. *Nursing Times*, Apr. 30, 1970, p. 551-2.

Menzies, I. E. P.
Communicating and counselling. *Occupational Health*, May/June 1963, p. 146-53.

Mitchell, Margaret
Interpreting nursing to the community: a paper given at the 12th Quadrennial Congress of the International Council of Nurses, Melbourne, 1961. *International Nursing Review* vol. 8, no. 3, 1961, p. 87-92.

Muntz, J.
Communication or conflict. *International Nursing Review*, vol. 12, no. 3, 1965, p. 47-52.

Noble, M.
Communications—an anthropological approach. *International Journal of Nursing Studies*, Feb. 1967, p. 29-35.

Noble, M.
Communications in the National Health Service—a survey of some of the published research findings. *International Journal of Nursing Studies*, Feb. 1967, p. 15-27.

Paynich, M. L.
Cultural barriers to nurse communication. *American Journal of Nursing*, Feb. 1964, p. 87-90.

Raphael, M., Sr.
The development and activities of a joint physician-nurse liaison committee. *Hospital Progress*, Aug. 1968, p. 80-3.

Reid, H. E.
Something to say . . . and how! *Canadian Nurse*, Mar. 1970, p. 52-4.

Revans, R. W.
Hospital attitudes and communications. Manchester College of Science and Technology, 1961.

Revans, R. W.
Hospital internal communications. *Nursing Times*, Mar. 15, 1968, Occasional Papers, p. 41-2.

Revans, R. W.
Hospital internal communications. Keeping the recruits. *Nursing Times*, Aug. 6, 1965, p. 1085-6.

Runck, Howard W.
Information systems need nurses. *Datamation*, Sept. 1968, p. 56-9.

Siggins, C. M.
A professor of English looks at communication skills. *Nursing Outlook*, Nov. 1961, p. 666-8.

Simpson, H. M.
Communication within the health team. *International Nursing Review*, vol. 12, no. 4, 1965, p. 40-2.

Skipper, J. K., and others
Some barriers to communication between patients and hospital functionaries. *Nursing Forum*, vol. II, no. 1, 1963, p. 15-23.

Skipper, J. K., and others
What communication means to patients. *American Journal of Nursing*, April 1964, p. 101-3.

NURSING AS A PROFESSION

THIS, LESLIE E.
The professional nurse looks at personal communication. Washington, Leadership Resources, 1966. [Leadership in Nursing series, no. 3.]

TOPF, M.
A behavioral checklist for estimating the development of communication skills. *Journal Nursing Education*, Nov. 1969, p. 29-34.

WAGNER, S. P.
The ABC's of communication. *American Association of Industrial Nurses Journal*, Aug. 1963, p. 8-11.

WEINER, H. N.
Making your public relations program work. *Nursing Outlook*, Sept. 1963, p. 654-5.

WENKERT, W., *and others*
Communications. Concepts and methodology in planning patient care services. *Medical Care*, July/Aug. 1969, p. 327-31.

WIELAND, G. F.
Evaluating the hospital internal communications project. The use of survey methods in evaluation. *International Nursing Review*, vol. 16, no. 2, 1969, p. 106-13.

ZACHARY, M. C.
Communication problems: nurse-employee-management-physician. *American Association of Industrial Nurses Journal*, Aug. 1963, p. 15-9.

Job Analysis

ALBERTA, DEPARTMENT OF HEALTH
A study of the activities of nursing personnel in ten health units and one city health department in the province of Alberta. Edmonton, 1968.

ALLEN, L.
A study of the activities of head nurses on twelve patient units, by ... and others. Saskatoon, Sask., University Hospital, 1965.

ARNDT, C., *and* LAEGER, E.
Role strain in a diversified role set: the director of nursing services. Part 1. *Nursing Research*, May/June 1970, p. 253-9.

ARNDT, C., *and* LAEGER, E.
Role strain in a diversified role set: the director of nursing services. Part 2. Sources of stress. *Nursing Research*, Nov./Dec. 1970, p. 495-501.

BAILEY, D. E.
Clinical inference in nursing: analysis of nursing action patterns. *Nursing Research*, Spring 1967, p. 154-60.

BENNIS, WARREN G., *and others*
The role of the nurse in the out-patient department: a preliminary report. New York, American Nurses' Foundation, 1961.
[Joint authors are Norman H. Berkowitz, Mary F. Malone and Malcolm W. Klein.]

BERGLIND, H.
Occupational activity of Swedish Registered Nurses. *International Journal of Nursing Studies*, vol. 2, no. 3, 1965, p. 251-60.

BOURNE, M. W.
The clinical assistant matron. *Nursing Times*, July 9, 1965, p. 934-6.

BOWDEN, EDGAR A. F.
Nurses' attitudes toward hospital nursing service. Implications for job satisfaction and transfers between services. *Nursing Research*, Summer 1967, p. 246-51.

BRITISH COLUMBIA. HOSPITAL INSURANCE SERVICE, CONSULTATION AND RESEARCH DIVISION
Report of functional nursing activity study at Surrey Memorial Hospital, Surrey, B.C., utilizing the consulting services of Health Insurance, Dept. of National Health and Welfare. Victoria, 1964.

BROWN, W. K.
An administrator's view of the head nurse's work. *Nursing Outlook*, Nov. 1963, p. 798-9.

CANADIAN HOSPITAL
Nursing activity study. *Canadian Hospital*, Mar. 1963, p. 36-40 and 56.

CANADIAN NURSES' ASSOCIATION
Guidelines for qualifications and functions, hospital nursing service personnel. Ottawa, The Association, 1966.

CLEVELAND UNIVERSITY HOSPITALS, OHIO
Position description for head nurses. The Hospitals, [1961].

COLLEDGE, M.
Is the ward sister a manager. *British Hospital Journal and Social Service Review*, July 10, 1970, p. 1342.

COMMISSION FOR ADMINISTRATIVE SERVICES IN HOSPITALS
Study of nursing time requirements for patients of various age groups. Los Angeles, The Commission, 1966.

CONNOR, R. J.
A work sampling study of variations in nursing work load. *Hospitals*, May 1, 1961, p. 40-1 and 111.

CRANE, K. H., *and* MACLEOD, VERNON
Analysis of nursing personnel utilization on patient care units. Ann Arbor, Mich., Community Systems Foundation, 1966.

DOWNEY, M. E., *and* LYNN, D. H.
Work study at Belfast City Hospital—1 and 2. *Nursing Times*, July 21, 1961, p. 939-41; July 28, 1961, p. 972-5.

FYKE, K. J.
Nursing utilization study. Regina, Sask., Regina Grey Nuns' Hospital, 1966.

GODDARD, H. A.
Work measurement in the nursing service. *Nursing Times*, June 15, 1962, p. 767-9.

GORHAM, W. A.
Methods for measuring staff nursing performance. *Nursing Research*, Winter, 1963, p. 4-11.

GROSS, P. A., *and* BROWN, R. A.
Contrasting job satisfaction elements shown for R.N.'s and L.P.N.'s. *Hospitals*, Feb. 1967, p. 73-81.

HANSEN, K. E.
How to measure nursing care time. *The Modern Hospital*, April 1963, p. 93-6.

HENRY, D. K.
Study of the non-nursing activities of the Evening Supervisor. Minneapolis, University of Minnesota, 1964.

HIBBERT, DOROTHY
A time study and activity analysis of the nursing personnel on eleven patient units and a comparison of these activities. Saskatoon, Sask., University Hospital, 1962.

HUFFMAN, VERNA
A study of the activities of nursing personnel in six health units and municipal health departments in one province of Canada; a report to the Research Committee of the Canadian Public Health Association. Toronto, Canadian Public Health Association, 1966.

JELINEK, R. C.
A new approach to the analysis of nursing activities. *Hospitals*, Oct. 1, 1966, p. 89-91.

LAMBERTSEN, E. C.
Toward a clearer definition of the nurse's function. *Hospitals*, July 16, 1961, p. 51-4 and 96.

MACDONNELL, J. ASA K.
Timing studies of nursing care in relation to categories of hospital patients by J. Asa K MacDonnell, Unnur Brown and Barbara Johannson. Ottawa, Department of Health, 1969.

New York State University
State Education Department. Division of Professional Education
Personal and employment characteristics of professional nurses registered in New York State. [New York, The University, 1966].

Notter, L.
How your time is spent. *American Journal of Nursing*, Feb. 1964, p. 115-7.

Ontario, Hospital Services Commission
Evaluation of the activities of nursing unit personnel, 1959-1965. Toronto, the Commission, 1968.

Robinson, S. S.
Is there a difference? A small study reveals wide variation in public health nurses' and social workers' perception of each other's specific and overlapping functions and areas of collaborative activities. *Nursing Outlook*, Nov. 1967, p. 34-6.

Saathoff, D. E., and Kurtz, R. A.
General duty nurses and aides—a study in roles. *Hospital Management*, July 1963, p. 60-8.

Schmieding, N. J.
Study of nurse activity after removal of management functions. *Journal of Psychiatric Nursing*, Nov./Dec. 1966, p. 531-9.

Scottish Hospitals Work Study Group
An investigation of nursing time devoted to clerical procedures in connection with supplies and services at ward and departmental level in Scottish hospitals. Edinburgh, The Group, 1964.

Singleton, Maria, and Smith, Aileen B.
How were supervisors spending their time? *Nursing Outlook*, Jan. 1962, p. 32-4.

Smith, Kathryn M.
Discrepancies in the role-specific values of head nurses and nurse educators. *Nursing Research*, Summer 1965, p. 196-202.

Spaziante, G.
Analysis of work in the wards of a general hospital, based on activity sampling. *World Hospitals*, Jan. 1968, p. 16-8.

Statts, H. A.
An activity analysis of the dual position of director of nursing service and nursing education. *Nursing Research*, Winter, 1963, p. 30-8.

Testoff, Arthur, and others
Analysis of part-time nursing in general hospitals. *Hospitals*, Sept. 1, 1963, p. 54, 56, 58 and 60.

Trites, D. K., and Schwartau, N. W.
Nursing or clerking? *Nursing Outlook*, Jan. 1967, p. 55-6.

United States Public Health Service, Division of Nursing
How to study nursing activities in a patient unit. Washington, Dept. of Health, Education and Welfare, 1964.

University of California School of Nursing
A functional analysis of nursing service in the University of California Hospital. San Francisco, The University [1966].

Vinall, R. P.
Measuring nursing care for nursing-home units. *Hospital Topics*, Oct. 1966, p. 49-52.

Nursing Service Organisation

American Hospital Association
An approach to organization of nursing services. *Practical Approaches to Nursing Service Administration*, Spring, 1970, p. 1-4.

American Nurses' Association
Standards of organized nursing services in hospitals, public health agencies, nursing homes, industries and clinics. New York, The Association, 1965.

Anderson, L. C.
Nursing service administration in a clinical research hospital. *International Journal of Nursing Studies*, Sept. 1969, p. 133-8.

Asperilla, P. F.
The role of nursing service administrator in leadership development. *The Philippine Journal of Nursing*, Nov./Dec. 1966, p. 335-8.

Aydelotte, Myrtle Kitchell
Survey of hospital nursing services: report. New York, National League for Nursing, 1968.

Ayers, R., and others
Action for change. An experiment in nursing service reorganization. *American Journal of Nursing*, April 1969, p. 783-6.

Benz, E. G.
Nursing service. *Hospitals*, April 1, 1969, p. 157-62.

Clark, M. A.
Nursing administration in a therapeutic community. *Nursing Mirror*, Oct. 13, 1967, p. 45-8.

Commonwealth Medical Conference
Nursing Services Committee
Commonwealth Medical Conference. Conclusions of Nursing Services Committee. *Nursing Mirror*, Oct. 15, 1965, p. 147.

Coulter, P. P.
Programing for nursing service. *Nursing Outlook*, Sept. 1967, p. 33-8.

De Stefano, G. M.
Management program increases nursing service effectiveness. *Hospital Progress*, Dec. 1968, p. 54-60.

Dunn, Helen W.
Nursing service; annual administrative reviews. *Hospitals*, April 1, 1964, p. 119-24.

Eng, Evelyn
Critical look at nursing service. *Hospital Topics*, June 1963, p. 51-3.

Germain, L. D.
Nursing service. *Hospitals*, April 1965, p. 135-8.

Glover, G., and Germaine, A.
Administrator and director of nursing can co-operate—if they communicate. *Hospital Administration in Canada*, April 1970, p. 76-7, 80 and 84.

Goldfarb, M.
Evaluation of the extension course in nursing unit administration. *The Canadian Nurse*, May 1966, p. 59-61.

Hauer, R. M.
Perspective on directing hospital nursing service. *American Journal of Nursing*, Dec. 1969, p. 2626-9.

Hawkins, J. L.
Ward manager system; a case study of the organization of hospital nursing care. Lafayette, Ind., Purdue University, 1964.

Howe, A.
Supervisors coordinate patient services. [A pattern by which even small hospitals can improve nursing efficiency]. *Modern Hospital*, July 1963, p. 77-81.

Ingbar, Mary L., and others
Differences in the costs of nursing service; a statistical study of community hospitals in Massachusetts. *American Journal of Public Health*, Oct. 1966, p. 1699-755.

Jameson, E. E., and Mackie, E. J.
Reorganization of a department of nursing. *The Canadian Nurse*, June 1964, p. 566-71.

Jensen, Deborah MacLurg, editor
Nursing service administration: principles and practice, by Edythe Alexander and others. St. Louis, Mosby, 1962.

JOHNSON, D. E.
Consequences for patients and personnel. Does the present organization of hospital nursing services do more harm than good? What change might solve the major problems which result from it? *The American Journal of Nursing*, May 1962, p. 96-100.

LUCKMAN, J., and others
Management policies for large ward units, by J. Luckman, M. Mackenzie and J. Stringer. Institute for Operational Research, 1969.
[Health report no. 1.]

MCGUINNESS, A. F.
Organization of the nursing service within the hospital. *Irish Nursing News*, May/June 1966, p. 9-14.

MERCADANTE, L. T.
Leadership development seminars. *Nursing Outlook*, Sept. 1965, p. 59-61.

MILLER, D. I.
Education for nursing service administration. *Nursing Forum*, vol. VII, no. 4, 1968, p. 375-85.

MOORE, L. F.
Problem recognition in nursing service administration. *Nursing Forum*, vol. VIII, no. 1, 1969, p. 94-102.

NATIONAL LEAGUE FOR NURSING
Is there a new design for the functions of nursing services? Papers presented at the Third Annual Meeting of Council of Hospital and Related Instructional Nursing Services. October 9-10, 1969, Cincinnati, Ohio. New York, The League, 1970.

NATIONAL LEAGUE FOR NURSING
DEPARTMNET OF HOSPITAL NURSING
Criteria for evaluating a hospital department of nursing services. New York, The League, 1965.

ORBELL, A.
Administration for nursing service. *The Australian Nurses' Journal*, May 1962, p. 108.

PURDY, FRANCES
Nursing service: annual administrative reviews. *Hospitals*, April 1, 1966, p. 113-6.

ROYAL COLLEGE OF NURSING and
NATIONAL COUNCIL OF NURSES OF THE UNITED KINGDOM
Administering the hospital nursing service—a review. The College, 1964.

ROYAL COLLEGE OF NURSING and
NATIONAL COUNCIL OF NURSES OF THE UNITED KINGDOM
Nursing service—supply and demand. Report of professional conference Annual General Meeting, July 1965. *Nursing Times*, July 16, 1965, p. 983-4.

SAREN, M., and STRAUB, A.
Nursing service effectiveness. *Hospitals*, Jan. 16, 1970, p. 45-50.
1968, p. 67-72.

SCHWIER, M. E., and GARDELLA, F. A.
Identifying the need for change in nursing service. *Nursing Outlook*, April 1970, p. 56-62.

SIMMS, LAURA L.
The role of the staff nurse in nursing service. New York, American Nurses Association, 1965.

SIMPSON, H. M.
Research for improvement of nursing service. *International Nursing Review*, Mar./April 1967, p. 21-8; *Queensland Nurses Journal*, Mar. 1969, p. 5-10.

SLEEPER, R.
Nursing service. *Hospitals*, April 1, 1967, p. 139-42.

SMITH, R., and others
Distribution of nursing service in a children's hospital. *Canadian Hospital*, July 1961, p. 38.

SOUTH AFRICAN NURSING ASSOCIATION
Report on nursing service in the republic of South Africa presented by the Board of the South African Nursing Association to the biennial congresses of the S.A.N.A., October 1966. [Pretoria, The Association, 1966].

SOTEJO, J. V.
Nursing research for improvement of nursing service. *The Philippine Journal of Nursing*, Nov./Dec. 1966, p. 329-34 and 339.

STEWART, D. Y.
The age of challenge must be faced by nursing service departments. *Hospital Administration in Canada*, Sept.

VENGER, M. J., and YOURMAN, J.
Modern management theory applied to nursing service. *Nursing Outlook*, Nov. 1966, p. 30-3.

WRIGHT, M. SCOTT
Administration of the nursing service. A lecture delivered at the Royal Society of Health Conference, 1965. *Nursing Mirror*, Oct. 15, 1965, p. 163-8.

YOUNG, E. G.
Nursing service budget. *Canadian Nurse*, Dec. 1963, p. 1149-54.

YOUNG, RACHAEL
Nursing service management study; based on a descriptive check list analysis. Edmonton, Alberta Association of Registered Nurses, Nursing Service Committee, 1966.

Staffing

ALONZO, B. S.
Nursing service staffing problems. *The Philippine Journal of Nursing*, Jan./Feb. 1967, p. 5-12.

ASSOCIATION OF NURSES OF THE PROVINCE OF QUEBEC.
AD HOC COMMITTEE ON NURSING NEEDS AND RESOURCES
Survey of nursing personnel in hospitals. Montreal, The Association, 1970.
[Report prepared by Barbara Kuhn.]

ASSOCIATION OF REGISTERED NURSES OF NEWFOUNDLAND.
COMMITTEE ON NURSING SERVICE
Survey of inactive nurses in Newfoundland, 1960-61. St. John's, The Association. 1961.

AULD, M.
A method by which the necessary nursing establishment of a hospital may be estimated. *International Journal of Nursing Studies*, Aug. 1970, p. 119-23.

BARTSCHT, K. G.
An analytical approach to nursing scheduling. *Hospital Topics*, Sept. 1963, p. 44-5.

BERZINS, G.
The elusive staff nurse. *Nursing Mirror*, May 23, 1969, p. 19-20.

BINKLEY, L., and others
AHA Survey Report. Fewer auxiliaries and volunteers are providing more—and more kinds—of service. *Hospitals*, Mar. 16, 1968, p. 60-4.

BLANSFIELD, MICHAEL G.
The professional nurse looks at appraisal of personnel. Washington, Leadership Resources, 1966.
[Leadership in Nursing series, no. 7.]

BLISHEN, BERNARD R.
Survey of nurses. Ottawa, Canadian Nurses' Association, 1964.

BOURNE, M. W.
Evaluation of services involving nursing staff at a new district general hospital. *Nursing Times*, Sept. 2, 1966, p. 1165-8.

BOURNE, M. W.
Finding and training staff for a new hospital. *Nursing Times*, Jan. 15, 1965, p. 100 and 102.

CANADIAN NURSES' ASSOCIATION
Historical overview of approaches to staffing the hospital nursing service department. Ottawa, The Association, 1966.
[French and English text.]

CAREY, M. C.
Staff disunity: a destructive force. *American Journal of Nursing*, Nov. 1969, p. 2375-81.

CHARTER, D.
How the Friesen concept effects nurse staffing. *Canadian Hospital*, Sept. 1970, p. 52-6.

CHRISTENSON, W. C.
Practical and college-degree nurses give longest employment, study shows. *Hospital Topics*, Feb. 1964, p. 30-2.

COMMISSION FOR ADMINISTRATIVE SERVICE IN HOSPITALS
Nursing service—staff utilization and control program. Los Angeles, The Commission, 1966.

CONNOR, R. J., *and others*
Effective use of nursing resources: a research report. *Hospitals*, May 1, 1961, p. 30-9.

COOPER, SIGNE S.
Activating the inactive nurse: a historical review. *Nursing Outlook*, Oct. 1967, p. 62-5.

CRANE, K. H., *and* MACLEOD, VERNON
Analysis of nursing personnel utilization on patient care units. Ann Arbor, Mich., Community Systems Foundation, 1966.

CUMING, M. W.
Shift working—an easier way? *Nursing Times*, Aug. 13, 1965, p. 1101.

DAHLSTEN, A. M., *and* FLOOD, R. F.
No evening or night supervisors. *Nursing Outlook*, Jan. 1970, p. 49-53.

DEARDEN, R. W.
Nursing staff structures: a compendium. *The Hospital*, Feb. 1967, p. 60-1; Mar. 1967, p. 95-8; April 1967, p. 133-4.

DEMARCO, J. P., *and* SNAVELY, S. A.
Nurse staffing with a data processing system. *The American Journal of Nursing*, Oct. 1963, p. 122-5.

DICKER, K.
Open forum. Straight shifts of duty. *Nursing Mirror*, Oct. 9, 1964, p. 41-2.

EAGEN, SR. MARY CECILIA
New staffing pattern allows for total individual quality care. *Hospital Progress*, Feb. 1970, p. 62-4 and 70.

FEYERHARM, A. M.
Nursing activity patterns; a guide to staffing. *Nursing Research*, Spring 1966, p. 124-33.

FRANCES, SISTER MARY ANN,
Implementing a program of cyclical scheduling of nursing personnel. *Hospitals*, July 16, 1966, p. 108-14.

FYKE, K. J.
Nursing utilization study. Regina, Sask., Regina Grey Nuns' Hospital, 1966.

GINZBERG, ELI
Nursing and manpower realities. *Nursing Outlook*, Nov. 1967, p. 26-9.

GREAT BRITAIN. DEPARTMENT OF HEALTH AND SOCIAL SECURITY NATIONAL NURSING STAFF COMMITTEE
National Health Service: a report . . . on the selection and appointment of senior nursing staff in the Hospital Service. Dept. of Health, 1969.

GREAT BRITAIN. DEPARTMENT OF HEALTH AND SOCIAL SECURITY *and* WELSH OFFICE
National Health Service: the selection and appointment of senior nursing staff in the Hospital Service. Dept. of Health, 1969.

GREAT BRITAIN. MINISTRY OF HEALTH
Nursing establishments: enquiry into ward staffing arrangements. (Reports of visits to 10 hospitals.) The Ministry, 1961.

HARTMANN, B.
Student nurse allocation. A planned programme—1 & 2. *Nursing Times*, Jan. 5, 1968, Occasional Papers, p. 1-4; Jan. 12, 1968, Occasional Papers, p. 5-8.

HATT, F. M.
Assessment of nursing staff arrangements in a General Hospital. *International Journal of Nursing Studies*, Aug. 1967, p. 201-6.

HOSPITAL COMPUTER CENTRE FOR LONDON
A computer-based nurse allocation and record system, undertaken by English Electric Leo Marconi Computers Ltd. The Centre, [1967?].

HOSPITAL COMPUTER CENTRE FOR LONDON
Nurse allocation and records system. Specification for the record program, undertaken by English Electric Leo Marconi Computers Ltd. The Centre, [1967?].

HOWELL, J. P.
Cyclical scheduling of nursing personnel. *Hospitals*, Jan. 16, 1966, p. 77-83.

JENKINSON, V. M.
Planning a duty rota in the ward. *Nursing Times*, April 26, 1963, p. 512-3.

JENSEN, F. T.
Four nursing patterns fit smaller hospitals. *Modern Hospital*, April 1961, p. 117.

KING EDWARD'S HOSPITAL FUND FOR LONDON
HOSPITAL CENTRE
Planned allocation for nurses in training. *Nursing Times*, April 12, 1968, Occasional Papers, p. 57-60.

KING EDWARD'S HOSPITAL FUND FOR LONDON
HOSPITAL CENTRE
Staff for non-nursing duties. Report of a conference held by the Hospital Centre. *Nursing Times*, Dec. 17, 1965, p. 1732-3.

KING EDWARD'S HOSPITAL FUND IN LONDON
HOSPITAL CENTRE
Staffing and teaching in intensive care units. *Nursing Times*, Dec. 9, 1966, p. 1610.

KNIGHT, J.
Are ward clerks of use? *Nursing Times*, Sept. 10, 1970, p. 1183.

LAMBERTSEN, E. C.
Availability of R.N.s affects responsibilities of others. *Modern Hospital*, Mar. 1970, p. 132.

LEEDS REGIONAL HOSPITAL BOARD
Work measurement as a basis for calculating nursing establishments: an analytical study. Harrogate, The Board, 1963.

LEICESTER ROYAL INFIRMARY
Short-stay surgery. Experimental five-day treatment scheme to defeat staff shortage. *Nursing Times*, Sept. 1, 1961, p. 1121-2.

LEVINE, E., *and others*
Diversity of nurse staffing among general hospitals. *Hospitals*, May 1, 1961, p. 42-8.

LIVENGOOD, L.
Planned shifts save nurses and dollars. *The Modern Hospital*, Feb. 1965, p. 101.

LUDWIG, D. J., *and* HUMPHREY, A.
Staffing by nursing hours per patient day. *Hospital Topics*, Sept. 1963, p. 46-8.

LYONS, T. F.
Research shows lack of supervisor influence in nursing turnover patterns. *Hospitals*, Oct. 16, 1970, p. 78-80.

McCartney, R. A., *and others*
Nurse staffing systems. *Hospitals*, Nov. 16, 1970, p. 102-5.

McGregor, Gladys
Realities of staffing. *American Journal of Nursing*, Nov. 1962, p. 56-63.

Martin, M., *and* Wild, R.
Society at work: the five-day ward. *New Society*, June 22, 1967, p. 920-1.

Mercadante, L. T.
Utilization of nursing personnel. [In continuity of care]. *Hospitals*, Dec. 1, 1970, p. 82-4.

Miller, Stephen J., *and* Bryant, W. D.
A division of nursing labour: experiments in staffing a municipal hospital. Kansas City, Community Studies, 1965.

Montag, M. L.
Utilization of graduates of associate degree programs. *Journal of Nursing Education*, April 1966, p. 5-10.

Mussallem, H. K.
Manpower problems in nursing. *The Canadian Nurse*, Aug. 1967, p. 25-8.

National League for Nursing
Research and Studies Service
Nurse-faculty census of 1966. New York, The League, 1966.

Newcastle Regional Hospital Board
Cherry Knowle Hospital Management Committee
Report of nurse establishment committee. The Board, 1963.

North Eastern Regional Hospital Board
Nursing workload per patient as a basis for staffing: report by the Work Study Department . . . on the development of a formula for calculating the day duty nurse staffing requirements of a hospital ward. Edinburgh, Scottish Home and Health Department, 1969.
[Scottish Health Service studies, no. 9.]

Oxford Regional Hospital Board
Optimal use of nursing staff: the patient and the nurse. Oxford, The Board, 1962.

Oxford Regional Hospital Board
Scheduling of student nurses with the aid of a computer. Oxford, The Board, 1965.

Pardee, G.
Classifying patients to predict staff requirements. *American Journal of Nursing*, Mar. 1968, p. 517-20.

Paetznick, Marguerite
A guide for staffing a hospital nursing service. Geneva, W.H.O., 1966.
[Public Health Papers, 31.]

Paulson, E., *and others*
Nursing care requirements for a polio unit. *The Canadian Nurse*, July 1963, p. 624-31.

Price, Elmina M.
Staffing for patient care: a guide for nursing services, based on a research report, by Elmina M. Price, Joyce M. Schowalter, Florence Marks and Hazel Johnson. New York, Springer, 1970.

Price, Elmina M.
Techniques to improve staffing [Shift systems]. *American Journal of Nursing*, Oct. 1970, p. 2112-5.

Rehm, D. A.
Design for staff growth. *American Journal of Nursing*, Sept. 1970, p. 1930-3.

Riddoch, M.
Internal rotation of student nurses on to night duty. *Nursing Times*, Aug. 4, 1967, p. 1025-8.

Royal College of Nursing and
National Council of Nurses of the United Kingdom *and*
King Edward's Hospital Fund for London.
Hospital Centre
Memorandum on nursing establishments: report of a joint working party . . . The Fund, 1966.

Ryan, J. R., *and* Boydston, G. B.
This flexible plan puts nurses in the right place at right times. *Modern Hospital*, Sept. 1965, p. 114-7.

Schechter, D. S.
Manpower for the smaller hospital: innovations in training and education. *Hospitals*, June 1, 1967, p. 55-8.

Smith, B. J.
The deployment of nurses in geriatric and general wards. *Nursing Times*, June 19, 1964, p. 802-4.

Smith, B. W., *and* Luckman, J.
The allocation of nurses: a feasibility report. Institute of Operational Research, 1968.

Stahl, Adele G.
Manpower Development and Training Act; concerns for nursing. *American Journal of Nursing*, June 1964, p. 112-5.

Steiner, B. H., *and* Lindquist, N. E.
Surprise find of staffing study: nurses have too much spare time. *Modern Hospital*, Feb. 1970, p. 108-10.

Testoff, A., *and others*
Analysis of part-time nursing in general hospitals. *Hospitals*, Sept. 1, 1963, p. 54, 56 and 58-60.

Testoff, A., *and others*
The part-time nurse. *American Journal of Nursing*, Jan. 1964, p. 88-9.

Watkin, B.
Nursing workload and staffing of wards. *British Hospital Journal and Social Service Review*, Oct. 17, 1969, p. 1938-9.

Weller, B. F.
The five-day ward in the children's hospital, an attempt to deal with staff shortage. *Nursing Times*, Mar. 16, 1962, p. 347-8.

Western Council on Higher Education for Nursing *and* Western Regional Council of State Leagues for Nursing
Utilization of nursing personnel. Boulder, Colorado, Western Interstate Commission for Higher Education, 1963.

Whitehead, J.
Student nurse allocation—1. *Nursing Times*, May 10, 1963, p. 585-7.

Whitehead, J.
Student nurse allocation—2. The Westminster Hospital Plan. *Nursing Times*, May 17, 1963, p. 609-10.

Wilson, L.
Nova Scotia study defines nurse utilization in health agencies. *Hospital Administration in Canada*, June 1969, p. 42-4.

Wolfe, Harvey, *and* Young, J. P.
Staffing the nurse-unit. Parts 1 and 2. *Nursing Research*, Summer 1965, p. 236-43; Fall 1965, p. 299-303.

Wright, M. J.
Staffing the nursing service [in smaller hospitals, maintaining standards of care]. *Hospitals*, June 16, 1963, p. 91-3, 96 and 99.

Zubkoff, Harry
Small improvements have a big effect on nurse utilization. *Hospitals*, Feb. 16, 1969, p. 56-8, 60 and 63-4.

AERO-SPACE NURSING

Bioastranautic Operational Support Unit
The stars beckon [Aerospace nursing]. *American Journal of Nursing*, Aug. 1967, p. 1650-3.

BYRNE, JACQUELINE
Space-age nursing. *Nursing Times*, Aug. 16, 1968, p. 1109-10.

GUNN, A. D. G.
Space Flight—1 and 2. *Nursing Times*, Jan. 6, 1967, p. 21-2; Jan. 13, 1967, p. 53-4.

MACH, E.
Nursing in the space age. *World Hospitals*, Jan. 1968, p. 27-30.

NURSING TIMES
To the Moon under medical supervision. *Nursing Times*, July 24, 1969, p. 947.

PIPER, D. A., *and* CORRADO, V. P.
Space age nursing. *International Nursing Review*, vol. 15, no. 4, 1968, p. 368-7.

RICHARDS, P. R.
Air travel and medical problems. *Nursing Mirror*, April 24, 1970, p. 29-32.

AUXILIARIES

ABDALLAH, MARY C.
Nurse's aide study manual. Philadelphia, W. B. Saunders, 1965.
2nd edn., by Mary E. Mayes, 1970.

AMERICAN NURSES' ASSOCIATION
Statement on auxiliary personnel in nursing service. *American Journal of Nursing*, July 1962, p. 72-3.

AMERICAN NURSES' ASSOCIATION, SPECIAL COMMITTEE ON ALLIED NURSING PERSONNEL
Health occupations supportive to nursing. *American Journal of Nursing*, Mar. 1966, p. 559-63.

BECK, F. S.
Auxiliary nursing personnel in the hospital nursing team. *World Hospitals*, July 1964, p. 31-42.

BECK, F. S.
Finding a new approach to the training and use of auxiliary nursing personnel. *International Nursing Review*, vol. 10, no. 1, 1963, p. 48-60.

BROWN, D. R.
The nursing assistant. *The Canadian Nurse*, Dec. 1962, p. 1101.

BROWN, ESTHER LUCILE
The nursing profession and auxiliary personnel. Reprinted from "Aspects of public health nursing", p. 9-34. Geneva, W.H.O., 1961.

BROWN, W. K.
The nurses' aide. A study of the selection, training, and utilization of nurses' aides in the general hospitals of Kentucky. *Hospital Topics*, May 1962, p. 45-8 and 56.

CARR, A. J.
When is a nursing auxiliary not a "nursing" auxiliary? *Nursing Times*, June 28, 1968, p. 863-4.

CHERESCAVICH, GERTRUDE D.
A textbook for nursing assistants. St. Louis, Mosby, 1964.
2nd edn., 1968.

CONWAY, M. M.
Training and use of the nursing auxiliary in the ward situation. *Irish Nurse*, April 1966, p. 399-402.

DIER, KATHLEEN A.
A survey of the educational problems in sixty English speaking schools for nursing auxiliaries in Canada. Montreal, McGill University, 1963.

DONOVAN, JOAN E., *and others*
The nurse aide, by Joan E. Donovan, Edith H. Belsjoe and Daniel C. Dillon. New York, McGraw-Hill, 1968.

ENSING, E.
Nursing auxiliaries. In service training. *Nursing Times*, Feb. 9, 1962, p. 159-61.

GILES, M. N.
Nursing auxiliaries/assistants in a Salmon pilot scheme. *Nursing Mirror*, Aug. 7, 1970, p. 30.

GRIFFIN, L. M., *and* GILMORE, R. F.
Training of nursing technicians. *Hospital Management*, Jan. 1962, p. 6.

HIBBERT, D.
Nurses' aides—are they needed? *Hospital Topics*, Oct. 1966, p. 103-4.

HOSPITAL TOPICS
Hospital trains army reservists as nursing-staff aides. *Hospital Topics*, Jan. 1970, p. 36-7.

HOSPITALS AND CHARITIES COMMISSION FOR NURSING AIDE TRAINING SCHOOLS IN VICTORIA
Handbook for nursing aides. Melbourne, The Commission, 1961.

INTERNATIONAL DIGEST OF HEALTH LEGISLATION
Training of auxiliary nurses and auxiliary male nurses. *International Digest of Health Legislation*, vol. 18, no. 1, 1967, p. 128-31.

ISLER, CHARLOTTE
The nurses' aide in the hospital. New York, Springer, 1968.

JANE, R.
Today's auxiliary in the modern hospital. *Canadian Hospital*, Aug. 1968, p. 44-6.

JODIAS, JANET
Personal care of paitents—a text for health assistants. Philadelphia, Saunders, 1970.

KERGIN, D. J.
Nursing assistants are here to stay. *Canadian Nurse*, Apr. 1969, p. 33.

KING, V. M.
Nursing aid service. *District Nursing*, Aug. 1963, p. 98-9 and 101.

LANG, P. A.
From brooms to blood pressures: a program to retrain housekeepers and janitors to become safe and productive nurses' aides and orderlies. *Nursing Outlook*, Oct. 1970, p. 25-7.

LEE, C. M.
Dependence on the auxiliary. *Nursing Times*, June 28, 1968, p. 865-6.

McFADDEN, GRACE M., *and others*
Employment of health aides in a tuberculosis program. *Public Health Reports*, Jan. 1966, p. 43-8.

McKEOWN, DOROTHY
The nursing assistant. *The Canadian Nurse*, Dec. 1962, p. 1111.

NICHOLSON, B. M.
Nursing assistants benefit by seminar approach in service. *Journal of Psychiatric Nursing*, July/Aug. 1970, p. 28-30.

OLDMEADOW, E.
The future of the nursing aide in the health service. *Australian Nurses' Journal*, Feb. 1970, |p. 28-30 and 32-3.

PAN AMERICAN SANITARY BUREAU REGIONAL OFFICE OF THE WORLD HEALTH ORGANIZATION
Report on a seminar on the training and utilization of auxiliary nursing personnel. Roseau, Dominica, 12th-23rd May 1969. Washington, The Bureau, 1969.
[Reports on nursing, no. 13.]

RAYNER, D. M.
Nursing auxiliaries in a maternity unit. *Nursing Mirror*, Mar. 11, 1966, p. 661-2.

RENNOLDSON, M.
The auxiliary nurse, her training and work. *Nursing Mirror*, Nov. 30, 1962, p. 193-4.

ROUTH, T. A.
Ancillary personnel in nursing homes. *The Journal of Practical Nursing*, Nov. 1969, p. 30-1, 35 and 46.

SCOTTISH HOME AND HEALTH DEPARTMENT
Auxiliary nursing personnel. Edinburgh, The Department, 1962.

SEYFFER, C.
Assistant nurse programmes as vocational education. *International Nursing Review*, vol. 14, no. 6, 1967, p. 36-40.

STEVENSON, N.
Curriculum development in practical nurse education. *American Journal of Nursing*, Dec. 1964, p 81-6.

STOCKMEYER, I.
Training of Red Cross nurses' aides in Germany. *Nursing Mirror*, Nov. 2, 1962, p. 107.

STRANK, R. A.
In-service training for auxiliaries. *Nursing Times*, May 15, 1969, p. 625-7.

SWANSON, A. L.
The organization of hospital auxiliaries. *Canadian Hospital*, Feb. 1963, p. 46-7.

WEDGERY, A. W.
One standard—or two? [Care of male patients by orderlies]. *The Canadian Nurse*, May 1970, p. 27-8.

WORLD HEALTH ORGANIZATION
Auxiliary personnel in nursing: a survey of existing legislation. Geneva, W.H.O., 1966.

WORLD HEALTH ORGANIZATION
REGIONAL OFFICE FOR EUROPE
The training and use of auxiliary nursing personnel: report on a seminar sponsored ... in collaboration with the government of Spain held at Escorial, 17-26 Oct. 1962. Copenhagen, W.H.O., 1963.

CLINICAL NURSE SPECIALIST

ANDERSON, L. C.
The clinical nursing expert. *Nursing Outlook*, July 1966, p. 62-4.

CAMPBELL, E. B.
The clinical nurse specialist: joint appointee. *American Journal of Nursing*, Mar. 1970, p. 543-6.

CHRISTMAN, L.
The nurse clinical specialist. *Hospital Progress*, Aug. 1968, p. 14-28.

CHRISTMAN, L.
Specialism and generalism in clinical nursing. *Hospitals*, Jan. 1, 1967, p. 83-6.

DILWORTH, A. S.
Joint preparation for clinical nurse specialists. *Nursing Outlook*, Sept. 1970, p. 22-5.

FAGIN, C. M.
The clinical specialist as supervisor. *Nursing Outlook*, Jan. 1967, p. 34-6.

GEORGOPOULOS, B. S., and CHRISTMAN, L.
The clinical nurse specialist: a role model. *American Journal of Nursing*, May 1970, p. 1030-9.

GEORGOPOULOS, B. S., and JACKSON, M. M.
Nursing Kardex behaviour on an experimental study of patient units with and without clinical nurse specialists. *Nursing Research*, May/June 1970, p. 196-218.

JOHNSON, E. A.
Nursing reorganization strengthens head nurse role, provides special nursing consultants. *Hospitals*, June 16, 1968, p. 85-90.

LEWIS, EDITH P., *compiler*
The clinical nurse specialist: a compilation of articles selected and reprinted from the *American Journal of Nursing, Nursing Research*, and *Nursing Outlook*. New York, American Journal of Nursing Company, 1970. [Contemporary nursing series.]

LITTLE, D.
The nurse specialist. *American Journal of Nursing*, Mar. 1967, p. 552-6.

MCINTYRE, H. M.
The nurse clinician—one point of view. *Nursing Outlook*, Sept. 1970, p. 26-9.

PALLIN, E.
The role of the clinical tutor. *The Australian Nurses' Journal*, Oct. 1968, p. 223-6.

RAMPHAL, M.
Clinical nursing supervision. *American Journal of Nursing*, Sept. 1968, p. 1900-2.

REITER, F.
The nurse-clinician. *International Nursing Review*, vol. 13, no. 4, 1966, p. 62-71; *American Journal of Nursing*, Feb. 1966, p. 274-80.

SCULLY, N. R.
The clinical nursing specialist: practical nursing. *Nursing Outlook*, Aug. 1965, p. 28-30.

SIMMS, L. L.
The clinical nursing specialist: an experiment. *Nursing Outlook*, Aug. 1965, p. 26-8.

STRONG, P. G.
The clinical tutor in a psychiatric hospital. *Nursing Times*, Jan. 22, 1970, Occasional Papers, p. 13-6.

STURZL, J. A.
More power to the nurse specialist. *Nursing Outlook*, Dec. 1970, p. 48-9.

TURK, HERMAN, and INGLES, THELMA
Clinic nursing: explorations in role innovation. Philadelphia, F. A. Davis, 1963.

WILLIAMS, M. A., and OLSEN, M. P.
Clinical teaching: a mutual education-service involvement. *Journal of Nursing Education*, April 1965, p. 5-14.

ENROLLED NURSE
[including the Practical nurse]

AMERICAN NURSES' ASSOCIATION
Statement of functions of the licensed practical nurse. *American Journal of Nursing*, Mar. 1964, p. 93.

AMERICAN NURSES' ASSOCIATION, and
NATIONAL FEDERATION OF LICENSED PRACTICAL NURSES
Statement of functions of the licensed practical nurse, and what's happening to proposed goal 111. *American Journal of Nursing*, Mar. 1964, p. 93.

ANDREWS, J. M.
Assessment of pupil nurses in psychiatric hospitals. *Nursing Mirror*, Mar. 10, 1967, p. 536-7.

BAGGOTT, E.
The SEN in psychiatric hospitals. *Nursing Times*, Oct. 29, 1965, p. 1478-80.

BECKER, BETTY GLORE, and HASSLER, SISTER RUTH ANN
Vocational and personal adjustments in practical nursing. St. Louis, C. V. Mosby, 1970.

BEDSIDE NURSE
The building of professional attitudes in students. [Salvation Army's William Booth Memorial Hospital School for Practical Nurse Education, Covington, Kentucky]. *Bedside Nurse*, Nov./Dec. 1969, p. 32-5.

BENEDIKT, L.
The social worker in practical nurse education. *Nursing Outlook*, Jan. 1965, p. 60-2.

BENNETT, B. A.
Britain's enrolled nurses an example to the world. *Hospital and Social Service Journal*, Dec. 15, 1961, p. 1447.

BENNETT, B. A.
Teaching pupil nurses with special reference to overseas students. *Nursing Times*, Feb. 21, 1964, p. 241-4.

BENNETT, MARGARET H.
Pupil nurses introductory course. Heinemann, 1967.
2nd edn., 1971.

BENTLEY, C.
The history of the NASEN. *Nursing Mirror*, April 17, 1964, p. vii-xiii.

BENTLEY, C.
The state enrolled nurse. *International Nursing Review*, vol. 16, no. 1, 1969, p. 69-79.

BLEIER, INGE J.
Maternity nursing: a textbook for practical nurses. Philadelphia, Saunders, 1961.

BURR, JOAN, *editor*
Swire's handbook of practical nursing. 6th edn. Bailliere Tindall, and Cassell, 1968.
[For earlier edns., see FARNOL, RUBY THORA. Swire's handbook for the enrolled nurse.]

BUSH, CHRISTINE H.
Personal and vocational relationships for practical nurses. Philadelphia, Saunders, 1961.
2nd edn., 1966.

BUTCHER, M. G.
History of the NASEN. *Nursing Times*, Mar. 20, 1964, p. 369-70.

CRAIG, J. B.
Post-enrolment education. *Nursing Mirror*, July 22, 1966, p. 379-80.

CROWLEY, D.
The LPN—today and tomorrow. *Journal of Practical Nursing*, Jan. 1969, p. 32-3.

CULVER, VIVIAN M., *and* BROWNELL, KATHRYN OSMOND
The practical nurse: textbook of nursing. 6th edn. Philadelphia, Saunders, 1964.

DAN MASON NURSING RESEARCH COMMITTEE
The work, responsibilities and status of the enrolled nurse. The Committee, 1962.

DAWSON, I. M.
The training of pupil nurses. *Nursing Times*, April 14, 1961, p. 474-6.

DAWSON, I. M.
The training of pupil nurses. *Nursing Times*, April 21, 1961, p. 505-6.

EDELSON, RUTH B.
Retraining project for preparing men practical nurses. *Nursing Outlook*, Aug. 1966, p. 33-4.

ENGEL, J.
Nurse's aide to LPN upgrading program. *Journal of Practical Nursing*, May 1970, p. 26-30.

FARNOL, RUBY THORA, *editor*
Swire's handbook for the enrolled nurse. 5th edn. Bailliere, Tindall and Cox, 1962.
[For later edns., see BURR, JOAN, Swire's handbook of practical nursing.]

FAWKES, B. N.
Twenty-one years of the Roll. *Nursing Times*, Mar. 20, 1964, p. 364-5.

FORREST, JANE
Practical nursing and anatomy for pupil nurses. Edward Arnold, 1966.
2nd edn., 1969.

FORREST, JANE
Questions and answers for pupil nurses. Edward Arnold, 1966.

FREEMAN, MARILYN GOTTEHRER, *and* HANNAN, JUSTINE
Clinical nursing workbook for practical nurses. 3rd edn. Philadelphia, Davis, 1968.
[*Note:* Previous edns. entitled—*Medical-surgical workbook for practical nurses.*]

GARDINER, G. O.
The importance of the SEN. in the nursing team. *Nursing Mirror*, Oct. 2, 1964, p. x-xii.

GENERAL NURSING COUNCIL FOR ENGLAND AND WALES
The assessment of pupil assistant nurses. *Nursing Mirror*, April 7, 1961, p. 57-8.

GREMP, ZELLA VON, *and* BROADWELL, LUCILLE
Practical nursing review: questions and situations. 2nd edn. Philadelphia, Lippincott, 1965.

HALL, E. D.
Surgical operating suite. A high school course in practical nursing trains personnel for hospital service. *Hospital Management*, Nov. 1964, p. 39 and 42.

HASLER, DORIS
The practical nurse and today's family. New York, Macmillan, 1964.

HIGHNETT, O. B.
The enrolled nurse in orthopaedic nursing. *Nursing Times*, Feb. 1, 1963, p. 127-8.

HOFFMAN, CLAIRE P., *and others*
Simplified nursing by Claire P. Hoffman, Gladys B. Lipkin, and Ella M. Thompson. 8th edn. Philadelphia, Lippincott, 1968.

ILLING, M.
Student assessment. *District Nursing*, Aug. 1970, p. 93-4.

JOHNSTON, DOROTHY F.
History and trends of practical nursing. St. Louis, C. V. Mosby, 1966.

JOHNSTON, DOROTHY F.
Medical-surgical nursing: workbook for practical nurses. St. Louis, Mosby, 1965.
2nd edn., 1969.

JOHNSTON, DOROTHY F.
Total patient care: foundations and practice. St. Louis, C. V. Mosby, 1964.
2nd edn., 1968.

JONES, N.
The licensed practical nurse and continuing education. *American Journal of Practical Nursing*, May 1965, p. 52-3.

KEANE, CLAIRE BRACKMAN
Saunders review for practical nurses. Philadelphia, W. B. Saunders, 1966.

KIRKHAM, I. L.
The Licensed Practical Nurse. *Nursing Mirror*, Sept. 25, 1970, p. 32-3.

KNOPF, LUCILLE, *and others*
Practical nurses: five years after graduation, nurse career-pattern study by Lucille Knopf, Barbara L. Tate and Sarah Patrylow. New York, National League for Nursing, 1970.

KUMAGAI, TSUTOMU
Study of the professional nursing staff's opinion of the licensed practical nurse's qualifications and its effects on appropriate employment and job satisfaction of the licensed practical nurse. Minneapolis, Minn., Program in Hospital Administration, University of Minnesota, 1962.

LANGDON, L. M.
The employed LPN and her job. *Bedside Nurse*, Nov. 1970, p. 20-3.

LOW, M.
The practical nurse and her education. *International Nursing Review*, vol. 16, no. 2, 1969, p. 180-2.

MARTIN, J. L.
West Indian pupil nurses and their problems in training. *Nursing Times*, Aug. 6, 1965, p. 1079-82.

MARTIN, R. G.
Our accrediting program—yesterday, to-day and to-morrow. *The Journal of Practical Nursing*, June 1968, p. 22-30.

NURSING AS A PROFESSION

MEADOW, L., and EDELSON, R. B.
Age and marital status and their relationship to success in practical nursing. *Nursing Outlook*, April 1963, p. 289-90.

MOCKETT, M.
Assessing the pupil nurse. *Nursing Times*, June 25, 1965, p. 869-72.

MOCKETT, M.
Teaching pupil nurses in ward and classroom. *Nursing Times*, Mar. 11, 1966, p. 321-3.

MOSBY, C. V., & Co.
Mosby's review of practical nursing. 3rd edn. St. Louis, Mosby, 1961.
4th edn., 1966.
5th edn., 1970.

NATIONAL ASSOCIATION OF STATE ENROLLED NURSES
Annual Meeting in Edinburgh, March 1968. *Nursing Mirror*, Mar. 22, 1968, p. 11-4.

NATIONAL ASSOCIATION OF STATE ENROLLED NURSES
Code of salaries, conditions of service, duties, responsibilities, ethical relationships, for State Enrolled Nurses employed in occupational health services. [The Association, 1969?]

NATIONAL ASSOCIATION OF STATE ENROLLED NURSES
Divided we fall. Report of the Winter Conference of NASEN. *Nursing Times*, Dec. 8, 1967, p. 1664-5.

NATIONAL ASSOCIATION OF STATE ENROLLED NURSES
Enrolled nurses in conference. [Report of 27th Annual General Meeting]. *Nursing Times*, June 4, 1970, p. 729.

NATIONAL ASSOCIATION OF STATE ENROLLED NURSES
Report of the Annual General Meeting held in London, May 1966. *Nursing Mirror*, June 10, 1966, p. 237.

NATIONAL ASSOCIATION OF STATE ENROLLED NURSES
Report of the 20th Annual Conference, Manchester, 1963. *Nursing Mirror*, May 31, 1963, p. 189-90.

NATIONAL ASSOCIATION OF STATE ENROLLED NURSES
Report of the Winter Conference of the National Association of State Enrolled Nurses. *Nursing Mirror*, Dec. 8, 1961, p. 194.

NATIONAL ASSOCIATION OF STATE ENROLLED NURSES
The state enrolled nurse in public health nursing services. [The Association, 1968.]

NATIONAL ASSOCIATION OF STATE ENROLLED NURSES
The state enrolled nurse: post-enrolment educational opportunities and preparation for special fields of nursing: a memorandum. The Association, 1962.

NATIONAL FEDERATION OF LICENSED PRACTICAL NURSES INC.
The LPN's. Who they are; where they work; what they do. Report of a recent study. *Bedside Nurse*, Jan./Feb. 1969, p. 29-31.

NURSING MIRROR
Nursing services: posts for senior enrolled nurses. *Nursing Mirror*, Aug. 21, 1964, p. 469-72.

O'BRIEN, MAUREEN J.
The role of the LPN in nursing homes. *The Journal of Practical Nursing*, May 1968, p. 21-2.

O'HARE, B.
Scheme for preparation of pupil nurses for enrolment. *Irish Nursing News*, Sept./Oct. 1967, p. 8-9 and 16.

PARRIS, E.
On an island paradise—the licensed practical nurse. *The Journal of Practical Nursing*, Jan. 1968, p. 22-7.

PEIMER, S. C., and others
Experiment in retraining unemployed men for practical nursing careers. *Hospitals*, Oct. 16, 1966, p. 87-90 and 164.

RAPIER, DOROTHY KELLEY, and others
Practical nursing: a textbook for students and graduates by Dorothy Kelley Rapier, Marianna Jones Koch, Louis Pearson Moran, J. R. Geronsin, Elwyn L. Cady and Deborah Maclurg Jensen. 2nd edn. St. Louis, Mosby, 1962.
3rd edn., 1966.
4th edn., 1970.
[For 1st edn. of this work see under Jensen, Deborah Maclurg, editor. Practical nursing . . .]

REA, J. N.
The nurse as an ancillary. *Nursing Mirror*, Nov. 22, 1963, p. 176-8.

REYNOLDS, P. L.
The state enrolled nurse. *Journal of Practical Nursing*, Mar. 1970, p. 31 and 54-5.

ROSS, CARMEN F.
Personal and vocational relationships in practical nursing. Philadelphia, Lippincott, 1961.
2nd edn., 1965.

ROYAL COLLEGE OF NURSING,
NURSE ADMINISTRATORS' SECTION
The enrolled nurse. Royal College of Nursing, 1962.

SMITH, E. M.
An evening program in practical nursing. *Journal of Practical Nursing*, May 1970, p. 31-3 and 47.

SPEELMAN, ARLENE
Examination review for practical nurses. New York, Putnam, 1962.

SPENCER, MAY, and TAIT, KATHERINE M.
Introduction to nursing. Oxford, Blackwell, 1965.
2nd edn., 1970.

STEVENSON, NEVA M.
Better utilization of licensed practical nurses. *Nursing Outlook*, July 1965, p. 34-7.

STEVENSON, NEVA M.
Roles of the licensed practical nurse should determine curriculum design. *Nursing Outlook*, Jan. 1962, p. 30-1.

SUTTON, AUDREY LATSHAW
Workbook for practical nurses. 3rd edn. Philadelphia, Saunders, 1969.

TAIT, K. M.
Where do we go from here? *Nursing Times*, Mar. 20, 1964, p. 383-4.

TOMLINSON, R. M.
Personal characteristics and employment profile of licensed practical nurses. *Bedside Nurse*, Mar./April 1969, p. 30-2.

TREECE, E. W.
An evaluation of practical nursing education. *Bedside Nurse*, Jan. 1970, p. 30-3.

ULLOM, M. M.
The challenge of the practical nurse in a climate of productivity. *Practical Nursing*, Mar. 1963, p. 40-1.

WAIN, O. M.
The Enrolled Nurses Committee. *Nursing Times*, Mar. 20, 1964, p. 381-2.

WEISS, OLGA
The practical nurse in Israel. *Journal of Practical Nursing*, Dec. 1968, p. 18-21 and 30.

WEST, MARGARET D., and CROWTHER, BEATRICE
Education for practical nursing, 1960: a report of the Committee on the questionnaire study of practical nursing schools. New York, National League for Nursing, 1962.

PRISON NURSING

BOORER, D.
Opportunities for men. Nursing those without liberty. *Nursing Times*, Oct. 2, 1964, p. 1289-92.

McCarrick, H.
Nursing behind bars—1. H.M. Prison, Holloway. *Nursing Times*, Dec. 4, 1969, p. 1546-8.

McCarrick, H.
Nursing behind bars—2. The surgical unit at Wormwood Scrubs. *Nursing Times*, Dec. 11, 1969, p. 1575-78.

Miles, B.
Nursing in prison. *Nursing Times*, April 30, 1965, p. 584-5.

PRIVATE NURSING

Gibbs, B. M.
Challenge of private nursing. *Nursing Mirror*, Feb. 20, 1970, p. 15-6.

Gibbs, B. M.
Private nursing—further training? *Nursing Times*, Feb. 17, 1967, p. 231.

Hacker, C.
Private duty—private choice. *The Canadian Nurse*, July 1969, p. 25-8.

Health Services Journal
A look at nursing agencies. *Health Services Journal*, July 1966, p. 4-5.

Royal College of Nursing and National Council of Nurses of the United Kingdom
Fees and conditions of service for private nurses. The College, 1969.
New edn., 1970.

TECHNIQUES OF NURSING
GENERAL WORKS

American Hospital Association
Hospital Research and Educational Trust
Nursing care plans: study program in nursing management. Chicago, The Trust, 1966.

American Medical Association *and*
American Nurses' Association
The sick person needs ... report of the third national conference for professional nurses and physicians, Coronado, California, February 23-25, 1967. Chicago, Illinois, American Medical Association, [1967?].

American Nurses' Association
Nursing of patients with loss of perceptions. New York, A.N.A., 1962.
[ANA Convention, 1962, clinical monograph no. 9.]

American Nurses' Association
Effects of stereotypes on nursing care. New York, A.N.A., 1962.
[ANA Convention, 1962, clinical monograph no. 11.]

Atkinson, W. J.
Posture of the unconscious patient. *Nursing Times*, May 28, 1970, p. 686-7.

Ayres, Stephen M., *and* Giannelli, Stanley, *editors*
Care of the critically ill. New York, Appleton-Century-Crofts, 1967.

Barton, J.
New fiber helps prevent bedsores. *The Modern Hospital*, May 1962, p. 104-6.

Bell, S.
Early morning temperatures? *American Journal of Nursing*, April 1969, p. 764-6.

Bray, R. E., *and* Bird, T. E.
Observation of the sick. *Nursing Times*, May 3, 1963, p. 544-6.

British Columbia, Department of Health Services and Hospital Insurance, Division of Public Health Nursing
A study of patient progress. Victoria, 1966.

British Medical Journal
Barrier nursing. *British Medical Journal*, April 9, 1966, p. 876.

Brownlowe, M. A., *and others*
New washable woolskins. *American Journal of Nursing*, Nov. 1970, p. 2368-70.

Burn, J. L.
Immunization by nurses. *Nursing Times*, Feb. 17, 1967, p. 202-3.

Burn, J. L.
Immunization by nurses in the home. *Nursing Times*, Feb. 24, 1967, p. 246-8.

Byers, Virginia B.
Nursing observation. Iowa, Wm. C. Brown, 1968.

Carr, A.
Blood sample survey. *Nursing Times*, Dec. 17, 1970, Occasional Papers, p. 191-2.

Charles Marie, Sister
The nurses orbit in relation to improved nursing care.
In
American Nurses' Association
Improvement of nursing practice. New York, The Association, 1961.

Clack, B.
Intravenous infusions: uses and contra-indications. *Nursing Times*, Aug. 11, 1967, p. 1068-9.

Clain, A.
Wound dressing. Modern methods. *Nursing Times*, April 13, 1962, p. 458-60.

Clarke, K. H., *and* Milne, J.
Principles and practice of radioactive nursing observed at the Peter MacCallum Clinic, Melbourne. *UNA Nursing Journal*, May 1962, p. 148-53.

Dann, T. C.
Routine skin preparation before injection—is it necessary? *Nursing Times*, Aug. 26, 1966, p. 1121-2.

Davitz, Lois Jean
Interpersonal processes in nursing case histories. New York, Springer, 1970.

Dickie, Helen M.
Pocket book on tray and trolley setting. 3rd edn. Livingstone, 1963.
4th edn., 1966.
5th edn., 1970.

Ewing, M. R., *and others*
A sheepskin as a nursing aid. *The Lancet*, Dec. 30, 1961, p. 1447-8.

Ewing, M. R., *and others*
Further experiences in the use of sheep skins as an aid in nursing. *Australian Nurses' Journal*, Sept. 1964, p. 215-8.

Fallows, P. B.
Bed warming in hospitals. *Nursing Times*, Mar. 4, 1966, p. 295-7.

Fenton, M.
What to do about thirst. *American Journal of Nursing*, May 1969, p. 1014-7.

Fiore, M., *and* Ramphal, M. M.
Prevention of decubitus ulcers. *Bedside Nurse*, Sept./Oct. 1968, p. 13-5.

Flores, A. M., *and* Zohman, L. R.
Energy cost of bedmaking to the cardiac patient and the nurse. *American Journal of Nursing*, June 1970, p. 1264-7.

Gardner, A. M. N.
Feeding the ill and weak. *Nursing Times*, Feb. 17, 1967, p. 205-6.

GARROW, C.
Report of the Perth Chest Hospital on the use of sheep skins. *Journal of the West Australian Nurses*, Aug. 1962, p. 12-3.

GORICK, G. M.
Sheepskin boots in the prevention of pressure sores. *Nursing Times*, Dec. 24, 1965, p. 1749-51.

HENDERSON, VIRGINIA
Basic principles of nursing care. Rev. edn. Geneva, I.C.N., 1969.

HODKINSON, M. A.
Treatment and care of pressure areas. *Nursing Mirror*, June 8, 1962, p. 183, 184 and 186.

INTERNATIONAL WOOL SECRETARIAT *and others*
Sheepskins for and against. *Nursing Mirror*, July 14, 1967, p. 343-5.

KEARNS, B.
Tracheotomy suctioning technique. *The Canadian Nurse*, Feb. 1970, p. 44-8.

KOZIER, BARBARA BLACKWOOD, *and* DU GAZ, BEVERLY WITTER
Fundamentals of patient care: a comprehensive approach to nursing. Philadelphia, Saunders, 1967.

LARSON, KENNETH H., *and others*
Direct care nursing: a teaching program for psychiatric nurses. New York, Macmillan, 1968.

LITTLE, DOLORES E., *and* CARNEVALI, DORIS L.
Nursing care planning. Philadelphia, Lippincott, 1969.

LOWTHIAN, P. T.
Bedsores—the missing links? *Nursing Times*, Nov. 12, 1970, p. 1454-8.

MCHUGH, N.
Sheepskins as an aid to nursing. *Nursing Mirror*, Sept. 28, 1962, p. 513-4.

MCLAREN, C. G.
Case closed—wound open. [A survey by district nurses of patients discharged from hospital with infected wounds and pressure sores.] *Nursing Times*, Nov. 12, 1970, p. 1452-3.

MEDICAL DEFENCE UNION *and* ROYAL COLLEGE OF NURSING AND NATIONAL COUNCIL OF NURSES OF THE UNITED KINGDOM
Joint memorandum on safeguards against failure to remove swabs etc. from patients. M.D.U. and Rcn, 1966.
Rev. 1968.
Rev. 1969.

MEDICAL DEFENCE UNION *and* ROYAL COLLEGE OF NURSING AND NATIONAL COUNCIL OF NURSES OF THE UNITED KINGDOM
Joint memorandum on safeguards against wrong operations. M.D.U. and Rcn, 1966.
Rev. edn., 1969.

MEDICAL DEFENCE UNION *and* ROYAL COLLEGE OF NURSING AND NATIONAL COUNCIL OF NURSES OF THE UNITED KINGDOM
Joint memorandum on steps that might be taken to minimise the risk of a foreign body being inadvertently left in a patient following surgical procedures. M.D.U. and Rcn, 1963.

MEINHART, N. T., *and* ASPINALL, M. J.
Nursing interventions in hypovigilance. *American Journal of Nursing*, May 1969, p. 994-8.

MOSS, F. T., *and* MEYER, B.
The effects of nursing interaction upon pain relief in patients. *Nursing Research*, Fall 1966, p. 303-6.

MOUNTJOY, PAMELA, *and* WYTHE, BARBARA
Nursing care of the unconscious patient. Bailliere, 1970.

NEW ZEALAND NURSING JOURNAL
Wool sheepskins for hospital use. *New Zealand Nursing Journal*, April 1963, p. 19-20.

NEW ZEALAND WOOL BOARD
Sheepskins in nursing. *International Nursing Review*, vol. 11, no. 1, 1965, p. 10-6.

NORTON, D.
Preventing lesions of the pressure areas. *Nursing Mirror*, July 14, 1967, p. 341-3.

PRINGLE, D. M.
Early ambulation and discharge—the problems and dangers. *Nursing Mirror*, Mar. 16, 1962, p. 475.

PUTT, A. M.
One experiment in nursing adults with peptic ulcers. *Nursing Research*, Nov./Dec. 1970, p. 484-94.

RIDLEY, M.
Barrier nursing. *Nursing Times*, Mar. 16, 1962, p. 340-1.

ROBERTS, G. W.
Use of silicone aerosol in prevention and treatment of bedsores. *Nursing Mirror*, Feb. 2, 1962, p. 347-8.

ROYAL COLLEGE OF NURSING
Steps that might be taken to obviate the risk of an operation being performed on the wrong patient, side, limb, or digit. The College, 1961.

RUDD, T. N.
Pressure sores; their origin and management. *Nursing Mirror*, May 26, 1961, p. 743-5.

SHAW, BARBARA A.
The new site for intramuscular injection.
In
AMERICAN NURSES' ASSOCIATION
Technical innovations in health care: nursing implications. New York, The Association, 1962.

SMITH, DOROTHY W., *and* GIPS, CLAUDIA D.
Care of the adult patient: medical-surgical nursing. Philadelphia, Lippincott, 1963.
2nd edn., 1966.

SPORNE, P.
Barrier nursing. *Nursing Times*, Jan. 26, 1962, p. 93, and 113-4.

TATE, G. V., *and others*
Correct use of electric thermometers. *American Journal of Nursing*, Sept. 1970, p. 1898-9.

THORNE, M. E.
Sorbo boots. A new idea in the prevention of pressure sores of the heels. *Nursing Times*, Sept. 13, 1963, p. 1135.

TRYON, PHYLLIS A.
The effect of patient participation in decision making on the outcome of a nursing procedure.
In
AMERICAN NURSES' ASSOCIATION
Nursing and the patient's motivations. New York, The Association, 1962.

VERHONICK, P. J.
Decubitus ulcer observations measured objectively. *Nursing Research*, Fall, 1961, p. 211-4.

WADDY, F. F.
Intravenous injections and infusions. *Nursing Times*, Oct. 13, 1967, p. 1361-4.

ZIMMERMAN, C. E.
Techniques of patient care: a manual of bedside procedures for students, interns, and residents. Boston, Little, Brown & Co., 1970.

INTENSIVE CARE

ADAMS, R. E.
Intensive care research—1. *Canadian Hospital*, Oct. 1963, p. 57-65.

ADAMS, R. E.
Intensive care research—2. Evaluation of six more intensive care units from a survey of hospitals on the west coast of the USA. *Canadian Hospital*, Jan. 1964, p. 57-61.

ADAMS, R. E.
Recommendations for an intensive care unit. *Canadian Hospital*, Jan. 1964, p. 62.

ARMSTRONG, D. M.
Organization of an intensive care unit. *AORN Journal*, April 1970, p. 50-4.

ASHWORTH, P. M.
Intensive care. *Nursing Mirror*, Feb. 23, 1968, p. 20-1.

BAILEY, I. C.
Intensive care ward in a neurosurgical unit. *Nursing Times*, Feb. 23, 1968, p. 244-6.

BASSEY, P.
Intensive care unit, Lagos University Teaching Hospital. *Nigerian Nurse*, Jan. 1970, p. 65-7.

BLUMBERG, M. S.
Where intensive patient care is heading. *The Modern Hospital*, Jan. 1963, p. 106.

BRITISH MEDICAL ASSOCIATION PLANNING UNIT
Report of the working party on intensive care. The Association, 1967.

BROMPTON HOSPITAL
Intensive care at the Brompton Hospital. *Nursing Times*, May 1, 1969, p. 551-2.

BURN, J. M. B.
Intensive care: its purpose and practice. *Health*, Summer 1970, p. 40-2.

BURN, J. M. B.
Design and staffing of an intensive care unit. *Lancet*, May 16, 1970, p. 1040-3.

BURRELL, ZEB L., and BURRELL, LENETTE OWENS
Intensive nursing care. St. Louis, Mosby, 1969.

CAM, J. F., and others
Organization and record-keeping in intensive-care wards. *The Lancet*, Nov. 28, 1964, p. 1168-9.

CHARING CROSS HOSPITAL, LONDON
Acute care ward. *Nursing Times*, Aug. 26, 1966, p. 1126-7.

CHOW, RITA
Developments in intensive care nursing. *AORN Journal*, Nov. 1969, p. 37-42.

CLARE MARIE, SISTER
Intensive care unit. *The Canadian Nurse*, Feb. 1965, p. 112-3.

CRAFT, N. B., and PERRY, D. A.
Has intensive care planning been wrong? *The Modern Hospital*, Jan. 1963, p. 92-3.

CRAIG, J. S.
A study on the intensive care unit in general hospitals. *Canadian Hospital*, Jan. 1962, p. 42.

DAVIDSON, R.
A medical intensive care unit. *American Journal of Nursing*, Dec. 1964, p. 79-80.

DEMEYER, J.
The environment of the intensive care unit. *Nursing Forum*, vol. VI, no. 3, 1967, p. 262-72.

FITZWATER, J.
Planning an intensive care unit. *American Journal of Nursing*, Feb. 1967, p. 310-4.

GALBALLY, B.
The planning and organization of an intensive care unit. *UNA Nursing Journal*, Nov./Dec. 1965, p. 369-72.

GARDNER, ERIC K., and SHELTON, BRENDA
The intensive therapy unit and the nurse. Faber, 1967.

GARNHAM, P. D.
Nursing in connection with anaesthetics and intensive care. *Nursing Times*, June 14, 1968, p. 789-91.

GARRETT, S. A. G., and others
The need for intensive nursing care. *British Journal of Preventive and Social Medicine*, Jan. 1966, p. 34-41.

GINSBERG, F.
Intensive care units are not an unmixed blessing. *The Modern Hospital*, Jan. 1963, p. 112.

HARPER, J. R.
Children in a district hospital ITU. *Nursing Times*, Nov. 5, 1970, p. 1417-9.

JOURNAL OF PRACTICAL NURSING
The LPN in the intensive care unit. *Journal of Practical Nursing*, Nov. 1966, p. 30-4.

KELLOGG, W. K., FOUNDATION
The planning and operation of an intensive care unit: an experience brochure. Battle Creek, Michigan, The Foundation, 1961.

KING EDWARD'S HOSPITAL FUND FOR LONDON, THE HOSPITAL CENTRE
Manuals, courses and equipment [For intensive therapy units]. *Nursing Times*, Sept. 13, 1968, p. 1246.

KIRK, G. M.
A post-registration course in intensive nursing care [at Edinburgh Royal Infirmary]. *Nursing Times*, Feb. 26, 1970, p. 261-4.

KIRK, G. M.
Training for intensive care. *Nursing Times*, Dec. 16, 1966, p. 1657-8.

KORNFELD, D. S., and others
Psychological hazards of the intensive care unit. Nursing care aspects. *The Nursing Clinics of North America*, March 1968, p. 41-51.

LAMBERTSEN, E. C.
Intensive patient care nurses should be expert generalists. *The Modern Hospital*, Jan. 1963, p. 118.

LAMBERTSEN, E. C.
The nature and objectives of intensive care nursing. *The Nursing Clinics of North America*, Mar. 1968, p. 3-6.

MCCARRICK, H.
A manual of intensive therapy. *Nursing Times*, Nov. 24, 1967, p. 1584 and 1586.

MCGEE, J. E.
The nurse in intensive therapy. *The Australian Nurses' Journal*, Feb. 1970, p. 26-7 and 36.

MCINTYRE, M. C.
The intensive care unit. *Nursing Outlook*, Nov. 1966, p. 39-43.

MELTZER, LAWRENCE E., and others, eds.
Concepts and practices of intensive care for nurse specialists. Editors: Lawrence E. Meltzer, Faye G. Abdellah and J. Roderick Kitchell. Philadelphia, Charles Press, 1969.

MINCKLEY, B. B.
The multiphasic human-to-human monitor (ICU model). Nursing observation in the intensive care unit. *The Nursing Clinics of North America*, Mar. 1968, p. 29-39.

MODERN HOSPITAL
How to provide the best intensive patient care. *Modern Hospital*, Jan. 1, 1963, p. 67-102 and 106.

MORLEY, A., and SPARK, M.
Resuscitation and the nurse. 1—Measures she can take. 2—The nurse and machine-dependent patient. *Nursing Times*, June 25, 1970, p. 814-5; July 2, 1970, p. 849-52.

MORTIMER, K.
Intensive care units—their implications for the nurse. A review of a small-scale sociological study in the North East Metropolitan Region. *Nursing Mirror*, Jan. 12, 1968, p. viii-ix.

NORTH EAST METROPOLITAN REGIONAL HOSPITAL BOARD
WORK STUDY UNIT
Attitude survey of nurses to intensive therapy units, by Kendrick Mortimer. The Board, [1966].

ROYAL COLLEGE OF NURSING AND NATIONAL COUNCIL OF NURSES OF THE UNITED KINGDOM. HOSPITALS DEPARTMENT. INTENSIVE THERAPY NURSING GROUP
The function and staffing of intensive therapy units and the preparation of nurses to work in the units. The College, 1969.

ST. THOMAS'S HOSPITAL
Intensive therapy unit: Mead Ward. *Nursing Times*, Nov. 18, 1966, p. 1519-22.

SALTER, M. E.
Nursing in an intensive therapy unit. *Nursing Times*, April 16, 1970, p. 486-7.

SMITH, J.
Developments in intensive nursing care. *Health Bulletin*, Jan. 1, 1962, p. 11.

STORLIE, FRANCES, *and others*
Principles of intensive nursing care, by Frances Storlie, Elizabeth Rambousek and Eutha Shannon. New York, Appleton-Century-Crofts, 1970.

STRAUSS, A.
The intensive care unit: its characteristics and social relationships. *The Nursing Clinics of North America*, Mar. 1968, p. 7-15.

TAN, N. C.
The intensive care unit. *Berita Jururawat*, Nov. 1965, p. 23-5.

THOMAS, E. B. J., *and* MITCHELL, M. LE Q.
Intensive care units. *Monthly Bulletin of the Ministry of Health and the Public Health Laboratory Service*, Oct. 1965, p. 310-9.

THOMS, E. J.
The intensive care unit. *The Journal of Practical Nursing*, June 1965, p. 18-22.

VREELAND, R., *and* ELLIS, G. L.
Stresses on the nurse in an intensive-care unit. *AORN Journal*, Sept. 1969, p. 54-6.

WELLENKAMP, D.
Planning and administering the intensive care unit. *The Nursing Clinics of North America*, Mar. 1968, p. 17-28.

WESSEX REGIONAL HOSPITAL BOARD
Experimenting with intensive care. *Nursing Times*, Nov. 9, 1962, p. 1443.

WHEELER, D. V.
How we trained intensive care nurses. *The Modern Hospital*, Jan. 1963, p. 90-1.

WHITTALL, K.
Intensive care of severe head injury: the role of the nurse. *Nursing Times*, July 30, 1970, p. 965-6.

ZSCHOCHE, D., *and* BROWN, L. E.
Intensive care nursing: specialism junior doctoring, or just nursing? *American Journal of Nursing*, Nov. 1969, p. 2370-4.

PAIN

AMERICAN JOURNAL OF NURSING
Pain. Part 1—Basic concepts and assessment. Programmed instruction. *American Journal of Nursing*, May 1966, p. 1085-108.

AMERICAN JOURNAL OF NURSING
Pain. Part 2—Rationale for intervention. Programmed instruction. *American Journal of Nursing*, June 1966, p. 1345-68.

BAER, EVA, *and others*
Inferences of physical pain and psychological distress, by Eva Baer, C. Lenburg and others. *Nursing Research*, Sept./Oct. 1970, p. 388-401.

BALME, H. W.
The relief of pain. *Nursing Mirror*, Feb. 7, 1969, p. 22-3.

BLAYLOCK, J.
The psychological and cultural influences on the reaction to pain: a review of the literature. *Nursing Forum*, Vol. VII, No. 3, 1968, p. 262-74.

BOCHNAK, MARY A.
The comparison of two types of nursing activity on the relief of pain.
In
AMERICAN NURSES' ASSOCIATION
Innovations in nurse-patient relationships: automatic or reasoned nurse actions. New York, The Association, 1962.

BRAIN, RUSSELL
Pain, its causes and treatment. Inaugural Lecture given at the Professional Nurses & Midwives Conference, 1961. *Nursing Mirror*, Oct. 20, 1961, p. 50-2; Oct. 27, 1961, p. 67-8; Nov. 3, 1961, p. 85-6.

COLES, M. D.
Pain intensity. *Nursing Mirror*, Aug. 25, 1961, p. 1487.

DAVITZ, L. J., *and others*
Nurses' inferences of suffering. *Nursing Research*, Mar./April 1969, p. 100-7.

EWING, G.
Pain. *The Canadian Nurse*, June 1965, p. 443-5.

LEWIS, M. R., *and others*
How do you measure pain? *Nursing Times*, June 17, 1966, p. 792-4.

LISHMAN, W. A.
The psychology of pain. *Nursing Times*, Dec. 10, 1970, p. 1577-8

McBRIDE, M. A. B.
Nursing approach, pain and relief: an exploratory experiment. *Nursing Research*, Fall 1967, p. 337-41.

MARKHAM, M. M.
The relief of pain. *Nursing Times*, Dec. 10, 1970, p. 1579-81.

OHIO STATE UNIVERSITY SCHOOL OF NURSING
A study of nurse action in relief of pain, by Mildred E. Newton and others. Columbus, The University, 1964.

SMILEY, DOROTHY M.
Nursing the patient who is experiencing chronic pain.
In
AMERICAN NURSES' ASSOCIATION
Nursing of patients with loss of perceptions. New York, The Association, 1962.

SMITH, MARY MARGO
Nursing knowledge and activity in relation to the period of anticipation of pain in the adult.
In
AMERICAN NURSES' ASSOCIATION
Solving "difficult" problems in nursing care. New York, The Association, 1962.

MONITORING

ABREU, XENIA A.
An experience in nursing care of selected patients on electronic monitors.
In
AMERICAN NURSES' ASSOCIATION
Technical innovations in health care: nursing implications. New York, The Association, 1962.

AMERICAN NURSES' FOUNDATION
An experimental approach to vigilance in nurse-patient monitoring. *Nursing Research*, June 1968, p. 1, 3-4 and 7.

BEAN, M. A., and others
Monitoring patients through electronics. *American Journal of Nursing*, April 1963, p. 65-9.

BERGIN, M. A.
Monitoring the fetal heart. *Nursing Clinics of North America*, Dec. 1966, p. 559-67.

BROWN, C., and others
Body function monitoring. *Nursing Clinics of North America*, Dec. 1966, p. 569-76.

CHOW, R.
Patient monitoring is more than just a dream. *Berita Jururawat*, April 1962, p. 37.

CROCKETT, G. S.
Patient monitoring. *Nursing Times*, May 7, 1970, p. 581-3.

GEORGE, J.
Monitoring the myocardial infarction patient. *Nursing Clinics of North America*, Dec. 1966, p. 549-57.

HARRIS, RUBY M.
Laying the right lines for electronic monitoring. *Nursing Outlook*, Aug. 1963, p. 573-6.

HOWLAND, D.
Approach to nurse-monitor research. *American Journal of Nursing*, Mar. 1966, p. 556-8.

JENKINS, A. C.
Successful cardiac monitoring. *Nursing Clinics of North America*, Dec. 1966, p. 537-47.

KING EDWARD'S HOSPITAL FUND FOR LONDON HOSPITAL CENTRE
Monitoring in intensive care units. *Nursing Times*, Sept. 16, 1966, p. 1227-8.
[Report of a ward-sister's conference.]

KING EDWARD'S HOSPITAL FUND FOR LONDON HOSPITAL CENTRE
Patient-monitoring. Report of a conference held at the Hospital Centre, Oct. 5, 1966. *Nursing Times*, Oct. 14, 1966, p. 1373-4.

RICHARDSON, G. A.
Patient monitoring. *Nursing Times*, Dec. 2, 1966, p. 1584-7.

PATIENT CARE

ABDELLAH, FAYE G., and LEVINE, EUGENE
Better patient care through nursing research. *International Journal of Nursing Studies*, April 1965, p. 1-12.

ABDELLAH, FAYE G., and LEVINE, EUGENE
Patients and personnel speak: a method of studying patient care in hospitals. Washington, U.S. Dept. of Health, Education and Welfare, 1964.

ADAMS, J. M.
The Dryburn experiment. Describes the experimental pre-discharge ward which has been in use at Dryburn Hospital for the past four years. *Nursing Mirror*, Nov. 18, 1966, p. ix-xi.

AIKEN, L. H.
Patient problems are problems in learning. *American Journal of Nursing*, Sept. 1970, p. 1916-8.

ALBERTA NURSING CARE SURVEY COMMITTEE
Nursing care in Alberta hospitals. Edmonton, Hospitals Division, Department of Public Health, 1961.

ALFORD, DOLORES M.
Caring for the individual patient: a student-centered, patient-centered approach to fundamentals of nursing. Philadelphia, Davis, 1962.

ALLEY, JANET ANN
Nurse actions during hemorrhage in the child.
In
AMERICAN NURSES' ASSOCIATION
Emergency intervention by the nurse. New York, The Association, 1962.

ALTSCHUL, A. T.
Go and talk to the patients [based on a lecture entitled Systems of Communication between Nurses and Patients]. *Nursing Mirror*, April 10, 1970, p. 41-6.

AMERICAN HOSPITAL ASSOCIATION
Patients over 65 receive more nursing care, early results in AHA study indicate. *Hospitals*, Feb. 16, 1967, p. 23a-23b.

AMERICAN MEDICAL ASSOCIATION and
AMERICAN NURSES' ASSOCIATION
Nurse-physician collaboration toward improved patient care; papers from the second national conference for professional nurses and physicians, Denver, Sept. 30-Oct. 2, 1965. New York, A.N.A., 1966.

AMERICAN NURSES' ASSOCIATION
Effects of continuity in nursing care on patient welfare. New York, A.N.A., 1962.
[ANA Convention 1962, clinical monograph no. 17.]

AMERICAN NURSES' ASSOCIATION
Nursing in relation to the impact of illness upon the family. New York, A.N.A., 1962.
[ANA Convention, 1962, clinical monograph no. 2.]

AMERICAN NURSES' ASSOCIATION
Solving "difficult" problems in nursing care. New York, A.N.A., 1962.
[ANA Convention, 1962, clinical monograph no. 20.]

ANDERSON, MAJA C.
Better patient care: a programmed introduction to nursing fundamentals. Philadelphia, W. B. Saunders, 1965.

ANGRIST, S.
Nursing care: the dream and the reality. *American Journal of Nursing*, April 1965, p. 66-9.

ARCHIBALD, R.
Patient and impatient in hospital. *Nursing Times*, Sept. 4, 1964, p. 1145-6.

ARMIGER, SISTER BERNADETT,
Reprise and dialogue. *Nursing Outlook*, Oct. 1968, p. 22-8.

BAGGOTT, E.
Back to the community—is the patient prepared? *Nursing Times*, Oct. 30, 1964, p. 1443.

BARNES, ELIZABETH
Changing hospital attitudes. *International Journal of Nursing Studies*, Dec. 1963, p. 11-6.

BARNES, ELIZABETH
People in hospital. Macmillan, 1961.

BARTON, J.
Good nursing is core of Panorama Plan. The circular arrangement of nursing units keeps nurses close to the patients and visitor traffic out of nursing work areas. *The Modern Hospital*, Nov. 1962, p. 85.

BARTON, R.
Unrestricted visiting. *Nursing Times*, Feb. 23, 1962, p. 233-5.

BEAN, W. B.
Some historic sidelights on medicine's forgotten man—the patient. *Nursing Forum*, vol. II, no. 1, 1963, p. 47-68.

BERKOWITZ, N. H., and others
Patient follow-through in the outpatient department. *Nursing Research*, Winter 1963, p. 16-22.

BLUMBERG, JEANNE E., and DRUMMOND, ELEANOR E.
Nursing care of the long term patient. New York, Springer, 1963.

BORDICKS, KATHERINE J.
Patterns of shock: implications for nursing care. New York, Macmillan, 1965.

BRACKETT, MARY E., and FOGT, JOAN R.
Is comprehensive nursing care a realistic goal? *Nursing Outlook*, July 1961, p. 402-4.

NURSING AS A PROFESSION

BRATTON, J. K.
A definition of comprehensive nursing care. *Nursing Outlook*, August 1961, p. 481.

BRIM, ORVILLE G., *and others, editors*
The dying patient: edited by Orville G. Brim, Howard E. Freeman, Sol Levine, and Norman A. Scotch. New York, Russell Sage Foundation, 1970.

BRITISH MEDICAL ASSOCIATION
So you are going into hospital. The Association, [1968].

BROWN, ESTHER LUCILLE
Newer dimensions of patient care. Part 1: the use of the physical and social environment of the general hospital for therapeutic purposes. New York, Russell Sage Foundation 1961.

BROWN, ESTHER LUCILLE
Newer dimensions of patient care. Part 2: improving staff motivation and competence in the general hospital. New York, Russell Sage Foundation, 1962.

BROWN, ESTHER LUCILLE
Newer dimensions of patient care. Part 3: Patients as people. New York, Russell Sage Foundation, 1964.

BUTLER, C.
Some practical results of recording nursing care in gynaecological wards.
In
MCLACHLAN, GORDON, *editor*
Problems and progress in medical care. O.U.P. (for Nuffield P.H.T.) 1964, p. 93.

BUERKI, R. C.
Changing patterns of patient care. *Hospitals*, July 16, 1963, p. 68-70 and 196.

BUTLER, R. M.
Patient studies: student nurse. Edinburgh, Livingstone, 1968.

CENTRAL HEALTH SERVICES COUNCIL
The pattern of the in-patient's day. H.M.S.O., 1961.

CENTRAL HEALTH SERVICES COUNCIL
STANDING NURSING ADVISORY COMMITTEE
Control of noise in hospitals. Ministry of Health, 1961.

CHILDS, E. M.
Nursing involves the care of the whole patient. *Nursing Times*, Sept. 2, 1966, p. 1153-5.

CHRISTMAN, L.
Assisting the patient to learn the "patient role". *The Journal of Nursing Education*, April 1967, p. 17-21.

CLWYD AND DEESIDE HOSPITAL MANAGEMENT COMMITTEE
How well were you looked after in hospital? *The Hospital*, February 1968, p. 59-60.

COLUMBIA UNIVERSITY TEACHERS COLLEGE.
DIVISION OF NURSING EDUCATION
Nursing of adults: a plan for teaching care of adults, by Dorothy W. Smith. New York, Columbia University, 1962.
Nursing education monographs, no. 1.]

COPELAND, O. E.
To know is to understand [Caring for patients from India and Pakistan]. *Nursing Times*, Feb. 26, 1970, Occasional Papers, p. 36.

COSTELLO, C. G.
It's depressing! [Effects of hospitalization]. *Canadian Nurse*, Sept. 1969, p. 43-5.

COVE-SMITH, R.
The patient and his illness. *Nursing Mirror*, July 13, 1962, p. 284-6.

DAN MASON NURSING RESEARCH COMMITTEE
"Home from hospital" the results of a survey conducted among recently discharged hospital patients, by Muriel Skeet. The Committee, 1970.

DONOVAN, H. M.
Determining priorities of nursing care. *Nursing Outlook*, January 1963, p. 44-5.

DUDGEON, M. Y., *and* DAVIDSON, T. W.
Some reactions of patients to their stay in hospital. Belfast Hospital Management Committee, 1965.

EASSON, WILLIAM M.
The dying child: the management of the child or adolescent who is dying. Springfield, Illinois, Thomas, 1970.

ELDER, R. G.
What is the patient saying? *Nursing Forum*, vol. II, no. 1, 1963, p. 25-37.

FADDIS, M. O.
This I believe ... about education's responsibility for patient care. *Nursing Outlook*, Dec. 1965, p. 26-8.

FIELD, MINNA
Patients are people: a medical-social approach to prolonged illness. 3rd edn. New York, Columbia University Press, 1967.

FITZ-GIBBON, A. J.
Development of a patients' committee. *Nursing Mirror*, Feb. 8, 1963, p. 417-8.

FLORENCE NIGHTINGALE INTERNATIONAL NURSES
ASSOCIATION CONFERENCE
Key to better nursing care. *International Nursing Review*, vol. 14, no. 5, 1967, p. 11-8.

FOLTA, JEANNETTE R., *and* DECK, EDITH S., *editors*
A sociological framework for patient care. New York, Wiley, 1966.

FRANCIS, SISTER J.
"Mini-care" at "maxi" demand. *Hospital Topics*, Oct. 1970, p. 21-5.

FREEMAN, R. B., *and others*
Patient care research: report of a symposium. *Medical Care*, July/Sept. 1963, p. 161-3.

FROST, M.
Talking and listening to relatives. *Nursing Times*, Sept. 3, 1970, Occasional Papers, p. 129-32.

FUJIKI, SUMIKO
Identification of patient's needs in nursing care of a mute patient.
In
AMERICAN NURSES' ASSOCIATION
Innovations in nurse-patient relationships: nursing the patient with problems of response. New York, The Association, 1962.

GEORGOPOULOS, BASIL S., *and* MANN, FLOYD C.
Assessment of patient care.
See
GEORGOPOULOS, BASIL S., *and* MANN, FLOYD C.
The community general hospital. New York, Macmillan, 1962.

GOODLAND, N. L.
Clatter does matter. *Nursing Times*, Oct. 19, 1962, p. 1346-7.

GOODLAND, N. L.
Putting the patient in the picture. *Nursing Mirror*, Dec. 31, 1965, p. vii and x.

GUNTER, L., *and others*
A study of three types of nursing care assignments. *Nursing Research*, Winter 1964, p. 20-8.

HARTNETT, W. F., *and others*
Time for nursing care. *American Journal of Nursing*, Aug. 1965, p. 98-101.

HASLAM, P.
Caring for the total patient. Noise in hospitals; its effect on the patient. *Nursing Clinics of North America*, Dec. 1970, p. 715-24.

HAYS, JOYCE SAMHAMMER, *and* LARSON, KENNETH H.
Interacting with patients. New York, Macmillan, 1963.

HENDERSON, C.
Can nursing care hasten recovery? *American Journal of Nursing*, June 1964, p. 80-3.

HIGSON, J.
Patiently waiting. *International Journal of Nursing Studies*, Nov. 1969, p. 189-202.

HUNT, L. W., *and others*
Pre-discharge ward: a step nearer home. *Nursing Times*, June 2, 1967, p. 723-5.

HURST, T. W.
Is noise important in hospitals? *International Journal of Nursing Studies*, Sept. 1966, p. 125-33.

INDIANA UNIVERSITY MEDICAL CENTER
Ritualism in nursing and its effect on patient care: a final report to the Public Health Service, by Virginia H. Walker, Eugene D. Selmanoff and James L. Hawkins. Indianapolis, the University, 1964.

JAMES, IRENE
Nursing, research and patient care.
See
MCLACHLAN, GORDON, *editor*
Problems and progress in medical care. . . . 1964, p. 73.

JOHNSON, J. E., *and others*
Interpersonal relations: the essence of nursing care. *Nursing Forum*, vol. VI, no. 3, 1967, p. 324-34.

JOHNSON, J. E., *and others*
Psychosocial factors in the welfare of surgical patients. *Nursing Research*, Jan./Feb. 1970, p. 18-29.

JOHNSTON, DOROTHY F.
Total patient care: foundations and practice. St. Louis, C. V. Mosby, 1964.
2nd edn., 1968.

KAUFMANN, MARGARET A.
Comfort measures: stereotypes or flexible elements of comprehensive patient care.
In
AMERICAN NURSES' ASSOCIATION
Effects of sterotypes on nursing care. New York, The Association 1962.

KENNEDY, M. J.
An exploratory study of the responses of the patient to the cancellation of his surgery. *International Journal of Nursing Studies*, Sept. 1969, p. 121-31.

LAMBERTSEN, ELEANOR C.
Improving the nursing care of the patient.
In
AMERICAN NURSES' ASSOCIATION
Improvement of nursing practice. New York The Association, 1961.

LAMBERTSEN, ELEANOR C.
Nurses have been trained to nurse people, not machines. (Modern Nursing Practice Department). *Modern Hospital*, Oct. 1965, p. 144.

LAMBERTSEN, ELEANOR C.
Nursing care plan should reflect present and future patient needs. *The Modern Hospital*, Oct. 1964, p. 128.

LEVINE, M. E.
The intransigent patient. *American Journal of Nursing*, Oct. 1970, p. 2106-11.

LEVINE, M. E.
This I believe . . . about patient-centered care. *Nursing Outlook*, July 1967, p. 53-5.

LEY, P., *and* SPELMAN, M. S.
Communicating with the patient. Staples Press, 1967.

LOOMIS, M. E., *and* DODENHOFF, J .T.
Working with informal patient groups. *American Journal of Nursing*, Sept. 1970, p. 1939-44.

LUDEMANN, R. S.
Empathy—a component of therapeutic nursing. *Nursing Forum*, vol. VII, no. 3, 1968, p. 275-88.

LUNT, J.
Bridging the gap in continuity of care. Liaison schemes between hospital and district nurses in Liverpool. *Nursing Times*, Mar. 19, 1970, p. 372.

MACDONALD, F. G.
Longer visiting hours? *Nursing Times*, June 4, 1970, p. 730.

MCGHEE, ANNE
The patient's attitude to nursing care. Livingstone, 1961.

MACKEITH, RONALD
Empathy in the hospital. *Nursing Times*, Feb. 6, 1969, p. 170-2.

MCNULTY, B.
Discharge of the terminally-ill patient. *Nursing Times*, Sept. 10, 1970, p. 1160-2.

MCWALTERS, BEVERLY H.
The relationship of attitudes to nursing practice.
In
AMERICAN NURSES' ASSOCIATION
Effects of sterotypes on nursing care. New York, The Association, 1962.

MADDISON, D.
The nurse and the dying patient. *Nursing Times*, Feb. 27, 1969, p. 265-6.

MARQUAND, C. J.
Planned nursing care applied. *New Zealand Nursing Journal*, May 1970, p. 11 and 13-4.

MATHENEY, RUTH V., *and others*
Fundamentals of patient-centered nursing, by Ruth V. Matheney, Breda T. Nolan, Alice M. Ehrhart, Gerald J. Griffin and Joanne King Griffin. St. Louis, C. V. Mosby, 1964.
2nd edn., 1968.

MAUKSCH, HANS O., *and* TAGLIACOZZO, DAISY M.
The patient's view of the patient role. Part 1: Analysis of interviews. 2nd edn. Chicago, Illinois Institute of Technology, 1963.

MAUREEN, SISTER
Attainment of goals for patients through changes in the nurse-patient-doctor relationship.
In
AMERICAN NURSES' ASSOCIATION
The nurse-patient-doctor triadic relationships: effects on nursing care of the patient. New York, The Association, 1962.

MAY, P. R. A., *and* WILKINSON, M.
Admitting a patient is therapy. The nursing role changes when the admission procedure in a psychiatric hospital recognizes the individual worth of each patient and makes of his admission a therapeutic process. *Nursing Outlook*, June 1963, p. 447-9.

MERCADANTE, L. T.
Unit manager plan gives nurses time to care for the patients. *The Modern Hospital*, August 1962, p. 73.

MERTZ, HILDA
Nurse actions that reduce stress in patients.
In
AMERICAN NURSES' ASSOCIATION
Emergency intervention by the nurse. New York, The Association, 1962.

MIDDLETON, B. M.
Use of assessment charts—in patient care. *Nursing Mirror*, Nov. 9, 1962, p. 131-2.

MINCKLEY, B. B.
A study of noise and its relationship to patient discomfort in the recovery room. *Nursing Research*, May/June 1968, p. 247-50.

NURSING AS A PROFESSION

MODERN HOSPITAL
Patient gives needle back to nurses (a critical appraisal of nursing care). *Modern Hospital*, June 1963, p. 69-70, 72-4, 146 and 147.

MOON, W. R.
Direct patient care by nursing personnel. *Hospital Management*, Jan. 1967, p. 68-70.

MOORE, J. S.
All rooms are private in this compact nursing unit plan. *Hospitals*, Oct. 1, 1963, p. 35-6 and 39-41.

MUECKE, M. A.
Overcoming the language barrier. *Nursing Outlook*, April 1970, p. 53-4.

NATIONAL LEAGUE FOR NURSING
Continuity of nursing care from hospital to home; a study in a voluntary general hospital. New York, The League, 1966.

NELSON, KATHERINE R.
How will individualized care, based on the patient's nursing needs, be provided?
In
AMERICAN NURSES' ASSOCIATION
Improvement of nursing practice. New York, The Association, 1961.

NEWSOM, BETTY H.
Nursing intervention in panic. 1962.
In
AMERICAN NURSES' ASSOCIATION
Emergency intervention by the nurse. New York, The Association, 1962.

NURSING CLINICS OF NORTH AMERICA
Symposium on the ambulatory patient. *Nursing Clinics of North America*, June 1970, p. 195-275.

NURSING CLINICS OF NORTH AMERICA
Symposium on nursing in long-term illness. *Nursing Clinics of North America*, Mar. 1970, p. 1-84.

NURSING MIRROR
Solving the problem of Noise in Hospital. *Nursing Mirror*, Sept. 8, 1961, p. 1542-3.

NURSING TIMES
The needs of the dying. *Nursing Times*, Nov. 13, 1969, p. 1450-1.

NURSING TIMES
Nursing care studies (second series): eight outstanding nursing care studies reprinted from the Nursing Times, with an introduction on how to write a nursing care study. Macmillan, 1966.

OXFORD REGIONAL HOSPITAL BOARD
Nursing care in a modern hospital. Oxford, The Board, 1962.
[Operational Research Unit, no. 2.]

PATTERSON, THORA K.
Patient-centered nursing. *Hospitals*, Nov. 1, 1966, p. 80, 82 and 84.

PEARSON, LEONARD, *editor*
Death and dying: current issues in the treatment of the dying person. Cleveland, Ohio, Chase Western Reserve University, 1969.

PEPLAU, H. E.
Professional closeness ... as a special kind of involvement with a patient, client or family group. *Nursing Forum*, vol. VIII, no. 4, 1969, p. 342-60.

PERCY, D. M.
Organized home care—a new-old dimension in patient care (Family and patient). *International Nursing Review*, vol. 9, no. 3, 1963, p. 31-7.

PETERSON, GRACE
Working with others for patient care. Dubuque, Iowa, Wm. C. Brown, 1968.

PLATT, D. M.
Illness and dying seen as status changes. *The Australian Nurses' Journal*, May 1969, p. 92 and 94-6.

POLAND, M., *and others*
PETO. A system for assessing and meeting patient care needs. *American Journal of Nursing*, July 1970, p. 1479-82.

PRENTICE, W. E.
Assessment of needs of patient care. *The Hospital*, July 1965, p. 378-82.

PRIDE, L. F.
An adrenal stress index as a criterion measure for nursing. *Nursing Research*, July/Aug. 1968, p. 292-303.

QUINT, J. C.
The threat of death: some consequences for patients and nurses. *Nursing Forum*, vol. VIII, no. 3, 1969, p. 286-300.

RAPHAEL, W.
Do we know what the patients think? A survey comparing the views of patients, staff and committee members. *International Journal of Nursing Studies*, Aug. 1967, p. 209-22.

RAPHAEL, W.
"If I could alter one thing ..." *Mental Health*, April 1965, p. 64-8.

RAPHAEL, W.
Patient care—1. *Nursing Times*, Nov. 26, 1965, p. 1606-8.

RAPHAEL, W.
Patient Care—2. Patients and staff—their likes and dislikes. *Nursing Times*, Dec. 3, 1965, p. 1654-6.

RAPHAEL, W.
Patient Care—3. "Nurse, nurse, for better or worse". *Nursing Times*, Dec. 10, 1965, p. 1686-7.

RAPHAEL, W.
Patient Care—4. Priorities in reconditioning old-fashioned wards. *Nursing Times*, Dec. 17, 1965, p. 1725-7.

RAPHAEL, W.
Patient Care—5. "A little of what you fancy ..." *Nursing Times*, Dec. 24, 1965, p. 1759-61.

RAYNER, C.
Opening the doors. Unrestricted visiting. *Nursing Times*, Mar. 31, 1961, p. 414-5.

REID, M., *and* WADDICOR, P. E. E.
Continuity of patient care (in Wythenshawe). *Nursing Times*, June 18, 1970, p. 786-8.

RIEDEL, DONALD C., *and* FITZPATRIC, THOMAS B.
Patterns of patient care: a study of hospital use in six diagnoses. Ann Arbor, University of Michigan, 1964.

RITVO, M. M.
Who are "Good" and "Bad" patients? *The Modern Hospital*, June 1963, p. 79-81.

ROBINSON, LISA
Psychological aspects of the care of hospitalized patients. Philadelphia, Davis, 1968.

ROEMER, M. I., *and* ARNOLD, L. M.
How to measure patient-centered service. *The Modern Hospital*, Aug. 1962, p. 81.

ROWE, A.
On being a patient: characteristics of hospital care. *Nursing Times*, Oct. 23, 1969, p. 1376-7.

RUSSELL, S.
The patient and the relative. *Nursing Times*, Nov. 23, 1962, p. 1484-5.

SANAZARO, P. J.
Seminar on research in patient care. *Medical Care*, Jan./Mar. 1966, p. 43-50.

SCHINDALL, H.
Better nursing supervision brings better patient care. *The Modern Hospital*, Feb. 1964, p. 102-3 and 148.

SCHWARTZ, D. R.
Research in patient care. A fruitful learning experience for selected students of nursing. *Nursing Outlook*, Feb. 1962, p. 108-10.

SHEPARD, M. W.
This I believe ... about questioning the right to die. *Nursing Outlook*, Oct. 1968, p. 22-5.

SHONE
The young chronic sick. *Nursing Mirror*, June 28, 1968, p. 21-5.

SIEGEL, N. H.
What is a therapeutic community? Some revealing thought on what is and is not "good" for patients. *Nursing Outlook*, May 1964, p. 49-51.

SIMON, J. RICHARD
Nurses' ratings of patient welfare as criterion measures in the health sciences. *Occupational Psychology*, Jan. and April 1961, p. 10-22.

SIMON, J. RICHARD
Systematic ratings of patient welfare: nurses' ratings of their patients' condition and progress can lead to improved patient care. *Nursing Outlook*, July 1961, p. 432-6.

SKIPPER, JAMES K., *and* LEONARD, ROBERT C., editors
Social interaction and patient care. Philadelphia, Lippincott, 1965.

SLATER, P.
Maximum patient care. *International Nursing Review*, vol. 10, no. 1, 1964, p. 37-42.

SMITH, A.
The patient in the community. *Nursing Times*, May 17, 1968, Occasional Papers, p. 77-9.

SMITH, D. M.
A clinical nursing tool [A guide to eliciting and organizing data that can be used to plan and evaluate nursing care]. *American Journal of Nursing*, Nov. 1968, p. 2384-8.

SMITH, D. W.
Patienthood and its threat to privacy. *American Journal of Nursing*, Mar. 1969, p. 509-13.

SORENSON, G.
Dependency—a factor in nursing care. *American Journal of Nursing*, Aug. 1966, p. 1762-3.

TAGLIACOZZO, D. M.
Patient expectations and the patient role. *The Canadian Nurse*, Sept. 1963, p. 840-6.

TAYLOR, C. D.
The hospital patient's social dilemma. *American Journal of Nursing*, Oct. 1965, p. 96-9.

TEWINKLE, M. B.
What do our patients tell us? *Journal of Practical Nursing*, Aug. 1970, p. 24-6 and 37-8.

TRITES, D. K., *and* GREEN, R. M.
Hospital visiting: the patients' point of view. *Nursing Outlook*, Aug. 1970, p. 44-5.

TRYON, P. A.
Patient participation vs. patient passivity. *Nursing Forum*, vol. II, no. 2, 1963, p. 48-57.

VELAZQUEZ, JANET M.
Alienation [in patients]. *American Journal of Nursing*, Feb. 1969, p. 301-4.

WALLACE, C. M.
Institutional neurosis and the nurse. *Nursing Mirror*, Feb. 21, 1969, p. 30.

WATKIN, B. V.
Noisy vacuum cleaners. Is this the answer? *Nursing Times*, Nov. 9, 1962, p. 1432-3.

WENSLEY, EDITH
Nursing service without walls: a call to action to all communities coast to coast. New York, National League for Nursing, 1963.

WERNER, ANITA M.
The angry patient.
In
AMERICAN NURSES' ASSOCIATION
Innovations in nurse-patient relationships: automatic or reasoned nurse actions. New York, The Association, 1962.

WHITE, RUTH PRESTON
Patient care classification: methods and application by Ruth White, Dana Quade and Kerr L. White. Washington, U.S. Public Health Service, 1967.

WILLIAMS, G. W.
Illness and personality. *American Journal of Nursing*, June 1963, p. 85-7.

WILSON, ALBERTA B.
Long-term nursing care in rural Minnesota. *Nursing Outlook*, Oct. 1964, p. 68-70.

WOODS, M. F.
Measuring a patient's needs and progress. *Nursing Outlook*, October 1966, p. 38-41.

ZERBE, RUTH A.
Nursing intervention in rejection.
In
AMERICAN NURSES' ASSOCIATION
Innovations in nurse-patient relationships: nursing the patient with problems of response. New York, The Association, 1962.

PROGRESSIVE PATIENT CARE

ANDERSON, M. H.
The influence of progressive patient care on central service. *Hospital Management*, Oct. 1961, p. 92, and 94.

BIRMINGHAM REGIONAL HOSPITAL BOARD
Progressive patient care. Report of a symposium held on 16 and 17 June 1962. *Nursing Times*, June 29, 1962, p. 849.

DEVRIES, R. A.
Progressive patient care. *Hospitals*, June 16, 1970, p. 43-8.

EDGEWORTH, DOROTHA *and others*
Progressive patient care—part 1—what is it? What does it involve? What should your hospital do about it? *Hospital Administration in Canada*, March 1963, p. 26-32; part II. *Hospital Administration in Canada*, April 1963, p. 29-36.

EXTON-SMITH, A. N.
Progressive patient care for geriatric patients. *Nursing Mirror*, June 29, 1962, p. ii, iii and iv.

GREAT BRITAIN. MINISTRY OF HEALTH
Progressive patient care: interim report of a departmental working group. H.M.S.O., 1962.

GROVE, W. A.
Why Chicago Hospital is expanding its progressive patient care planning. *The Modern Hospital*, April 1966, p. 99-102.

IRVINE, M.
Progressive patient care in Northern Ireland. *Nursing Times*, Nov. 29, 1968, Occasional Papers, p. 185-6.

LEES, W., *and* BIDDULPH, C.
Progressive patient care—1. *Nursing Times*, Jan. 26, 1968, Occasional Papers, p. 13-6.

LEES, W., *and* BIDDULPH, C.
Progressive patient care—2. *Nursing Times*, Feb. 2, 1968, Occasional Papers, p. 17-20.

LEES, W., *and* BIDDULPH, C.
Survey of progressive patient care. [Ministry of Health], 1966[?].

MCCUTCHEON, M. I.
Progressive patient care surveys—1. *Nursing Times*, May 14, 1965, p. 661-2.

McCutcheon, M. I.
Progressive patient care surveys—2. Preparation and method. *Nursing Times*, May 21, 1965, p. 692-5.

Magherafelt Hospital, Ulster
Progressive patient care in an Irish hospital. *Nursing Times*, Oct. 27, 1961, p. 1386-8.

Morgan, H.
Progressive nursing care. *Hospital Management Planning and Equipment*, Jan. 1965, p. 41-3.

O'Connor, V.
Patient handling in progressive care. *British Hospital Journal and Social Service Review*, April 3, 1970, p. 622.

Pennington, M.
Continuity of care. A responsibility of the professional nurse. *Occupational Health Nursing*, Sept. 1969, p. 14-6.

Rorem, C. R.
Progressive patient care. *World Hospitals*, July 1969, p. 143-7.

St. Helen's Hospital, Hastings
Progressive patient care in a geriatric department. *Nursing Times*, June 1, 1962, p. 701-2.

United States Public Health Service
Division of Hospital and Medical Facilities
Elements of progressive patient care. Rev. edn. Washington, Govt. Printing Office, 1962.

United States Public Health Service
Division of Hospital and Medical Facilities
The progressive patient care hospital: Estimating bed needs. Washington, U.S. Dept. Health, Education and Welfare, 1963.

Weeks, Lewis K.
The complete gamut of progressive patient care in a community hospital: an experience brochure. Battle Creek, Michigan, W. K. Kellogg Foundation, [1967].

Weeks, Lewis E., *and* Griffith, John R., editors
Progressive patient care: an anthology. Ann Arbor, University of Michigan, 1964.

Wren, G. R.
Progressive patient care. *Practical Nurses Digest*, May 1963, p. 78-9.

QUALITY OF CARE

American Nurses' Association
Establishing standards for nursing practice. *American Journal of Nursing*, July 1969, p. 1458-63.

Barr, Alex
Measuring nursing care.
In
McLachlan, Gordon, editor
Problems and progress in medical care. O.U.P. (for Nuffield P.H.T.) 1964, p. 77.

Blumberg, M. S., *and* Drew, J. A.
Methods for assessing nursing care quality. *Hospitals*, Nov. 1, 1963, p. 72, 74, 76-7 and 80.

Brodt, D. E., *and* Anderson, E. H.
Validation of a patient welfare evaluation instrument. *Nursing Research*, Spring 1967, p. 167-9.

Campion, F. Lillian
A report on the project for the evaluation of the quality of nursing service. Ottawa, Canadian Nurses' Association, 1966.

Canadian Nurse
Quality patient care. *Canadian Nurse*, Dec. 1965, p. 975-8.

Charles Marie Frank, Sister
The effect of diversity of preparation of nursing personnel on the quality of patient care. *International Nursing Review*, vol. 9, no. 4, 1963, p. 48-55.

Daniels, R. R.
Can hospitals measure the quality of nursing care? Here's the program at Sequoia. *Hospital Topics*, April 1964, p. 35-7 and 47.

Davis, K. G.
Give nurses the chance to explore these twelve routes to better care. *Modern Hospital*, Oct. 1968, p. 82-5.

Densen, P. M.
Problems in the development of adequate criteria. *Nursing Research*, Fall, 1962, p. 207-8.
See also
Hasselmeyer, E. G.
Schlotfeldt, R. M.

Donabedian, A.
Promoting quality through evaluating the process of patient care. *Medical Care*, May/June 1968, p. 181-202.

Drew, J.
Determining quality of nursing care. *American Journal of Nursing*, Oct. 1964, p. 82-5.

Dunn, Helen W., *and* Morgan, Elizabeth M.
The nursing audit. New York, National League for Nursing, 1968.

Dunn, M. A.
Development of an instrument to measure nursing performance. *Nursing Research*, Nov./Dec. 1970, p. 502-10.

Durham, R. C.
How to evaluate nursing performance. *Hospital Management*, May 1970, p. 24-5, 28 and 32.

Dwyer, J. M., *and* Schmitt, J. A.
Using the computer to evaluate clinical performance. *Nursing Forum*, vol. VIII, no. 3, 1969, p. 266-75.

Edgecumbe, R. H.
How the Commission for Administrative Services in Hospitals (CASH) helps nurses improve care. *The Modern Hospital*, May 1966, p. 97-9.

Ewell, C. M.,
What patients really think about their nursing care. *Modern Hospital*, December 1967, p. 106-8.

Feisel, K.
What quality nursing means today. *International Nursing Review*, vol. 9, no. 6, 1963, p. 37-45.

Georgopoulos, Basil S., *and* Mann, Floyd C.
Factors affecting the quality of patient care.
In
Georgopoulos, Basil S., *and* Mann, Floyd C.
The community general hospital. New York, Macmillan, 1962.

Goldstein, J.
Exploring attitudes that affect nursing care. *Nursing Outlook*, June 1968, p. 50-1.

Graham, L. E.
Planning priorities in *quality* nursing care. *Journal of Nursing Education*, Nov. 1969, p. 9-18 and 44.

Greenough, K.
Determining standards for nursing care. *American Journal of Nursing*, Oct. 1968, p. 2153-7.

Grosicki, J. P., *and others*
Nursing care plans: survey of status and opinions about current usage. *Journal of Psychiatric Nursing*, Nov./Dec. 1967, p. 567-79 and 582-5.

Hasselmeyer, E. G.
Problems in the development of adequate criteria [in assessing the quality of nursing care]. *Nursing Research*, Fall 1962, p. 208-11.
See also
Densen, P. M.
Schlotfeldt, R. M.

HERRING, SISTER CARREN,
Ohio hospitals' quality control and staff utilization program. *Hospital Progress*, July 1970, p. 38-44.

HOWLAND, D., and MCDOWELL, W. E.
The measurement of patient care: a conceptual framework. *Nursing Research*, Winter 1964, p. 4-7.

HUTTON, G. A.
It all began with talk. *International Nursing Review*, vol. 10, no. 4, 1964, p. 13-5.

LAMBERTSEN, ELEANOR C.
Evaluating the quality of nursing care. *Hospitals*, Nov. 1, 1965, p. 61-6.

LAMBERTSEN, ELEANOR C.
Graduate nurses' duty to define standards of good nursing care. *The Modern Hospital*, Aug. 1964, p. 130.

LAMBERTSEN, ELEANOR C.
Nurses need an intelligent definition of what good nursing care really is. *The Modern Hospital*, Oct. 1962, p. 110.

LAMBERTSEN, ELEANOR C.
Nursing research should emphasize improving the quality of patient care. *The Modern Hospital*, April 1967, p. 158.

LANDDECK, J. R.
Efficiency and quality of patient care. *Hospitals*, Sept. 16, 1970, p. 41-4.

LOWRY, MURIEL V.
A survey to determine the nursing care needs of patients in certain standard welfare wards (indigent) of the Ottawa Civic Hospital following their discharge from the hospital. Ottawa, 1962.

MCFARLANE, J. K.
Study of nursing care—the first two years of a research project. *International Nursing Review*, vol. 17, no. 2, 1970, p. 101-8.

MCKENZIE, H.
In pursuit of quality nursing. *The Australian Nurses' Journal*, April 1967, p. 80-2.

MINCKLEY, B. B.
Justification for a trial-and-error theory of nursing. *Nursing Research*, Nov./Dec. 1970, p. 526-9.

MYERS, R. S.
Lack of liaison in hospital can impair the quality of patient care. *The Modern Hospital*, Feb. 1966, p. 122.

NADLER, G., and SAHNEY, V.
A descriptive model of nursing care. [Development of a mathematical model of measuring care by an interdisciplinary group coordinated by industrial engineers at the University of Wisconsin Hospitals]. *American Journal of Nursing*, Feb. 1969, p. 336-41.

NATIONAL LEAGUE FOR NURSING
Criteria for quality. New York, The League, 1967.

NATIONAL LEAGUE FOR NURSING
DEPARTMENT OF HOSPITAL NURSING
Quest for quality: a self evaluation guide to patient care. New York, The League, 1966.

ORLEANS, DONALD
The use of managerial tools in evaluating and improving the quality of nursing care: a survey of selected hospitals in New Jersey. New York, National League for Nursing, 1970.
[The League exchange, no. 92.]

ORTELT, J. A.
The development of a scale for rating clinical performance. *The Journal of Nursing Education*, Jan. 1966, p. 15-7.

OXFORD REGIONAL HOSPITAL BOARD
OPERATIONAL RESEARCH UNIT
Measurement of nursing care. Headington, The Board, 1967.

PHANEUF, M. C.
A nursing audit method. Appraisal of patient care from the records of service can be developed by nurses into a specific method of audit. *Nursing Outlook*, May 1964, p. 42-5.

POWELL, M. B.
The modern health service and the nurse.
In
COLLEGE OF GENERAL PRACTITIONERS
The quality of medical care; report of a symposium. . . . *Journal of the College of G.P.s, Supplement*, no. 3, May 1966, p. iii-36.

POWELL, M. B.
Nursing training and standards of care. *Nursing Times*, Aug. 30, 1963, p. 1081-2.

QUINT, J. C.
Delineation of qualitative aspects of nursing care. *Nursing Research*, Fall 1962, p. 204-6.

REITER, FRANCES
Choosing the better part. *American Journal of Nursing*, Dec. 1964, p. 65-8.

REITER, FRANCES, and KAKOSH, MARGUERITE E.
Quality of nursing care: a report of a field study to establish criteria, conducted at Division of Nursing Education, Teachers College, Columbia University, 1950-1954. New York, Graduate School of Nursing, New York Medical College, 1963.

ROYAL COLLEGE OF NURSING AND NATIONAL COUNCIL OF NURSES OF THE UNITED KINGDOM. RESEARCH DISCUSSION GROUP
A record of the proceedings of group discussions on methods of assessing standards of nursing care, held at High Wycombe, 12th-14th June 1964. The College, 1964.

SCHLOTFELDT, R. M.
Problems in the development of adequate criteria. *Nursing Research*, Fall 1962, p. 211-3.
See also
DENSEN, P. M.
HASSELMEYER, E. G.

SCHWARTZ, DORIS
Quality in nursing service. *Nursing Times*, June 30, 1967, p. 862.

SCHWARTZ, DORIS
Some thoughts on quality in nursing service. *International Nursing Review*, vol. 13, no. 2, 1967, p. 29-34.

SCHWARTZ, DORIS
Some thoughts on quality in nursing service. [Geneva], W.H.O., 1967[?].

SCHWARTZ, DORIS
Toward more precise evaluation of patients' needs. *Nursing Outlook*, May 1965, p. 42-4.

SEIVWRIGHT, M. J.
Some observations on quality nursing care. *The Jamaican Nurse*, Aug./Sept. 1964, p. 34-5.

SMITH, D. B., and METZNER, C. A.
Differential perceptions of health care quality in a prepaid group practice. *Medical Care*, July/Aug. 1970, p. 264-75.

SMITH, D. W.
Deterrents to quality. *The Canadian Nurse*, June 1965, p. 458-60.

TATE, BARBARA L.
Test of a nursing performance evaluation instrument. New York, National League for Nursing, 1964.

UNITED STATES PUBLIC HEALTH SERVICE
Toward quality in nursing: needs and goals: report of the Surgeon General's Consultant Group on Nursing. Washington, U.S. Government Printing Office, 1963.

WALKER, VIRGINIA H.
Nursing and ritualistic practice. New York, Macmillan, 1967.

WEIL, T. P.
Will computer installations improve quality of patient care? *Hospital Management*, Sept. 1967, p. 40-3.

WEISS, JAMES M. A., *editor*
Nurses, patients and social systems: the effects of skilled nursing intervention upon institutionalized patients. Columbia, University of Missouri Press, 1968.

WESTERN COUNCIL ON HIGHER EDUCATION FOR NURSING *and*
WESTERN REGIONAL COUNCIL OF STATE LEAGUES FOR NURSING
Development of personnel toward quality nursing care. Colorado, Western Interstate Commission for Higher Education, 1964.

YURA, HELEN, *and* WALSH, MARY B., *editors*
The nursing process: assessing, planning, implementing, and evaluating: the proceedings of the Continuing Education series, conducted at The Catholic University of America ... 1967. Washington, D.C., The University, 1967.

TEAM NURSING

ALLEN, G.
Team nursing's not new but its satisfying. *The New Zealand Nursing Journal*, Sept. 1970, p. 5-9.

AULD, M. G.
Team nursing in a maternity hospital. *International Journal of Nursing Studies*, June 1970, p. 57-65.

BELTRAN, HELEN G., *and others*
Guide for leadership in team nursing. New York, National League for Nursing, 1961.

BROOKS, E. A.
Team Nursing—1961. *American Journal of Nursing*, April 1961, p. 87-91.

BROWN, ELAINE, *and* ROCHE, JOHN
Methods study shaped team nursing plan. *Modern Hospital*, Sept. 1966, p. 121-3.

CORONA, D. F., *and* BLACK, E. E.
One hospital's approach to team nursing. *Nursing Outlook*, July 1963, p. 506-7.

CRUMPTON, E., *and* ROGERS, E. P.
Some effects of team nursing on a psychiatric ward. *Nursing Research*, Summer 1963, p. 181-2.

DOUGLAS, LAURA MAE, *and* BEVIS, EM OLIVIA
Team leadership in action: principles and application to staff nursing situations. St. Louis, Mosby, 1970.

ETHERINGTON, A.
Team nursing in the USA. Reactions of an observer. *Nursing Times*, Jan. 22, 1970, p. 110-2.

FIELDING, V. V.
New team plan frees nurses to nurse. *The Modern Hospital*, May 1967, p. 122-4.

FOSBERG, G. C.
Teaching management skills in a team nursing setting. *Nursing Outlook*, April 1967, p. 67-8.

GERARD, SISTER MARY.
Recognizing the nursing service director as an administration team member. *Hospital Progress*, Mar. 1969, p. 100-5.

GERMAINE, A.
Problems of producing an effective nursing team. *Hospital Administration in Canada*, Mar. 1970, p. 36, 38 and 40.

JENKINSON, V. M.
Team Nursing. *Nursing Times*, Mar. 3, 1961, p. 264-6.

KILOURIE, C. W.
Relationship of the head nurse to team nursing. *Hospital Management*, Feb. 1967, p. 47-51.

KRON, THORA
Nursing team leadership. Philadelphia, Saunders, 1961. 2nd edn., 1966.

MERCY HOSPITAL, PITTSBURGH
Manual for team nursing. St. Louis, Catholic Hospital Association, 1968.

POTTER, T. I.
The health-team approach to total patient-care. *Hospital Administration in Canada*, Nov. 1969, p. 53-6.

REGINA ELIZABETH, SISTER
The team assignment plan. *Hospital Progress*, Feb. 1965, p. 76-82 and 104.

SWANSBURG, RUSSELL C.
An experiment in team nursing. *Nursing Outlook*, Aug. 1968, p. 45-7.

SWANSBURG, RUSSELL C.
Team nursing: a programmed learning experience. New York, Putman, 1968.

WAR AND DISASTER NURSING

AMERICAN NURSES' ASSOCIATION
The role of the nurse in disaster. New York, The Association, 1964.

AMERICAN NURSES' ASSOCIATION
Three approaches to disaster preparedness; a symposium. ... New York, The Association, 1966.

AMERICAN NURSES' ASSOCIATION *and*
NATIONAL FEDERATION OF LICENSED PRACTICAL NURSES
The role of the licensed practical nurse in disaster. New York, A.N.A., 1966.

FIEDLER, D. E.
Medical care in Viet Nam. *Occupational Health Nursing*, Mar. 1969, p. 11-4.

HERRMANN, J. B.
Thermal injuries and their treatment in disaster. *American Association of Industrial Nurses Journal*, May 1963, p. 11-5.

MAHONEY, ROBERT F.
Emergency and disaster nursing. 2nd edn. Collier-Macmillan, 1969.

MURRAY, V. P.
Disaster planning. *New Zealand Nursing Journal*, Feb. 1970, p. 10-2.

NATIONAL LEAGUE FOR NURSING
Disaster nursing preparation: report of a pilot project conducted in four schools of nursing and one hospital service, prepared by Mary V. Neal. New York, National League for Nursing, 1963.

NEAL, MARY V.
Progress report on NLN project on instruction in nursing in national defense in the basic program.
In
AMERICAN NURSES' ASSOCIATION
Report of a conference for State Boards of Nursing. New York, The Association, 1961.

NURSING JOURNAL OF INDIA
Emergency care for accident victims. *Nursing Journal of India*, Aug. 1969, p. 273-4.

NURSING MIRROR
New "Department of nuclear medicine" established in the U.S. *Nursing Mirror*, Sept. 1, 1967, p. 506.

SEXTON, H. M.
Morgue duty. [Nurses involved identifying victims of an air crash.] *American Journal of Nursing*, May 1970, p. 1054-6.

SULLIVAN, CATHERINE M.
The place of nursing in civil defense and defense mobilization.
In
AMERICAN NURSES' ASSOCIATION
Report of a conference for State Boards of Nursing. New York, The Association, 1961.

TRITES, D. K., *and others*
Radio nursing units prove best in controlled study. *Modern Hospital*, April 1969, p. 94-9.

VERHONICK, P. J.
Nursing care of traumatic injuries. *American Association of Industrial Nurses Journal*, May 1963, p. 7-10.

WALLIN, JUDITH
ANA program on nursing in national defense.
In
AMERICAN NURSES' ASSOCIATION
Report of a conference for State Boards of Nursing. New York, The Association, 1961.

SPECIALITIES OF KNOWLEDGE AND PRACTICE

ALLERGIES

FIELDER, R. E.
Food allergies. *District Nursing*, Sept. 1968, p. 118-9.

MILNER, F. H.
Some unusual cases of allergy. *Nursing Mirror*, June 7, 1963, p. 204-6.

ROBERTS, T. E.
Hay fever—a forgotten allergy? *District Nursing*, Sept. 1968, p. 121-2.

GARLAND, H.
Neurological problems. Special investigations—1. *Nursing Times*, Jan. 12, 1968, p. 39-41.

GARLAND, H.
Neurological problems. Special investigations—2. *Nursing Times*, Jan. 19, 1968, p. 89-91.

ANATOMY AND PHYSIOLOGY

ANTHONY, CATHERINE PARKER
Basic concepts in anatomy and physiology: a programmed presentation. St. Louis, Mosby, 1966.
2nd edn., 1970.

ARMSTRONG, KATHARINE F.
Aids to anatomy and physiology for nurses. 7th edn. Bailliere, Tindall and Cassell, 1964.

BOCOCK, E. J., and HAINES, R. WHEELER
Applied anatomy for nurses. 3rd edn. Edinburgh, Livingstone, 1965.

BROOME, W. E.
Fluid balance chart for teaching student nurses. *Nursing Mirror*, July 29, 1966, p. 402-3.

BURDON, IAN M., and MACDONALD, S., editors
Anatomical atlas for nurses and students. 4th edn., rev. by John Mackenzie. Faber, 1962.

BURGESS, AUDREY
The nurse's guide to fluid and electrolyte balance. New York, McGraw-Hill, 1970.

BURGESS, R. E.
Fluids and electrolytes. *American Journal of Nursing*, Oct. 1965, p. 90-5.

CAIRNEY, JOHN, and CAIRNEY, J.
The human body: a survey of structure and function. Christchurch, N.Z., Peryer, 1966.
[Supersedes "First studies in anatomy and physiology", *q.v.*]

CHAFFEE, ELLEN E.
Laboratory manual in physiology and anatomy, with study guide questions and practical applications. 2nd edn. Philadelphia, Lippincott, 1963.

CHAFFEE, ELLEN E., and GREISHEIMER, ESTHER M.
Basic physiology and anatomy. Philadelphia, Lippincott, 1964.

DEAN, W. B., and others
Basic concepts of anatomy and physiology: a programmed study, by W. B. Dean, G. E. Farrar and A. J. Zoldos. Philadelphia, Lippincott, 1966.

DICKENS, MARGARET L.
Fluid and electrolyte balance: a programmed text. Philadelphia, Davis, 1967.
2nd edn., 1970.

DODD, I. A.
Programmed physiology. Methuen, 1967.

DODDS, CHARLES
The nurse and the biochemist. *Nursing Mirror*, Oct. 18, 1963, p. 52-4; Oct. 25, 1963, p. 84.

DUTCHER, ISABEL E., and FIELO, SANDRA B.
Water and electrolytes: implications for nursing practice. New York, Macmillan, 1967.

FIELO, SANDRA B.
Teaching fluid and electrolyte balance. *Nursing Outlook*, March 1965, p. 43-4.

FORREST, JANE
Questions and answers in anatomy and physiology for pupil nurses. Edward Arnold, 1967.

FORREST, JANE
Practical nursing and anatomy for pupil nurses. Edward Arnold, 1966.

FOURMAN, P.
Water, thirst and polyuria. *Nursing Mirror*, July 26, 1963, p. 355-6.

GIBSON, JOHN
Human biology: an elementary anatomy and physiology for students and nurses. 2nd edn. Faber, 1967.

GLENISTER, T. W. A., and ROSS, JEAN R. W.
Anatomy and physiology for nurses. Heinemann, 1965.

GOWLAND, W. P., and CAIRNEY, JOHN
Anatomy and physiology for nurses. 6th edn. Christchurch, New Zealand, Peryer, 1961.
7th edn., 1965.

GRUNHUT, I.
Water and electrolyte balance—1. *Nursing Times*, Sept. 21, 1962, p. 1203.

GRUNHUT, I.
Water and electrolyte balance—2. *Nursing Times*, Sept. 28, 1962, p. 1237.

HOLMES, MARGUERITE C., and GOTTLIEB, MARVIN I., editors
Anatomy and physiology: 1,500 multiple choice questions and referenced answers. New York, Medical Examination Publishing Co., 1966. [Nursing examination review book, vol. 5.]
2nd edn., 1969.

KIMBER, DIANA CLIFFORD, and GRAY, CAROLYN E.
Textbook of anatomy and physiology, revised by Caroline E. Stackpole and Lutie C. Leavell. 14th edn. New York, Macmillan, 1961.
15th edn., 1966.

LAMBERT, K., and BLAIR, E.
Pathophysiology and management of bacteremic shock. *AORN Journal*, Nov. 1969, p. 67-71.

LANGLEY, L. L., and others
Dynamic anatomy and physiology, by L. L. Langley, E. Cheraskin and Ruth Sleeper. 2nd edn. New York, McGraw-Hill, 1963.

MCNAUGHT, ANN B.
Companion to "Illustrated Physiology". Edinburgh, Livingstone, 1965.
2nd edn., 1970.

MCNAUGHT, ANN B., and CALLANDER, ROBIN
Illustrated physiology. Edinburgh, Livingstone, 1963.
2nd edn., 1970.

METHENY, NORMA MILLIGAN, and SNIVELY, WILLIAM D.
Nurses' handbook of fluid balance. Philadelphia, Lippincott, 1967.

SPECIALITIES

PEARCE, EVELYN C.
Anatomy and physiology for nurses: a complete textbook for the preliminary state examination. 14th edn. Faber, 1962.
14th edn., revised 1966.
15th edn., 1968, entitled: Anatomy and physiology for nurses, including notes on their clinical application.

PEARSON, J. B.
Water and electrolyte balance. *Nursing Times*, Mar. 31, 1967, p. 415-8.

RICHES, H. R. C.
Lung function tests. *Nursing Times*, Feb. 28, 1964, p. 280-2.

RIDDLE, JANET T. E.
Elementary textbook of anatomy and physiology applied to nursing. Edinburgh, Livingstone, 1961.
2nd edn., 1966.
3rd edn., 1969.

ROPER, NANCY
Man's anatomy, physiology and health. Edinburgh, Livingstone, 1963.
2nd edn., 1965.
3rd edn., 1969.

ROSS, JANET S., *and* WILSON, KATHLEEN J. W.
Foundations of anatomy and physiology. Edinburgh, Livingstone, 1963.
2nd edn., 1966.
3rd edn., 1968.

ROWE, JOYCE W., *and* WHEBLE, VICTOR H.
A concise textbook of anatomy and physiology applied for orthopaedic nurses. 2nd edn. Edinburgh, Livingstone, 1967.

SCHWALM, SISTER MARY ELISE
Applied physiological chemistry. Philadelphia, Davis, 1964.

SEARS, WILLIAM GORDON
Anatomy and physiology for nurses. 4th edn. Arnold, 1965.

SIMPSON, K.
Moment of death. *Nursing Times*, Dec. 1, 1967, p. 1604-6.

SNIVELY, W. D.
Toward a better understanding of body fluid disturbances. *Nursing Forum*, vol. III, no. 1, 1964, p. 61-77.

SYLVESTER, PETER E.
Applied anatomy and physiology for nurses. Oxford, Blackwell, 1964.

TAVERNER, DERYCK
Physiology for nurses. E.U.P., 1961.

VODA, A. M.
Body water dynamics: a clinical application. *American Journal of Nursing*, Dec. 1970, p. 2594-601.

WARREN, C. P.
Fluid balance, water and salt balance. *Nursing Times*, June 9, 1961, p. 722-4; June 16, 1961, p. 759-62; June 23, 1961, p. 793-6; June 30, 1961, p. 826-9.

ARITHMETIC

BUTTON, DOROTHY
Mathematics for nurses, a course for pre-nursing students. 3rd edn. Faber, 1966.

FERSTER, MARILYN B.
Arithmetic for nurses: programmed for class use and home study. New York, Springer, 1961.

FITCH, GRACE E.
Arithmetical review and drug therapy for practical nurses. New York, Macmillan, 1961.

FREAM, WILLIAM C.
Aids to arithmetic in nursing. 3rd edn. Bailliere, Tindall and Cox, 1964.

GOOSTRAY, STELLA
Mathematics and measurements in nursing practice. 3rd edn. New York, Macmillan, 1963.
[Earlier editions entitled: Problems in solutions and dosage.]

HODGSON, R. W.
Every student's guide to the metric system. *Nursing Mirror*, July 20, 1962, p. 305-7.

JESSEE, RUTH W.
Self-teaching tests in arithmetic for nurses. 7th edn. St. Louis, Mosby, 1967.

LEVINE, E.
Statistics: a tool for nurses. *International Nursing Review*, vol. 15, no. 3, 1968, p. 224-34.

LIPSEY, SALLY IRENE
Mathematics for nursing sciences: a programmed review. New York, John Wiley, 1965.

MCCLAIN, M. ESTHER
Simplified arithmetic for nurses. 3rd edn. Philadelphia, Saunders, 1966.

NAST, MINETTE
Simplified drugs and solutions for nurses, including arithmetic. 3rd edn. St. Louis, Mosby, 1964.

PRICE, GERALDINE G.
Self-study guide of mathematics used in nursing. New York, Putnam, 1963.

ROSIER, MARGARET
Nursing mathematics. Oxford University Press, 1967.

SACKHEIM, GEORGE I.
Applied mathematics for nurses. New York, Macmillan, 1961.

SAXTON, DOLORES F., *and* WALTER, JOHN F.
Programmed instruction in arithmetic, dosages and solutions. St. Louis, Mosby, 1966.

SHAMESS, D.
Plan your change to metric. *The Canadian Nurse*, Sept. 1968, p. 50-2.

WEAVER, MABEL E., *and* KOEHLER, VERA J.
Programmed mathematics of drugs and solutions. 2nd edn. Philadelphia, Lippincott, [1964].
3rd edn., [1966].

BACTERIOLOGY

BOCOCK, E. JOAN, *and* ARMSTRONG, KATHERINE F.
Aids to bacteriology for nurses. 2nd edn. Bailliere, Tindall and Cassell, 1962.
3rd edn., entitled Microbiology for nurses, 1968.

BROOME, W. E.
An introduction to nursing bacteriology. Butterworths, 1969.

HARE, RONALD
Bacteriology and immunity for nurses. Longmans, 1961.
2nd edn., 1967.

HATCHER, J.
A bunch of grapes: the discovery of staphylococci. *Nursing Times*, Dec. 24, 1970, p. 1654.

KARMINSKY, DANIEL, *and others*
Microbiology, 1,500 multiple choice questions and referenced answers, edited by Daniel Karminsky, Alice M. Ehrhart and Arlene L. Levey. Flushing, N.Y., Medical Examination Publishing Company, 1966.
[Nursing examination review book, vol. 7.]

MARSHALL, STANLEY
Elementary bacteriology and immunity for nurses. 4th edn. Lewis, 1965.

RICHARDSON, S., and WILLIAMS, R. F.
The meaning of antibiotic resistance in bacteria. *Nursing Times*, July 3, 1969, p. 839-42; July 10, 1969, p. 884-6; July 17, 1969, p. 911-3.

TAYLOR, GEOFFREY
Bacteriology for nurses. Heinemann, 1964.
2nd edn., 1968.

WHITE, LIDA S., and NELSON, SIGRID L.
Practical approach to microbiology for nurses. 2nd edn. Philadelphia, Davis, 1964.

WINNER, H. I.
Microbiology in modern nursing. English Universities Press, 1969.

BIOLOGY AND GENETICS

FREAM, WILLIAM C.
Applied human biology for nurses. Bailliere, Tindall and Cassell, 1964.
2nd edn., 1970.

HILLSMAN, G. M.
Genetics and the nurse. *Nursing Outlook*, Jan. 1966, p. 34-9.

ROBERTS, T.
Background notes to the study of human biology for nurses. Arnold, 1970.

WILSON, MARION E., and MIZER, HELEN ECKEL
Microbiology in nursing practice. New York, Macmillan, 1969.

CANCER NURSING

AIRD, IAN
Operable cancer in the abdomen—1. The patient and his cancer. *Nursing Times*, Oct. 19, 1962, p. 1320-2.

AIRD, IAN
Operable cancer in the abdomen. 2—The stomach. *Nursing Times*, Oct. 26, 1962, p. 1366-9.

AIRD, IAN
Operable cancer in the abdomen. 3—The colon and rectum. *Nursing Times*, Nov. 2, 1962, p. 1399-1402.

AIRD, IAN
Operable cancer of the abdomen. 4—The bladder and prostate gland. *Nursing Times*, Nov. 9, 1962, p. 1422-4.

AIRD, IAN
Operable cancer in the abdomen. 5—The liver and the gall bladder. *Nursing Times*, Nov. 16, 1962, p. 1455-6.

AIRD, IAN
Operable cancer in the abdomen. 6—The pancreas and small intestine. *Nursing Times*, Nov. 23, 1962, p. 1486-8.

AMERICAN CANCER SOCIETY
Guidelines for cancer content in refresher courses for registered nurses. New York, American Cancer Society, 1967.

AMERICAN CANCER SOCIETY and THE NATIONAL ASSOCIATION FOR PRACTICAL NURSE EDUCATION AND SERVICE
Lung cancer: implications for nursing care. Report of a symposium. *The Journal of Practical Nursing*, Aug. 1968, p. 20-6.

AMERICAN CANCER SOCIETY and THE NATIONAL ASSOCIATION FOR PRACTICAL NURSE EDUCATION AND SERVICE
Nursing care of patients with cancer of the head and neck. *Journal of Practical Nursing*, July 1970, p. 22-4.

ANDERSON, J.
The dangers of smoking. *Nursing Times*, April 6, 1962, p. 424-6.

ANSTICE, E.
The emotional operation [Mastectomy]. *Nursing Times*, July 2, 1970, p. 837-8; July 9, 1970, p. 882-3.

ANTOFT, K.
Cancer *can* be beaten. *Canadian Nurse*, April 1970, p. 39-40.

AXELROD, A. R.
Cancer chemotherapy—an historical review. *American Association of Industrial Nurses' Journal*, Jan. 1968, p. 17-20.

BARCKLEY, V.
Crises in cancer. *Nursing Mirror*, April 12, 1968, p. 41-2.

BARCKLEY, V.
Occupational health and cancer: a pair with potential. *Occupational Health Nursing*, Aug. 1969, p. 9-12.

BARCKLEY, V.
A visiting nurse specializes in cancer nursing. *American Journal of Nursing*, Aug. 1970, p. 1680-3.

BASSFORD, P. A.
Cancer health education in industry. *Nursing Times*, June 12, 1969, p. 748-9.

BERGEL, F.
Current advances in cancer research. *Nursing Times*, Dec. 1, 1967, p. 1609-11.

BERRY, D. M.
Support from nursing staff helps nurse-patient cope with cancer. *Hospital Topics*, Oct. 1970, p. 60-2.

BIGNALL, J. R.
Lung cancer. *Nursing Times*, June 10, 1966, p. 758-9.

BODENHAM, D. C.
A plastic surgeon looks at skin cancer. *Nursing Times*, May 29, 1969, p. 683-6.

BOUCHARD, ROSEMARY
Cancer of the head and neck. *Journal of Practical Nursing*, July 1970, p. 25-6, 32, and 34-5.

BOUCHARD, ROSEMARY
Nursing care of the cancer patient. St. Louis, Mosby, 1967.

BOUCHIER, I. A. D.
Cancer of the pancreas. *Nursing Mirror*, Jan. 16, 1970, p. 25-7.

BOYLAND, E.
Environmental factors in cancer. *Nursing Times*, Jan. 3, 1964, p. 4-6.

BROWN, M. KENNEDY
Malignant melanoma. *Nursing Times*, Jan. 30, 1969, p. 135-7.

BRUDENELL, M.
Cervical screening for carcinoma of the uterine cervix. *District Nursing*, July 1969, p. 68-9.

CHAMBERLAIN, GEOFFREY
The cervical smear—is it worth while? *Nursing Times*, Mar. 27, 1969, p. 391-3.

CRAGG, C. E.
The child with leukemia. *Canadian Nurse*, Oct. 1969, p. 30-4.

CRAYTOR, J. K.
Talking with persons who have cancer. *American Journal of Nursing*, April 1969, p. 744-8.

DAVISON, R. L.
Opinion of nurses on cancer, its treatment and curability. A survey among nurses in public health service. *British Journal of Preventive and Social Medicine*, Jan. 1965, p. 24-9.

DEVLIN, H. B.
Abdominoperineal resection of the rectum. *Nursing Times*, Oct. 11, 1968, p. 1364-8.

EGERTON, M. E.
Detecting cancer by means of smears. *Nursing Mirror*, June 21, 1963, p. 252-4.

SPECIALITIES

ELLISON, R. R.
Treating cancer with antimetabolites. *The American Journal of Nursing*, Nov. 1962, p. 79.

EVERETT, ANNA E.
Nursing care of the patient receiving radiation-cobalt 60.
In
AMERICAN NURSES' ASSOCIATION
Technical innovations in health care: nursing implications. New York, The Association, 1962.

FITZPATRICK, G.
Caring for the patient with cancer of the breast. *Bedside Nurse*, Feb. 1970, p. 20-4; Mar. 1970, p. 19-28.

FRANCIS, G. M.
Cancer: the emotional component. *American Journal of Nursing*, Aug. 1969, p. 1677-81.

GRIBBONS, C. A., and ALIAPOULIOS, M. A.
Early carcinoma of the breast. *American Journal of Nursing*, Sept. 1969, p. 1945-50.

HARRISON, D. F. N.
Hypothermia: an aid to cancer chemotherapy. *Nursing Times*, Nov. 17, 1967, p. 1536-8.

HIRSKYJ, L.
Immunotherapy in advanced malignant disease. *Nursing Times*, April 16, 1970, p. 497-8.

HOBBS, P.
Cancer education through industry. *District Nursing*, Sept. 1963, p. 129-30.

HOBBS, P.
Changing attitudes to cancer. *Nursing Mirror*, May 10, 1963, p. v-vi.

HOBBS, P.
Changing attitudes to cancer. *Nursing Mirror*, May 17, 1963, p. xi-xii.

HOHLOCH, F. J., and COULSON, M. E.
Developing an attitude inventory. [Student nurses' attitudes to cancer patients.] *Journal of Nursing Education*, Aug. 1968, p. 9-13.

HOWKINS, J.
Cancer of the body of the uterus. *Nursing Times*, Jan. 4, 1963, p. 21-3.

HUEPER, W. C.
Lung cancer. Air pollutants as a cause. *American Journal of Nursing*, April 1961, p. 64-5 and 68-9.

ILLINGWORTH, C.
Breast cancer. *Nursing Times*, Mar. 12, 1970, p. 328-9.

JOHNSTON, R. N.
Lung cancer. *Nursing Times*, Jan. 16, 1969, p. 73-5.

JOINER, J. P.
The role of the industrial nurse in cancer education. *American Association of Industrial Nurses' Journal*, June 1964, p. 14-5.

JOURNAL OF PRACTICAL NURSING
Cancer of the gastrointestinal tract: implications for nursing care. *Journal of Practical Nursing*, July 1969, p. 23-5 and 53-4.

LEVITT, E. E.
Obstacles to the prevention and treatment of cancer: a critical summary of a crucial investigation. *Occupational Health Nursing*, Jan. 1970, p. 19-22.

MCKELVIE, P.
Cancer of the larynx and pharynx. *Nursing Mirror*, Dec. 5, 1969, p. 20-3.

MARIE CURIE MEMORIAL FOUNDATION
Domiciliary care of the patient with cancer. [Report of a symposium held at the Royal College of Surgeons, London, 28 May 1969.] *Nursing Times*, June 5, 1969, p. 729.

MEMORIAL HOSPITAL FOR CANCER AND ALLIED DISEASES. NURSING DIVISION
A handbook of nursing care for head and neck patients. *The Hospital*, 1967.

MEURER, SISTER MARY CHRISTOPHER
Working with the mother to improve nursing care of the child with leukaemia.
In
AMERICAN NURSES' ASSOCIATION
Nursing in relation to the impact of illness upon the family. New York, The Association, 1962.

NURSING TIMES
Cervical smear tests. *Nursing Times*, April 26, 1968, p. 572-3.

PLATT, L. I., and ZACHARY, M. C.
An experience with annual pelvic examinations in 290 women workers. *Occupational Health Nursing*, Feb. 1970, p. 13-5.

RAVEN, R. W.
The prevention of cancer. *Nursing Mirror*, June 26, 1970, p. 21-3; July 3, 1970, p. 25-7.

ROUALLE, H. L. M.
Management of breast cancer. *Nursing Mirror*, Sept. 12, 1969, p. 45-8.

SHAW, H. J.
Social problems involved in treating cancer of the larynx. *Nursing Mirror*, June 27, 1969, p. 26-7.

SMITH, S. E.
How drugs act: Drugs and cancer. *Nursing Times*, Mar. 3, 1967, p. 283-4.

STEWART, M. A.
Radiotherapy of malignancy and the nursing problems. *District Nursing*, Jan. 1963, p. 219-20.

STEWART, M. J.
Evaluation of a home test for cervical cancer. *Occupational Health Nursing*, Feb. 1970, p. 20, 22 and 40.

STOKER, M. G. P.
Modern trends in cancer research. *Nursing Mirror*, Oct. 2, 1970, p. 19-22.

TANSLEY, DORIS A.
The young wife with choriocarcinoma.
In
AMERICAN NURSES' ASSOCIATION
Technical innovations in health care: nursing implications. New York, The Association, 1962.

THOMSON, W.
Cancer of the scrotum. *Nursing Times*, Sept. 3, 1970, p. 1129-30.

UNITED STATES. BUREAU OF DISEASE PREVENTION AND ENVIRONMENTAL CONTROL
Cancer manual for public health nurses. Virginia, The Bureau, 1963.

WILTSHAW, E.
Leukaemia and chemotherapy. *Nursing Mirror*, Oct. 12, 1962, p. 27.

CARDIAC NURSING

AMERICAN COLLEGE OF CARDIOLOGY and BAPTIST HOSPITAL, NASHVILLE, TENNESSEE
Advanced cardiac nursing. Philadelphia, Charles Press 1970.

AMERICAN HEART ASSOCIATION and AMERICAN NURSES' ASSOCIATION
Nursing care of the cardiac patient. [New York], American Heart Association, 1965.

ANDERSON, BERNICE E.
Legal aspects of nursing care for cardiac patients. *Cardiovascular Nursing*, Mar./April 1969, p. 5-8.

ANDREOLI, KATHLEEN G.
The cardiac monitor. *American Journal of Nursing*, June 1969, p. 1238-43.

ANDREOLI, KATHLEEN G., *and others*
Comprehensive cardiac care: a handbook for nurses and other paramedical personnel, by Kathleen G. Andreoli, Virginia K. Hunn, Douglas P. Zipes and Andrew G. Wallace. Saint Louis, Mosby, 1968.

BESTERMAN, EDWIN
Cardiac resuscitation. *Nursing Times*, Mar. 27, 1969, p. 396-8.

BETT, J. H. N.
Cardiac pacemaking. *NATNews*, Autumn 1968, p. 27-9.

BETTICE, D., *and others*
Cardiac patients' feelings about monitors. *American Journal of Nursing*, Sept. 1970, p. 1950-2.

BOISVERT, C.
Intensive care unit in cardiovascular surgery. *The Canadian Nurse*, Jan. 1967, p. 36-8.

BOOTH, S., *and* MATHER, H. G.
Treating coronary thrombosis in an intensive care unit. *Nursing Times*, May 10, 1968, p. 618-20.

BRAUN, HAROLD A., *and others*
Coronary care unit nursing, by Harold A. Braun, Gerald A. Diettert and Vera E. Wills. 2 vols. Missoula, Mountain Press Publishers, 1968, 1969.
Part I. Programmed text in electrocardiography.
Part II. Workbook in clinical aspects.

BRIGGS, L. W., *and* MORTENSEN, J. D.
Nursing care of the patient with a prosthetic heart valve. *American Journal of Nursing*, Oct. 1963, p. 66-70.

BURN, J. L.
Cardiovascular and chronic neurological disease. *Nursing Times*, Nov. 2, 1962, p. 1393.

BUSBY, E. R.
Artificial cardiac pacing. *Nursing Mirror*, Dec. 4, 1964, p. iv-vi.

CASSEM, N. H., *and others*
Reactions of coronary patients to the CCU nurse. *American Journal of Nursing*, Feb. 1970, p. 319-25.

CEDARS-SINAI MEDICAL CENTER. DEPARTMENT OF NURSING
Aggressive nursing management of acute myocardial infarction: a symposium . . . Philadelphia, Charles Press, 1968.

CHAVIGNY, K. H.
Palpation of the pulse in the cardiac care unit. *International Journal of Nursing Studies*, Aug. 1970, p. 167-74.

CHEST AND HEART ASSOCIATION
Some nursing homes accepting patients suffering from chest, heart and "stroke" illness. The Association, 1970.

CHILDERS, E. D.
The nursing care of patients with myocardial infarction. *Journal of Practical Nursing*, Oct. 1969, p. 39-40.

CHONG, S.
The cardio-thoracic unit, Tan Tock Seng Hospital. *Berita Jururawat*, April 1970, p. 33-4.

CLEMENT, A. J.
Emergency treatment of cardiac arrest. *Nursing Times*, Nov. 2, 1962, p. 1395-8.

CLEMENT, A. J.
The treatment of cardiac arrest. *Nursing Times*, Nov. 5, 1965, p. 1513-8.

CROPPER, C. F. J.
Heart-lung resuscitation, "When seconds count". *Nursing Times*, Aug. 28, 1969, p. 1095-7.

DAWBER, T. R., *and others*
Risk factors in coronary heart disease. *Cardio-Vascular Nursing*, Jan./Feb. 1970, p. 29-33.

DAWSON-BUTTERWORTH, K.
Heart-block and the nurse's role in treatment. *Nursing Mirror*, July 21, 1967, p. 372-4.

DOBSON, M.
The coronary care unit: patients' attitudes and the role of the nurse. *Nursing Times*, July 9, 1970, p. 869-71.

DOLMAN, S., *and others*
Prinzmetal's variant angina in a coronary unit. *Canadian Nurse*, June 1970, p. 23-5.

EDDY, J. D., *and* SINGH, S. P.
Nursing posture after acute myocardial infarction. *The Lancet*, Dec. 27, 1969, p. 1378-82.

FEELEY, E. McN.
The new graduate in cardiopulmonary resuscitation. *American Journal of Nursing*, June 1970, p. 1304-7.

FERRIGAN, M.
A new nursing horizon. The cardiac nurse specialist. *International Nursing Review*, vol. 13, no. 2, 1966, p. 19-20.

FLEMING, J. S.
New methods of treatment in cardiac disease. *Nursing Mirror*, Aug. 5, 1966, p. 424-6.

FOSTER, S., *and* ANDREOLI, K. G.
Behavior following acute myocardial infarcation. *American Journal of Nursing*, Nov. 1970, p. 2344-8.

FRY, J.
Coronary heart disease. *Nursing Times*, April 3, 1963, p. 444-6.

FULLER, E. D., *and* DISMUKES, L. M.
An open-chest preparation in the laboratory for teaching coronary care. *Nursing Forum*, vol. VIII, no. 3, 1969, p. 302-10.

GILSTON, A.
Cardiac resuscitation: some questions and answers. *Nursing Mirror*, June 2, 1967, p. vii-xii.

GOODLAND, NORMAN L.
Coronary care. Bristol, Wright, 1970.

GRACE, WILLIAM J., *and* KEYLOUN, VICTOR
The coronary care unit. Butterworths, 1970.

GRAHAM, L. E.
Patients' perceptions in the CCU. *American Journal of Nursing*, Sept. 1969, p. 1921-2.

GRUHL, V. R.
Some basic considerations about myocardial infarction. *Journal of Practical Nursing*, Oct. 1969, p. 27-8 and 39.

HALLIDAY, N. P.
Management of cardiac arrest. *Nursing Times*, Mar. 10, 1967, p. 308-10.

HAHN, A., *and* DOLAN, N.
After coronary care—what then? *American Journal of Nursing*, Nov. 1970, p. 2350.

HARRIS, A.
Cardiac pacing. *Nursing Mirror*, Feb. 6, 1970, p. 25-30.

HARTLEY, I. D.
Cardiovascular disease: implications for LPN/LVNs. *Journal of Practical Nursing*, Mar. 1970, p. 26-8.

HELLER, A. F.
Nursing the patient with an artificial pacemaker. *American Journal of Nursing*, April 1964, p. 87-92.

HOLDER, B. J.
Cardiopulmonary resuscitation. Implications and responsibilities for the occupational health nurse. *Occupational Health Nursing*, Aug. 1970, p. 13-5.

HONEY, M., *and* SIMON, G.
Cardiac catheterization and angiocardiography. *Nursing Times*, Jan. 13, 1961, p. 57 and 59-61.

SPECIALITIES

HUBNER, P. J. B.
Nursing guide to cardiac monitoring.
1. Introduction, monitors and electrodes.
2. The normal ECG trace.
3-5. Arrhythmias.
6. Cardiac pacing.
7. General notes and hints on monitor observation.
Nursing Mirror, Aug. 21, 1970, p. 13-5; Aug. 28, 1970, p. 9-11; Sept. 4, 1970, p. 32-4; Sept. 11, 1970, p. 48-9; Sept. 18, 1970, p. 32-4; Sept. 25, 1970, p. 41-4; Oct. 2, 1970, p. 34-5.

HUNN, V. K.
Cardiac pacemakers. *American Journal of Nursing*, April 1969, p. 749-54.

JENKINSON, V. M.
Congestive heart failure. *Nursing Times*, Sept. 28, 1962, p. 1220-2.

JONES, B.
Inside the coronary care unit. The patient and his responses. *American Journal of Nursing*, Nov. 1967, p. 2313-20.

JOSEPH, M.
Severe congenital heart disease in the neonate. *Nursing Mirror*, Aug. 28, 1970, p. 32-5.

KERNICKI, JEANETTE, *and others*
Cardiovascular nursing: rationale for therapy and nursing approach, by Jeanette Kernicki, Barbara L. Bullock and Joan Matthews. New York, Putman, 1970.

KOS, B. A., *and* CULBERT, P. A.
Teaching the patient with a pacemaker. *Cardio Vascular Nursing*, Nov./Dec. 1970, p. 57-60.

LANE, C.
Intra-aortic phase-shift balloon pumping in cardiogenic shock. *American Journal of Nursing*, Aug. 1969, p. 1654-9.

LARGE, HELEN, *and others*
In the first stroke intensive care unit. *American Journal of Nursing*, Jan. 1969, p. 76-80.

LASSERS, B. W.
Coronary arteriography. *Nursing Times*, Nov. 15, 1968, p. 1551-3.

LOFTIN, SISTER ELIZABETH
A new dimension in the nursing care of coronary patients. *Hospital Progress*, Oct. 1968, p. 104-7.

MCKENZIE, F. L.
Oscilloscope tracing of the cardiac cycle. *Nursing Times*, Jan. 2, 1969, p. 18-20.

MCLOUGHLIN, M. J.
Pericarditis. *Nursing Times*, June 28, 1963, p. 800-2.

MARINO, BEATRICE, *editor*
Nursing challenges in cardiovascular and metabolic disease. Philadelphia, Saunders, 1969.
[*Nursing Clinics of North America*, vol. 14, no. 1, March, 1969.]

MARTIN, M.
Traumatic rupture of aorta. *Nursing Times*, Aug. 14, 1969, p. 1031-4.

MATHER, G.
Advances in the management of heart disease. *Nursing Mirror*, April 2, 1965, p. xi-xiii.

MELTZER, LAWRENCE E., *and others*
Intensive coronary care—a manual for nurses, by Lawrence E. Meltzer, Rose Pinneo and J. Roderick Kitchell. Philadelphia, Charles Press (for the Coronary Care Unit Fund), 1965.

MERKEL, R., *and* BROWN, C. M.
Evaluating feeding activities in a CCU. *American Journal of Nursing*, Nov. 1970, p. 2348-50.

MERKEL, R., *and* SOVIE, M. D.
Electrocution hazards with transvenous pacemaker electrodes. *American Journal of Nursing*, Dec. 1968, p. 2560-3.

MODELL, WALTER
Handbook of cardiology for nurses: the disease, the patient, modern concepts of treatment. 4th edn. New York, Springer, 1962.
5th edn., 1966.

MORRIS, D. G.
The patient in cardiogenic shock. *Cardio-Vascular Nursing*, July/Aug. 1969, p. 15-7.

NITE, GLADYS, *and* WILLIS, FRANK N.
The coronary patient: hospital care and rehabilitation. New York, Macmillan, 1964.

NURSING CLINICS OF NORTH AMERICA
Symposium on care of the cardiac patient. *Nursing Clinics of North America*, Dec. 1969, p. 561-649.

NURSING MIRROR
Multi-patient cardiac monitor. *Nursing Mirror*, May 30, 1969, p. 9.

PENTECOST, B. L.
Complications of acute myocardial infarction. *District Nursing*, Nov. 1970, p. 150 and 156.

PERRINE, G., *and* BOUDREAU, SISTER M. C.
CCU nurse specialists: [training programs]. *Hospitals*, Mar. 1, 1970, p. 49-52.

PINNEO, R.
A new dimension in nursing. Intensive coronary care. *American Association of Industrial Nurses' Journal*, Feb. 1967, p. 7-10.

PINNEO, R.
The nurse's responsibilities in cardiac emergencies. *Hospital Topics*, Nov. 1966, p. 59-61.

PITORAK, ELIZABETH FORD, *and others*
Nurses' guide to cardiac surgery and nursing care, by Elizabeth Ford Pitorak, Carolyn Hudak, Joan O'Gureck and Patricia Prendergast Hanusz. New York, McGraw-Hill, 1969.

POWELL, C.
Cardiograms for nurse.
1. A simple introduction.
2. Normal and abnormal rhythms.
3. Ventricular abnormal rhythms.
4. The nurse, the patient, the machine.
Nursing Times, Sept. 10, 1970, p. 1157-9; Sept. 17, 1970, p. 1202-4; Sept. 24, 1970, p. 1229-31; Oct. 1, 1970, p. 1267-70.

POWERS, MARYANN, *and* STORLIE, FRANCES
The cardiac surgical patient: pathophysiologic considerations and nursing care. Macmillan, 1969.

RAE, N. M.
Caring for patients following open heart surgery. *American Journal of Nursing*, Nov. 1963, p. 77-82.

REDWOOD, D. R.
Heart block and cardiac pacemakers. *Nursing Times*, May 12, 1967, p. 614-6.

REYNOLDS, M.
Cardiac emergencies in industry—nursing implications for the occupational health nurse. *American Association of Industrial Nurses Journal*, Feb. 1967, p. 11-7.

RITCHIE, MIGNON
The nurse's responsibility in cardiac arrest.
In
AMERICAN NURSES' ASSOCIATION
Emergency intervention by the nurse. New York, The Association, 1962.

ROBERTS, S. L.
The patient's adaptation to the coronary care unit. *Nursing Forum*, vol. IX, no. 1, 1970, p. 56-63.

ROYAL COLLEGE OF NURSING *and* NATIONAL COUNCIL OF NURSES OF THE UNITED KINGDOM. WARD AND DEPARTMENTAL SECTION
: Resuscitation—the nurse's responsibility. *Nursing Times*, Nov. 11, 1966, p. 1496-7.

SCHMITT, Y.
: Armchair treatment in the coronary care unit: effect on blood pressure and pulse. *Nursing Research*, Mar./April 1969, p. 114-8.

SHARP, LaVAUGHN, *and* RABIN, BEATRICE
: Nursing in the coronary care unit. Philadelphia, Lippincott, 1970.

SHILLINGFORD, J. P.
: Intensive coronary care. *Nursing Times*, Nov. 11, 1966, p. 1481-3.

SMITH, B. C.
: Congestive heart failure. *American Journal of Nursing*, Feb. 1969, p. 278-82.

SOBEL, DAVID E.
: Personalization on the coronary care unit. *American Journal of Nursing*, July 1969, p. 1439-42.

SPANDAU, M. M.
: Insertion of temporary cardiac pacemakers without fluoroscopy. *American Journal of Nursing*, May 1970, p. 1011-3.

STANTON, A.
: Cardiac catheterization in Scandinavia. *Nursing Times* Oct. 15, 1970, p. 1331-3.

SUMMERFORD, R. V.
: Myocardial infarction. *Nursing Times*, May 3, 1968, p. 592-5.

TORRENS, P. R., *and* HANCHETT, E. S.
: Public health nursing and the congestive heart failure patient. *Cardio-Vascular Nursing*, July/Aug. 1967, p. 15-8.

UNITED STATES. PUBLIC HEALTH SERVICE
: Outlook for coronary nursing: proceedings of a conference at Wheaton, Maryland, May 23-24, 1968. Washington, U.S. Government Pring Office, [1969].

UNITED STATES PUBLIC HEALTH SERVICE. DIVISION OF NURSING
: Nursing and summary papers: second National Conference on Cardiovascular Diseases, November 22-24, 1964. Washington, United States, Department of Health, Education and Welfare, 1965.

VAN DER HORST, R. L., *and* GOTSMAN, M. S.
: Patient care after cardiac catheterization. *S.A. Nursing Journal*, Jan. 1970, p. 7-10.

YOKES, J. A.
: The clinical specialist in cardiovascular nursing. *American Journal of Nursing*, Dec. 1966, p. 2667-70.

YU, P. N.
: Future trends in coronary care. *Journal of Practical Nursing*, Oct. 1969, p. 31-3 and 51.

CHEMISTRY

BIDDLE, HARRY C., *and* FLOUTZ, VAUGHAN W.
: Chemistry for nurses: including certain essential principles from inorganic, organic and biochemistry. 6th edn. Philadelphia, Davis, 1963.

BROOKS, STEWART M.
: Basic chemistry: a programmed presentation. St. Louis, Mosby, 1966.

GOOSTRAY, STELLA, *and* SCHWENCK, J. RAE
: A textbook of chemistry. 8th edn. New York, Macmillan, 1961.

GRILLOT, GERALD F.
: A chemical background to nursing and other paramedical programs. New York, Harper and Row, 1964.

JONES, GRACE KELLER
: Experimental chemistry for student nurses. Philadelphia, Saunders, 1961.

MARMOR, SOLOMON
: General and biological chemistry: a textbook for students of nursing. Philadelphia, Saunders, 1961.

SACKHEIM, GEORGE I., *and* SCHULTZ, RONALD M.
: Chemistry for the health sciences. New York, Macmillan, 1969.

SCHWALM, SISTER MARY ELISE
: Applied physiological chemistry. Philadelphia, Davis, 1964.

CIRCULATORY DISEASES

AMERICAN JOURNAL OF NURSING
: Correcting common errors in blood pressure measurement. Programmed instruction. *American Journal of Nursing*, Oct. 1965, p. 133-64.

BECHTOLDT, A. A.
: Blood transfusion and transfusion reactions. *Journal of the American Association of Nurse Anesthetists*, Dec. 1969, p. 450-9.

BROWSE, N. L.
: Deep vein thrombosis. *Nursing Times*, Mar. 20, 1969, p. 369-71.

CARR, A.
: Blood sample survey. *Nursing Times*, Dec. 17, 1970, Occasional Papers, p. 191-2.

CARTER, L.
: Canada's rare blood bank. *Canadian Nurse*, Mar. 1969, p. 35-6.

CARTIER, GEORGE-E.
: Vascular diseases of the limbs. *The Canadian Nurse*, Mar. 1964, p. 224-32.

CLEGHORN, T. E.
: Uses and abuses of blood transfusion. *Nursing Mirror*, June 28, 1968, p. 26-9.

COLES, M.
: Haemophilia to-day. *Nursing Times*, Nov. 6, 1969, p. 1415-6.

DUNN, G. C.
: Positive pressure oxygen in treatment of leg ulcers. *Nursing Mirror*, Aug. 21, 1970, p. 23-5.

EVANS, D. S.
: The diagnosis of deep vein thrombosis by ultrasound. *Nursing Times*, Oct. 16, 1969, p. 1319-20.

FEGAN, W. G.
: Compression sclerotherapy in the treatment of varicose veins. *Nursing Times*, Nov. 8, 1968, p. 1509-11.

FEGAN, W. G.
: Continuous compression technique of injecting varicose veins. *The Lancet*, July 20, 1963, p. 109-13.

GRANT, J.
: Complications of blood transfusion. *Nursing Mirror*, April 21, 1967, p. 60-2.

GUNN, A. D. G.
: Venous pressure—man's compensation. *Nursing Times*, July 30, 1970, p. 976-7.

HANDLEY, A. J.
: Anticoagulant therapy. *Nursing Mirror*, July 25, 1969, p. 20-2.

HIRSKYJ, L.
: Innovations in blood transfusion techniques. *Nursing Times*, Aug. 6, 1970, p. 997-1000.

ILLINGWORTH, C.
: Postoperative thrombosis and pulmonary embolism. *Nursing Times*, April 9, 1970, p. 459-60.

SPECIALITIES

ILLINGWORTH, C.
Vascular diseases of the lower limbs. *Nursing Times,* May 7, 1970, p. 591-2.

KARNICKI, J.
Prenatal transfusion. *Nursing Times,* April 7, 1967, p. 445-7.

LEHMANN, H., *and* HUNTSMAN, R. G.
Sickle-cell anaemia. *Nursing Times,* April 17, 1969, p. 491-4.

MALPAS, J. S.
The functions of the spleen. *Nursing Times,* Sept. 13, 1968, p. 1224-5.

MARSHALL, J.
Measuring cerebral blood-flow. *Nursing Mirror,* Feb. 27, 1970, p. 19-21.

MEYER, P. F.
Arteriosclerosis. *Nursing Mirror,* Nov. 29, 1968, p. 28-32.

NEWCOMB, P.
Wolff-Parkinson-White syndrome. *Nursing Times,* Jan. 5, 1968, p. 18-9.

PEACOCK, J. H.
Raynaud's disease. *Nursing Times,* Sept. 28, 1962, p. 1229-31.

PENNINGTON, G. W.
Modern trends in the diagnosis of Rhesus incompatibility. *Nursing Mirror,* April 12, 1968, p. 8-11.

PHILLIPS, T. T. B.
The blood group reference laboratory. *Nursing Times,* Jan. 30, 1969, p. 146-8.

REICH, T.
Implantation of a carotid sinus nerve simulator. *AORN Journal,* Dec. 1969, p. 53-6.

RIVLIN, S.
A new way with old leg ulcers. *Nursing Mirror,* Aug. 16, 1963, p. vii-x.

SAWYER, H. P.
Central venous pressure. *Journal of the American Association of Nurse Anesthetists,* Dec. 1970, p. 448-58.

SCOPES, J. W.
Intraperitoneal transfusion as a means of giving whole blood to babies. *Nursing Mirror,* Mar. 20, 1964, p. 557-8.

SCOTT, B. O.
The physical treatment of varicose ulcers. *Nursing Mirror,* Aug. 9, 1963, p. vii-xi.

SHEAHAN, J.
Frostbite. *Nursing Times,* Jan. 4, 1963, p. 12.

SMITH, S. E.
How drugs act. Drugs and the blood. *Nursing Times,* Feb. 3, 1967, p. 153-5.

TINDALL, V. R.
Pulmonary embolism and deep vein thrombosis in the puerperium. *Midwives' Chronicle and Nursing Notes,* June 1969, p. 204-7.

TOVEY, G. H.
Nursing care during blood transfusion. *Nursing Mirror,* April 14, 1967, p. 35-7.

WILKINSON, R.
Gamma globulins in health and disease. *Nursing Times,* May 31, 1968, p. 725-8.

DENTAL NURSING

BRERETON, GWENDOLEN
Introduction to dental nursing. Mills & Boon, 1969.

COULTAS, ROMA
Dental nurses' digest. British Dental Nurses' and Assistants' Society, [1962].

DYER, M. R.
Care of the teeth: dentures. *Nursing Times,* Dec. 17, 1970, p. 1609-10.

JAMES, P. M. C.
Dental decay: how nurses can help. *Nursing Times,.* Mar. 5, 1970, p. 303-5.

KLOCKE, J. M., *and* SUDDUTH, A. G.
Oral hygiene instruction and plaque formation during hospitalization. *Nursing Research,* Mar.-April 1969, p. 124-30.

LEVISON, H.
Textbook for dental nurses. 2nd edn. Oxford, Blackwell, 1963.
3rd edn., 1969.

PARRY, W. H.
Fluoridation: a major controversy. *Nursing Times,* Jan. 21, 1964, p. 118-20.

PORRITT, J. L.
Oral surgery [in relation to occupational health]. *American Association of Industrial Nurses' Journal,* July 1968, p. 27-44.

WALTERS, E.
Dental office anesthesia: pre-induction precautions. *Journal of the American Association of Nurse Anesthetists,* Aug. 1969, p. 285-96.

WEYMAN, J.
Tetracycline and children's teeth. *Nursing Mirror,* Jan. 5, 1968, p. viii-x.

DERMATOLOGY

ASHURST, P. J. C.
Dermatology for nurses. 1—Psoriasis vulgaris. *Nursing Mirror,* Mar. 29, 1963, p. 563-4.

ASHURST, P. J. C.
Dermatology for nurses. 2—Lichen planus and bullous diseases. *Nursing Mirror,* April 5, 1963, p. 9-11.

BETTLEY, F. R.
Effects of soap on the skin. *Nursing Mirror,* April 14, 1967, p. i-v.

BIDDLECOMBE, A., *and* WEBB, F. W. S.
A water immersion bed in the management of patients with pressure sores. *Nursing Times,* July 24, 1969, p. 942-4.

BIRMINGHAM, D. J.
Skin hygiene and dermatitis in industry. *American Association of Industrial Nurses' Journal,* Aug. 1967, p. 20-3.

BLISS, M. R., *and* McLAREN, R.
Preventing pressure sores in geriatric patients. *Nursing Mirror,* Jan. 27, 1967, p. 379-84.

BLISS, M. R., *and* McLAREN, R.
Preventing pressure sores in geriatric patients. *Nursing Mirror,* Feb. 3, 1967, p. 404-8.

BLISS, M. R., *and* McLAREN, R.
Preventing pressure sores in geriatric patients. *Nursing Mirror,* Feb. 10, 1967, p. 434-7 and 444.

BOR, SIMON
Some aspects of dermatology. Varicose dermatitis and varicose ulcers. *Nursing Times,* July 5, 1968, p. 905-7.

BORRIE, P.
Xanthomatosis. *Nursing Mirror,* Sept. 20, 1963, p. x-xii.

BOURNE, L. B.
Unusual cases of industrial skin disease. *Nursing Mirror,* Mar. 15, 1968, p. 29-31.

BROCKLEHURST, J. C.
Geriatric nursing. Pressure sores. *Nursing Times,* Aug. 4, 1967, p. 1033-5.

CARNEY, R. G.
The aging skin. *The American Journal of Nursing*, June 1963, p. 110-2.

CRONIN, E.
Allergic skin condition. *Nursing Mirror*, April 17, 1970, p. 21-3.

CROWTHER, H. A. H., *and* LISBOA, J.
Control of ammonical dermatitis. *Health Visitor*, April 4, 1970, p. 118-21.

DIXON, W. M.
Care of the skin in industry. *Nursing Mirror*, Jan. 20, 1967, p. 361-2.

FEIWEL, MICHAEL
Some aspects of dermatology. The skin and some of its diseases in the young. *Nursing Times*, June 7, 1968, p. 759-62.

HELLIER, F. F.
Caterpillar dermatitis. *Nursing Mirror*, Sept. 1, 1967, p. ix-x.

HODKINSON, L.
Contact dermatitis and the orthopaedic patient. *Nursing Journal of India*, June 1970, p. 191 and 202.

INGRAM, JOHN T.
The nursing care of the patient with skin disease. Heinemann, 1970.

KELLY, E. A.
Dermatological nursing—1. *Nursing Times*, May 25, 1962, p. 683-4.

KELLY, E. A.
Dermatological nursing—2. *Nursing Times*, June 1, 1962, p. 722-3.

MACDONALD, ANGUS
Some aspects of dermatology. Infectious diseases of the skin—I. *Nursing Times*, June 14, 1968, p. 799-800.

MACDONALD, ANGUS
Some aspects of dermatology. Infectious diseases of the skin—II. Viral diseases. *Nursing Times*, June 21, 1968, p. 831-4.

MACDONALD, ANGUS
Some aspects of dermatology. Drug eruptions. *Nursing Times*, July 12 1968, p. 933-4.

MACKAY, J.
Emotion and the skin. *Nursing Times*, June 1, 1962, p. 699-700.

MACKENNA, R. M. B.
Skin diseases in the elderly. *Nursing Mirror*, Jan. 5, 1968, p. i-iv.

MACKENNA, R. M. B.
Skin diseases in the elderly. *Nursing Mirror*, Jan. 12, 1968, p. x-xii.

MELNYK, EMILY
Epidermolysis bullosa. *Canadian Nurse*, Feb. 1969, p. 33-6.

MOYNAHAN, E. J.
Some common skin disorders in infancy and childhood. *Nursing Mirror*, May 3, 1968, p. 29-31.

MUNRO, D. D.
Some aspects of dermatology. Psoriasis. *Nursing Times*, June 28, 1968, p. 867-71.

MUNRO-ASHMAN, DONALD
Some aspects of dermatology. Contact dermatitis as a nursing hazard. *Nursing Times*, July 19, 1968, p. 974-6.

NEWHOUSE, M. L.
Industrial dermatitis—I. *Nursing Mirror*, April 22, 1966, p. v-vii.

NEWHOUSE, M. L.
Industrial dermatitis—II. *Nursing Mirror*, April 29, 1966, p. xiv-xv.

POL, MADELINE L.
Nursing care of the patient with psoriasis.
In
AMERICAN NURSES' ASSOCIATION
Solving "difficult" problems in nursing care. New York, The Association, 1962.

SAMUEL, H. S.
Detergent dermatitis. *Nursing Times*, Jan. 19, 1962, p. 68-71.

SCOTT, O.
The skin in the elderly. *Midwife and Health Visitor*, Feb. 1970, p. 61-7.

SILVERTHORN, A.
Psoriasis—the stubborn malady. *The Canadian Nurse*, Nov. 1969, p. 38-40.

SNEDDON, I. B., *and* CHURCH, R. E.
Nursing skin disease. Arnold, 1968.

SNEDDON, J.
The management of hand infection. *Nursing Times*, Sept. 11, 1969, p. 1172-4.

THORNE, N.
Cosmetics and dermatology. *Nursing Mirror*, April 1, 1966, p. vii-x.

THORNE, N.
The problem of the black skin. *Nursing Times*, Aug. 7, 1969, p. 999-1002.

WILKINSON, D. S.
The nursing and management of skin diseases. 3rd edn. Faber, 1969.

WILSON, H. T. H.
Rubber glove dermatitis. *Nursing Mirror*, May 12, 1961, p. x.

WOODS, B.
Plant dermatitis. *Nursing Mirror*, Nov. 1, 1963, p. ii-iv.

DIABETES

ARNOLD, H. M.
Elderly diabetic amputees. *American Journal of Nursing*, Dec. 1969, p. 2646-9.

BOWEN, RHODA G.
Effects of organized instruction given by registered professional nurses for patients with the diagnosis of diabetes mellitus.
In
AMERICAN NURSES' ASSOCIATION
The nurse and groups of patients or clients. New York, The Association, 1962.

BRITISH DIABETIC ASSOCIATION
The care of the elderly diabetic: a booklet issued by the B.D.A. to help matrons and wardens of old people's homes who may have diabetics in their care. British Diabetic Association, 1969.

CANTRELL, E. G.
The diabetic in pregnancy. *Nursing Mirror*, Aug. 9, 1963, p. 401-2.

CARNELL, C. M.
Diabetic primigravida. *Nursing Mirror*, Aug. 9, 1963, p. ii-iii.

DERR, S. D.
Testing for glycosuria. *American Journal of Nursing*, July 1970, p. 1513-5.

GARNET, J. D.
Pregnancy in women with diabetes. *American Journal of Nursing*, Sept. 1969, p. 1900-2.

HECTOR, WINIFRED
Food for the diabetic: a text specially prepared for programmed learning. Heinemann, [1964].

SPECIALITIES

HICKS, J. B.
A diabetic undergoes operation. *Nursing Times*, July 5, 1963, p. 831-2.

HOPKINS, S. J.
Diabetes and insulin resistance. *Nursing Times*, May 28, 1970, p. 677-9.

HOWELLS, L.
Diabetic emergencies in the home. *Nursing Mirror*, Nov. 7, 1969, p. 43-5.

KEEN, H.
Finding diabetics. *District Nursing*, June 1970, p. 56-7.

KEEN, H.
The modern approach to diabetes mellitus. *District Nursing*, June 1965, p. 64-7.

LAWRENCE, ROBERT DANIEL
The diabetic ABC: a practical book for patients and nurses. 13th edn. Lewis, 1964.
14th edn., 1967.

NORTH DAKOTA NUTRITION AND DIABETES WORKSHOP
Continuing education in diabetes. *Bedside Nurse*, Dec. 1970, p. 14-9.

ORMEROD, T. P., *and* STONES, P.
The treatment of diabetes.
1. Coma.
2. Diet.
3. Insulin and oral hypoglycaemic drugs.
4. Complications.
Nursing Times: May 29, 1969, p. 679-82; June 5, 1969, p. 713-5; June 12, 1969, p. 750-2; June 19, 1969, p. 786-7.

UNITED STATES PUBLIC HEALTH SERVICE. DIVISION OF CHRONIC DISEASES. DIABETES AND ARTHRITIS PROGRAM
Diabetes mellitus: a guide for nurses. Washington, U.S. Government Printing Office, 1962.

WARREN, B.
Night shift workers in diabetic study. *Occupational Health Nursing*, Jan. 1970, p. 23-5.

DIAGNOSIS AND DIAGNOSTIC TECHNIQUES

BROWN, CHARLES H., editor
Diagnostic procedures in gastroenterology with nurse's notes and supplements on instructions to patients and dietary treatment. St. Louis, Mosby, 1967.

BULLOCK, M. W.
The volemetron. *Nursing Times*, Feb. 21, 1964, p. 237.

CHESNEY, D. N.
Scintiscanning: a new light on diagnosis. *Nursing Times*, Aug. 18, 1967, p. 1093-5.

DURAND, M., *and* PRINCE, R.
Nursing diagnosis: process and decision. *Nursing Forum*, vol. V, no. 4, 1966, p. 50-64.

FRENCH, RUTH M.
Nurse's guide to diagnostic procedures. N.Y., McGraw-Hill, 1962.
2nd edn., 1967.

GARB, SOLOMON
Laboratory tests in common use.
3rd edn. New York, Springer, 1963.
4th edn. 1966.

GARB, SOLOMON, *and* SPORNE, P.
Nurses' manual of laboratory tests. Heinemann, 1962.

HUNT, P. J.
Thermography in medicine. *District Nursing*, April 1970, p. 2-4.

McLAUGHLIN, L.
Nursing in telediagnosis. *American Journal of Nursing*, May 1969, p. 1006-8.

SEEDOR, MARIE M.
Aids to diagnosis: a programmed unit in fundamentals of nursing. New York, Columbia University, 1964.

DIGESTIVE SYSTEM

BEVAN, P. G.
Intestinal obstruction. *Nursing Mirror*, Sept. 26, 1969, p. 24-6.

BOLAM, R. F.
Intestinal obstruction. *Nursing Times*, June 26, 1969, p. 813-5.

BOND, M. R.
The effects of vagotomy and a drainage procedure on nutrition. *Nursing Times*, Mar. 31, 1967, p. 410-2.

BROATCH, D. L., *and others*
The treatment of constipation in the elderly. *Nursing Times*, Nov. 29, 1968, p. 1631-2.

COX, E. V.
Medical complications of partial gastrectomy. *Nursing Times*, June 28, 1963, p. 810-2.

CREAMER, B.
Crohn's disease. *Nursing Times*, Jan. 31, 1964, p. 130-1.

DEVLIN, H. B., *and* PLANT, J. A.
Colostomy and its management. *Nursing Times*, Feb. 20, 1969, p. 231-4.

DOLL, R.
Medical treatment of gastric ulcers. *Nursing Times*, Aug. 12, 1966, p. 1056-8.

DOWNS, H. S.
The control of vomiting. *Nursing Mirror*, Jan. 19, 1968, p. 388-90.

EDWARDS, H. C.
Crohn's disease. *Nursing Mirror*, Feb. 13, 1970, p. 24-31.

GUNN, A. D. G.
Pancreatitis. *Nursing Times*, June 5, 1969, p. 724-6.

HARGREAVES, T.
Jaundice in pregnancy and in the neonate. *Nursing Mirror*, April 17, 1970, p. 27-9.

HAYTER, J.
Impaired liver function and related nursing care. *American Journal of Nursing*, Nov. 1968, p. 2374-9.

HUDSON, E.
Bowel management. *Nursing Times*, Dec. 8, 1961, p. 1597.

HUME, B.
Nursing a patient with a gastric fistula. *Nursing Times*, Jan. 26, 1968, p. 106-8.

JOHNSTON, G. W.
The management of bleeding oesophageal varices. *Nursing Times*, Nov. 29, 1968, p. 1618-20.

KATONA, E. A.
Learning colostomy control. *American Journal of Nursing*, Mar. 1967, p. 534-41.

KITZES, G.
What the nurse should know about peptic ulcers. *Journal of Practical Nursing*, Jan. 1970, p. 20-1.

LEONARD, M.
The constipation problem. *District Nursing*, Sept. 1970, p. 114-5.

McCALLISTER, J.
Nursing care of a patient with bleeding oesophageal varices. *Nursing Times*, Nov. 29, 1968, p. 1621-2.

MAINGOT, R.
Pancreatic fistulae. *Nursing Times*, Nov. 13, 1969, p. 1447-9.

MAY, R. E., and REYNOLDS, K. W.
Extraperitoneal perforation of the rectum with a rubber rectal tube. *Nursing Times*, Mar. 6, 1969, p. 295-6.

PARK, W. D.
Peptic ulceration. *Nursing Times*, Mar. 31, 1967, p. 408-9.

PARRY, W. H.
Infant gastro-enteritis. *Nursing Times*, Aug. 12, 1966, p. 1062-4.

PATON, A.
Jaundice. *Nursing Times*, Oct. 11, 1968, p. 1375-6.

PLANT, J. A., and DEVLIN, H. B.
Ileostomy and its management. *Nursing Times*, May 24, 1968, p. 711-4.

PUTT, A. M.
One experiment in nursing adults with peptic ulcers. *Nursing Research*, Nov./Dec. 1970, p. 484-94.

ROSE, J. F.
The medical treatment of gastric and duodenal ulcers. *Nursing Times*, Aug. 14, 1969, p. 1038-40.

SECOR, S. M.
Colostomy rehabilitation. *American Journal of Nursing*, Nov. 1970, p. 2400-1.

SEARGEANT, P. W.
Management of a colostomy. *Nursing Times*, Jan. 12, 1968, p. 36-8.

SHEPHERD, J. A.
Perforated peptic ulcer. *Nursing Times*, Oct. 8, 1970, p. 1299-1304.

WATKINSON, G.
Peptic ulcer—1. Pathology, causation, clinical features and complications. *Nursing Times*, Sept. 15, 1961, p. 1186-9.

WATKINSON, G.
Peptic ulcer. 2—Medical and surgical treatment. *Nursing Times*, Sept. 22, 1961, p. 1215-7.

ZUIDEMA, G. D., and KLEIN, M. K.
A new esophagus. *American Journal of Nursing*, Sept. 1961, p. 69.

EAR, NOSE AND THROAT

ANDREWS, E. M.
Understanding the world of deaf children. *Nursing Mirror*, May 24, 1968, p. 38-9.

ARGAMASO, R. V.
Care of cleft lip and palate patients. *Bedside Nurse*, Nov./Dec. 1969, p. 28-31.

BIRCH, M. G.
Instruments and procedures used in ENT examinations. *Nursing Times*, Aug. 27, 1965, p. 1163-5.

BOORER, D.
Barrier of silence. *Nursing Times*, Dec. 31, 1965, p. 1787-9.

CARTER, B. S.
Treatment of ear, nose and throat conditions. Dysphagia. *Nursing Mirror*, July 5, 1963, p. i-ii and xiv-xv.

COLES, R. R. A.
Research into deafness. *District Nursing*, Dec. 1968, p. 188-9 and 191.

CRABTREE, N. L.
Treatment of ear, nose and throat conditions. Deafness. *Nursing Mirror*, July 26, 1963, p. x-xii and xvi.

DARWIN, JOAN, and MARKHAM, JOAN
Eye, nose, throat and ear nursing: an introduction. Heinemann, 1966.

DAVIS, R. W.
Care of the patient with laryngectomy. *Bedside Nurse*, Nov. 1970, p. 13-7.

DELANEY, R. E.
Stapedectomy. *American Journal of Nursing*, Nov. 1969, p. 2406-9.

DIX, M. R.
Hearing tests in modern clinical practice. *Nursing Mirror*, Feb. 28, 1969, p. 30-5.

DOUGHERTY, A. L., and COHEN, J. L.
Auditory screening for infants and preschoolers; a new technique ... *Nursing Outlook*, May 1961, p. 310-2.

EDWARDS, R.
Deafness in children. What it means to be deaf—and the educational facilities we are providing. *Nursing Times*, Dec. 20, 1968, p. 1718-20.

EDWARDS, R.
Deafness in children. Helping them to help their children. *Nursing Times*, Dec. 27, 1968, p. 1759-61.

EDWARDS, R.
Deafness in children. Deaf, not dumb—teaching deaf children to speak. *Nursing Times*, Jan. 2, 1969, p. 12-4.

FISCH, L.
A modern hearing clinic. *Nursing Times*, Aug. 21, 1964, p. 1083-6.

FOX, M. S.
Industrial hearing loss—conservation and compensation aspects. *Occupational Health Nursing*, May 1969, p. 18-24.

GIBB, A. G.
Syringeing the ear. *Nursing Times*, Oct. 1, 1970, p. 1264-6.

GIBB, A. G.
Tympanoplasty. *Nursing Times*, Oct. 25, 1968, p. 1434-7.

GROSS, C. W.
Initial evaluation of the patient with otologic problems. *Occupational Health Nursing*, May 1969, p. 11-4.

HARPMAN, J. A.
Treatment of ear, nose and throat conditions. *Nursing Mirror*, June 28, 1963, p. ii-vi.

HARVEY, R. M.
Deafness in children.
1. The causes.
2. How deaf?
3. Treatment.
Nursing Times, Nov. 29, 1968, p. 1623-5; Dec. 6, 1968, p. 1659-61; Dec. 13, 1968, p. 1694-5.

HAVENER, WILLIAM H., and others
Nursing care in eye, ear, nose and throat disorders by William H. Havener, William H. Saunders and Betty S. Bergerson. St. Louis, C. V. Mosby, 1964.

HUMENIK, P.
Audiological management of adults. *The Canadian Nurse*, Aug. 1966, p. 38-9.

HUMENIK, P.
Audiological management of children. *The Canadian Nurse*, Aug. 1966, p. 41-2.

KEYSELL, P.
Teaching the deaf to mime. *Nursing Mirror*, Sept. 20, 1963, p. 533-4.

KORKIS, F. BOYES
Ear, nose and throat nursing. 2nd edn. Churchill, 1965.

LUDMAN, HAROLD
Ear, nose and throat diseases: principles of patient care. Pitman, 1969.

McCAULEY, J. M.
Nursing care in microsurgery of the ear. *Nursing Times*, Mar. 20, 1969, p. 361-2.

McKENZIE, W.
Stapes surgery. *Nursing Mirror*, Feb. 10, p. i-iii.

SPECIALITIES

MARSHALL, SUSANNA
Aids to ear, nose and throat nursing. 3rd edn. Bailliere, Tindall and Cox, 1962.
4th edn., 1967.

MAWSON, S.
Problem of the born-deaf child. *Nursing Mirror*, April 26, 1968, p. 30-1.

MORRISON, A. W.
Ultrasonic therapy in ear, nose and throat surgery. *Nursing Times*, Nov. 10, 1967, p. 1504-6.

NURSING CLINICS OF NORTH AMERICA
Symposium on patients with sensory defects. *Nursing Clinics of North America*, Sept. 1970, p. 449-547.

NURSING MIRROR
Seeing sound. New visual aid for the deaf. *Nursing Mirror*, Sept. 16, 1966, p. viii-ix.

PARSONS, H. M.
Surgery for diseases of the mastoid process. *Nursing Times*, July 23, 1970, p. 942-5.

RILEY, E. C.
Preventing deafness from industrial noise. *American Journal of Nursing*, May 1963, p. 80-4.

ROBIDOUX-POIRIER, H.
Esophageal manometry. *Canadian Nurse*, Dec. 1970, p. 37-8.

ROLAND, P. E.
Treatment of ear, nose and throat conditions. Hoarseness and stridor. *Nursing Mirror*, July 12, 1963, p. x-xii.

ST. CLAIRE-VERNAN, J.
Screening for hearing in infancy. *District Nursing*, Dec. 1968, p. 186-7.

SAUNDERS, WILLIAM H., *and others*
Nursing care in eye, nose and throat disorders, by William H. Saunders, William H. Havener, Carol J. Fair and Josephine T. Hickey. 2nd edn. St. Louis, Mosby, 1968.

SMYTH, G. D. L.
Microsurgical treatment of deafness. *Nursing Times*, Mar. 20, 1969, p. 359-61.

WALKER, A. SMITH
Hearing aids. *Nursing Times*, Oct. 2, 1964, p. 1286-8.

ENDOCRINE, METABOLIC AND NUTRITIONAL DISEASES

BROWN, A.
Obesity. A modern social problem. *Nursing Times*, July 5, 1963, p. 846-7.

CARSON, N. A. J.
Phenylketonuria and its detection in mass screening surveys. *Nursing Mirror*, Mar. 27, 1964, p. vii and x.

CHINQUE, K. M.
The management of children with phenylketonuria. *Nursing Outlook*, May 1962, p. 328-31.

DAVIO, E. L.
Nursing management of patients with thyroid dysfunction. *Journal of Practical Nursing*, Sept. 1969, p. 33, and 46-7.

GREENE, R.
Occult hypothyroidism. *Nursing Mirror*, June 13, 1969, p. 36-7.

HARGREAVES, T.
Inborn errors of metabolism. *Nursing Mirror*, July 3, 1970, p. 30-1.

HOLT, K. S.
The dietary treatment of phenylketonuria. *Nursing Mirror*, July 14, 1961, p. 1372.

HUDSON, F. P., *and* MORDAUNT, V. L.
Opinions of health visitors and mothers on screening for phenylketonuria. *The Medical Officer*, Oct. 11, 1968, p. 205-7.

KIRMAN, B. H.
Phenylketonuria. *Nursing Times*, Mar. 27, 1964, p. 396-8.

MACGUINNISS, O.
Albinos—our unknown minority. *Nursing Outlook*, Jan. 1962, p. 26-9.

MONCRIEFF, A., *and others*
Method for feeding the phenylketonuric infant. *Nursing Mirror*, Jan. 22, 1965, p. 381-2.

MONTFORD, A. A. W.
Classical phenylketonuria. *Nursing Times*, July 24, 1969, p. 938-41.

O'FLYNN, M. E.
Diet therapy in phenylketonuria. *American Journal of Nursing*, Aug. 1967, p. 1658-60.

RICHARDS, I. D. G.
Rickets in Britain. *Nursing Mirror*, Jan. 17, 1969, p. 26-7.

ROXBURGH, R. A.
Splenectomy and the indications for it. *Nursing Times*, Sept. 13, 1968, p. 1227-9.

SCHNEE, B.
A child with phenylketonuria. *The Canadian Nurse*, July 1964, p. 665-7.

STEPHENSON, J. B. P.
Screening for phenylketonuria. *Mother and Child*, May, 1968, p. 7-14.

STEVENS, V.
Homocystinuria. Recent research into cause and treatment. *Nursing Times*, Feb. 16, 1968, p. 210-2.

TAUBER, I. J.
A metabolic approach to mental disorders at Hollymoor Hospital, Birmingham. *Nursing Times*, Sept. 11, 1964, p. 1172-4.

UNITED STATES. NATIONAL INSTITUTES OF HEALTH. CLINICAL CENTER
Nursing care of patients with cystinosis: a nursing clinical conference. Washington. [U.S. Department of Health, Education and Welfare, 1969.]

UNITED STATES. NATIONAL INSTITUTES OF HEALTH. CLINICAL CENTER
Nursing care of patients with homocystinuria. Washington, U. S. Department of Health, 1970.

WAKELEY, SIR CECIL
Glands in the neck.
1. The thyroid gland.
2. Goitre.
3. Thyroid swellings.
4. Neoplasms of the thyroid.
5. Operations of the thyroid gland.
6. The parathyroid gland.
Nursing Mirror, Oct. 23, 1970, p. 44-5; Oct. 30, 1970, p. 26-9; Nov. 6, 1970, p. 31; Nov. 13, 1970, p. 42-3; Dec. 11, 1970, p. 29-30; Dec. 18, 1970, p. 38-9.

GENITO-URINARY SYSTEM

ALBERS, J.
Evaluation of blood volume in patients on hemodialysis. *American Journal of Nursing*, Aug. 1968, p. 1677-9.

ASHWORTH, A.
1. Hydronephrosis.
2. Diagnostic investigations.
Nursing Times, Mar. 29, 1968, p. 427-8; April 5, 1968, p. 460-2.

BEVIS, G.
Obtaining a midstream specimen of urine. *Nursing Times*, Sept. 4, 1969, p. 1135-6.

BIBLIOGRAPHY OF NURSING

BLAINEY, J. D.
Acute renal failure. *Nursing Times*, July 12, 1963, p. 862-4.

BLISS, M. R.
New nursing aid for incontinent female patients. *Nursing Mirror*, Jan. 29, 1965, p. 399-400 and 402.

BOIS, M. S., and others
Nursing care of patients having kidney transplants. *American Journal of Nursing*, June 1968, p. 1238-9 and 1242-7.

BURROWS, K.
Peritoneal dialysis. *Nursing Times*, Feb. 12, 1970, p. 206-8.

BURROWS, K.
Treatment of acute renal failure. *Nursing Times*, Jan. 6, 1967, p. 8-10.

CAMERON, J. S., and RUSSELL, ALISON M. E.
Nephrology for nurses: a modern approach to the kidney. Heinemann Medical, 1970.

CATTELL, W. R.
Peritoneal dialysis. *Nursing Mirror*, Nov. 8, 1968, p. 24-6; Nov. 15, 1968, p. 26-8.

CATTELL, W. R.
Substitution of kidney function by artificial means—1. 2—Dialysis therapy and peritoneal dialysis. *Nursing Times*, Sept. 18, 1969, p. 1191-3; Sept. 25, 1969, p. 1236-8.

CATTELL, W. R.
Substitution of kidney function by artificial means. 3—Problems of chronic dialysis. *Nursing Times*, Oct. 2, 1969, p. 1263-4.

CHISHOLM, G. D.
Renal calculi. *Nursing Mirror*, Sept. 5, 1969, p. 33-6.

CLARIDGE, Martin
Abnormalities of the urinary tract in pregnancy. *Nursing Mirror*, May 16, 1969, p. 31-5.

CLARK, J.
An introduction to home dialysis. *Nursing Times*, Sept. 22, 1967, p. 1269-70.

CRASSWELLER, P. O.
Benign hyperplasia of the prostate. *Canadian Nurse*, Dec. 1968, p. 32-4.

DELEHANTY, L., and STRAVINO, V.
Achieving bladder control. *American Journal of Nursing*, Feb. 1970, p. 312-8.

DENT, M. J. W.
Administration of diuretics. *Nursing Mirror*, June 27, 1969, p. 41-3.

DEMPSTER, W. J.
Kidney transplantation. *Nursing Times*, April 10, 1964, p. 456-7.

DLIN, B. M., and others
Psychosexual response to ileostomy and colostomy. *AORN Journal*, Nov. 1969, p. 77-84.

DOWNING, S. R.
Nursing support in early renal failure. *American Journal of Nursing*, June 1969, p. 1212-6.

ECKSTEIN, H. B.
Urinary infection in children. *Nursing Mirror*, July 22, 1966, p. x-xiii.

EDMUNDS, C.
Haemodialysis. A social and psychological problem? *Nursing Times*, Sept. 3, 1970, p. 1150-1.

FERGUSON, J.
New approach to the X-ray examination of the male uretha. *Nursing Mirror*, Jan. 13, 1967, p. viii-ix.

FRYE, C.
Chemotherapy in hemodialysis. *Canadian Nurse*, Dec. 1970, p. 32-6.

FRYE, C.
The nurse is a specialist in the artificial kidney unit. *Canadian Nurse*, Dec. 1969, p. 33-6.

GIBBS, GERTRUDE E.
Perineal care of the incapacitated patient. *American Journal of Nursing*, Jan. 1969, p. 124-5.

GREGG, E.
Home dialysis. *Nursing Times*, July 19, 1968, p. 959-61.

GREVILLE, R.
Haemodialysis in the treatment of renal failure. *Irish Nursing News*, Mar./April 1968, p. 7-8.

GROSICKI, J. P.
Effect of operant conditioning on modification of incontinence in neuropsychiatric geriatric patients. *Nursing Research*, July/Aug. 1968, p. 304-11.

GUNN, A. D. G.
Renal dialysis. *Nursing Times*, Jan. 6, 1967, p. 3-4.

HALL, A.
Nursing care of patient following prostatectomy. *Canadian Nurse*, Dec. 1968, p. 35-7.

HEAN, LING MIE
The responsibility of the renal nurse in a dialysis unit. *Berita Jururawat*, Nov. 1968, p. 43-9.

HOPEWELL, J.
Prostatectomy—1. *Nursing Times*, Aug. 11, 1961, p. 1022-5.

HOPEWELL, J.
Prostatectomy—2. *Nursing Times*, Aug. 18, 1961, p. 1060-2.

HOWAT, H. T.
1. Chronic pancreatitis.
2. Diagnosis and treatment.
Nursing Times, Aug. 27, 1970, p. 1093-4; Sept. 3, 1970, p. 1133-6.

HUTCHINGS, M. T.
Mid-stream specimens of urine from female patients. *Nursing Times*, Oct. 13, 1961, p. 1317.

KING EDWARD'S HOSPITAL FUND FOR LONDON. HOSPITAL CENTRE
Renal dialysis: the home, the help, the hazards. *Nursing Times*, April 16, 1970, p. 506-7.

KOSSORIS, P.
Family therapy. An adjunct to hemodialysis and transplantation. *American Journal of Nursing*, Aug. 1970, p. 1730-3.

LEGAULT, JEAN-PAUL
Urology in review. *Canadian Nurse*, Sept. 1963, p. 821-4.

LEYSHON, G. E.
Renal dialysis at home. *District Nursing*, June 1970, p. 51-4.

LLOYD-DAVIES, R. W.
Renal transplantation. *Nursing Times*, Oct. 4, 1968, p. 1326-8.

LLOYD-DAVIES, R. W., and ROSS, S. G.
Haemodialysis. *Nursing Times*, May 10, 1968, p. 627-30.

LLOYD-DAVIES, R. W., and ROSS, S. G.
Peritoneal dialysis. *Nursing Times*, May 3, 1968, p. 587-91.

MACDONALD, J.
Nursing care in renal transplantation. *The Canadian Nurse*, Oct. 1967, p. 35-9.

MARCUS, C. M., and BRENNAN, K. S. W.
Nursing the incontinent patient. *Nursing Mirror*, Feb. 28, 1969, p. 18-21.

METCALFE, J. T., and GODFREY, J. M.
Peritoneal dialysis. *Nursing Mirror*, Nov. 22, 1968, p. 37-9.

MITCHELL, J. P.
Urology for nurses. Bristol, John Wright, 1965.
2nd edn., 1969.

SPECIALITIES

NASSEN, A.
Arteriovenous shunt implantation. An adolescent's perception and response [in haemodialysis]. *American Journal of Nursing*, Oct. 1970, p. 2171-6.

NESBITT, L.
Nursing the patient on long-term hemodialysis. *The Canadian Nurse*, Oct. 1967, p. 40-1.

NEWMAN, J. L.
How to prevent wet beds. *Nursing Times*, Nov. 23, 1962, p. 1482-3 and 1485.

NEWMAN, J. L.
Old folk in wet beds. *British Medical Journal*, June 30, 1962, p. 1824-7.

NURSING TIMES
Viral hepatitis—an occupational hazard? *Nursing Times*, June 11, 1970, p. 753.

PARTON, IAN
Urology for nurses. Wellington, Butterworths, 1968.

PATON, A.
Hepatic coma. *Nursing Times*, Oct. 23, 1969, p. 1351-2.

POLLEY, M.
Renal transplantation. *Nursing Times*, Oct. 6, 1967, p. 1382-3.

RAWNSLEY, P. A.
Haemodialysis: the social problem. *Nursing Times*, June 18, 1970, p. 783-5.

RAWNSLEY, P. A.
The management of renal failure. *Nursing Times*, June 18, 1970, p. 780-2.

ROBINSON, JAMES O.
Modern urology for nurses. Heinemann, 1968.

SAWYER, JANET R.
Nursing care of patients with urologic diseases. St. Louis, Mosby, 1963.

SAYERS, B. P. C., *and* HODGSON, R. W.
Urological nurse teaching unit at St. Peter's, St. Paul's and St. Philip's Hospitals, London. *Nursing Mirror*, June 28, 1963, p. vii-ix.

SCHLOTTER, L.
Dialysis for kidney failure. *Journal of Practical Nursing*, Sept. 1970, p. 24-7 and 42-6.

SCHLOTTER, L.
What do you teach the dialysis patient? *American Journal of Nursing*, Jan. 1970, p. 83.

SCHOFIELD, D.
Management of urinary incontinence. *Nursing Mirror*, Aug. 21, 1970, p. 39-40.

SEARLE, D. J.
Bowel management in the elderly and disabled. *Nursing Mirror*, Jan. 2, 1970, p. 11-3.

SHALDON, S.
Home-maintenance haemodialysis. *Nursing Mirror*, May 10, 1968, p. 19-22.

SHALDON, S., *and* ABRAHAMS, C.
Independence concept of haemodialysis. *Nursing Times*, Oct. 4, 1968, p. 1329-31.

SIEGGREEN, MARY
The closed urinary drainage system: an illustrated guide to correct procedures. New York, American Journal of Nursing Company, 1970.

TUDOR, L. L.
Bladder and bowel retraining. *American Journal of Nursing*, Nov. 1970, p. 2391-3.

WAKELEY, J.
Urinary outflow obstruction in the male. *Nursing Mirror*, April 26, 1968, p. 17-21.

WALLACE, D. M.
Ileal conduits for carcinoma of the bladder. *Nursing Mirror*, July 18, 1969, p. 38-41.

WHITEHEAD, E.
Coping with female incontinence. *Nursing Mirror*, Aug. 14, 1970, p. 38-9.

WHITEHEAD, SYLVIA L.
Nursing care of the adult urology patient. New York, Appleton-Century-Crofts, 1970.

WILLIAMS, D. I.
Urinary infections in the elderly. *Nursing Mirror*, Jan. 3, 1964, p. v-vi.

WINTER, CHESTER C., *and* ROEHM, MARILYN M.
Sawyer's nursing care of patients with urologic diseases. 2nd edn. Saint Louis, Mosby, 1968.

WOOD, S.
Hemodialysis in the home. *Canadian Nurse*, April 1969, p. 42-4.

WOODWARD, SISTER M. HILARY
Urinary incontinence in the physically handicapped child. *Nursing Times*, Aug. 27, 1970, p. 1098-1101.

WRIGHT, F. K.
Principles of haemodialysis. *Nursing Times*, Jan. 6, 1967, p. 5-7.

GERIATRICS

ADAMS, G. F., *and* McILWRAITH, P. L.
Geriatric nursing: a study of the work of geriatric ward staff. O.U.P. for the Nuffield Provincial Hospitals Trust, 1963.

AGATE, J. N.
Geriatric care at Ipswich and East Suffolk Hospital. *Nursing Mirror*, Feb. 21, 1969, p. 33-5.

AGATE, JOHN
Preparation for retirement. Looking towards the nurses' retirement. *Nursing Mirror*, July 17, 1964, p. 347-9.

AMERICAN NURSES' ASSOCIATION
Exploring progress in geriatric nursing practice. New York, The Association, 1966.

AMERICAN NURSES' ASSOCIATION. COMMITTEE ON STANDARDS FOR GERIATRIC NURSING PRACTICE
Standards for geriatric nursing practice. *American Journal of Nursing*, Sept. 1970, p. 1894-7.

ANDERSON, C. J.
Instituting change in psychiatric geriatric settings. *Journal of Psychiatric Nursing*, July/Aug. 1970, p. 13-8.

ANSTICE, E.
So many old people need not be in hospital. *Nursing Times*, Sept. 24, 1970, p. 1239-40.

ANTON-STEPHENS, D.
Psychology of old age. *Nursing Mirror*, May 26, 1967, p. 172-4.

ARNOLD, H. M.
Elderly diabetic amputees. *American Journal of Nursing*, Dec. 1969, p. 2646-9.

ASHLEY, P. J.
Nursing aspects of geriatric rehabilitation. *Nursing Times*, Aug. 1970, p. 1102-5.

BARBER, R. M.
Setting up a day centre [for rehabilitation of the elderly sick]. *Health Visitor*, July 1970, p. 232-4.

BATTEN, L. W.
Terminal illness at home. *Nursing Mirror*, Feb. 27, 1970, p. 28-31.

BERESFORD, C. C.
Senile dementia. *Nursing Times*, July 6, 1962, p. 861-4.

BIER, RUTH
Motivation of the chronically ill aged patient.
In
AMERICAN NURSES' ASSOCIATION
Culture, atmosphere and social organization: effects on nursing care of the patient. New York, The Association, 1962.

BLISS, M. R., *and others*
Day clothing for geriatric patients. *Nursing Times*, May 5, 1967, p. 598-600.

BLISS, M. R., *and* MCLAREN, R.
Preventing pressure sores in geriatric patients. *Nursing Mirror*, Feb. 10, 1967, p. 434-7 and 444.

BOUCHER, C. A.
What is geriatrics. *Nursing Mirror*, Nov. 15, 1968, p. 20-3.

BOURNE, J.
Ageing and old age. *Nursing Times*, April 26, 1968, p. 550-2.

BROCKLEHURST, J. C.
A geriatric long-stay research unit. *Nursing Mirror*, Aug. 21, 1964, p. i-iii.

BROCKLEHURST, J. C.
Geriatric nursing. 1—Cerebrovascular disease. *Nursing Times*, July 7, 1967, p. 880-2.

BROCKLEHURST, J. C.
Geriatric nursing. 2—Mental confusion. *Nursing Times*, July 14, 1967, p. 937-8.

BROCKLEHURST, J. C.
Geriatric nursing. 3—Incontinence of urine. *Nursing Times*, July 21, 1967, p. 954-6.

BROCKLEHURST, J. C.
Geriatric nursing. 4—Faecal incontinence. *Nursing Times*, July 28, 1967, p. 995.

BROCKLEHURST, J. C.
Geriatric nursing. 5—Pressure sores. *Nursing Times*, Aug. 4, 1967, p. 1033-5.

BROCKLEHURST, J. C.
Geriatric nursing. 6—Various problems in geriatric medicine. *Nursing Times*, Aug. 11, 1967, p. 1072-4.

BROCKLEHURST, J. C.
Geriatric nursing. 7—Ward equipment. *Nursing Times*, Aug. 18, 1967, p. 1088-91.

BROCKLEHURST, J. C.
Geriatric nursing. 8—More equipment for geriatric nursing. *Nursing Times*, Aug. 25, 1967, p. 1137-40.

BROCKLEHURST, J. C., *and* FRANKLIN, G.
Life in a geriatric long-stay ward. *Nursing Mirror*, Jan. 20, 1967, p. xi-xv.

BURN, J. L.
Senile dementia. *Nursing Times*, Nov. 23, 1962, p. 1491-3.

BURNSIDE, I. M.
Crisis intervention with geriatric hospitalized patients. *Journal of Psychiatric Nursing and Mental Health Services*, March-April 1970, p. 17-20.

BURNSIDE, I. M.
Grief work in the aged patient. *Nursing Forum*, vol. VIII, no. 4, 1969, p. 417-27.

BURNSIDE, I. M.
Group work among the aged. *Nursing Outlook*, June 1969, p. 68-71.

CALNAN, M. F., *and* HANRON, J. B.
Young nurse—elderly patient. *Nursing Outlook*, Dec. 1970, p. 44-6.

CAPE, R. D. T., *and others*
Modern geriatrics. *Nursing Times*, Jan. 24, 1964, p. 105-7.

CARR, A. J.
Training nurses to care for the elderly. *Nursing Times*, Dec. 10, 1965, p. 1679-80.

CARRIER, P. J., *and others*
Notes on geriatric anesthesia. *Journal of the American Association of Nurse Anesthetists*, Aug. 1969, p. 273-83.

CHENERY, J. L.
Geriatric nursing. *Occupational Therapy*, Mar. 1969, p. 37-40.

CLEMENTS, G.
A geriatric day hospital serving a rural community. *Nursing Times*, July 5, 1968, p. 908-9.

COOPER, S.
A day hospital for elderly persons. *The Canadian Nurse*, Feb. 1970, p. 41-3.

CORBY, PATRICIA, *and others*
The elderly patient in Guy's by Patricia Corby, Mary Baker-Rogers, Mary Elford, Jean Meyric-Hughes and Anne Venus. *Guy's Hospital Gazette*, Nov. 13, 1965, p. 544-52.

CRAMOND, W. A.
Psychiatry and old age.
I. The psychiatric hospital and the aged patient.
II. Prevention of mental illness in old age.
Nursing Mirror, Mar. 17, 1961, p. xi-xii; Mar. 24, 1961, p. 2301-2.

CROPPER, C. F. J.
The psychogeriatric patient. *Nursing Times*, May 17, 1968, p. 667-9.

DAVID, J. D. P.
Modern geriatric care. *Nursing Times*, Dec. 20, 1963, p. 1594-6.

DAVIS, B. M.
Rehabilitation of the crippled elderly. *Nursing Mirror*, April 17, 1970, p. 24-5.

DAVIS, R. W.
Psychologic aspects of geriatric nursing. *American Journal of Nursing*, April 1968, p. 802-6.

DAWSON-BUTTERWORTH, K.
Modern gerontology—1.
Modern gerontology—2.
Nursing Times, Jan. 8, 1970, p. 37-9; Jan. 15, 1970, p. 75-6.

DEIBEL, A. W.
Geriatrics [in the USSR]. *Journal of Psychiatric Nursing and Mental Health Services*, Sept./Oct. 1968, p. 308-9.

DELARGY, J.
The rocking chair in old age. *Nursing Mirror*, Sept. 29, 1961, p. vi.

DEVAS, M. B.
A geriatric orthopaedic unit. *Nursing Mirror*, Feb. 2, 1968, p. 23-5.

DRANSFIELD, G. A.
Emotional problems of the elderly and chronic sick. *Nursing Mirror*, Oct. 6, 1961, p. x-xii.

ELIZABETH, SISTER REGINA
The dignity of aging: reminders for nursing service. *Hospital Progress*, Mar. 1967, p. 110-5.

ELLIOTT, J.
St. Francis' Hospital, Dulwich. *Nursing Times*, Oct. 25, 1968, p. 1447-9.

EXTON-SMITH, A. N.
Progressive patient care for geriatric patients. *Nursing Mirror*, June 29, 1962, p. ii-iv.

FADDIS, M. O.
What is different about geriatric nursing? *The Journal of Nursing Education*, June 1963, p. 13-5.

SPECIALITIES

FAULKNER, H.
Clinics for geriatric patients. *Midwife and Health Visitor*, Oct. 1966, p. 421-2.

FELSTEIN, I.
Mental illness and mordant information. *Midwife and Health Visitor*, Feb. 1970, p. 55-7.

FENNESSY, C. M.
Nursing care of the aged patient. *Hospital Progress*, Jan. 1970, p. 46-50.

FINE, W.
Sphincteric disorders in the elderly. *Nursing Mirror*, Dec. 5, 1969, p. 30-1 and 34.

FORBES, J. A.
Locating the elderly in a general practice. *Nursing Times*, Aug. 21, 1969, p. 1063-5.

GLASGOW RETIREMENT COUNCIL
The Glasgow Retirement Council. *Nursing Mirror*, April 12, 1963, p. v-vi.

GUNN, A. D. G.
Lonely old people. *Nursing Times*, Oct. 15, 1965, p. 1405-6.

GUNTER, L. M.
A new look at the older patient in the community through the eyes of nursing students. *Nursing Forum*, vol. VIII, no. 1, 1969, p. 50-63.

HARDY, S.
Residential accommodation for the elderly. *Nursing Mirror*, Nov. 13, 1970, p. 20.

HARRISON, M.
Hypothermia in the elderly. *Nursing Mirror*, Oct. 25, 1968, p. 18-9.

HARROLD, J. M.
Liaison work and geriatric services. *District Nursing*, July 1970, p. 75-6.

HAYTER, M.
An experiment in the care of the disabled elderly. [Ealing Day-treatment Centre.] *Nursing Mirror*, April 3, 1964, p. iv-vi.

HERD, L.
A chairleg-elevator solves a problem. *Nursing Times*, Feb. 12, 1970, p. 203.

HILLIAM, IRIS E. O.
Practical problems in the care of the elderly [incontinence and pressure sores]. *Nursing Times*, Feb. 13, 1969, p. 207-9.

HODKINSON, MARY A.
The future of geriatric nursing. *Nursing Mirror*, Jan. 12, 1962, p. iii-iv.

HODKINSON, MARY A.
Nursing the elderly. Oxford, Pergamon, 1966.

HOWELL, T. H.
Geriatrics and geriatric nursing. *British Hospital Journal and Social Service Review*, July 23 1965 p. 1397-9.

HOWELL, T. H.
The medicine of old age. *District Nursing*, July 1970, p. 70-1.

HULICKA, I. M.
Fostering self-respect in aged patients. *American Journal of Nursing*, Mar. 1964, p. 84-9.

HURR, W. A.
Bathing the elderly and infirm. *Nursing Mirror*, Mar. 6, 1970, p. 42-3.

HYAMS, D. E.
A realistic look at geriatrics—1. *Nursing Times*, Nov. 3, 1967, p. 1477-9.

HYAMS, D. E.
A realistic look at geriatrics. 2—The art of geriatric nursing. *Nursing Times*, Nov. 10, 1967, p. 1507 and 1509.

INGLIS, D., and SAYERS, L. A.
An active treatment geriatric ward. *Canadian Nurse*, Dec. 1963, p. 1136-41.

IRVINE, E. D.
Community care for the elderly mentally deteriorated. *District Nursing*, May 1967, p. 34-5.

IRVINE, R. E.
Nursing the elderly sick. *Nursing Times*, Mar. 20, 1964, p. 371-3.

JOSHI, JAYANT B.
Nursing of tomorrow in geriatrics. *Nursing Journal of India*, Jan. 1970, p. 11 and 32.

KEMP, R.
A positive approach to old age. *Nursing Times*, Sept. 7, 1962, p. 1128-30.

KING EDWARD'S HOSPITAL FUND FOR LONDON. THE HOSPITAL CENTRE
Comprehensive care for the elderly. *Nursing Times*, July 19, 1968, p. 983.

KINOY, S. K.
Home health services for the elderly. *Nursing Outlook*, Sept. 1969, p. 59-62.

KLEIN, Sister M. AMADEUS
Understanding the aged: a basis for nursing care. *Hospital Progress*, June 1969, p. 106, 110, 114 and 116-7.

KLUGMAN, H. B.
Nutrition in the aged. *South African Nursing Journal*, Mar. 1964, p. 7-9.

LAMB, DOROTHY E.
Nurse-geriatric patient relationships in a stress situation. *In*
AMERICAN NURSES' ASSOCIATION
Phases in human development: relevance in nursing. New York The Association, 1962.

LLOYD, W. H.
Medical problems of old age and final rehabilitation in comprehensive unit. *Nursing Mirror*, Dec. 15, 1961, p. 201-2.

McCALL, J.
Attitudes to health in the elderly. *Nursing Times*, April 30, 1970, p. 562-4.

MICHELL, B.
Advanced clinical work [in the care of the elderly]. *Nursing Times*, May 15, 1969, Occasional Papers, p. 77-80.

MITCHELL, J.
Communication in the geriatric unit—1. *Nursing Times*, April 3, 1969, p. 423-5.

MITCHELL, J.
Communication in the geriatric unit—2. *Nursing Times*, April 10, 1969, p. 465-6.

MITCHELL, J.
Communication in the geriatric unit—3. *Nursing Times*, April 17, 1969, p. 495-6.

NATIONAL NURSES' ASSOCIATION OF THE NETHERLANDS
Nursing services for the aged and chronic sick. *International Nursing Review*, vol. 8, no. 1, 1961, p. 28-39.

NEVILLE, R.
Psychogeriatric day hospitals. *Nursing Mirror*, Aug. 11, 1967, p. ix-x.

NEW ZEALAND, DEPARTMENT OF HEALTH. RESEARCH AND PLANNING UNIT
Patient-nurse dependency: geriatrics; an analysis of survey data from three public hospitals in Christchurch, 1962. Wellington, Owen, 1964.

NEWTON, KATHLEEN, *and* ANDERSON, HELEN C.
Geriatric nursing. 4th edn. St. Louis, Mosby, 1966.

NOBBS, K. L. G.
Confusion in the elderly. *Nursing Times*, Sept. 21, 1962, p. 1190-2.

NORTON, DOREEN
Concept of geriatric nursing. *Nursing Mirror*, Oct. 15, 1965, p. 167-8.

NORTON, DOREEN
Effects of ward temperatures on the elderly. *Nursing Times*, June 29, 1962, p. 826-8.

NORTON, DOREEN
The elderly patient and the student nurse. *Nursing Times*, July 27, 1962, p. 950-1.

NORTON, DOREEN
Geriatric nursing problems. *Nursing Times*, Feb. 23, 1962, p. 236-8.

NORTON, DOREEN, *and others*
An investigation of geriatric nursing problems in hospital, by Doreen Norton, Rhoda McLaren and A. N. Exton-Smith. National Corporation for the Care of Old People [1962].

NURSING TIMES
L.C.C. homes for old people. *Nursing Times*, Mar. 31, 1961, p. 403.

OLSON, EDITH V.
The nurse and the repersonalization of the aged.
In
AMERICAN NURSES' ASSOCIATION
Effects of stereotypes on nursing care. New York, The Association, 1962.

PARRY, W. H.
Growing old in the Welfare State. *Nursing Times*, Mar. 13, 1964, p. 346-8.

PESZCZYNSKI, M.
Why old people fall. *American Journal of Nursing*, May 1965, p. 86-8.

PRITCHARD, J. G.
Reaction to long-term illness in the elderly. *Nursing Mirror*, Aug. 21, 1970, p. 19-21.

PLYMOUTH COUNCIL OF SOCIAL SERVICE
The kindest people. Boarding out old people in Plymouth. *Nursing Times*, June 26, 1964, p. 831-3.

RAE, M.
Nursing training in geriatrics. *Nursing Times*, Nov. 24, 1967, p. 1587-8.

RAINSBURY, J. P.
Preparation for retirement. *District Nursing*, June 1970, p. 58-9.

RICHARDSON, D. K.
Cold is a killer. *Nursing Times*, Sept. 24, 1970, p. 1234-6.

ROBERTSON, H.
Dentures: their significance in psychogeriatric nursing. *Nursing Mirror*, Feb. 6, 1970, p. 42-3.

ROSIN, A. J.
Aspects of geriatrics today. *District Nursing*, April 1970, p. 6-8.

ROSIN, A. J.
Long-stay care and its problems. *Nursing Times*, Oct. 9, 1969, p. 1287-90.

ROSIN, A. J.
Modern approach to the care of the elderly. *Nursing Mirror*, Mar. 17, 1967, p. 560-2.

ROYAL COLLEGE OF NURSING *and* NATIONAL COUNCIL OF NURSES OF THE UNITED KINGDOM
Care of the elderly. The College, 1969.

ROYAL COLLEGE OF NURSING *and* NATIONAL COUNCIL OF NURSES OF THE UNITED KINGDOM
Living longer! living happier! Report of a conference held in London, March 1965. *Nursing Times*, Mar. 12, 1965, p. 373-4.

RUDD, T. N.
Geriatric long-stay wards as therapeutic communities. *Nursing Times*, Sept. 8, 1961, p. 1156 and 1160-1.

RUDD, T. N.
Human relations in old age: a handbook for health visitors, social workers and others. Faber, 1967.

RUDD, T. N.
The nursing of the elderly sick: a practical handbook of geriatric nursing. 4th edn. Faber, 1964.
5th edn., 1966.
6th edn., 1970.

RUDD, T. N.
Preparation for retirement.
1. Philosophical and psychological aspects.
2. Pre-retirement training schemes.
Nursing Mirror, July 3, 1964, p. 303-4; July 10, 1964, p. 331-2.

RUDD, T. N.
Return to nursing. Geriatric nursing today. *Nursing Mirror*, May 9, 1969, p. 38-41.

SAUNDERS, C.
Care of patients suffering from terminal illness. *Nursing Mirror*, Feb. 14, 1964, p. vii-x.

SAUNDERS, C.
The last stages of life. *Nursing Times*, July 30, 1965, p. 1028-32.

SAX, S.
The modern approach to the nursing care of the aged. *The Australian Nurses' Journal*, Dec. 1967, p. 240-4.

SCHAPIRA, K.
Mental disorders in the elderly. *Nursing Times*, Nov. 6, 1969, p. 1426-9.

SCHWARTZ, DORIS, *and others*
The elderly ambulatory patient: nursing and psychosocial needs, by Doris Schwartz, Barbara Henley and Leonard Zeitz. New York, Macmillan, 1964.

SEARLE, D. J.
The psychogeriatric services. Report of a conference held at the Hospital Centre, London, on Sept. 9, 1970. *Nursing Mirror*, Sept. 25, 1970, p. 10-11.

SEPPELT, I. H.
The elderly at home in Ealing. *Nursing Times*, Jan. 15, 1965, p. 87-90.

SHAW, A.
Hypothermia in the elderly. *District Nursing*, July 1970, p. 78-9.

SHEEN, E. M., *and* DUNCAN, E. H. L.
The health visitor's work among the chronic sick and aged. *Nursing Times*, Aug. 18, 1961, p. 1057-9.

SKRIMSHIRE, M.
On approaching retirement. *Occupational Health*, Aug. 1970, p. 241-3.

SMITH, B. J.
Geriatric nursing. *Nursing Mirror*, Mar. 31, 1967, p. iv-viii.

SMITH, EMILY M.
Nursing services for the aged in housing projects and day centers. *American Journal of Nursing*, Dec. 1965, p. 72-4.

SNEDDON, R.
Psychiatric geriatric assessment unit at Crichton Royal Hospital. *Nursing Mirror*, April 7, 1967, p. x-xv.

STAFFORD, N. H.
Bowel hygiene of aged patients. *American Journal of Nursing*, Sept. 1963, p. 102-3.

STEVENS, MARION KEITH
Geriatric nursing for practical nurses. Philadelphia, Saunders, 1965.

STONE, V.
Give the older person time. *American Journal of Nursing*, Oct. 1969, p. 2124-7.

STOTSKY, BERNARD A., *editor*
The nursing home and the aged psychiatric patient. New York, Appleton-Century-Crofts, 1970.

TAYLOR, JOSEPHINE, *and* GAITZ, CHARLES M.
Obstacles encountered in the rehabilitation of geriatric patients. *Nursing Forum*, vol. VIII, no. 1, 1969, p. 64-73.

TEWARI, S. N., *and* BLENKIRON, C. H.
A comparison of non-barbiturate sedatives in elderly patients. *Nursing Times*, Feb. 5, 1970, p. 178-80.

THOMPSON, J. D., *and others*
Age a factor in amount of nursing care given, AHA study shows. *Hospitals*, Mar. 1, 1968, p. 33-9.

TURNER, W. J.
The home care program. Modern approaches to the care of the elderly in the home environment. *Bedside Nurse*, Feb. 1970, p. 15-9.

WARD, P. M.
The purpose and work of geriatric day hospitals. *Nursing Times*, June 23, 1967, p. 819-21.

WHITAKER, A.
The aged. *District Nursing*, July 1964, p. 92-4.

WIGNALL, E. W.
Helping old people to keep warm. *District Nursing*, Oct. 1965, p. 170-2.

WILKINS, P. S. W.
Hazards of the electric blanket for the elderly. *Nursing Times*, Feb. 1, 1963, p. 135.

WILLINGTON, F. L.
Dietary factors in the maintenance of health in the elderly. *District Nursing*, July 1970, p. 72-4.

WILSON, M.
A guide for the public health nurse to assist elderly patients in the achievement of selected functional tasks at home. *International Journal of Nursing Studies*, Nov. 1970, p. 243-6.

YALOM, I. D., *and* TERRAZAS, F.
Group therapy for psychotic elderly patients. *American Journal of Nursing*, Aug. 1968, p. 1690-4.

ZEMAN, F. D.
Guidelines for the professional nurse in geriatric drug therapy. *Hospitals*, Mar. 1, 1967, p. 67-70.

GYNAECOLOGY

BREWER, JOHN I., *and others*
Gynecologic nursing, by John I. Brewer, Doris M. Molbo and Albert B. Gerbie. St. Louis, Mosby, 1966.

CAIRNEY, JOHN
Gynaecology for senior students of nursing. 2nd edn. Christchurch, N.Z., Peryer, 1961.
3rd edn., 1963.

DODDS, GLADYS H.
Gynaecology: a handbook for nurses. 4th edn. Faber, 1962.
5th edn., 1967.

FISHER, A. M.
Introduction to laparoscopy in gynaecology. *NATNews*, Autumn 1970, p. 21-3.

FITZPATRICK, GENEVIEVE M.
Gynecologic nursing. New York, Macmillan, 1965.

HECTOR, WINIFRED, *and* BOURNE, GORDON
Modern gynaecology with obstetrics for nurses. 3rd edn. Heinemann, 1963.
4th edn., 1969.

LERCH, CONSTANCE, *and* WAGNER, JOANNE K.
Workbook for gynecologic nursing. St. Louis, Mosby, 1967.

LEYSHON, V. N.
Taking cervical smears in the home. *Nursing Times*, Mar. 18, 1966, p. 361-2.

MILLER, NORMAN F., *and* AVERY, HAZEL
Gynecology and gynecologic nursing: with a chapter on the gynecology operating room by Molly Kowal. 5th edn. Philadelphia, Saunders, 1965.

PATTULLO, A. W., *and* BARNARD, K. E.
Teaching menstrual hygiene to the mentally retarded. *American Journal of Nursing*, Dec. 1968, p. 2572-5.

PLATT, L. I., *and* ZACHARY, M. C.
An experience with annual pelvic examinations in 290 women workers. *Occupational Health Nursing*, Feb. 1970, p. 13-5.

SNAITH, L.
Childlessness. *District Nursing*, July 1969, p. 62-3.

INFECTIOUS AND PARASITIC DISEASES

COLE, A. C. E.
Parasitic infection in the U.K.—1.
Parasitic infection in the U.K.—2.
Nursing Times, Aug. 16, 1968, p. 1106-8; Aug. 23, 1968, p. 1147-8 and 1151.

CORRIGAN, MARJORIE J., *and* CORCORAN, LUCILLE E.
Epidemiology in nursing: the proceedings of the workshop on epidemiology in nursing, conducted at the Catholic University of America, June 10 to 21, 1960. Washington, Catholic University of America Press, 1961.

JAMIESON, W. M.
Return to nursing. Communicable disease in its modern setting. *Nursing Mirror*, May 2, 1969, p. 33-6.

JOHNSTON, DOROTHY F.
Essentials of communicable diseases, with nursing principles. St. Louis, Mosby, 1968.

JUDD, E.
Herpes Zoster: a nursing challenge. *Journal of Practical Nursing*, Nov. 1969, p. 27 and 47-8.

PEARMAN, E.
Teaching communicable diseases. *Nursing Mirror*, May 8, 1970, p. 30-1.

LEPROSY

CHEUNG, P. L.
Leprosy—1 and 2. *Nursing Times*, Mar. 26, 1970, p. 389-91; April 2, 1970, p. 427-9.

SWEENEY, SISTER CATHERINE
Advance against leprosy in Pakistan. *Nursing Mirror*, May 8, 1970, p. 36-9.

SWEENEY, SISTER CATHERINE
Some social aspects of leprosy. *Nursing Mirror*, June 5, 1970, p. 40-3.

POLIOMYELITIS

JAMIESON, S. R.
Poliomyelitis. *Nursing Times*, Jan. 4, 1963, p. 9-11.

PEACH, A. M.
Poliomyelitis—a conquered fear? *Nursing Times*, Jan. 22, 1970, p. 107-9.

TYPHOID

NAIRN, M.
Health visitors in the Aberdeen typhoid epidemic. *Nursing Times*, Jan. 8, 1965, p. 59-60.

LOCOMOTOR SYSTEM

CHARTERED SOCIETY OF PHYSIOTHERAPY
Lifting patients in hospital. The Society [1962].

CHARTERED SOCIETY OF PHYSIOTHERAPY
Lifting patients in the home. The Society [1963].

CLARK, WILLIAM S.
Arthritis: a challenge to excellence in nursing care. *The Journal of Practical Nursing*, May 1968, p. 23-4.

COPEMAN, W. S. C., and BOWLER, K.
The chronic rheumatic diseases. 1—Rheumatoid arthritis. *Nursing Mirror*, Nov. 8, 1963, p. i-iv and vi.

COPEMAN, W. S. C., and BOWLER, K.
The chronic rheumatic diseases. 2—Drugs used in treatment of rheumatoid arthritis. *Nursing Mirror*, Nov. 15, 1963, p. 161-2.

CYRIAX, J.
Posture and pain. *District Nursing*, Nov. 1969, p. 154-5 and 158.

DAVIS, P. R.
The nurse and her back. *Nursing Times*, Oct. 20, 1967, p. 1403-4.

DOWNIE, W. W.
Rheumatoid arthritis—1. *Nursing Times*, April 24, 1969, p. 529-30.
See
WHALEY, K., for part 2.

EMERY, A. E. H.
Muscular dystrophies. *Nursing Mirror*, Mar. 1, 1968, p. 26-8.

GRAVELING, B.
Physiotherapy for replacement of arthritic hip. *Nursing Times*, Sept. 27, 1968, p. 1297-9.

GUTTMAN, Sir LUDWIG
Nursing problems in traumatic tetraplegia. *International Journal of Nursing Studies*, Sept. 1969, p. 151-60.

HART, F. D.
Analgesics in rheumatic disorders. *Nursing Mirror*, Mar. 17, 1961, p. 2197-8.

HOLT, P. J. L.
Surgery in rheumatoid arthritis. *Nursing Times*, Oct. 30, 1969, p. 1393-6.

HOLT, P. J. L.
Surgery in rheumatoid arthritis—2. *Nursing Times*, Nov. 6, 1969, p. 1417-8.

KINNAIRD, L. S.
Preserving skeletal muscle tone in inactive patients. *American Journal of Nursing*, Dec. 1969, p. 2662-3.

MACRAE, I.
Some aspects of nursing care in rheumatic diseases. *Nursing Times*, Mar. 13, 1969, p. 327-9.

MATTHEWS, W. B.
Facial myokymia. *Nursing Mirror*, Oct. 18, 1968, p. 34-5.

NICOLL, KATHLEEN B.
Skin traction: its management and nursing care. *Nursing Times*, Oct. 4, 1963, p. 1239-42.

NICOLL, KATHLEEN B.
Understanding traction. *Nursing Times*, 1963.
[A series of articles which appeared in the *Nursing Times* from Sept. to Nov. 1963.]

NUKI, G., and KEMPSILL, C. D.
The treatment of rheumatoid arthritis. *Nursing Times*, Oct. 18, 1968, p. 1411-2.

SIMMONS, J. Q.
Nursing the multiple sclerosis patient. *The Journal of Practical Nursing*, Nov. 1968, p. 22-4.

STEEL, V.
"Nurses' back injuries need not occur." Report of a conference held by Royal Australian Nursing Federation, West Australian Branch. *Journal of the West Australian Nurses*, Nov. 1969, p. 3-4 and 6-8.

VALENTINE, L. R.
Self-care through group learning [arthritic patients taught by a multi-disciplinary team]. *American Journal of Nursing*, Oct. 1970, p. 2140-2.

VAUGHAN-JACKSON, O. J.
The rheumatoid hand. *Nursing Mirror*, Oct. 15, 1970, p. 26-9.

WALSH, E. G.
Physiology of standing. *Nursing Times*, May 22, 1964, p. 659-60.

WHALEY, K.
Rheumatoid arthritis and the cervical spine. *Nursing Times*, May 8, 1969, p. 596-8.
See
DOWNIE, W. W.
for part I.

WOOD, H. L. C.
Treatment of arthritis of the hip. *Nursing Mirror*, Mar. 10, 1961, p. iv-vi.

YEOMAN, W.
The chronic rheumatic diseases. *Nursing Mirror*, Nov. 16, 1962, p. 143-4 and 150.

MEDICINE

ASHER, PATRIA
Modern medicine for nurses. Heineman, 1961.
[Previous title, "An introduction to medicine for nurses".]

CABLE, JAMES VERNEY
Principles of medicine: an integrated textbook for nurses. 2nd edn. Christchurch, New Zealand, Peryer, 1963.
3rd edn., 1966.
4th edn., 1969.

COOKE, R. GORDON
A summary of medicine for nurses for use in revision. 4th edn. Faber, 1963.
5th edn., 1966.

COOPER, PHILIP
Ward procedures and techniques. New York, Appleton-Century-Crofts, 1967.

DAVID, H. P.
Some criteria of clinical change and measurement. *Journal of Psychiatric Nursing*, Nov./Dec. 1967, p. 550-4.

GIBBS, D. D.
Some changes in the face in relation to general disease. *Nursing Times*, July 12, 1963, p. 871-4.

GIBSON, JOHN
Modern medicine for nurses. Oxford, Blackwell, 1970.

HECTOR, WINIFRED, and FAIRLEY, G. HAMILTON
Textbook of medicine for nurses. Heinemann, 1967.

JOULE, J. W.
Textbook of medicine for nurses. 3rd edn. Lewis, 1962.

SEARS, W. GORDON
Medicine for nurses. 9th edn. Arnold, 1963.
10th edn., 1966.
11th edn., 1970, by W. G. Sears and R. S. Winwood.

TOOHEY, M.
Medicine for nurses, with a chapter on psychological medicine by Henry R. Rollin. 6th edn., ed. by A. Bloom. Edinburgh, Livingstone, 1963.
7th edn., 1965.
8th edn., 1967.
9th edn., 1969.

SPECIALITIES

FIRST AID AND DOMESTIC MEDICINE

BURKE, M.
Gastric lavage in the treatment of poisoning. *Nursing Times*, Dec. 3, 1970, p. 1545-8.

FLEMING, MARY OWERS, *and* BENSON, MARION C.
Home nursing handbook. [2nd edn.] Boston, Heath, 1966.

GIDSEG, LUCILLE, *and* SARA, DOROTHY
Home nursing care: a self-instruction guide to techniques and equipment. New York, Collier Books, 1965.

KENDALL, JAMES S.
Medicine for home, factory, and first aid post. Birmingham, K & M Printing and Publishing Company, 1961.

LAWSON, A. A. H.
The basic management of acute poisoning. *Nursing Times*, Oct. 29, 1965, p. 1475-7.

LONDON, P. S.
Advances in first aid. *Nursing Times*, April 15, 1966, p. 494-6.

PEARSON, L.
Poison control as a nursing function. *The Canadian Nurse*, May 1967, p. 35-7.

ROSS, D. S.
First aid bags for doctors and nurses and a motorist's first aid kit. *Occupational Health*, Nov. 1970, p. 355-7.

RUSLINK, Doris
Family health and home nursing. New York, Macmillan, 1963.

SEARGEANT, P. W.
Netelast. *Nursing Times*, Sept. 15, 1967, p. 1248-50.

SMITH, R. A. GORDON
Essentials of first aid treatment. *Nursing Mirror*, July 20, 1962, p. ii-iv and xvi.

TAYLOR-YOUNG, S.
First aid for district nurses. Emergency resuscitation. *District Nursing*, Sept. 1968, p. 126-7 and 129.

THOMSON, W.
Teaching first aid. *Nursing Times*, Feb. 26, 1970, p. 271-3.

WATKIN, B.
First-aid and the S.R.N. *Nursing Mirror*, Jan. 28, 1966, p. 506.

WINGATE, D.
Gastric lavage in acute poisoning. *Nursing Times*, May 21, 1970, p. 648-9.

TROPICAL MEDICINE

ADAMS, A. R. D., *and* MAEGRAITH, B. G.
Tropical medicine for nurses. 2nd edn. Oxford, Blackwell, 1963.
3rd edn., 1970, by B. G. Maegraith and H. M. Gilles.

FREAM, WILLIAM C.
Aids to tropical hygiene and nursing. 5th edn. Bailliere, Tindall and Cassell, 1964.

GILLES, H. M.
Tropical diseases. The schistosomiases. *Nursing Times*, April 26, 1968, p. 565-7.

ROWLAND, H. A. K.
Here from the Tropics; management of recently arrived patients. *Nursing Times*, Nov. 19, 1970, p. 1481-4.

MENTAL HEALTH

AMERICAN NURSES' ASSOCIATION
Community mental health nursing. *American Journal of Nursing*, May 1970, p. 1019-21.

BATEMAN, D. J., *and* SACKETT, H. G.
The Mental Health Act 1959. Notes for nurses—1. *Nursing Times*, July 22, 1966, p. 963-4.

BATEMAN, D. J., *and* SACKETT, H. G.
The Mental Health Act, 1959. Notes for nurses—2. *Nursing Times*, July 29, 1966, p. 1010-2.

BAVIN, J.
Mental handicap—the role of the health visitor. *Midwife and Health Visitor*, July 1970, p. 248-51.

BELL, K. K.
The nursing consultant in a suicide prevention center. *Nursing Clinics of North America*, Dec. 1970, p. 687-97.

BROCKMEIER, M. J.
Who are the significant others? [Community mental health.] *Nursing Outlook*, Oct. 1969, p. 34-7.

BROCKOPP, G. W.
Assessment of suicide. *The Pennsylvania Nurse*, Dec. 1970, p. 2-4 and 21.

BULBULYAN, A.
Nurses in a community mental health center. *American Journal of Nursing*, Feb. 1969, p. 328-31.

BURN, J. L.
Health begins at home. Mental health in the home. *Nursing Times*, July 29, 1966, p. 1007-9.

CANADIAN NURSES' ASSOCIATION
Mental health nursing in Canada—an emerging role. *International Nursing Review*, vol. 16, no. 2, 1969, p. 173-7.

ELWELL, R.
Community mental health centres. *American Journal of Nursing*, May 1970, p. 1014-8.

EVANS, FRANCES MONET CARTER
The role of the nurse in community mental health. New York, Macmillan, 1968.

FARBEROW, N. L., *and* PALMER, R. A.
The nurse's role in the prevention of suicide. *Nursing Forum*, vol. III, no. 1, 1964, p. 93-103.

FISCHER, L. R.
Symposium on the nurse in community mental health. *Nursing Clinics of North America*, Dec. 1970, p. 631-712.

HARE, E. H.
Do new housing estates endanger mental health? *Nursing Mirror*, April 21, 1967, p. viii-x.

HORSLEY, S.
Key people in community mental welfare. 1—Introduction. *Nursing Mirror*, Jan. 5, 1968, p. 325-6.

HORSLEY, S.
Key people in community mental welfare. 2—Janus and the health visitor. *Nursing Mirror*, Jan. 12, 1968, p. 359 and 368.

HORSLEY, S.
Key people in community mental welfare. 3—Communication through psychodrama. *Nursing Mirror*, Jan. 19, 1968, p. xi-xii.

HORSLEY, S.
Key people in community mental welfare. 4—Emotional factors in midwifery. *Nursing Mirror*, Jan. 26, 1968, p. 20.

HORSLEY, S.
Key people in community mental welfare. 5—A glimpse into the future. *Nursing Mirror*, Feb. 2, 1968, p. 37-9.

KNIGHT, G.
Chronic depression and drug addiction treated by stereotactic surgery. *Nursing Times*, May 8, 1969, p. 583-6.

KRATTER, F. E.
Mental health services in the United States. *Nursing Mirror*, Feb. 10, 1967, p. vii-xiii.

LEWIS, R. V.
The nurse in a community mental health center. *Journal of Psychiatric Nursing*, May 1963, p. 228-32.

McGuire, J.
A cry for help: suicide and accident proneness. *Journal of Psychiatric Nursing*, Sept./Oct. 1964, p. 500-8.

Mackworth, J.
Religion and mental health—1 and 2. *Nursing Times*, Dec. 1, 1961, p. 1577; Dec. 8, 1961, p. 1603.

May, A. R., and Moore, S.
The mental nurse in the community. *The Lancet*, Jan. 26, 1963, p. 213-4.

Meldman M. J. and others
Nurse psychotherapists in a private practice. *American Journal of Nursing*, Nov. 1969, p. 2412-5.

Moss, B. J. L.
Stress a hazard of modern living. *Nursing Times*, Jan. 7, 1966, p. 7-9.

Popkin, D. R.
Coordination of field work experience in a course in community mental health. *Nursing Outlook*, Oct. 1969, p. 41-3.

Poulos, J.
Suicide. *Bedside Nurse*, Jan. 1970, p. 27-9.

Rae-Grant, Q.
Broad horizons of community mental health. *Journal of Psychiatric Nursing*, Mar./April 1967, p. 109-20.

Rees, J. R.
The nurse's contribution to mental health. *Nursing Mirror*, Nov. 23, 1962, p. 175.

Roberts, W. L.
Mental ill-health—the school child at risk. *Midwife and Health Visitor*, Mar. 1969, p. 101-3.

Robinson, Sister John Mary
Integrating mental health concepts in nursing care in six diploma schools of nursing; report of pilot study, July 1962-66 St. Vincent's Hospital Psychiatric Nursing Program, St. Louis, Missouri. St. Louis, St. Vincent's Hospital, 1966.

Satchell, B. M., and others
Are five weeks enough? [A course in community mental health care.] *Nursing Outlook*, July 1970, p. 38-40.

Shneidman, E. S.
Preventing suicide. *American Journal of Nursing*, May 1965, p. 111-6.

Stobo, Elizabeth C., and others
Report of the nurse in the elementary school: promotion of mental health, by Elizabeth C. Stobo, Dorothy Shoobs, Rosemary McKevitt and Grace Matsunage. New York, Teachers' College, Columbia University, 1968.

Torrie, A.
The health visitor and the new Mental Health Act. *Nursing Mirror*, Feb. 9, 1962, p. 367.

Torrie, A.
The health visitor and the new Mental Health Act. *Nursing Mirror*, Feb. 16, 1962, p. v.

University of California Extension and The School of Nursing
Community mental health concepts for nurse leaders. Conference held at Las Vegas, Nevada, November 13-18, 1966. Los Angeles, The University, 1966.

Wallace, C. M.
Another look at suicide. *Nursing Mirror*, Nov. 21, 1969, p. 27-8.

World Health Organization
The nurse in mental health practice. *Who Chronicle*, Jan. 1964, p. 9-13.

MENTAL SUBNORMALITY

Adams, M.
Community care for the mentally subnormal. *Nursing Times*, Aug. 18, 1961, p. 1053-6.

Arenillas, L.
Mental subnormality: clinical types, early detection and prevention. *District Nursing*, Mar. 1970, p. 242-4.

Bavin, J. T. R.
Aspects of care of mentally subnormal. 1—Biochemical disorders in mental deficiency. *Nursing Mirror*, June 15, 1962, p. ii-iv.

Bavin, J. T. R.
Aspects of care of mentally subnormal. 1—Biochemical disorders in mental deficiency (conclusion). *Nursing Mirror*, June 22, 1962, p. vi-vii.
See
Roswell D. Part 2.
Williams, R. M., Part 3.

Bavin, J. T. R.
The nurse in the subnormality hospital. The time for revolution is now. *Nursing Times*, May 8, 1969, p. 590-2; May 15, 1969, p. 628-30; May 22, 1969, p. 654-6.

Corfmat, P. T.
Aspects of care of mentally subnormal. The deaf and dumb subnormal person. *Nursing Mirror*, July 27, 1962, p. xi-xii; Aug. 3, 1962, p. xi.

Dittman, Laura
The nurse in home training programs for the retarded child. Washington, U.S. Department of Health, 1961.

Duncan, A. C.
Nursing care of the mentally subnormal. *Nursing Times*, May 25, 1962, p. 669-72.

Dunham, P. E.
The use of Plastazote, in a subnormality hospital. *Nursing Mirror*, Feb. 13, 1970, p. 40-1.

Dunsdon, E.
Care for the mentally retarded: nursing service in a large institution. *American Journal of Nursing*, Sept. 1963, p. 75-7.

Evagorou, D.
Kushlick: a wizard at Wessex [care of subnormal children]. *Nursing Times*, Nov. 26, 1970, p. 1530-2.

Fell, J. H.
Treating the mentally subnormal—a deputy charge nurse's original method. *Nursing Mirror*, Dec. 8, 1967, p. 247-8.

Garrety, C.
Social aspects of mental subnormality in the community. *District Nursing*, Mar. 1970, p. 245-6.

Gibson, John, and French, Thomas
Nursing the mentally retarded. 2nd edn. Faber, 1967.
[Previously titled "Mental deficiency nursing".]

Graham, P.
Psychopaedic nursing. Training the mentally defective child. *The New Zealand Nursing Journal*, June 1969, p. 26 and 28-9.

Gunzburg, H. C., and Gunzburg, A. L.
The nurse and institutional design in mental subnormality hospitals. *Nursing Times*, Aug. 20, 1970, Occasional Papers, p. 121-4.

Hallas, Charles H.
Nursing the mentally subnormal. 2nd edn. Bristol, Wright, 1962.
3rd edn. entitled "Care and training of the mentally subnormal", 1967.
4th edn., 1970.

Handley, P. R.
Activity nursing of severely subnormal children with gross physical handicaps. *Nursing Mirror*, Oct. 4, 1963, p. v-vii.

SPECIALITIES

Harris, L. E.
Attitudes of nurses in mental subnormality to their work and patients. *International Journal of Nursing Studies*, vol. 2 no. 1 1965 p. 13-22.

Haynes, Una
Sixteen thousand nurses ask for help (nursing problems relating to care of patients who sustain brain damage early in life).
In
American Nurses' Association
Phases in human development: relevance in nursing. New York, The Association, 1962.

Hill, N. J. W.
Nursing the disturbed, severely subnormal child. *Nursing Mirror*, April 30, 1965, p. vi-ix.

Hodges, B. E.
The future of mental subnormality hospitals. *Nursing Mirror*, Mar. 22, 1968, p. 22-4.

Holtgrewe, Marian M.
A guide for public health nurses working with mentally retarded children. Washington, U.S. Dept. of Health, 1964.

Holtgrewe, Marian M.
The role of the public health nurse in mental retardation. St. Louis, Missouri, Child Development Clinic, 1961.

Johnson, M. L.
Training centres for the mentally subnormal. *Nursing Mirror*, Dec. 19, 1969, p. 31-3.

Kahn, J. H.
Social factors affecting mentally subnormal children. *Nursing Mirror*, Nov. 10, 1967, p. 139-41.

Kirman, B.
The retarded child. *Nursing Times*, July 24, 1969, p. 935-7; July 31, 1969, p. 976-8.

Kushlick, A.
Mental subnormality—three patterns of care. *Nursing Times*, July 9, 1970, p. 889.

Leslie, E. A., *and* Ritchie, J. B.
Training of the subnormal patient—2. *Nursing Mirror*, June 10, 1966, p. vi-viii.
See
Robinson, J. R., Part 1.

Lockett, J.
Training the severely subnormal child in hospital. *Nursing Times*, June 19, 1969, p. 775-6.

Manning, M.
Nurse for the mentally subnormal. *Nursing Mirror*, June 17, 1966, p. 264-6.

Metson, B. H.
Mental subnormality nursing—the need for change. *Nursing Times*, Dec. 30, 1966, p. 1714-5.

Murison, J.
Limitations and possibilities in the care of the mentally handicapped. *Nursing Times*, Mar. 6, 1969, Occasional Papers, p. 37-40; Mar. 13, 1969, Occasional Papers, p. 41-4.

Murray, M.
Nursing and the mentally subnormal. *Nursing Mirror*, Nov. 29, 1968, p. 35-8.

National Association for Mental Health
Services for the mentally subnormal: a brief survey of community and residential facilities, with information on statutory and voluntary provisions. The Association, 1962.

National Society for Mentally Handicapped Children
Children out of touch. *Nursing Mirror*, Jan. 9, 1970, p. 31-2.

National Society for Mentally Handicapped Children
Needs of the backward child. *Nursing Mirror*, Jan. 16, 1970, p. 14-5.

Noble, M. A.
Nursing's concern for the mentally retarded is overdue. *Nursing Forum*, vol. IX, no. 2, 1970, p. 192-201.

Patterson, E. G., *and* Rowland, G. T.
Towards a thoery of mental retardation nursing. An educational model. *American Journal of Nursing*, Mar. 1970, p. 531-5.

Pilkington, T.
The growing problem of subnormality—1. *Nursing Times*, June 2, 1967, p. 732-3.

Pilkington, T.
The growing problem of subnormality—2. *Nursing Times*, June 9, 1967, p. 764-6.

Pilkington, T.
Subnormality in perspective. 1—What is mental subnormality? *Nursing Times*, Nov. 24, 1967, p. 1577-8.

Pilkington, T.
Subnormality in perspective. 2—What causes subnormality? *Nursing Times*, Dec. 1, 1967, p. 1623-5.

Pilkington, Thomas
Subnormality in perspective. 3—What can be done? *Nursing Times*, Dec. 8, 1967, p. 1657-8.

Pilkington, Thomas
Subnormality in perspective. 4—Pseudo-subnormality. *Nursing Times*, Dec. 15, 1967, p. 1677-9.

Pilkington, Thomas
Subnormality in perspective. 5—Prevention and research. *Nursing Times*, Dec. 22, 1967, p. 1725-7.

Pilkington, T.
Subnormality in perspective. 6—The hospital. *Nursing Times*, Dec. 29, 1967, p. 1755-6.

Pinfield, Ivan N.
Domestic training unit for mentally subnormal patients. *Nursing Mirror*, June 13, 1969, p. 21-3.

Pothier, P. C.
The developmental concepts of Piaget applied to nursing assessment and interventions with atypical children. *Journal of Psychiatric Nursing and Mental Health Services*, Jan./Feb. 1970, p. 30-6.

Pounds, V. A.
Play therapy [with subnormal children]. *Nursing Times*, June 12, 1969, p. 769.

Pozz, L. W.
The child who is mongoloid. *Bedside Nurse*, Jan. 1970, p. 17-20.

Quigley, C. J. P., *and* Barnes, A. L.
The importance of ward design in the socialization of subnormal patients. *Nursing Times*, May 14, 1970, Occasional Papers, p. 67-8.

Rajokovich, M.
Meeting the needs of parents with a mentally retarded child. *Journal of Psychiatric Nursing and Mental Health Services*, Sept./Oct. 1969, p. 207-11.

Robinson, J. R.
Training of the subnormal patient—1. The special training unit. *Nursing Mirror*, June 3, 1966, p. vii-ix.
See
Leslie, E. A. *and* Ritchie, J. B.—Part 2.

Roswell, D.
Aspects of care of mentally subnormal. 2—Some aspects of learning. *Nursing Mirror*, June 29, 1962, p. xi-xiii; July 6, 1962, p. x-xii.
See
Bavin, J. T. R., Part 1
Williams, R. M., Part 3

Royal College of Nursing *and* National Council of Nurses of the United Kingdom
The function, scope and training of nurses in England and Wales for the mentally subnormal. Rcn, 1967.

ROYAL MEDICO-PSYCHOLOGICAL ASSOCIATION
Nursing the mentally handicapped. *British Hospital Journal and Social Service Review*, June 5, 1970, p. 1070.

ST. CLAIRE-VERNON, J.
Problems of the mentally handicapped child in the family. *Midwife and Health Visitor*, May 1969, p. 192-5.

SMITH, J. P.
Care of the mentally subnormal in Scandinavia. *Nursing Mirror*, July 12, 1968, p. 27-8.

SMITH, M. C.
Mental retardation nursing: children with a difference. *Australian Nurses' Journal*, Mar. 1969, p. 48-52.

SPENCER, D. A.
100 points for the hospital for the mentally subnormal. *Nursing Times*, May 28, 1970, p. 695.

TUTT, N. S.
Nurse or teacher? [Nurses for the subnormal.] *Nursing Times*, Sept. 4, 1969, p. 1140-1.

VEVANG, B., *and others*
Experience in mental retardation for basic nursing students. *Nursing Forum*, vol. VI, no. 2, 1967, p. 183-94.

VON SCHILLING, K.C.
Needed: a positive approach to the mentally retarded. *Canadian Nurse*, June 1970, p. 30-2.

WATSON, G.
Out of a dark cellar. *Nursing Times*, June 18, 1970, p. 786-8.

WEAVER, S.
Through night to light [group activities with mentally subnormal patients to encourage mental activity]. *Nursing Mirror*, June 26, 1970, p. 40-3.

WEIR, T. W. H.
Experiment in nurse-teacher collaboration in care of mentally subnormal. *Nursing Mirror*, Feb. 7, 1964, p. iv-vi.

WHITE, EVELYN L.
Group teaching of mental retardates by nursing personnel.
In
AMERICAN NURSES' ASSOCIATION
The nurse and groups of patients or clients. New York, The Association, 1962.

WILLIAMS, RONA M.
Aspects of care of mentally subnormal. 3—Speech therapy and subnormality. *Nursing Mirror*, July 20, 1962, p. v-vi.
See
BAVIN, J. T. R.,—Part 1.
ROSWELL, D.,—Part 2.

WILMORE, S. B.
A mongol baby in the family. *Nursing Times*, July 16, 1970, p. 922-3.

WOLFF, ILSE S.
Nursing role in counselling parents of mentally retarded children. Washington, U.S. Department of Health, 1964.

WOLLEN, W.
Progress in medical aspects of mental subnormality. *Nursing Mirror*, May 19, 1967, p. vii-xii.

WOLLEN, W.
Psychiatric illness among the subnormal. *Nursing Mirror*, Sept. 4, 1970, p. 28-31.

WOOD, T.
Nursing the mentally subnormal: the facts and the future. *Nursing Mirror*, Feb. 6, 1970, p. 20-1.

WOODFALL, RUTH E.
Care for the mentally retarded: a retarded child at home. *American Journal of Nursing*, Sept. 1963, p. 80-2.

WOODFALL, RUTH E.
The nurse, the mentally retarded child and his family.
In
AMERICAN NURSES' ASSOCIATION
Nursing approaches to denial of illness. New York, The Association, 1962.

WRIGHT, M. W.
Care for the mentally retarded: scope of the problem. *American Journal of Nursing*, Sept. 1963, p. 70-4.

NEUROLOGY

ASHER, P.
The man and the disease. Harvey Cushing and Cushing's syndrome. *Nursing Mirror*, June 14, 1963, p. 236-8.

BICKERSTAFF, EDWIN R.
Brain-stem tumours. *Nursing Times*, Nov. 20, 1969, p. 1488-91.

BICKERSTAFF, EDWIN R.
Neurology for nurses. English Universities Press, 1965.

BORSAY, MARIA
A nursing challenge—caring for an adult patient with renal shutdown and neurological dysfunction [following laminectomy].
In
AMERICAN NURSES' ASSOCIATION
Phases in human development: relevance in nursing. New York, The Association, 1962.

BROMPTON, A. W.
"Stroke" rehabilitation. *Nursing Times*, July 5, 1963, p. 828-30.

BURT, M. M.
Perceptual deficits in hemiplegia. *America Journal of Nursing*, May 1970, p. 1026-9.

BURTIS, MARY B.
Dependency-independency conflicts of the quadriplegic patient.
In
AMERICAN NURSES' ASSOCIATION
Phases in human development: relevance in nursing. New York, The Association, 1962.

CHIVERS, R. J.
Patients with hemiplegia in the care of district nurses. *Nursing Times*, 1968, p. 1604-6.

COOK, J. B., *and others*
Traumatic tetraplegia. *Nursing Mirror*, Sept. 15, 1967, p. i-vii.

DAVIS, R. W.
Communication with the stroke victim. *Bedside Nurse*, Dec. 1970, p. 24-6.

GRAHAM, J. G.
Acute disseminated encephalomyelopathy. *Nursing Mirror*, Aug. 28, 1964, p. i-ii.

HANLEY, J.
Testing for epilepsy—at home. *Nursing Mirror*, Nov. 13, 1970, p. 17.

HENSON, R. A.
Neurological manifestations of malignant disease. *Nursing Mirror*, Sept. 26, 1969, p. 29-31.

HICKS, M. L.
Acoustic nerve tumors. *Nursing Science*, April 1963, p. 14-31.

HILKEMEYER, R., *and others*
Nursing care of patients with brain tumors. *American Journal of Nursing*, Mar. 1964, p. 81-3.

HORSLEY, S.
Conflicts and harmonies of normal stress. 1—Traumatic silence. *Nursing Times*, June 23, 1967, p. 816-8.

SPECIALITIES

HORSLEY, S.
Conflicts and harmonies of normal stress. 2—Creative tension. *Nursing Times*, June 30, 1967, p. 867-9.

HORSLEY, S.
Conflicts and harmonies of normal stress. 3—Echoes of neglected stress. *Nursing Times*, July 7, 1967, p. 898-901.

JACOBS, ERWIN M., and DENAULT, PHYLLIS M.
Neurology for nurses, including nursing technics in neurology. Springfield, Charles C. Thomas, 1964.

KIMBER, P. M., and MORGAN, G. A.
Cerebral angiography by arterial catheterization. *Nursing Times*, Sept. 3, 1970, p. 1137-40.

KRENZEL, JUDITH R., and ROHRER, LOIS M.
Paraplegic and quadriplegic individuals (handbook of care for nurses). Chicago, The National Paraplegia Foundation, 1966.

LEISTEN, D. P.
Rehabilitation of hemiplegics in the home. *Nursing Times*, July 23, 1965, p. 1004-6.

LIDDELL, D.
The care of paraplegic and quadriplegic patients.
1. The treatment begins.
2. The period of mobilization begins.
3. Towards full rehabilitation.
Nursing Times, Mar. 1, 1968, p. 281-4; Mar. 8, 1968, p. 319-21; Mar. 15, 1968, p. 360-3.

MCKENZIE, B.
Dysphasia, the patient, his family and the nurse. *Cardio Vascular Nursing*, Sept./Oct. 1970, p. 51-5.

MARSHALL, JOHN and MAIR, JEAN
Neurological nursing: a practical guide. 2nd edn. Oxford, Blackwell Scientific Publications, 1967.

MARTIN, M. A.
Nursing management of a patient with cerebral aneurysm. *The Journal of Nursing Education*, Aug. 1967, p. 27-39.

MEYER, R. G.
Caring for the spastic child at home. *Nursing Mirror*, Jan. 18, 1963, p. 341-3.

NEWTON, E. J.
Syringomyelia. *Nursing Mirror*, May 8, 1970, p. 21-5.

PARSONAGE, M.
Modern management of epilepsy. *Nursing Mirror*, Oct. 3, 1969, p. 34-8.

PARSONAGE, M.
Treatment and management of epilepsy. *District Nursing*, Aug. 1968, p. 94-5.

POUNDS, V. A.
Managing the subnormal epileptic. *Nursing Mirror*, Oct. 16, 1970, p. 38.

POWELL, MARY
Modern concepts in the nursing of paraplegia. *International Journal of Nursing Studies*, July 1969, p. 99-104.

PRATT, R.
Caring for the paralysed. *District Nursing*, June 1970, p. 48-50.

PRATT, R.
Caring for the paralysed—II. *District Nursing*, July 1970, p. 83-4.

RAMEY, I. G.
The stroke patient *is* interesting. *Nursing Forum*, vol. VI, no. 3, 1967, p. 273-9.

RAMSAY, A. M.
Infections of the central nervous system.
1—Acute suppurative meningitis.
2—Acute aseptic meningitis, meningoencephalitis and acute encephalitis.
Nursing Mirror, July 27, 1962, p. iv-vii; Aug. 3, 1962, p. iii-vi and xii.

RUBIN, S.
Home care of the "stroke" patient. *Nursing Times*, Oct. 6, 1967, p. 1339 and 1342-3.

SOUTHWOOD, J.
Obsessional neurosis. *Nursing Mirror*, Oct. 8, 1965, p. 27-9.

THOMPSON, B.
Parkinson people and others. Basic nursing of patients with mid-brain damage. *Nursing Times*, Aug. 6, 1970, p. 1004-6.

TRIGIANO, L. L.
Independence is possible in quadriplegia. *American Journal of Nursing*, Dec. 1970, p. 2610-3.

WHITE, P. D.
Strokes—prevention, diagnosis and patient care. *The Journal of Practical Nursing*, Oct. 1965, p. 24-7.

SPEECH DISORDERS

ADLER, S.
Speech after laryngectomy. *American Journal of Nursing*, Oct. 1969, p. 2138-41.

FOX, J.
Let the silent be heard [communication devices for people without speech]. *Nursing Times*, Oct. 15, 1970, p. 1326-8.

GREENE, M. C. L.
Early detection of speech difficulty.
1. The role of the health visitor.
2. Danger signals.
Nursing Times, Sept. 4, 1969, p. 1138-9; Sept. 11, 1969, p. 1170-1.

LECHE, P.
Speech therapy with adult brain-damaged patients. *Nursing Times*, Nov. 20, 1969, p. 1485-7.

MILLER, B. E.
Assisting aphasic patients with speech rehabilitation. *American Journal of Nursing*, May 1969, p. 983-5.

MOSER, D.
An understanding approach to the aphasic patient. *American Journal of Nursing*, April 1961, p. 52.

OWEN, E. N.
Treatment of ear, nose and throat conditions. Speech disabilities and their treatment. *Nursing Mirror*, Aug. 16, 1963, p. xi-xiii.

WALCHER, S. D.
Stuttering: the phenomenon, feelings and the nurse. *International Journal of Nursing Studies*, Sept. 1968, p. 185-91.

WOHL, M. T.
Disorders of communication. *Nursing Mirror*, Mar. 14, 1969, p. 20-1.

OBSTETRICS

BAILEY, ROSEMARY E.
Obstetric and gynaecological nursing. Bailliere, Tindall and Cassell, 1969.

BALL, H.
Relieving pain in labour. *Nursing Times*, May 7, 1965, p. 638-9.

BARNARD, J. E.
Peer group instruction for primigravid adolescents. *Nursing Outlook*, Aug. 1970, p. 42-3.

BETHEA, DORIS C.
Introductory maternity nursing. Pitman, 1968.

BLEIER, INGE J.
Maternity nursing: a textbook for practical nurses. Philadelphia, Saunders, 1961.

BLEIER, INGE J.
Workbook in bedside maternity nursing. Philadelphia, Saunders, 1969.

BURNETT, C. W. F.
A textbook of obstetric nursing. Oxford, Blackwell, 1964.

BURNETT, C. W. F.
Foetal distress during labour. *Nursing Times*, Dec. 11, 1969, p. 1579-81.

BURNETT, C. W. F.
Post-partum haemorrhage. *Nursing Times*, Dec. 18, 1969, p. 1618-20.

BURNETT, C. W. F.
Prolonged first stage of labour. *Nursing Times*, Dec. 4, 1969, p. 1553-5.

CHALMERS, J. A.
New concepts in the management of labour. *Nursing Mirror*, Nov. 22, 1968, p. 20-2.

CHERSTERMAN, J. N.
Intra-natal care. *Australian Nurses' Journal*, March 1961, p. 56-61.

CLARIDGE, M.
Abnormalities of the urinary tract in pregnancy. *Nursing Mirror*, May 16, 1969, p. 31-5.

CLARKE, C. A.
Prevention of Rh-haemolytic disease. *Nursing Mirror*, Jan. 16, 1970, p. 17-21.

COOKE, E. M.
Control of infection in maternity units. *Nursing Mirror*, Sept. 25, 1970, p. 23-4.

CROXFORD, E. A.
Focus on the maternity services. *Nursing Times*, Sept. 13, 1968, Occasional Papers, p. 141-4.

DAVIS, M. EDWARD, and RUBIN, REVA
Obstetrics for nurses. 17th edn. Philadelphia, Saunders, 1962.
For earlier editions see
DE LEE, JOSEPH BOLIVAR, and CARMON, MABEL C.

DUDGEON, J. A.
Intra-uterine infections—I, II and III. *Nursing Times*, July 23, 1970, p. 939-41; July 30, 1970, p. 973-5; Aug. 6, 1970, p. 1007-9.

DUNSTON, B. N.
Pica practice: its relationship to hemoglobin level and perinatal casualties. *Nursing Science*, April 1963, p. 32-9 and 64-9.

DWYER, J. M.
Transplantation immunity and the human placenta. *American Journal of Nursing*, Aug. 1968, p. 1712-5.

EDELSTON, H.
The psychological approach in childbirth. *Nursing Mirror*, April 19, 1963, p. 54-5.

EDWARDS, J.
Combined OB-gyn units: implications for nursing. *Hospital Topics*, April 1970, p. 95 and 98-9.

EDWARDS, J.
Needed: patient-oriented nursing in the maternity unit. *Hospital Topics*, Mar. 1970, p. 83-4 and 86.

FAIRWEATHER, D. V. I.
Intra-uterine transfusion of the foetus. *Nursing Mirror*, May 3, 1968, p. 19-22.

FELL, M. R.
Placenta praevia. *Nursing Times*, April 16, 1970, p. 494-6.

FITZPATRICK, ELSIE, and others
Maternity nursing. 11th edn., by Elsie Fitzpatrick, Nicholson J. Eastman and Sharon R. Reeder. Philadelphia, Lippincott, 1966.
For earlier editions see
ZABRISKIE, LOUISE, and EASTMAN, NICHOLSON J., "Nurses' handbook of obstetrics."

GARLAND, GORDON W., and QUIXLEY, JOAN M. E.
Obstetrics and gynaecology for nurses. 2nd edn. E.U.P., 1966.

GARNET, J. D.
Pregnancy in women with diabetes. *American Journal of Nursing*, Sept. 1969, p. 1900-2.

GODBER, GEORGE
The changing pattern in maternity care. *Nursing Mirror*, July 20, 1962, p. 301-3; July 27, 1962, p. 321-2.

GRANT, A.
Intranatal care in hospital. *Nursing Mirror*, Aug. 1, 1969, p. 18-9.

GRAY, H. H.
Anaesthesia and drugs in management of labour. *New Zealand Nursing Journal*, Aug. 1969, p. 20-2.

GREEN, G. H.
Introduction to obstetrics: a theory and practice for obstetric nurses. Christchurch, N.Z., Peryer, 1962. 2nd edn., 1963.

GREEN, G. H.
Multiple pregnancy. *Nursing Mirror*, Feb. 2, 1968, p. 13-4.

GRIFFIN, JOANNE K., and others, editors
Maternal and child health nursing: 1,500 multiple choice questions and referenced answers, edited by Joanne K. Griffin, Agnes V. Murray, Estelle B. Resnick and Jean W. Tease. 2nd edn. New York, Medical Examination Publishing Co., 1968.
[*Nursing Examination Review Book*, vol. 3.]

GUNN, A. D. G.
The normal pregnancy. *Nursing Times*, Jan. 15, 1970, p. 69-71.

GUNN, A. D. G.
The prevention of haemolytic disease of the newborn—the final steps. *Nursing Times*, July 17, 1969, p. 907-9.

HAMILTON, C. M.
Mothers and babies in a psychiatric unit. *Nursing Mirror*, Dec. 26, 1969, p. 28-30.

HAMILTON, PERSIS MARY
Basic maternity nursing. Saint Louis, C. V. Mosby, 1967.

HARGREAVES, T.
Jaundice in pregnancy and in the neonate. *Nursing Mirror*, April 17, 1970, p. 27-9.

HEHRE, F. W.
Obstetrical anesthesia: some physiological responses and common problems. *Journal of the American Association of Nurse Anesthetists*, Dec. 1970, p. 441-7.

HOFF, FLORENCE E.
Natural childbirth—how any nurse can help. *American Journal of Nursing*, July 1969, p. 1451-3.

HOMMEL, FLORA
Natural childbirth—nurses in private practice as monitrices. *American Journal of Nursing*, July 1969, p. 1446-50.

IORIO, JOSEPHINE
Principles of obstetrics and gynecology for nurses. St. Louis, Mosby, 1967.

JACKSON, R. J. A.
Prevention of prolonged labour. *Nursing Times*, Oct. 16, 1969, p. 1331-2.

JEFFERISS, D.
The sequelae of childbirth. *Nursing Mirror*, June 28, 1963, p. 283-4.

KAPLAN, A.
Obstetrics and gynecology: a text book for nurses. Moscow, Foreign Languages Publishing House, [1963?].

KELLY, D.
Painless childbirth. *Nursing Times*, Sept. 17, 1970, p. 1192-5.

SPECIALITIES

KITZINGER, S.
A fresh look at antenatal exercises. *Nursing Mirror*, Sept. 5, 1969, p. 14-6.

KLOPPER, A.
Obstetric disasters—pre-eclamptic toxaemia. *Nursing Times*, Jan. 26, 1968, p. 116-7.

KUZUCU, E. Y.
Anesthesia for obstetrics and resuscitation of the newborn. *Journal of the American Association of Nurse Anesthetists*, June 1969, p. 212-9.

LERCH, CONSTANCE
Maternity nursing. St. Louis, Mosby, 1970.

LUNDSTROM, P.
Monitoring the foetus in utero. *Nursing Mirror*, Jan. 23, 1970, p. 20.

LUSCHINSKY, L.
Breathing patterns and the relief of childbirth pain. *Practical Nursing*, Mar. 1963, p. 14 and 33.

MACDONALD, R. R.
Complications of abortion. *Nursing Times*, Mar. 10, 1967, p. 306-7.

NELSON, M. M.
Amniotic fluid. Its use in antenatal diagnosis. *Nursing Times*, Aug. 27, 1970, p. 1106-8.

PATEL, N. B., *and* MACNAUGHTON, M. C.
Premature labour—a new technique. *Nursing Times*, May 22, 1969, p. 650-1.

PHILLIPP, ELLIOT E., *and* CRISP, EVA
Midwifery for nurses. Lewis, 1962.

ROSENHEIM, G., *and* BRANSON, H. K.
The nurse and placenta praevia and abruptio. *Bedside Nurse*, Dec. 1970, p. 31-2.

RUSSELL, J. K.
Mothers—at risk. *Nursing Times*, Aug. 28, 1969, p. 1106-7.

RUSSELL, J. K.
The nurse as a member of the obstetric research team. *Nursing Times*, Sept. 13, 1968, p. 1230-2.

SCHNEIDER, M.
Automation and new techniques in obstetric nursing. *The Australian Nurses' Journal*, Sept. 1968, p. 200-7.

SMITH, CHRISTINE SPAHN
Maternal-child nursing. Philadelphia, Saunders, 1963.

SMITHELLS, R. W.
Paediatric aspects of therapeutic abortion. *Nursing Mirror*, April 28, 1967, p. 77-80.

STEVENS, B.
Post-partum psychoses: a changing pattern. *Nursing Times*, Oct. 1, 1970, p. 1257-9.

TINDALL, V. R.
Pulmonary embolism and deep vein thrombosis in the puerperium. *Midwives' Chronicle and Nursing Notes*, June 1969, p. 204-7.

ULIN, P. R.
Changing techniques in psychoprophylactic preparation for childbirth. *American Journal of Nursing*, Dec. 1968, p. 2587-91.

WATSON, M.
The present position of pain relief in labour. *Nursing Mirror*, Aug. 16, 1963, p. 431-2.

WILLIAMS, B.
48-hour maternity discharge—good or bad? *Nursing Mirror*, Oct. 11, 1968, p. 33-5.

WILLIAMS, B. L., *and* RICHARDS, S. F.
Fetal monitoring during labour. *American Journal of Nursing*, Nov. 1970, p. 2384-8.

WILLIAMS, G.
Reversal of sterilization in the female. *Nursing Times*, July 31, 1969, p. 973-5.

WILLIS, T.
Monitoring the mother and fetus during labor. *Canadian Nurse*, Dec. 1970, p. 28-31.

WOODWARD, HENRY L., *and* GARDNER, BERNICE
Obstetric management and nursing. 7th edn. Philadelphia, Davis, 1964.

YEAWORTH, R. C.
Identification and maternity nursing. *Nursing Forum*, vol. VII, no. 3, 1968, p. 249-61.

YUNEK, M. J.
Postpartum care is more than a routine. *Nursing Outlook*, Jan. 1969, p. 50-2.

ZUCK, D.
Epidural analgesia in obstetrics. *Nursing Times*, Nov. 15, 1968, p. 1548-50.

OCCUPATIONAL HEALTH NURSING

ALEXY, B. J., *and* CONDRON, C. A.
Treatment and nursing care of patients with contact dermatitis from epoxy resins. *American Association of Industrial Nurses' Journal*, May 1964, p. 6-7.

AMERICAN MEDICAL ASSOCIATION
Guiding principles and procedures for industrial nurses in care of eye injuries. *American Journal of Nursing*, Sept. 1961, p. 86.

AMERICAN NURSES' ASSOCIATION. OCCUPATIONAL HEALTH NURSES' SECTION
Selected areas of knowledge or skill basic to effective practice of occupational health nursing. New York, The Association, 1966.

ARCHIBALD, R. McL.
Nursing problems in the coal mining industry. *Nursing Mirror*, May 6, 1966, p. x-xii.

ARCHIBALD, R. McL.
Protective clothing—some random thoughts. *Occupational Health*, Sept. 1970, p. 275-9.

ATKINSON, E. J.
The work of the industrial nurse. *Nursing Times*, Oct. 20, 1967, p. 1405-6.

AVERY, H. P.
The industrial nurse—the person and the challenge. *American Association of Industrial Nurses' Journal*, Nov. 1961, p. 28-30.

BASSFORD, P. A.
Cancer health education in industry. *Nursing Times*, June 12, 1969, p. 748-9.

BIDEN-STEELE, K.
Some occupational disease hazards. 5—Infections in relation to occupation. *Occupational Health*, Jan./Feb. 1963, p. 3-9.
See
Part 1. MALCOLM, M.
Part 2. COOKE, M. A.
Part 3. BIDSTRUP, P. L.
Part 4. BROWNING, E.
Part 6. EDSON, E. F.

BIDSTRUP, P. L.
Chemical hazards in industry. *Nursing Mirror*, June 10, 1966, p. 225-7.

BIDSTRUP, P. L.
Some occupational disease hazards.
Part 3. The newer metals. *Journal for Industrial Nurses*, July/Aug. 1962, p. 173-85.
See
Part 1. MALCOLM, M.
Part 2. COOKE, M. A.
Part 4. BROWNING, E.
Part 5. BIDEN-STEELE, K.
Part 6. EDSON, E. F.

BLAIR, M.
The care of women employees in a general hospital. *American Association of Industrial Nurses' Journal*, May 1967, p. 9-11.

BLAKELEY, M.
Today's occupational health nurse. *Nursing Mirror*, May 3, 1968, p. 16 and 52-3.

BLAKELEY, M.
Today's occupational health nurse. *Nursing Mirror*, May 10, 1968, p. 41-2.

BLANEY, L.
Perspectives on lasers. *American Association of Industrial Nurses' Journal*, July 1968, p. 13-6.

BOND, H. M.
The hand in industry. *Occupational Health*, May 1970, p. 137-40.

BONNELL, J. A.
Radiation protection in nuclear power stations. *Nursing Times*, Mar. 1, 1968, p. 278-81.

BOURNE, L. B.
Synthetic resin dermatitis. *Nursing Mirror*, Aug. 7, 1964, p. v-vi.

BOURNE, L. B.
Unusual cases of industrial skin disease. *Nursing Mirror*, Mar. 15, 1968, p. 29-31.

BROWN, M. L.
A profile of occupational health nursing. *Occupational Health Nursing*, Feb. 1970, p. 16-8.

BROWN, M. L.
The role of the nurse in occupational mental health. *Occupational Health*, Mar./April 1969, p. 66-80.

BROWNING, E.
Early signs of industrial poisoning. *Nursing Mirror*, Aug. 2, 1963, p. 383-4.

BROWNING, E.
Ionising radiations.
Part 2. *Journal for Industrial Nurses*, Mar./April 1961, p. 57-65.
See
Part 1. CHAVE, S. P. W.
Part 3. JONES, B. E.
Part 4. HUGHES, J. P. W.
Part 5. DUNCAN, K. P.
Part 6. BURNETT, M. K.

BROWNING, E.
Some occupational disease hazards.
Part 4 (1). Solvents—the hydrocarbons. *Journal for Industrial Nurses*, Sept./Oct. 1962, p. 241-6.
Part 4 (2). Solvents—other important toxic solvents. *Journal for Industrial Nurses*, Nov./Dec. 1962, p. 287-94.
See
Part 1. MALCOLM, M.
Part 2. COOKE, M. A.
Part 3. BIDSTRUP, P. L.
Part 5. BIDEN-STEELE, K.
Part 6. EDSON, E. F.

BRUEGGEN, S. L.
Eye health in industry. *American Journal of Nursing*, Sept. 1961, p. 83.

BUNDLE, N.
The nurse and industrial accident prevention. *Occupational Health*, May/June 1967, p. 164-70.

BURN, J. L.
Modern threats to health—Radiation hazards. *Nursing Times*, Oct. 19, 1962, p. 1314.

BURNETT, M. K.
Ionising radiations.
Part 6. The role of the occupational health nurse in an industry with a radiation hazard. *Journal for Industrial Nurses*, Nov./Dec. 1961, p. 283-8.
See
Part 1. CHAVE, S. P. W.
Part 2. BROWNING, E.
Part 3. JONES, B. E.
Part 4. HUGHES, J. P. W.
Part 5. DUNCAN, K. P.

BUSBY, J.
Epoxy resins—practical control. *Occupational Health*, Mar./April 1965, p. 97 and 99.

CAMERON, J. D.
Accident prevention in relation to the work of the occupational health nurse. *Nursing Mirror*, Sept. 4, 1964, p. x-xii.

CHADWICK, D. L.
Care of the ear in industry. *Occupational Health*, May/June 1963, p. 135-43.

CHAVE, S. P. W.
Ionising radiations.
Part 1. Introduction to radiation. *Journal for Industrial Nurses*, Jan./Feb. 1961, p. 3-10.
See
Part 2. BROWNING, E.
Part 3. JONES, B. E.
Part 4. HUGHES, J. P. W.
Part 5. DUNCAN, K. P.
Part 6. BURNETT, M. K.

COOKE, M. A.
Some occupational disease hazards.
Part 2. The older metals and metalloids. *Journal for Industrial Nurses*, May/June 1962, p. 119-28.
See
Part 1. MALCOLM, M.
Part 3. BIDSTRUP, P. L.
Part 4. BROWNING, E.
Part 5. BIDEN-STEELE, K.
Part 6. EDSON, E. F.

COOLEY, C. E.
Occupational health nursing and rehabilitation. *Rehabilitation*, Oct./Dec. 1968, p. 21-6.

DAVIES, B. M.
Airport nurse. *Nursing Times*, Oct. 29, 1970, p. 1392-4.

DAVIES, D.
Coalworkers' pneumoconiosis. *Nursing Times*, Aug. 3, 1962, p. 981-3.

DAWES, J.
Inspection for chrome ulceration. *Occupational Health*, Jan. 1970, p. 13-5.

DIXON, W. M.
Care of the skin in industry. *Nursing Mirror*, Jan. 20, 1967, p. 361-2.

DORAN, W. T.
Occupational health nursing and the nuclear age. *Occupational Health Nursing*, July 1970, p. 26-8.

DOWNIE, A. P.
Lung function tests and their application in industrial pulmonary disease. *Occupational Health*, Nov./Dec. 1966, p. 297-307.

SPECIALITIES

DUNCAN, K. P.
Ionising radiations.
Part 5. Clinical effects of exposure to ionizing radiations. *Journal for Industrial Nurses*, Sept./Oct. 1961, p. 225-9.
See
Part 1. CHAVE, S. P. W.
Part 2. BROWNING, E.
Part 3. JONES, B. E.
Part 4. HUGHES, J. P. W.
Part 6. BURNETT, M. K.

ECKARDT, R. B.
The toxicological aspects of petroleum distillates. *American Association of Industrial Nurses' Journal*, July 1967, p. 13-5.

EDSON, E. F.
Some occupational disease hazards.
Part 6. Chemical pesticides. *Occupational Health*, Mar./April, 1963, p. 61-70.
See
Part 1. MALCOLM, M.
Part 2. COOKE, M. A.
Part 3. BIDSTRUP, P. L.
Part 4. BROWNING, E.
Part 5. BIDEN-STEELE, K.

EKDAWI, M. Y., *and* DICKER, J.
Psychiatric emergencies in industry. *Nursing Mirror*, May 16, 1969, p. 28 and 35.

FEURTADO, M.
Occupational health nursing in a bauxite industry. *Occupational Health*, July 1970, p. 205-20.

FLY, O. A., *and* McGOVERN, J. P.
Epoxy resins in industry. Allergic reactions and their control. *American Association of Industrial Nurses' Journal*, April 1964, p. 23-5.

FRASER, M.
Report on First Industrial Safety Course for Women held at Paraparaumu, New Zealand, 13-16 April 1964. *The New Zealand Nursing Journal*, Mar. 1965, p. 10-1.

GALLAHER, H. L., *and* WYATT, G. M.
The occupational health nurse and the patient with trauma. *Nursing Clinics of North America*, Dec. 1970, p. 609-19.

GHEI, P. N., *and* SIVARAMAN, P.
Nurse and noise. *The Nursing Journal of India*, Dec. 1969, p. 431 and 442.

GRACE, H. K.
The work setting as a mental health system. *Occupational Health Nursing*, July 1970, p. 13-7 and 44.

GUCKIAN, J. C.
Aiding your employees' physical fitness. *Occupational Health Nursing*, Aug. 1969, p. 23-6.

HALLAHAN, J. D.
The industrial nurse as a medical evaluator. *American Association of Industrial Nurses' Journal*, Aug. 1968 p. 20-1.

HAMILTON, V.
Preventing hearing loss in industry. *Canadian Nurse*, Sept. 1970, p. 37-40.

HAWTHORNE, V. M.
Multiphasic screening. *Occupational Health*, June 1970, p. 178-82.

HINE, C. H.
The role of the industrial nurse in the detection and prevention of drug abuse. *Occupational Health Nursing*, April 1969, p. 15-7.

HIRSCHFELD, A. H.
What to do until the psychiatrist comes. *American Association of Industrial Nurses' Journal*, May 1961, p. 12-8.

HOLDER, B. J.
Cardiopulmonary resuscitation. Implications and responsibilities for the occupational health nurse. *Occupational Health Nursing*, Aug. 1970, p. 13-5.

HOLGATE, P. D., *and* KNIGHT, K. L.
The control of trichloroethylene hazards: the nurse's role. *Occupational Health*, Jan. 1970, p. 3-12.

HUGHES, J. P. W.
Ionising radiations. Part 4. Protection of workers exposed to ionising radiations from radioactive isotopes used in industry. *Journal for Industrial Nurses*, July/Aug. 1961, p. 169-74.
See
Part 1. CHAVE, S. P. W.
Part 2. BROWNING, E.
Part 3. JONES, B. E.
Part 5. DUNCAN, K. P.
Part 6. BURNETT, M. K.

HUGHES, J. P. W.
Role of the occupational health nurse today and tomorrow. *Nursing Mirror*, Oct. 20, 1967, p. 72-6.

HUTCHINS, J.
Orientation of the aerospace nurse to occupational health. *American Association of Industrial Nurses' Journal*, July 1968, p. 7-12.

INTERSOCIETY COMMITTEE ON NOISE EXPOSURE CONTROL
Noise exposure control. *American Association of industrial Nurses' Journal*, May 1968, p. 17-21.

JONES, B. E.
Ionising radiations. Part 3. Some applications of ionising radiations. *Journal for Industrial Nurses*, May/June 1961, p. 113-20.
See
Part 1. CHAVE, S. P. W.
Part 2. BROWNING, E.
Part 4. HUGHES, J. P. W.
Part 5. DUNCAN, K. P.
Part 6. BURNETT, M. K.

KELLER, M. J.
The occupational health nurse and short-term illness absences. *Nursing Outlook*, Sept. 1968, p. 32-4.

KRUGER, D. G.
Occupational health nursing—Rx for tomorrow. The Catherine R. Dempsey Lecture. *Occupational Health Nursing*, July 1970, p. 9-12.

LEATHART, G. L.
Asbestos. A medical hazard of the 20th century. *Occupational Health*, May/June 1964, p. 119-31.

LEE, W. R.
Towards the prevention of electric shock. *Nursing Mirror*, Jan. 28, 1966, p. 507-8.

McCALLUM, R. I.
Decompression sickness: the complications of work in compressed air. *Nursing Times*, Aug. 28, 1969, p. 1108-10.

McCANN, J. K.
The safe use of epoxy resins in industry. *Occupational Health*, Mar./April 1965, p. 90-6.

McCATTY, B. E.
An industrial nurse in an ore processing plant. *The Jamaican Nurse*, April/May 1969, p. 12.

McLAUGHLIN, A. I. G.
Preventing dust disease. *Nursing Mirror*, Feb. 1, 1963, p. 383-5.

MAAS, R. B.
Personal hearing protection—the occupational health nurse's challenge and opportunity. *Occupational Health Nursing*, May 1969, p. 25-7.

MALCOLM, M.
Some occupational disease hazards.
Part 1. Lead: inorganic and organic. *Journal for Industrial Nurses*, Jan./Feb. 1962, p. 3-11.
See
Part 2. COOKE, M. A.
Part 3. BIDSTRUP, P. L.
Part 4. BROWNING, E.
Part 5. BIDEN-STEELE, K.
Part 6. EDSON, E. F.

MELNICK, W.
Ear protectors. *Occupational Health Nursing*, May 1969, p. 28-31.

MOORE, W. K. S.
Occupational health nursing in the pharmaceutical industry. *Nursing Mirror*, July 29, 1966, p. xi-xiii.

MORANT, P. E.
Protective clothing: then and now. *Occupational Health*, Sept. 1970, p. 285-90.

MUNRO, L. B.
Preplacement health screening by nurses in industry. *Canadian Nurse*, Nov. 1970, p. 29-32.

MURPHY, A. J.
The identity of the nurse in an industrial hearing conservation program. *Occupational Health Nursing*, May 1969, p. 32-4 and 36.

NILO, E. R.
Audiometers. *Occupational Health Nursing*, May 1969, p. 15-7.

O'CONNOR, K. J. R.
The mysteries of radiation. 1—Hazards. *Nursing Times*, Oct. 28, 1966, p. 1414-6.

O'CONNOR, K. J. R.
The mysteries of radiation. 2—Effects and treatment of over-radiation. *Nursing Times*, Nov. 4, 1966, p. 1452-3.

OWENS, F. M.
The human cost of accidents. *Occupational Health*, May 1970, p. 141-4.

PARRY, W. H.
Farmer's lung. *Nursing Times*, Feb. 23, 1968, p. 261-2.

PEMBERTON, DOREEN
Essentials of occupational health nursing. Arlington Books, 1965.

PLATT, L. I., and ZACHARY, M. C.
An experience with annual pelvic examinations in 290 women workers. *Occupational Health Nursing*, Feb. 1970, p. 13-5.

PORRITT, J. L.
Oral surgery (in relation to occupational health). *American Association of Industrial Nurses' Journal*, July 1968, p. 27-44.

POSNER, E.
Health conditions in the ceramic industry. *Occupational Health*, July/Aug. 1968, p. 218-24.

RAJA, G. L. P.
Health hazards in refractory work. *The Nursing Journal of India*, June 1967, p. 142-3.

RALPHS, D.
Industrial nursing. *Nursing Mirror*, April 4, 1969, p. 35.

RENNIE, R. S.
Epoxy resins as an industrial health hazard. *Occupational Health*, May/June 1969, p. 147-53.

RILEY, E. C.
Preventing deafness from industrial noise. *American Journal of Nursing*, May 1963, p. 80-4.

ROACH, E. G.
The occupational health sister. Paper given at the Royal Australian Nursing Federation Third Biennial Convention held at Brisbane 13th-16th October 1964. *Journal of the West Australian Nurses*, July 1965, p. 17-21.

ROCHE, L.
The nurse in industry. *The Canadian Nurse*, Aug. 1964, p. 749-50.

ROSS, D. S.
Investigation of a storeman's exposure to X-ray radiation. *Occupational Health*, Oct. 1970, p. 329-32 and 335.

ROYAL COLLEGE OF NURSING *and* NATIONAL COUNCIL OF NURSES OF THE UNITED KINGDOM
A hospital occupational health service. *Nursing Times*, Nov. 27, 1964, p. 1582-3.

ROYAL COLLEGE OF NURSING *and* NATIONAL COUNCIL OF NURSES OF THE UNITED KINGDOM. OCCUPATIONAL HEALTH COMMITTEE
Occupational health nursing. Rcn, 1966.
Rev. edn., 1968.

RUMMERFIELD, P. S., *and* RUMMERFIELD, M. J.
Noise induced hearing loss. *Occupational Health Nursing*, Nov. 1969, p. 23-9, 43-4 and 46.

SATALOFF, J.
The ear and the industrial nurse. *American Association of Industrial Nurses' Journal*, July 1965, p. 11-4.

SIEGEL, G. S.
Occupational health nursing. *American Association of Industrial Nurses' Journal*, June 1968, p. 22-4.

SINNOTT, M. B.
A health interview program. *American Association of Industrial Nurses' Journal*, April 1964, p. 6-10.

SKRIMSHIRE, M. J.
Occupational health nursing. *Rehabilitation*, July/Sept. 1968, p. 19-24.

SLANEY, B.
Broad aspects of occupational health nursing. *Occupational Health*, Sept./Oct. 1969, p. 256-66.

SMITH, E. J.
Functions of an occupational health nurse [with the Public Utility Transportation Corporation in Johannesburg]. *South African Nursing Journal*, Nov. 1970, p. 26.

SMITH, V. L.
Industrial nursing. *Bedside Nurse*, Dec. 1970, p. 20-3.

STEELE, MARGARET L.
The difference in industrial nursing. *Nursing Outlook*, April 1961, p. 234-5.

STEELE, MARGARET L.
Standard procedures for the nurse in industry. *American Association of Industrial Nurses' Journal*, Oct. 1961, p. 16-7.

STEELE-BODGER, A.
Hazards of animal handling. *Occupational Health*, Feb. 1970, p. 43-51.

STEMBRIDGE, J.
A survey of hand injuries. *Occupational Health*, July/Aug. 1967, p. 222-6.

STOVES, V.
What is occupational health nursing? *Nursing Times*, July 29, 1966, p. 995.

TEPLOW, L.
Industrial nursing; skill or profession. *American Association of Industrial Nurses' Journal*, Nov. 1962, p. 10-3.

THOMAS, S. M. G.
The use of protective gloves. *Occupational Health*, Sept. 1970, p. 281-4.

THOMSON, W.
Leptospirosis—an occupational hazard. *Nursing Times*, July 2, 1970, p. 847-8.

THOMSON, W.
The problems of asbestos. *Nursing Times*, Nov. 12, 1970, p. 1449-51.

TRANSACTIONS OF THE SOCIETY OF OCCUPATIONAL MEDICINE
Nurses in industry. *Transactions of the Society of Occupational Medicine*, Oct. 1966, p. 93.

TYRER, F. H.
Occupational health nursing. Bailliere, Tindall and Cassell, 1961.

SPECIALITIES

UNITED STATES. BUREAU OF DISEASE PREVENTION AND ENVIRONMENTAL CONTROL
Nursing practices and occupational mental health. Cincinnati, Ohio, U.S. Department of Health, Education and Welfare, 1967.

VOELZ, G. L.
Industrial nursing in the nuclear reactor industry. *American Association of Industrial Nurses' Journal*, Nov. 1961, p. 18-21.

WALKER, GRACE G.
Dressing techniques in industry. *Occupational Health*, Mar./April 1963, p. 71.

WALKER, GRACE G.
Dressing techniques in industry. *Nursing Mirror*, Nov. 1, 1963, p. v-vii.

WALLACE, S. A.
The occupational health nursing consultant service in Ontario. *Occupational Health Nursing*, June 1969, p. 29-30.

WEST, MARION M.
A handbook for occupational health nurses, with contributions by Brenda M. Slaney and H. F. Chard. 3rd edn. Arnold, 1962.
[Previously "A handbook for industrial nurses".]

WEST, R.
Factory workers and their health. *Nursing Times*, Oct. 22, 1965, p. 1438-40.

WHITE, R.
Health and the worker. *Nursing Times*, July 19, 1963, p. 898-9.

WIENER, A. D.
Control of occupational disease in small plants. *American Association of Industrial Nurses' Journal*, Dec. 1961, p. 23-6.

WILCOX, F. W.
Radiation safety. *Occupational Health Nursing*, Oct. 1970, p. 14-7.

WILLIAMS, M. MARGARET
Dressing techniques in industry. *Nursing Times*, Dec. 1, 1961, p. 1568-70.

WILLIAMS, M. MARGARET
Report of a survey of some current surgical dressing techniques in industry. Rcn, 1961.

WILLIAMS, N.
Automation and health. *The Canadian Nurse*, May 1965, p. 360-2.

WILSON, P. D.
Industrial and medical emergencies. *Occupational Health*, Jan./Feb. 1967, p. 5-12.

WRIGHT, B. J.
Occupational health nurse or welfare officer? *Nursing Mirror*, Mar. 1, 1968, p. 32-4.

ADMINISTRATION

AHERN, MARGUERITE S.
The occupational health nurse's role in absentee control. How to collect and provide meaningful data. *American Association of Industrial Nurses' Journal*, May 1968, p. 7-10.

AHERN, MARGUERITE S.
Reflections of an occupational health nurse as "safety engineer." *Occupational Health Nursing*, Oct. 1969, p. 22-3.

AHLERS, M. E.
Occupational health nursing in the Republic of South Africa. *Occupational Health*, Jan./Feb. 1967, p. 3-4.

ALLARDICE, J. T.
A reference system in an occupational health unit. *Occupational Health*, May/June 1969, p. 154-6.

AMERICAN ASSOCIATION OF INDUSTRIAL NURSES
The American Association of Industrial Nurses. *American Association of Industrial Nurses' Journal*, Dec. 1961, p. 8.

AMERICAN ASSOCIATION OF INDUSTRIAL NURSES
Principles of the nurse-physician relationships in industry. *American Association of Industrial Nurses' Journal*, Sept. 1962, p. 22.

AMERICAN NURSES' ASSOCIATION
Functions and qualifications for an occupational health nurse in a one-nurse service. New York, The Association, 1968.

AMERICAN NURSES' ASSOCIATION. OCCUPATIONAL HEALTH NURSES' SECTION
Functions, standards and qualifications for occupational health nurses. New York, The Association, [196?]

AMERICAN NURSES' ASSOCIATION. OCCUPATIONAL HEALTH NURSES' SECTION
Guide for the development of a manual for an employee health program. New York, American Nurses' Association, 1962.

BELL, A.
Occupational health. The pattern in Australia with particular reference to New South Wales. *International Nursing Review*, vol. 8, no. 5, 1961, p. 23-30.

BLACKLAWS, D. M.
Industrial nursing in South Africa. *Occupational Health Nursing*, June 1969, p. 11-2.

BLACKLAWS, D. M.
The occupational health nurse [at Lever Brothers, Transvaal]. *South African Nursing Journal*, Nov. 1970, p. 31-2.

BLAKELEY, M.
The specialty of occupational health and the nurse's role within it. *Australian Nurses' Journal*, Nov. 1969, p. 241-3.

BLAKELEY, M.
The specialty of occupational health and the nurse's role within it. [cont.] *Australian Nurses' Journal*, Dec. 1969, p. 254-7.

BOORER, D.
Opportunities for men. The challenge of industry. *Nursing Times*, Sept. 11, 1964, p. 1185-8.

BOUCOT, K. R.
The future of occupational health. *American Association of Industrial Nurses' Journal*, Sept. 1961, p. 18.

BRIDGER, H., and others
The doctor and sister in industry—1. *Occupational Health*, Sept./Oct. 1963, p. 235-50.

BRIDGER, H., and others
The doctor and sister in industry—2. A study of change. *Occupational Health*, Nov./Dec. 1963, p. 293-308.

BROGAN, MILDRED M.
What is worth doing is worth recording. [Medical records in industry.] *Occupational Health Nursing*, Jan. 1969, p. 9-14.

BROWN, M. L.
Data on occupational health nurses. *American Journal of Nursing*, May 1965, p. 120-3.

CAFFREY, C. A.
Toward enlarging the role of the industrial nurse in the company. *American Association of Industrial Nurses' Journal*, Nov. 1964, p. 14-7.

CHARD, S. D.
Analysing the work pattern of S.R.N.s in industry. *Nursing Mirror*, Oct. 2, 1964, p. 5-7.

CHRISTIE, E. J.
Occupational health nursing in Northern Ireland. *Occupational Health*, Sept./Oct. 1966, p. 225-6.

COUNCIL ON OCCUPATIONAL HEALTH, CHICAGO
Medical directives for occupational health nurses. *American Association of Industrial Nurses' Journal*, Nov. 1963, p. 15-21.

DAVIES, M. K., and RHODES, C. E.
Occupational health in civil aviation. *Nursing Mirror*, May 1, 1970, p. 30-1.

DE KRETSER, A. J. H.
Working with the safety officer. *Journal for Industrial Nurses*, May/June 1962, p. 129.

DIXON, W. M.
Place of the nurse in a group industrial health service. *Nursing Mirror*, Sept. 3, 1965, p. x-xii.

DONOVAN, J.
Occupational health nursing in Great Britain. *Occupational Health*, Sept./Oct. 1966, p. 223-5.

DOYLE, M.
Why the one-nurse unit? *American Association of Industrial Nurses' Journal*, June 1964, p. 20-2 and 30.

EDWARDS, K. E.
Occupational health nursing. *The Jamaican Nurse*, April/May 1969, p. 9-11.

EDWARDS, K. E.
Occupational health nursing and the Jamaican environment. *Occupational Health*, Sept./Oct. 1968, p. 238-51.

FELTON, J. S.
Medical direction in occupational health nursing. *American Journal of Nursing*, Sept. 1966, p. 2019-22.

FELTON, J. S., and PLEASANTS, I.
Men in occupational health nursing. *Occupational Health Nursing*, Jan. 1970, p. 9-18.

FISHBEIN, MORRIS
Communication on industrial nursing. *Occupational Health Nursing*, July 1969, p. 11-2.

FLUNDER, D. J.
What the employer expects from the occupational health nursing service. *Occupational Health*, Jan./Feb. 1969, p. 21-4.

GILHESPY, M.
Hospital casualty department and the works surgery. *Nursing Mirror*, Oct. 4, 1963, p. 9.

GILLIN, E. F.
The occupational health sister's contribution to the economic structure of an organization. *The Lamp*, Jan. 1969, p. 19-22.

HALLAM, J.
Human relations and the occupational health nurse. *Nursing Mirror*, Sept. 13, 1963, p. 511-2.

HARRIS, A. M.
Measuring the nurse's effectiveness. *American Association of Industrial Nurses' Journal*, Nov. 1968, p. 9-12.

HEALEY, J. T.
Microfilming industrial medical records. *Occupational Health Nursing*, Sept. 1970, p. 19-20.

HEFETZ, G.
The industrial health nurse in Israel. *Occupational Health*, Sept./Oct. 1966, p. 227-9.

HENRIKSEN, H. L.
Satisfactions and challenges in occupational health nursing. *American Association of Industrial Nurses' Journal*, May 1961, p. 20-5.

HINE, C. H., and WRIGHT, J. A.
A program for control of drug abuse in industry. *Occupational Health Nursing*, April 1970, p. 17-8 and 41.

HOWARD, L. S.
Community resources—how the occupational nurse can use them. *American Association of Industrial Nurses' Journal*, Sept. 1965, p. 7-10.

HUNTER, W.
The doctor's view on the development of the occupational health nurse's role. *Occupational Health*, Jan./Feb. 1969, p. 10-6.

HUNTER, W.
Modern role of the occupational health nurse. *Nursing Mirror*, July 25, 1969, p. 29-31.

JAMES, M. J.
Survey of occupational health practices by nurses in Victoria, Australia. *Occupational Health Nursing*, Feb. 1970, p. 11-2.

JOHNSON, D. R.
Today and tomorrow. *American Association of Industrial Nurses' Journal*, June 1968, p. 17-9.

KELLER, M. J.
An overview of occupational health nursing in an era of change. *Occupational Health Nursing*, April 1970, p. 19-21 and 44.

KELLY, J.
A co-operative program between hospital and industrial nurses. *Occupational Health Nursing*, Sept. 1970, p. 13-4.

KNABE, H.
The occupational health nurse in the German Democratic Republic. *Occupational Health*, Sept./Oct. 1968, p. 252-3.

KUHLI, R.
The management of industrial safety. *American Association of Industrial Nurses' Journal*, July 1967, p. 9-12.

LEE, DOROTHY M.
Training and organization of first aiders in industry. *Occupational Health*, Mar./April, 1963, p. 94.

LEE, J. A.
The occupational health nurses' responsibilities to the employee. *Occupational Health Nursing*, April 1969, p. 18-21.

McCAULEY, S.
Part-time nursing service in small industry. *American Association of Industrial Nurses' Journal*, Sept. 1967, p. 7-12.

McHENRY, R. W.
The importance of good leadership. *American Association of Industrial Nurses' Journal*, Nov. 1968, p. 13-7.

McNAUGHTON, N.
Employee health service. *The Canadian Nurse*, Dec. 1967, p. 45-6.

MEIKLEJOHN, A.
The future of health in industry. *Occupational Health*, Sept./Oct. 1965, p. 233-54.

MURPHY, D. C.
Industrial hygiene. *Nursing Mirror*, May 27, 1966, p. x-xii.

NADEL, L.
Management cares. *American Association of Industrial Nurses' Journal*, Sept. 1968, p. 19-21.

NURSING MIRROR
Occupational health nurses at the BBC. *Nursing Mirror*, Oct. 11, 1968, p. 41-3.

O'BRIEN, M. E.
Widening horizons in occupational health nursing. *International Nursing Review*, vol. 15, no. 3, 1968, p. 280-4.

ONTARIO. DEPARTMENT OF HEALTH. ENVIRONMENTAL HEALTH BRANCH
Occupational health nursing in Ontario: a report on results from a questionnaire prepared by M. I. Hardy. Toronto, The Department, 1967.

RAFFLE, P. A. B.
Human factors in automation. *Occupational Health*, July/Aug. 1966, p. 190-204.

SPECIALITIES

REYNARD, W. A.
The wider responsibilities of the occupational health nurse. *Occupational Health*, Jan./Feb. 1963, p. 12-9.

RHODES, C. E.
The Trade Union Movement. An extract from a day book prepared during the O.H.N.C. Course, Rcn, 1965-66. *Occupational Health*, May/June 1967, p. 157-63.

ROGAN, J.
Automation: social changes for which we should prepare. *Occupational Health*, Sept./Oct. 1966, p. 251-61.

ROYAL COLLEGE OF NURSING. OCCUPATIONAL HEALTH SECTION
Nursing service to industry and commerce: salaries and conditions of service, duties and responsibilities and ethical relationships. New edn., The College, 1961.

ROYAL COLLEGE OF NURSING and NATIONAL COUNCIL OF NURSES OF THE UNITED KINGDOM. OCCUPATIONAL HEALTH COMMITTEE
Occupational health nursing structure. Rcn, 1968.

RUSH, H. C.
The role of the industrial nurse re-examined. *American Association of Industrial Nurses' Journal*, Mar. 1967, p. 10-1.

RUSSO, A. M.
The focus of the occupational health nurse in a changing environment. *Occupational Health Nursing*, July 1970, p. 18-9.

SASDI, M.
Industrial health services in Hungary. *Occupational Health*, Sept./Oct. 1966, p. 233-7.

SAYANJARVI, R.
Occupational health nursing in Finland. *Occupational Health Nursing*, June 1969, p. 18-20.

SCHMIDT, M. D.
The administration and supervision of multiple nursing services within an industry. *American Association of Industrial Nurses' Journal*, April 1961, p. 26-7.

SHERMAN, A. W.
Working together in business. *American Association of Industrial Nurses' Journal*, Aug. 1963, p. 20-3.

SKRIMSHIRE, M.
The new occupational health nursing structure. *Occupational Health*, Jan./Feb. 1969, p. 4-9.

SLANEY, B. M.
Healthy at work? Employed Persons (Health and Safety) Bill. *Nursing Times*, April 23, 1970, p. 528-30.

SLANEY, B. M.
Occupational health nursing in international associations. *International Nursing Review*, vol. 16, no. 4, 1969, p. 340-52.

SLANEY, B. M.
Principles of occupational health nursing. *Journal for Industrial Nurses*, Nov./Dec. 1961, p. 308.

STOVES, V.
The support of the professional organization to the occupational health nurse. *Occupational Health*, Mar./April 1969, p. 104-14.

STRIEGEL, BERNADINE
Correlation—a new dimension. *Occupational Health*, Mar./April 1963, p. 79.

SUMMERS, M.
An industrial nurse's role in the conservation of labor. *American Association of Industrial Nurses' Journal*, Jan. 1962, p. 12.

TAYLOR, J.
The changing pattern of occupational health. *Queensland Nurses' Journal*, May 1969, p. 9-11.

TAYLOR, J.
Occupational health. The factory is a battlefield. *Australian Nurses' Journal*, Sept. 1969, p. 190-2.

UNITED STATES. PUBLIC HEALTH SERVICE. DIVISION OF OCCUPATIONAL HEALTH
Occupational health nurses: an initial survey, by Mary Lou Bauer and Mary Louise Brown. Washington, U.S. Department of Health, Education and Welfare, 1966.

UNITED STATES. PUBLIC HEALTH SERVICE. DIVISION OF OCCUPATIONAL HEALTH
Nursing part time in industry. Washington, U.S. Government Printing Office, 1965.

VANHOORNE, M.
Occupational medicine in Belgium. *Occupational Health*, Nov./Dec. 1968, p. 312-4.

WHITE, B. J.
Nursing in industry. 1—What to expect. *Nursing Mirror*, Dec. 27, 1963, p. 275-6.

WHITE, B. J.
Nursing in industry. 2—Professional ethics in the factory. *Nursing Mirror*, Jan. 3, 1964, p. 299-300.

WHITE, B. J.
Nursing in industry. 3—Professional relationships. *Nursing Mirror*, Jan. 10, 1964, p. 329.

WHITE, R.
A concept of occupational health nursing. *Nursing Mirror*, Oct. 22, 1965, p. 183-4.

WHITE, R.
A reappraisal of the nurse's role. *Occupational Health*, Jan./Feb. 1969, p. 17-20.

WHITE, R.
Reappraisal of the occupational health nurse's role. *Nursing Mirror*, Aug. 1, 1969, p. 40-1.

WILKINSON, L.
The enrolled nurse in industry. *Nursing Mirror*, April 4, 1969, p. 32-4.

WILLIAMS, E. V.
The 1st AAIN. *American Association of Industrial Nurses' Journal*, Jan. 1968, p. 7-9.

WOODMAN, M. M. L.
Some aspects of occupational health nursing in Australia. *Occupational Health Nursing*, June 1969, p. 21-3.

WOODS, J.
Occupational health nursing in Saskatchewan. *Journal for Industrial Nurses*, May/June 1962, p. 136.

ZACHARY, M. C.
Confidentiality of medical records. Role of the nurse. *Occupational Health Nursing*, Dec. 1969, p. 18-20.

EDUCATION

AMERICAN ASSOCIATION OF INDUSTRIAL NURSES
Committee on Education 1943-1968. *American Association of Industrial Nurses' Journal*, Jan. 1968, p. 10-1.

AMERICAN ASSOCIATION OF INDUSTRIAL NURSES
Recommended qualifications of an industrial nurse. *American Association of Industrial Nurses' Journal*, Sept. 1964, p. 24-8.

AMERICAN ASSOCIATION OF INDUSTRIAL NURSES
Report... of a survey to determine the number of schools of professional nursing in the United States which offer learning experiences related to occupational health. *American Association of Industrial Nurses' Journal*, Mar. 1962, p. 24-6.

BROWN, M. L.
Occupational health nursing in the United States: training and education. *Occupational Health Nursing*, Nov. 1969, p. 11-5.

FELTON, J. S.
A curriculum in occupational health for nurses. *American Association of Industrial Nurses' Journal*, Nov. 1968, p. 18-20.

HARRIS, A. M.
Education for tomorrow's industrial nurse. *American Association of Industrial Nurses' Journal*, Dec. 1961, p. 14-6.

INTERNATIONAL LABOUR ORGANISATION. INTERNATIONAL LABOUR OFFICE
The occupational health nurse. Proceedings of the symposium on the Training of Occupational Health Nurses held during the International Occupational Safety and Health Congress (Geneva, 30 June - 4 July 1969). Geneva, The Office, 1970.

JUNEL, I.
Education of the occupational health nurse in Sweden. *Occupational Health*, Mar./April 1969, p. 81-6.

KELLER, MARJORIE J.
Answer to an inquiry about education for occupational health nursing. *Occupational Health Nursing*, Mar. 1969, p. 11-4.

KELLER, MARJORIE J.
The student program: participation, not observation. *Occupational Health Nursing*, Nov. 1970, p. 17-9.

KELLER, MARJORIE J., and MAY, W. THEODORE
Occupational health content in baccalaureate nursing education. Cincinnati, Ohio, U.S. Department of Health, Education and Welfare, 1970.

KLUTAS, E. M.
Graduate education in occupational health nursing—an experiment. *American Association of Industrial Nurses' Journal*, Dec. 1964, p. 6-13.

LAMBERT, E. E.
Industrial nursing. *South African Nursing Journal*, Nov. 1966, p. 12-3.

NATIONAL LEAGUE FOR NURSING. INTERDIVISIONAL COUNCIL ON OCCUPATIONAL HEALTH NURSING
Occupational health nursing for the basic nursing student; a report of a workshop, July 2-6, 1962, University of Washington School of Nursing, by Edna May Klutas. New York, The League, 1966.

NOBLE, E.
An experimental course. *Occupational Health*, July/Aug. 1966, p. 188-9.

ORGAIN, F.
Education for occupational health nursing. *American Association of Industrial Nurses' Journal*, Oct. 1966, p. 22-3 and 27.

RASAK, E.
The new nurse. Orientation and in-service training. *American Association of Industrial Nurses' Journal*, Nov. 1968, p. 21-2.

ROBERTS, L.
Educational opportunities for industrial nurses. *American Association of Industrial Nurses' Journal*, Oct. 1966, p. 17-9.

SAYANJARVI, R.
Education of the occupational health nurse in Finland. *Occupational Health*, Mar./April 1969, p. 87-94.

SIMPSON, H. M.
Education and training of industrial nurses in various European countries. *American Association of Industrial Nurses' Journal*, Mar. 1961, p. 24-7.

SLANEY, B. M.
Education for occupational health nursing. *Occupational Health*, Mar./April 1969, p. 95-103.

SLANEY, B. M.
Education for occupational health nursing. *Occupational Health*, July/Aug. 1966, p. 170-4.

SLANEY, B. M.
My job—tutor in occupational health nursing. *Occupational Health Nursing*, June 1969, p. 31-3.

SLANEY, B. M.
Why take the Occupational Health Nursing Certificate? *Nursing Mirror*, Dec. 9, 1966, p. 221-3.

STOVES, V.
I.L.O. Symposium on the training of occupational health nurses. Report on United Kingdom, Finland, United States, USSR, East Germany, Spain, Brazil, Greece, Norway and Sudan. *Occupational Health*, Nov./Dec. 1969, p. 318-32.

WILLIAMS, M. M.
The need for specialist tutors in occupational health nursing education. *Occupational Health*, Nov./Dec. 1969, p. 333-5.

SPECIAL OCCUPATIONAL HEALTH SERVICES

BOAC Nursing Service, London Airport. *Nursing Times*, Aug. 23, 1963, p. 1057-60.

BURGESON, E. C.
Sixty-two years later. The philosophy and principles are the same ... only the people have changed. [Medical Department of Sears, Roebuck & Co., Chicago.] *Occupational Health Nursing*, Aug. 1970, p. 19-23.

CENTRAL MIDDLESEX INDUSTRIAL HEALTH SERVICE
Central Middlesex Industrial Health Service. *Occupational Health*, Sept./Oct. 1964, p. 245-52.

DUNDEE UNIVERSITY
Department of Social and Occupational Medicine. Ten years on. *Occupational Health*, Nov. 1970, p. 359-68.

GREAT BRITAIN. MINISTRY OF HEALTH. SCOTTISH HOME AND HEALTH DEPARTMENT
Central and Scottish Health Services councils. The care of the health of hospital staff. Report of the Joint Committee. H.M.S.O. 1968.
[Chairman: Professor Sir Ronald Tunbridge.]

HARTE, M. B., and HUNT, D.
Occupational health service for staff, Bedford General Hospital. *Occupational Health*, May/June 1968, p. 151-60.

HUDDERSFIELD COUNTY BOROUGH
A health service for the smaller industries. *Nursing Mirror*, Oct. 14, 1966, p. 42-4.

JARMAN, B. M.
A hospital occupational health service [St. George's Hospital]. *Occupational Health*, May/June 1969, p. 136-42.

KING EDWARD'S HOSPITAL FUND FOR LONDON. HOSPITAL CENTRE
Occupational health of hospital staff. *Nursing Times*, June 18, 1965, p. 845.

KNIGHT, M. C.
Unilever House health centre. *Occupational Health*, July/Aug. 1966, p. 177-85.

LAYCOCK, J.
People at risk in hospital. *Occupational Health*, Oct. 1970, p. 321-7.

RADWANSKI, D. M.
A health service for hospital employees. *Occupational Health*, Jan./Feb. 1963, p. 22-4.

RAFFLE, P. A. B.
London Transport Medical Service. *Nursing Times*, Nov. 27, 1969, p. 1514-6.

ROYAL COLLEGE OF NURSING and NATIONAL COUNCIL OF NURSES OF THE UNITED KINGDOM
Independent health service for hospital employees. *Nursing Mirror*, Nov. 20, 1964, p. 189 and 191.

WREFORD, B. M.
The five oases—I. A study of group occupational health in England. *Occupational Health*, July/Aug. 1967, p. 183-218.

WREFORD, B. M.
The five oases—II. *Occupational Health*, Sept./Oct. 1967, p. 253-92.

OPHTHALMIC NURSING

AISH, A.
A patient with cataracts. *The Canadian Nurse*, Sept. 1968, p. 44-6.

AMERICAN MEDICAL ASSOCIATION
Guiding principles and procedures for industrial nurses in care of eye injuries. *American Journal of Nursing*, Sept. 1961, p. 86.

BRIDGEMAN, G. J. O.
Squint in children. *Nursing Times*, Sept. 29, 1961, p. 1254-6.

BROCKHURST, R. J., *and* O'DONNELL, C. T.
Detachment of the retina. *American Journal of Nursing*, April 1964, p. 96-100.

BRUEGGEN, S. L.
Eye health in industry. *American Journal of Nursing*, Sept. 1961, p. 83.

BRUEGGEN, S. L.
Schiotz tonometry and the professional nurse. *American Association of Industrial Nurses' Journal*, Sept. 1968, p. 13-6.

CANADIAN NURSE
Entire issue devoted to ophthalmology. *Canadian Nurse*, Mar. 1961.

CARDONA, H.
Restoring vision by prosthokeratoplasty. *Nursing Mirror*, Nov. 24, 1967, p. iv-vii.

CHOYCE, D. P.
Intra-corneal plastic implants. *Nursing Times*, June 4, 1970, p. 715-8.

CHOYCE, D. P.
Intra-ocular implants. *Nursing Times*, May 28, 1970, p. 680-2.

COLLIER, L. H.
Trachoma: the Cinderella disease. *Nursing Times*, April 6, 1962, p. 428-30.

DALLAS, N. L.
Diseases of the eyelids. *Nursing Mirror*, July 7, 1967, p. v-viii.

EVANS, C.
Corneal graft. *Nursing Times*, Oct. 6, 1961, p. 1293-4.

EVANS, P. J.
Treatment of diseases of the cornea. *Nursing Mirror*, May 29, 1964, p. i-iii.

FREEMAN, M. H.
Ultrasonic techniques in ophthalmic examination. *Nursing Mirror*, June 12, 1964, p. x-xii.

GARLAND, P.
Emergency work in the casualty department of an eye hospital. *Nursing Times*, April 6, 1962, p. 435-8.

GARLAND, P.
Ophthalmic nursing. 4th edn. Faber, 1962.
5th end., 1966.

GREAVES, D. P.
Night blindness. *Nursing Mirror*, May 26, 1961, p. 733-4.

GURD, D. P., *and others*
Herpes simplex infections of the cornea. *Nursing Mirror*, Sept. 10, 1965, p. 577-8.

HAVENER, WILLIAM H., *and others*
Nursing care in eye, ear, nose and throat disorders by William H. Havener, William H. Saunders and Betty S. Bergerson. St. Louis, Mosby, 1964.
2nd edn., 1968, by Saunders, W. H., *and others*.

JENKINS, M.
Pack system for a small ophthalmic unit. *Nursing Mirror*, Mar. 8, 1968, p. 32-6.

MASON, R., *and others*
Doyne's honeycomb degeneration of the retina: a survey. *Nursing Times*, Oct. 27, 1967, p. 1446-8.

MILES, B.
Bowls therapy for the blind. *Nursing Mirror*, Feb. 9, 1968, p. 42-3.

ROPER-HALL, M. J.
Changes in ophthalmic nursing. *Nursing Mirror*, July 12, 1968, p. 23-5.

RUBEN, M.
The contact lens in current practice. *Nursing Times*, Nov. 15, 1963, p. 1449-53.

RUBEN, M.
Contact lenses today. *Nursing Mirror*, Jan. 19, 1968, p. vi-ix.

RUBINSTEIN, K.
Ophthalmic cryosurgery. *Nursing Times*, Dec. 8, 1967, p. 1640-2.

RYCROFT, P. V.
The modern management of retinal detachment. *Nursing Mirror*, Oct. 21, 1966, p. i-iii.

RYCROFT, P. V.
Modern trends of corneal grafting and its nursing problems. *Nursing Mirror*, April 5, 1968, p. 19-22.

SAUNDERS, WILLIAM H., *and others*
Nursing care in eye, ear, nose, and throat disorders, by William H. Saunders, William H. Havener, Carol J. Fair and Josephine T. Hickey. 2nd edn. St. Louis, C. V. Mosby, 1968.
1st edn., 1964, by Havener, W. H., *and others*.

SELLORS, P. J. H.
Senile cataract. *Nursing Times*, Oct. 4, 1968, p. 1337-9.

SIMPSON, N. L.
Acrylic implant: a new vision. *Nursing Times*, Feb. 9, 1968, p. 170-1.

SORSBY, A.
Blindness in childhood. *Nursing Times*, July 5, 1968, p. 903-4.

TONKIN, D.
The role of the nurse in preventing blindness. *South Australian Journal of Nursing*, Sept. 1969, p. 8-9.

WILLIAMS, C. E.
The Mary Sheridan Unit [for the study of blind psychiatrically disturbed children]. *Nursing Mirror*, Oct. 23, 1970, p. 57-8.

ZUGSMITH, G.
Eye emergencies. *American Association of Industrial Nurses' Journal*, Sept. 1968, p. 17-8.

PAEDIATRIC NURSING

ALLICK, H. D.
Artificial feeding: a new concept. The "Ready to feed" approach. *Nursing Times*, Aug. 21, 1969, p. 1071-2.

ANDERSON, J. A. D.
Child health centres. *Nursing Mirror*, Nov. 8, 1968, p. 36-7.

ANDERSON, NORMA J.
Workbook for pediatric nurses. St. Louis, Mosby, 1970.

ASHER, P.
Child health problems in the community. *Nursing Times*, July 19, 1968, p. 963-5.

ASSOCIATION OF BRITISH PAEDIATRIC NURSES
Why paediatric nurses? 1—An assessment of the past, present and future of this nursing specialty. *Nursing Times*, Nov. 12, 1970, Occasional Papers, p. 169-72.

BIBLIOGRAPHY OF NURSING

Association of British Paediatric Nurses
Why paediatric nurses? 2—Why paediatric nurses? *Nursing Times*, Nov. 19, 1970, Occasional Papers, p. 173-5.

Baldwin, E. M.
Nursing care in a fibrocystic disease. *Nursing Times*, Aug. 16, 1963, p. 1019-20.

Bethell, M. F.
Caring for children. *Nursing Times*, April 5, 1968, p. 457-9.

Blake, Florence G., *and others*
Nursing care of children, by Florence G. Blake, F. Howell Wright and Eugenia H. Waechter. 8th edn. Philadelphia, Lippincott, 1970.
[For 7th edn of this work see Essentials of pediatric nursing, by Florence G. Blake and F. Howell Wright.]

Blake, Florence G., *and* Wright, F. Howell
Essentials of pediatric nursing. 7th edn. Philadelphia, Lippincott, 1963.
[For later edition of this work see Nursing care of children, by Florence G. Blake and others.]

Bonine, Gladys N., *and* Pounds, Lois
Workbook in pediatric nursing. New York, Macmillan, 1962.

Broadribb, Violet
Foundations of pediatric nursing. Philadelphia, Lippincott, 1967.

Bromley, D., *and* Burston, W. R.
The Pierre Robin syndrome. *Nursing Times*, Dec. 30, 1966, p. 1717-20.

Coffin, Margaret A.
Nursing observations of the young patient. Dubuque, Iowa, Wm. C. Brown, 1970.

Conant, L. H.
What helps mothers to speak out. *American Journal of Nursing*, Dec. 1969, p. 2650-3.

Court, J.
The battered child syndrome. *Midwives' Chronicle and Nursing Notes*, July 1970, p. 212-6.

Crosby, Marian H.
The status of patient-contact as an experience in the preparation of teachers in the area of nursing of children. *Nursing Research*, Jan./Feb. 1969, p. 45-50.

Crow, R. A.
Child deaths in Manchester: a health visitor's study of deaths in children ages 1 to 14 years during 1964 and 1965. *International Journal of Nursing Studies*, Mar. 1969, p. 37-51.

Cunningham, P. J., *editor*
Nursery nursing. Faber and Faber, 1967.

Davidson, S.
Bereavement in children. *Nursing Times*, Dec. 16, 1966, p. 1650-2.

Duncombe, M. A.
Aids to paediatric nursing. Bailliere, Tindall & Cox, 2nd edn., 1965.
3rd edn., 1969.

Duncombe, M. A.
Challenge of change in the paediatric nursing field. *Nursing Mirror*, June 22, 1962, p. 225-6 and 228.

Erikson, F.
Nurse specialist for children. *Nursing Outlook*, Nov. 1968, p. 34-6.

Farrow, Raymond, *and* Forrest, Duncan
The surgery of childhood for nurses. 2nd edn. Edinburgh, Livingstone, 1964.
3rd edn., 1968.

Gibson, M., *and* Mann, T.
Barrier nursing for sick children. *Nursing Times*, June 26, 1969, p. 807-12.

Gozzi, E.
Pediatric nurse practitioner at work. [In a medical group practice.] *American Journal of Nursing*, Nov. 1970, p. 2371-6.

Gracey, M., *and* Anderson, C. M.
Some gastrointestinal disorders and enzyme deficiencies in childhood. *District Nursing*, May 1970, p. 24-6.

Graham, P.
Psychopaedic nursing. On being a member of a psychopaedic team. *The New Zealand Nursing Journal*, May 1969, p. 11 and 13-4.

Gruhl, V. R.
Some basic considerations about myocardial infarction. *Journal of Practical Nursing*, Oct. 1969, p. 27-8 and 39.

Haldane, J. D.
The functions, selection and training of the nurse in a residential psychiatric unit for children. *International Journal of Nursing Studies*, Dec. 1963, p. 27-36.

Hamilton, Persis Mary
Basic pediatric nursing. St. Louis, Mosby, 1970.

Hiller, R. B.
The battered child—a health visitor's point of view. *Nursing Times*, Oct. 2, 1969, p. 1265-6.

Honig, A.
The role of the nurse in stimulating early learning. *Journal of Nursing Education*, Jan. 1970, p. 11-6.

Hopkins, J.
The nurse and the abused child. *Nursing Clinics of North America*, Dec. 1970, p. 589-98.

Husband, P.
The child with repeated accidents. *Midwife and Health Visitor*, July 1969, p. 279 and 281-3.

Hymovich, Debra P.
Nursing of children: a guide for study. Philadelphia, Saunders, 1969.

Illingworth, R. S.
Sleep problems in children. *Nursing Mirror*, Mar. 7, 1969, p. 18-20.

Jackson, Q. M.
A handbook of paediatrics for nurses in general training. 3rd edn. Lewis, 1967.

Jaeger, Margaret Ann
Child development and nursing care. New York, Macmillan, 1962.

Kalafatich, Audrey J.
Pediatric nursing. New York, Putnam, 1966.

Kessel, I.
The essentials of paediatrics for nurses. 2nd edn. Edinburgh, Livingstone, 1963.
3rd edn., 1967.

King Edward's Hospital Fund for London. The Hospital Centre
The incontinent child. Report of a Conference held on 21 June 1970. *Nursing Times*, July 30, 1970, p. 985-6.

Latham, Helen C., *and* Heckel, Robert V.
Pediatric nursing. St. Louis, Mosby, 1967.

Lee, C. M.
"Feed me with food convenient for me." *Nursing Times*, Sept. 27, 1968, p. 1290-3; Oct. 4, 1968, p. 1340-3.

Leifer, Gloria
Principles and techniques in pediatric nursing. Philadelphia, Saunders, 1965.

SPECIALITIES

Levy, A. Harrison
Cardio-thoracic surgery in infancy and childhood.
1. Management of cardiac failure in infancy.
2. Lesions of the oesophagus, lungs and heart.
3. Diaphrogmatic and hiatus hernia in infancy.
4. Surgery of congenital heart disease.
5 (a). Tetralogy of Fallot and patent ductus arteriosus.
5 (b). Ventricular septal defects.
Nursing Mirror, Mar. 22, 1963, p. 533-6; Mar. 29, 1963, p. x-xii; April 5, 1963, p. v-vii; April 12, 1963, p. 34-6; April 19, 1963, p. iii-v; April 26, 1963, p. 71-2.

Lore, A.
Nursing students help children express their feelings. *Journal of Nursing Education*, Jan. 1970, p. 39-42.

Marlow, Dorothy R., *and* Sellew, Gladys
Textbook of pediatric nursing. Philadelphia, Saunders, 1961.
2nd edn., 1965.
3rd edn., 1968.

Mobbs, J.
Childhood obesity. *International Journal of Nursing Studies*, Mar. 1970, p. 3-16.

National League for Nursing
Seeking plus factors in nursing. New York, The League, 1967.
[NLN convention papers—1967, no. 1.]

Nelson, A. C.
How can you stand the crying? *American Journal of Nursing*, Jan. 1970, p. 66-9.

New Zealand. Department of Health. Operational Research Unit
Patient nurse dependency: paediatrics; an analysis of survey data from three public hospitals in Christchurch. Wellington, The Department, 1963.

Nursing Clinics of North America
Symposium on care of the infant and young child. *Nursing Clinics of North America*, Sept. 1970, p. 373-448.

Okell, C.
The battered child—a tragic breakdown in parental care? *Midwife and Health Visitor*, June 1969, p. 235-40.

Pask, E. G.
Collecting urine specimens from children. *Canadian Nurse*, Oct. 1969, p. 35-7.

Pomeroy, M. R.
Sudden death syndrome. *American Journal of Nursing*, Sept. 1969, p. 1886-90.

Raffensperger, John G., *and* Primrose, Rosellen Bohlen, editors
Pediatric surgery for nurses, by various authors. Boston, Little, Brown, 1968.

Reade, T., *and* Clow, C.
Home care of children with inborn errors of metabolism. *Canadian Nurse*, Oct. 1970, p. 41-3.

Reeves, K. R.
Children's reactions to head injuries. *American Journal of Nursing*, Jan. 1970, p. 108-11.

Sacharin, R. M., *and* Hunter, M. H. S.
Paediatric nursing procedures. Edinburgh, Livingstone, 1964.
2nd edn., 1969.

Sather, M. A.
Volunteer teachers for prospective parents. *American Journal of Nursing*, Aug. 1970, p. 1700-2.

Scahill, M.
Preparing children for procedures and operations. *Nursing Outlook*, June 1969, p. 36-8.

Seidl, Frederick W.
Pediatric nursing personnel and parent participation: a study in attitudes. *Nursing Research*, Jan./Feb. 1969, p. 40-4.

Shade, D. A.
Limits to service in child abuse. *American Journal of Nursing*, Aug. 1969, p. 1710-2.

Shrand, H.
Fibrocystic disease of the pancreas. *Nursing Times*, Aug. 16, 1963, p. 1016-9.

Shrand, H.
Hydrocephalus. *Nursing Times*, Sept. 13, 1963, p. 1136-8.

Stanley-Brown, Edward G.
Pediatric surgery for nurses. Philadelphia, Saunders, 1961.

Stephen, C. R
Pediatric anesthesia. *Journal of the American Association of Nurse Anesthetists*, Dec. 1970, p. 441-7.

Strachan, Isobel G.
A central milk kitchen. *Nursing Times*, April 17, 1964, p. 496-8.

Tanguay, J.
Infant care following cardiac surgery. *The Canadian Nurse*, Mar. 1964, p. 279-81.

Thomas, B. J.
How students perceive pediatric nursing. *Nursing Outlook*, Oct. 1970, p. 44-6.

Thompson, Eleanor Dumont
Pediatrics for practical nurses. Philadelphia, Saunders, 1965.
Saunders, 1965.
2nd edn., 1970.

Thompson, N. A., *and* Goodman, L.
Psychopaedic nurse training. *New Zealand Nursing Journal*, July 1969, p. 14-5.

Watt, James Michael
Practical paediatrics: a guide for nurses. Christchurch, N.Z., Peryer, 1961.
3rd edn., 1969.

Weinberg, Sheila, *and others*
Seminars in nursing care of the adolescent. *Nursing Outlook*, Dec. 1968, p. 18-23.

Wingert, P.
The pediatric nurse specialist in the community. *Nursing Outlook*, Dec. 1969, p. 28-31.

World Health Organization. Regional Office for Europe
Nursing education for child care; report on a seminar . . ., Vienna, Nov. 14-23, 1960. Copenhagen, W.H.O., 1965.

CHILDREN IN HOSPITAL

Abbott, N. C., *and others*
Dress rehearsal for the hospital. Nurses visit kindergartens to teach about hospital customs. *American Journal of Nursing*, Nov. 1970, p. 2360-2.

American Nurses' Foundation
Aggressive post-operative play responses of hospitalized pre-school children. *Nursing Research Report*, June 1969, p. 1 and 4-5.

Andrews, J., *and* Donaldson, J.
A children's psychiatric unit. *The Canadian Nurse*, Aug. 1965, p. 632-5.

Anstice, E.
Nurse, where's my mummy? *Nursing Times*, Nov. 26, 1970, p. 1513-8.

Aufhauser, T. R.
Parent participation in hospital care of children. *Nursing Outlook*, Jan. 1967, p. 40-2.

Bach, W. G.
Teen-age patients. *Hospital*, Jan. 16, 1970, p. 51-3.

BLAKE, F. G.
Immobilized youth. *American Journal of Nursing*, Nov. 1969, p. 2364-69.

BRANSTETTER, ELLAMAE
The young child's response to hospitalization—separation anxiety or lack of mothering care? Presented at the 95th annual meeting of the American Public Health Association, Public Health Nursing Section Meeting, Oct. 23, 1967. Tempe, Arizona, the Author, 1967.

CHALONER, L.
Play in hospital. *Nursing Mirror*, April 12, 1968, p. 23-5.

CONDON, M., and PETERS, C.
Family participation unit. *American Journal of Nursing*, Mar. 1968, p. 504-7.

DABRITZ, L., and others
Rescue fantasy in the nurse therapist relationship with a psychotic child. *Journal of Psychiatric Nursing*, Mar./April 1968, p. 71-8.

DOLCH, E. T.
Books for the hospitalized child. *American Journal of Nursing*, Dec. 1961, p. 66.

FAGIN, C. M.
Why not involve parents when children are hospitalized? *The American Journal of Nursing*, June 1962, p. 78.

FARRELL, DOLORES
Nursing a child with a long term illness.
In
AMERICAN NURSES' ASSOCIATION
Phases in human development: relevance in nursing. New York, The Association, 1962.

FLEMING, MILDRED
Constructive nursing approaches to disciplinary problems with hospitalized children. 1962.
In
AMERICAN NURSES' ASSOCIATION
Solving "difficult" problems in nursing care. New York, The Association, 1962.

FROMMER, E. A.
Children as individuals.
The child in the outpatient department—5.
Ward care of children—6.
Nursing Times, June 22, 1962, p. 811; June 29, 1962, p. 832-4.

FUSZARD, SISTER MARY BLAISE
Acceptance of authoritarianism in the nurse by the hospitalized teen-ager. *Nursing Research*, Sept./Oct. 1969, p. 426-32.

GIPS, CLAUDIA D.
The interpretation and misinterpretation by hospitalized school-age children of being sick; implications for nursing.
In
AMERICAN NURSES' ASSOCIATION
Phases in human development: relevance in nursing. New York, The Association, 1962.

GREEN, ALISON P.
Meeting the needs of a child in hospital. *Nursing Times*, Feb. 12, 1970, p. 210-2.

GREEN, ALISON P.
Nursing the young adolescent in hospital. *Nursing Times*, Sept. 9, 1968, p. 1242-3.

HARPER, J. R.
Children in a district hospital ITU. *Nursing Times*, Nov. 5, 1970, p. 1417-9.

ISBISTER, C.
The hospitalization of children. *The Australian Nurses' Journal*, Oct. 1961, p. 238.

JERMAN, B.
Playtime in hospital. *Nursery Journal*, Nov. 1970, p. 11-4.

KELLIE, G. A.
Children's ward in Nepal. *Nursing Times*, Feb. 12, 1970, p. 22-3.

LAWRIE, R.
Operating on children as day-cases. *Nursing Mirror*, Jan. 28, 1966, p. 509-10.

LAWSON, D.
Home or hospital for children who are ill. *Midwife and Health Visitor*, Oct. 1966, p. 441-3.

MCCLURE, M. J., and RYBURN, C.
Care-by-parent unit. *American Journal of Nursing*, Oct. 1969, p. 2148-52.

MACDONALD, E. M.
Parents participate in care of the hospitalized child. *Canadian Nurse*, Dec. 1969, p. 37-9.

MATIC, V.
A hospital without nurses. [Paediatric unit where mothers look after their children.] *Nursing Mirror*, July 19, 1963, p. iii-iv.

MEYER, H. L.
Predictable problems of hospitalized adolescents. *American Journal of Nursing*, Mar. 1969, p. 525-8.

MORGAN, B. D.
Mothers in hospital. The nurse's viewpoint. *The Lancet*, July 1, 1967, p. 38-9.

MORGAN, B. D.
Visiting in children's units: a changing pattern. *Nursing Times*, Dec. 22, 1967, p. 1711-3.

NATIONAL ASSOCIATION FOR THE WELFARE OF CHILDREN IN HOSPITAL
Coming into hospital. The Association, 1967.

PLANK, EMMA N.
Working with children in hospitals: a guide for the professional team. Cleveland, Ohio, Western Reserve University, 1962.

ROBINSON, D.
Parents' satisfaction with in-hospital information about their young children. *Nursing Times*, Oct. 25, 1968, Occasional Papers, p. 165-7.

SCHMALZRIED, GEORGIA L.
Effects of continuity in the nursing care of emotionally disturbed children.
In
AMERICAN NURSES' ASSOCIATION
Effects of continuity in nursing care on patient welfare. New York, The Association, 1962.

SHOPE, J.
Parental involvement program (at City of Hope Medical Center, Duarte, California). *Nursing Outlook*, April 1970, p. 32-4.

SMITH, J. D.
Psychological problems in children. 1—Personal problems for nursing staff. *Nursing Mirror*, Aug. 23, 1968, p. 28-9.

SMITH, J. D.
Psychological problems in children. 2—Patients have families. *Nursing Mirror*, Aug. 30, 1968, p. 22-3.

STACEY, MARGARET, *editor*
Hospitals, children and their families: the report of a pilot study, by Margaret Stacey, Rosemary Dearden, Roisin Pill and David Robinson. Routledge and Kegan Paul, 1970.

SUTTON, CAROLE
Mother and child experiment at Bolton: admitting mothers with children in the paediatric block. *Nursing Mirror*, April 26, 1963, p. xii.

TADDY, SISTER JOSEPH
How the nurse can help parents during the admission period of their child to the hospital.
In
AMERICAN NURSES' ASSOCIATION
Nursing in relation to the impact of illness upon the family. New York, The Association, 1962.

SPECIALITIES

THORNTON, M.
A play group in a children's ward. *Nursing Times*, April 28, 1967, p. 574-5.

HANDICAPPED CHILDREN

COOLEY, ELIZABETH J.
The child with autistic behavior.
In
AMERICAN NURSES' ASSOCIATION
Nursing of patients with loss of perceptions. New York, The Association, 1962.

FORD, H. A.
Care of the handicapped child. *Nursing Times*, July 21, 1967, p. 962-3.

FORD, H. A.
Nursing a spina bifida child in a general hospital. *Nursing Times*, Mar. 5, 1970, p. 293-5.

GILLIS, L.
Physically handicapped children. 1. The nurses approach to the mother. 2. Treatment and management. *Nursing Times*, March 19, 1965, p. 382-3; March 26, 1965, p. 428-30.

HEALY, H. T.
Variations in services to handicapped children. *American Journal of Nursing*, Aug. 1968, p. 1725-7.

HOLT, K. S.
Care of the handicapped child. *Nursing Mirror*, Apr. 11, 1969, p. 19-21.

KAPKE, K. A.
Spina Bifida: mother-child relationship. *Nursing Forum*, vol. IX, no. 3, 1970, p. 310-20.

KEATING, L.
Education of the epileptic child. *District Nursing*, Aug. 1968, p. 96-9.

LAURENCE, K. M.
Spina Bifida Cystica. *Nursing Times*, May 12, 1967, p. 620-3.

LINDSAY, A.
The handicapped child: the health visitor's role in the community care of the handicapped child. *Nursing Times*, Sept. 27, 1968, Occasional Papers, p. 151-2.

LORBER, J.
Children with spina bifida. *Nursing Mirror*, Sept. 20, 1968, p. 19-22.

ROAKE, D. P.
Caring for the handicapped child. *Nursing Mirror*, Aug. 24, 1962, p. 409.

WATERHOUSE, R. A.
Spina bifida: an ever increasing problem. *Nursing Times*, Dec. 24, 1970, p. 1646-8.

WHATLEY, E.
Helping parents of physically handicapped babies. *Nursing Mirror*, Jan. 11, 1963, p. 315-6.

WOOD, B. G., *and* KEVILL, G. A.
Nursing care of babies with cleft lip and palate. *Nursing Times*, Nov. 5, 1970, p. 1420-5; Nov. 12, 1970, p. 1459-61; Nov. 19, 1970, p. 1490-3.

WOODWARD, SISTER M. HILARY,
Urinary incontinence in the physically handicapped child. *Nursing Times*, Aug. 27, 1970, p. 1098-101.

MATERNAL CHILD HEALTH

ANKERS, E.
Mothers, babies and LPNs. *Practical Nursing*, Nov. 1970, p. 21-3, and 36.

BONHAM, D. G.
Perinatal mortality—the present and the future—I. *Nursing Mirror*, Sept. 20, 1963, p. 529-30.

BONHAM, D. G.
Perinatal mortality—the present and the future—II. *Nursing Mirror*, Sept. 27, 1963, p. 553-5.

CLARK, ANN L., *and others*
Patient studies in maternal and child nursing: a family-centered student guide, by Ann L. Clark, Hella M. Hakerem, Stephanie C. Basara and Diane A. Walano. Philadelphia, Lippincott, 1966.

COLLIS, W. R. F.
Infant feeding and hygiene in Nigeria. *Nursing Times*, Dec. 30, 1966, p. 1711-3.

DERASARI, A. J.
Infant feeding. Nurses' role in educating the mothers. *The Nursing Journal of India*, Feb. 1969, p. 47-8 and 66.

EPPINK, H.
An experiment to determine a basis for nursing decisions in regard to time of initiation of breastfeeding. *Nursing Research*, July/Aug. 1969, p. 292-9.

FOLEY, J.
The role of the nurse in maternal and child welfare. *Australian Nurses' Journal*, Dec. 1964, p. 291-3.

FROMMER, E. A.
Children as individuals.
1. Child, mother and nurse.
2. Development of the baby, and welfare work.
3. Symptoms of illness in babies.
4. Normal infant feeding.
Nursing Times, May 25, 1962, p. 662; June 1, 1962, p. 703; June 8, 1962, p. 733-4; June 15, 1962, p. 770-2.

INGALLS, A. JOY
Maternal and child health nursing. St. Louis, Mosby, 1967.

JOSLIN, E. E.
A future for the maternity service. *Nursing Mirror*, Aug. 20, 1965, p. v-viii.

MICHELSON, A.
Disposable feeding bottles. *Nursing Times*, Nov. 4, 1966, p. 1449-51.

NEWTON, N.
Decline of breast feeding: 1. Psychological implications—2. Social aspects of breast feeding—3. Psychophysical regulating mechanisms. *Nursing Times*, Sept. 22, 1967, p. 1267-8; Sept. 29, 1967, p. 1310-1; Oct. 6, 1967, p. 1346-8.

PRINGLE, D. M., *and* RUSSELL, J .K.
Maternity in Newcastle upon Tyne. A community study. *Nursing Mirror*, Dec. 6, 1963, p. 214-6.

REDDIN, M.
Evening infant welfare clinic. *Nursing Times*, Mar. 3, 1967, p. 285-7.

SCHMITT, M. H.
Superiority of breast-feeding, fact or fancy? *American Journal of Nursing*, July 1970, p. 1488-93.

SMITH, J. P.
Services for mothers and children in Scandinavia. *Nursing Mirror*, July 28, 1967, p. xi-xiii, and xvi.

PREMATURE & NEW BORN BABIES

BARRY, H.
Resuscitation of the newborn. *Nursing Times*, Sept. 20, 1968, p. 1265-7.

BAUM, J. DAVID
Prevention of hypothermia in the newborn. *Nursing Mirror*, Aug. 9, 1968, p. 31-3.

BETSON, CAROL, *and others*
Cardiac surgery in neonates: a chance for life. *American Journal of Nursing*, Jan. 1969, p. 69-73.

BOGDAN, ANDREW
An introduction to the newly born infant for nurses. [Leeds], Tutorial System Publications, 1963.

BRANSON, H. K.
When a defective infant is born. *Bedside Nurse*, Nov. 1970, p. 18-9.

CORNER, B.
Care of the newborn infant. *Nursing Mirror*, July 10, 1970, p. 20-2.

CRAIG, W. S.
Detecting neonatal morbidity. *Nursing Mirror*, July 17, 1970, p. 13-5.

DRILLIEN, C. M.
Prognosis for babies of very low birth weight. *Nursing Mirror*, June 14, 1963, p. 227-9.

GANS, B.
Perinatal paediatrics. *Nursing Times*, Nov. 20, 1969, p. 1482-4.

HALLIDAY, N. P.
Assessment of gestational ages of neonates. *Nursing Mirror*, Nov. 6, 1970, p. 26-30.

HART, E. W.
Haemorrhagic states in the newborn infant. *Nursing Mirror*, Oct. 25, 1968, p. 28-9.

JOSEPH, M.
Severe congenital heart disease in the neonate. *Nursing Mirror*, Aug. 28, 1970, p. 32-5.

MCKILLIGIN, HELEN R.
The first day of life: principles of neonatal nursing. New York, Springer, 1970.

MANN, T. P.
Hypothermia in the newborn. *Nursing Times*, Jan. 14, 1963, p. 15-8.

NEAL, M. V., *and* NAUEN, C. M.
Ability of premature infant to maintain his own body temperature. *Nursing Research*, Sept./Oct. 1968, p. 396-402

PARKE, PRISCILLA C.
Current trends in nursing care of the premature infant.
In
AMERICAN NURSES' ASSOCIATION
Technical innovations in health care: nursing implications. New York, The Association, 1962.

ROBINSON, R. J.
Low birthweight babies: premature and small-for-dates. *Nursing Mirror*, Sept. 6, 1968, p. 32-5.

STRUTHERS, J. N. M.
Early or late feeding of premature infants. *Nursing Times*, Nov. 19, 1965, p. 1577-9.

SYDOW, G. VON
Care of premature babies in Sweden. *Nursing Mirror*, Feb. 22, 1963, p. 455-6.

TORRANCE, J. T.
Temperature readings of premature infants. *Nursing Research*, July/Aug. 1968, p. 312-20.

UNITED STATES PUBLIC HEALTH SERVICE
DIVISION OF NURSING
Behaviour patterns of premature infants: a study of the relationship between a specific nursing procedure and general well-being of the prematurely born infant, by Eileen G. Hasselmeyer. Washington, U.S. Govt. Printing Office, 1961.

WALKER, A. H. C.
Ante-natal prediction of haemolytic disease in newborn. *Nursing Mirror*, May 10, 1963, p. ii-iv.

WHITLEY, N. N.
Breast feeding the premature. *American Journal of Nursing*, Sept. 1970, p. 1909.

WHITNER, W., *and* THOMPSON, M. C.
The influence of bathing on the new-born infant's body temperature. *Nursing Research*, Jan./Feb. 1970, p. 30-6.

WILKINSON, A. W.
Modern developments in surgery of the newborn. *Nursing Mirror*, June 24, 1966, p. 279-82.

PHYSICS

FLITTER, HESSEL HOWARD
An introduction to physics in nursing. 4th edn. St. Louis, Mosby, 1962.
5th edn., 1967.

KILGOUR, O. F. G.
An introduction to the physical aspects of nursing science. Heinemann, 1969.

SACKHEIM, GEORGE I.
Practical physics for nurses. 2nd edn., Philadelphia, Saunders, 1962.

PSYCHIATRIC NURSING

ACKNER, BRIAN, *editor*
Handbook for psychiatric nurses. 9th edn. Bailliere, Tindall and Cox (in conjunction with the Royal Medico-Psychological Association), 1964.
[For earlier editions see Royal Medico-Psychological Ass. "Handbook for mental nurses."]

AGUILERA, D. C.
Sociocultural factors: barriers to therapeutic intervention. *Journal of Psychiatric Nursing*, Sept./Oct. 1970, p. 14-8.

ALTSCHUL, A.
Aids to psychiatric nursing. 2nd edn. Bailliere, Tindall and Cox, 1964.
3rd edn., 1969.

ALTSCHUL, A.
Patient/nurse interaction in the psychiatric scene. *Nursing Mirror*, April 3, 1970, p. 37-41.

AMERICAN NURSES' ASSOCIATION
Exploring progress in psychiatric nursing practice. New York, the Association, 1966.

AMERICAN NURSES' ASSOCIATION
Nursing care of the disoriented patient. New York, The Association, 1962.
[ANA Convention, 1962, clinical monograph no. 13.]

AMERICAN NURSES' ASSOCIATION
DIVISION ON PSYCHIATRIC-MENTAL NURSING
Statement on psychiatric nursing practice. New York, the Association, 1967.

ANDERSON, D. B.
Nursing therapy with families. *Perspectives in Psychiatric Care*, Jan./Feb. 1969, p. 21-7.

ARMSTRONG, SHIRLEY W., *and* ROUSLIN, SHEILA
Group psychotherapy in nursing practice. New York, Macmillan, 1963.

BAGGOTT, E.
The SEN in psychiatric hospitals. *Nursing Times*, Oct. 29, 1965, p. 1478-80.

BALDWIN, A. H.
Psychiatric nursing in the future. Presidential address to annual conference of the National Association of Chief Male Nurses. *Hospital & Social Service Journal*, June 9, 1961, p. 669-70.

BALKONEN, I.
Psychiatric nursing in Finland. *Sairaanhoitajalehti*, no. 16, 1961, translated in *Nursing Mirror*, Mar. 1, 1963, p. x-xi.

BARKER, J. C.
Team work in the service of the mentally ill. *Nursing Mirror* Dec. 25, 1964, p. 285-7.

BARKER, P.
Child psychiatry and the health visitor. *Nursing Mirror*, Sept. 15, 1967, p. 549-51.

SPECIALITIES

BARNES, ELIZABETH, editor
Psychosocial nursing. [Studies from the Cassel Hospital.] Tavistock Publications, 1968.

BARRY, A. C.
Understanding the psychiatric patient. *Nursing Times*, Jan. 24, 1964, p. 102-4.

BARTON, WALTER E., and others
Traditions and developments in nursing.
In
BARTON, WALTER E., and others
Impressions of European psychiatry. Washington, American Psychiatric Association, 1961.

BAZLEY, M. C.
New ideas in psychiatric nursing. *New Zealand Nursing Journal*, Nov. 1970, p. 18.

BEAL, E., and others
Nursing care approaches for operant reinforcement with psychiatric patients. *Journal Psychiatric Nursing and Mental Health Services*, July/Aug. 1969, p. 157-9.

BOORER, DAVID, and BOORER, HEATHER
An introduction to psychiatric nursing. Oxford, Pergamon, 1966.

BRAY, R. E., and BIRD, T. E. J.
Observation of patients by the psychiatric nurse. *Nursing Times*, Dec. 6, 1963, p. 1532-4.

BRAY, R. E., and BIRD, T. E. J.
The practice of psychiatric nursing. Edinburgh, Livingstone, 1964.

BRESSLER, B.
The psychotherapeutic nurse. *The American Journal of Nursing*, May 1962, p. 87.

BROWN, D. I.
Nurses participate in group therapy. *The American Journal of Nursing*, January 1962, p. 68.

BROWN, MARTHA MONTGOMERY, and FOWLER, GRACE R.
Psychodynamic nursing. 2nd edn. Philadelphia, Saunders, 1961.
3rd edn., 1966.

BUDGE, U. V.
Security and restraint. *Nursing Mirror*, Oct. 9, 1970, p. 12-3

BULBULYAN, A. A.
The psychiatric nurse as family therapist. *Perspectives in Psychiatric Care*, Mar./April 1969, p. 58-68.

BURD, SHIRLEY F., and MARSHALL, MARGARET A., editors
Some clinical approaches to psychiatric nursing. New York, Macmillan, 1963.

BURKE, NANCY
Therapy—eight hours a day.
In
AMERICAN NURSES' ASSOCIATION
The nurse and groups of patients or clients. New York, The Association, 1962.

BURR, JOAN
Nursing the psychiatric patient. Bailliere, Tindall and Cassell, 1967.
2nd edn., 1970.

CAINE, T. M., and SMAIL, D. J.
Attitudes of psychiatric nurses to their work. *Nursing Times*, Dec. 29, 1967, p. 1747-8.

CAMP, R. P.
Person, group, and organization dimensions of nursing care. *Perspectives in Psychiatric Care*, vol. IV, no. 4, 1966, p. 10-7.

CARLETON, ESTELLE I.
Nursing intervention in dealing with problems of regression and hostility in the borderline psychiatric patient.
In
AMERICAN NURSES' ASSOCIATION
Innovations in nurse-patient relationships: automatic or reasoned nurse actions. New York, The Association, 1962.

CARTER, ELIZABETH WACKERMAN
A proposed technique of nursing intervention with patients who deny mental illness. 1962.
In
AMERICAN NURSES' ASSOCIATION
Nursing approaches to denial of illness.

CENTRAL HEALTH SERVICES COUNCIL. JOINT SUB-COMMITTEE OF THE STANDING MENTAL HEALTH AND THE STANDING NURSING ADVISORY COMMITTEES
Psychiatric nursing, today and tomorrow: report. H.M.S.O., 1968.

CHEADLE, J.
The psychiatric nurse as a social worker. *Nursing Times*, Nov. 26, 1970, p. 1520-2.

CLACK, JANICE
An interpersonal technique for handling hallucinations.
In
AMERICAN NURSES' ASSOCIATION
Nursing care of the disoriented patient. New York, The Association, 1962.

CONOVER, C. L.
Motion picture therapy in a mental hospital. *Hospitals*, June, 1963, p. 56-8.

COPE, H. J.
Psychiatric nursing—need for change. *British Hospital Journal and Social Service Review*, Jan. 23, 1970, p. 160.

CRAWFORD, A. L.
Trends in psychiatric nursing—implications for the profession. *Journal of Psychiatric Nursing*, July/Aug. 1964, p. 384-8 and 393-6.

CRAWFORD, ANNIE LAURIE, and BUCHANAN, BARBARA BORING
Psychiatric nursing: a basic manual. Philadelphia, Davis, 1961.
3rd edn., 1970.
[Previously titled "Nursing manual for psychiatric aides", by Crawford, A. L., and Kilander, V. C.]

CRITCHLEY, DEANE L.
A description of a nurse-patient relationship with a hospitalized psychotic boy.
In
AMERICAN NURSES' ASSOCIATION
Phases in human development: relevance in nursing. New York, The Association, 1962.

CUBBIN, J. K.
Mechanical restraints: to use or not to use them? *Nursing Times*, June 11, 1970, p. 752.

CUNDELL, R.
Unit for autistic children. *Nursing Mirror*, Aug. 28, 1970, p. 26-7.

DAWSON, R.
No "magic" about mental nursing. *Nursing Mirror*, Aug. 14, 1970, p. 30-1.

DEACON, C. E.
Nursing the long-stay psychiatric patient. An experiment at Moorhaven Hospital. *Nursing Times*, April 3, 1964, p. 428-30.

DEWAR, JOHN, and JONES, MAXWELL
Whither psychiatric nursing. *Nursing Times*, June 5, 1964, p. 731-3.

DEWHURST, J.
Nursing restraints. 1. Past and present. 2. New methods of restraint. *Nursing Times*, June 4, 1970, p. 709-11; June 11, 1970, p. 749-51.

DICKER, J. R.
Assessing the mental nurse. *Nursing Times*, Aug. 14, 1964, p. 1042-4.

DONNER, G.
Treatment of a delusional patient. *American Journal of Nursing*, Dec. 1969, p. 2642-4.

Downey, D.
Public health nurses' attitudes toward patients with a psychiatric diagnosis. *Nursing Research*, May/June 1969, p. 244-50.

Duran, F. A., and Errion, G. D.
Perpetuation of chronicity in mental illness. *American Journal of Nursing*, Aug. 1970, p. 1707-9.

Earle, A., *and others*
The role of the psychiatric nurse in the rehabilitation of the schizophrenic patient. *Journal of Psychiatric Nursing and Mental Health Services*, Jan./Feb. 1970, p. 16-23.

Edwards, J., and Hults, M. S.
"Open" nursing stations on psychiatric wards. *Perspectives in Psychiatric Care*, Sept./Oct. 1970, p. 209-17.

Ekdawi, M. Y., and Dicker, J.
Psychiatric emergencies in industry. *Nursing Mirror*, May 16, 1969, p. 28 and 35.

Ellsworth, R. B., and Ellsworth, J.
The psychiatric aide; therapeutic agent or lost potential? *Journal of Psychiatric Nursing*, Sept./Oct. 1970, p. 7-13.

Emens, A.
Psychiatric nursing. Challenge of the future. *Nursing Times*, Jan. 8, 1970, p. 45-6.

Emens, A.
New approach to psychiatric care. 2. A home of their own. *Nursing Mirror*, Nov. 28, 1967, p. 196-8.
Pt. 1: *see* Forrest, Colin.
Pt. 3: *see* Leopoldt, H.

Fagerhaugh, S. Y.
Mental illness and the tuberculosis patient. *Nursing Outlook*, Aug. 1970, p. 38-41.

Fagin, C. M.
Psychotherapeutic nursing. *American Journal of Nursing*, Feb. 1967, p. 298-304.

Field, W. E., and Dayton, M.
Psychiatric nursing and combat casualties. *Perspectives in Psychiatric Care*, vol. IV, no. 4, 1966, p. 38-42.

Forrest, A. D., and Ritson, E. B.
Role of the nurse as therapist. [Group techniques in the psychiatric unit]. *Nursing Mirror*, Dec. 6, 1968, p. 22-3.

Forrest, Colin
New approach to psychiatric care. 1. St. Clement's psychogeriatric day hospital. *Nursing Mirror*, Nov. 17, 1967, p. 167-8 and 171.
Pt. 2: *see* Emens, A.
Pt. 3: *see* Leopoldt, H.

Foster, J.
Industrial unit in a mental hospital. *Nursing Times*, Aug. 6, 1963, p. 1024-6.

Frame, H. B. P.
Industrial therapy in the Netherlands. *Nursing Mirror*, Sept. 13, 1968, p. 23-6.

Frommer, E.
Physical treatments in psychiatric nursing. Some principles. *Nursing Times*, Mar. 22, 1963, p. 350-1.

Getty, C., and Shannon, A. M.
Co-therapy as an egalitarian relationship. *American Journal of Nursing*, April 1969, p. 767-71.

Gibson, John
Psychiatry for nurses. Oxford, Blackwell, 1962. 2nd edn., 1965.

Gibson, J.
Wider scope for nurses. *Nursing Times*, Sept. 2, 1966, p. 1169-70.

Glover, B. H.
A psychiatrist calls for a new nurse therapist. *American Journal of Nursing*, May 1967, p. 1003-5.

Gosney, K. G., and Brennan, K. S. W.
Community psychiatry. *Nursing Times*, Jan. 22, 1970, p. 105-6.

Gowell, E. C.
An experience with the use of group work methods and process with student nurse groups over a period of 5 years. *Journal of Psychiatric Nursing*, July/Aug. 1966, p. 351-62.

Graham, Peter
Psychopaedic nursing. On being a psychopaedic nurse *The New Zealand Nursing Journal*, April 1969, p. 9-10 and 16.

Graham, Peter
Psychopaedic nursing. On being a member of a psychopaedic team. *The New Zealand Nursing Journal*, May 1969, p. 11, and 13-4.

Greene, J.
Changes in nursing the mentally sick. *International Journal of Nursing Studies*, Dec. 1963, p. 37-43.

Greene, J.
The improved outlook in psychiatry and psychiatric nursing. *Nursing Mirror*, Feb. 9, 1968, p. 40-2.

Greene, J.
The psychiatric nurse in the community nursing service. *International Journal of Nursing Studies*, Sept. 1968, p. 175-83.

Gregory, E.
Society at work. Psychiatric nursing. *New Society*, Oct. 16, 1969, p. 595-6.

Group for the Advancement of Psychiatry Committee on Therapeutic Care
Toward therapeutic care: a guide for those who work with the mentally ill. 2nd edn. New York, Springer, 1970.

Gunn, M.
District nursing and the mentally ill. *Nursing Times*, April 17, 1969, p. 497.

Haffey, V. A.
Behavior modification utilizing a token economy program. *Journal of Psychiatric Nursing and Mental Health Service*, Mar./April 1970, p. 31-5.

Haldane, J. D., and Smith, J. D.
Psychiatric in-patient facilities for children and adolescents. *Nursing Times*, Mar. 5, 1970, p. 299-302.

Hargreaves, W. A.
Rate of interaction between nursing staff and psychiatric patients. *Nursing Research*, Sept./Oct. 1969, p. 418-25.

Hargreaves, W. A., and Runyon, N.
Patterns of psychiatric nursing: role differences in nurse-patient interaction. *Nursing Research*, July/Aug. 1969, p. 300-7.

Haward, L. R. C.
Nursing and psychosis. Does nursing provide a source of stress which makes psychosis more likely? *Nursing Mirror*, Feb. 24, 1961, p. 1903.

Hawkins, E., *and others*
Nursing dress, an experimental evaluation of its effect on psychiatric patients. *Journal of Psychiatric Nursing*, Mar./April 1966, p. 148-57.

Hays, J. S.
The psychiatric nurse as sociotherapist. *The American Journal of Nursing*, June 1962, p. 64.

Hemphill, R. E.
Infanticide and puerperal mental illness. *Nursing Times*, Nov. 3, 1967, p. 1473-5.

Hess, G.
Perception of nursing role in a developing mental health center. *Journal of Psychiatric Nursing and Mental Health Services*, Mar./April 1969, p. 77-81.

SPECIALITIES

HOLMES, MARGUERITE J., *and* WERNER, JEAN A.
Psychiatric nursing in a therapeutic community. New York, Macmillan, 1966.

HOPKINS, T. D.
Integration of the sexes in a psychiatric hospital. *Nursing Mirror*, June 23, 1961, p. xi.

HORSLEY, S.
The nurse and family psychiatry. *Nursing Mirror*, May 28, 1965, p. 217-8.

HOULISTON, MAY
The practice of mental nursing. 3rd edn. Edinburgh, Livingstone, 1961.
4th edn., 1965.

HUNTER, P.
The evolving role of the mental nurse. *Nursing Mirror*, Mar. 2, 1962, p. 427.

HYDE, N.
Changing horizons in psychiatric nursing. *The Canadian Nurse*, Mar. 1970, p. 49-51.

JACK, A.
Changing pattern of care of the intellectually handicapped. *New Zealand Nursing Journal*, Nov. 1970, p. 5-7.

JACOBS, L. M.
Beginning practitioner's adjustment to a psychiatric unit. *Nursing Outlook*, Oct. 1970, p. 28-31.

JACOBSON, S.
A therapeutic community in an acute admission ward. *Nursing Mirror*, May 13, 1966, p. v-vii.

JOHN, AUDREY L.
A study of the psychiatric nurse. Edinburgh, Livingstone, 1961.

JOHN, AUDREY L., *and others*
The nurse in mental health practice: report on a technical conference, Nov. 1961, by Audrey L. John, Maria O. Leite-Ribeiro and Donald Buckle. Geneva, W.H.O., 1963.

JOHNSON, J.
New drugs in the treatment of mental illness. *Nursing Mirror*, Nov. 24, 1961, p. 151.

JOHNSON, J.
Recent advances in psychiatric treatment. 1. The role of the psychiatric nurse. *Nursing Mirror*, July 5, 1963, p. 303-4

JOHNSON, J.
Recent advances in psychiatric treatment. 2. Psychological methods of treatment. *Nursing Mirror*, July 12, 1963, p. 325-6.

JOHNSON, J.
Recent advances in psychiatric treatment. 3. Physical methods of treatment. *Nursing Mirror*, July 19, 1963, p. 346-8.

JOHNSON, K.
Hyperkinetic syndrome in children. *Nursing Mirror*, May 23, 1969, p. 21-4.

JONES, L.
Mental illness and the work of the district nurse. *Nursing Mirror*, Jan. 21, 1966, p. 481-2.

JONES, MAXWELL
Psychiatric nursing is out of tune in the U.S.A. *American Journal of Nursing*, Jan. 1964, p. 103-5.

JONES, MAXWELL
What is psychiatric nursing? *The Lancet*, Nov. 23, 1963, p. 1108-10.

JONES, M., *and* MULLEN, C.
What psychiatric nursing is about. *Nursing Times*, June 7, 1963, p. 701-3.

KALKMAN, MARION E., *and others*
Psychiatric nursing. 3rd edn. New York, McGraw-Hill, 1967.
[Previously entitled "Introduction to psychiatric nursing".]

KARLIN, MARGARET MCCORKINDALE
Nursing management of adolescent patients in a psychiatric hospital.
In
AMERICAN NURSES' ASSOCIATION
Effects of continuity in nursing care on patient welfare. New York, The Association, 1962.

KARNOSH, LOUIS J., *and* MERENESS, DOROTHY
Essentials of psychiatric nursing. 6th edn. Kimpton, 1962.
7th edn., 1966.
8th edn., 1970.
[Previously entitled, "Psychiatry for nurses".]

KELSEY, F. D.
Early signs of mental illness—1 and 2. *Nursing Times*, Mar. 31, 1967, p. 413-4; April 7, 1967, p. 463-4.

KENNEDY, MARION
The wrong side of the door. (The story of a trainee nurse in a mental hospital). Harrap, 1963.

KIDD, H. B.
Work of nursing and medical teams in a psychiatric hospital. *Nursing Mirror*, Dec. 7, 1962, p. ii.

KIMBALL, LENORE
Psychiatric nursing: syllabus and work book for student nurses. 3rd edn. Kimpton, 1962.

KINSLER, D.
The nurse therapist. *Journal of Psychiatric Nursing*, Mar./April 1968, p. 86-7.

KIRKPATRICK, W. J. A.
Some thoughts on psychiatric nursing. *Nursing Times*, July 10, 1964, p. 903-4.

KIRKPATRICK, W. J. A.
The in and out nurse: Thoughts on the role of the psychiatric nurse in the community and the preparation required. *International Journal of Nursing Studies*, Aug. 1967, p. 225-30.

KLACHAN, J., *and* KALWINSKI, H.
The nurse's role in the informal group. *Journal Psychiatric Nursing and Mental Health Services*, Sept./Oct. 1968, p. 267-73.

KUPKA, M. E., *and* MELLOR, V.
A learning experience in the care of geriatric psychiatric patients. *Journal of Psychiatric Nursing*, May 1963, p. 199-206.

LANDESBERG, A., *and* KOCH, L.
Psychiatric nursing in a unique environment. *Journal of Psychiatric Nursing and Mental Health Services*, July/Aug. 1969, p. 164-8.

LARSON, R., *and* ELLSWORTH, R. B.
The nurse's uniform and its meaning in a psychiatric hospital. *Nursing Research*, Spring 1962, p. 100.

LAWSON, W. G. A.
Experimental unit for treatment of schizophrenia. *Nursing Times*, Jan. 5, 1962, p. 19-21.

LEIB, E.
A student looks at the psychosocial aspects of patient care. *Nursing Outlook*, Dec. 1962, p. 799-800.

LEININGER, MADELEINE M.
Changes in psychiatric nursing: a reflection of the impact of sociocultural forces. *Canadian Nurse*, Oct. 1961, p. 938.

LEININGER, MADELEINE M.
Community psychiatric nursing: trends, issues, and problems. *Perspectives in Psychiatric Care*, Jan./Feb. 1969, p. 10-20.

LEITCH, A.
Treatment of depression—1 and 2. *Nursing Times*, Jan. 11, 1963, p. 43; Jan. 18, 1963, p. 69-71.

LEOPOLDT, H.
Industrial therapy in psychiatric hospitals. *Nursing Mirror*, June 27, 1969, p. 16-8.

LEOPOLDT, H.
New approach to psychiatric care. 3. The group-home. *Nursing Mirror*, Dec. 1, 1967, p. x-xiii.
Pt. 1: *see* Forrest, C.
Pt. 2: *see* Emens, A.

LOOMIS, M. E.
Nursing management of acting-out behavior. *Perspectives in Psychiatric Care*, July/Aug. 1970, p. 168-73.

LOOMIS, M. E., *and* DODENHOFF, J. T.
Working with informal patient groups. *American Journal of Nursing*, Sept. 1970, p. 1939-44.

LYON, G. G.
Trust in the non-hospitalized group. *Perspectives in Psychiatric Care*, Mar./April 1970, p. 64-72.

MACARTHUR, C. H.
Designing a behaviour graph. *Nursing Times*, July 16, 1970, p. 911-4.

MCBRIEN, M.
What is wrong with psychiatric nursing? *Nursing Mirror*, May 10, 1968, p. 31-3.

MCGUINNESS, A. F.
The nurse's part in the psychiatric service. *Nursing Mirror*, Aug. 11, 1961, p. ii.

MACINNES, D., *and* MACAULAY, K.
Pattern for tomorrow. *Nursing Times*, July 12, 1963, p. 868-70.

MACLEOD, W. G.
Domiciliary psychiatric nursing observed—1 and 2. *Nursing Times*, Dec. 10, 1970, Occasional Papers, p. 185-8; Dec. 17, 1970, Occasional Papers, p. 189-90.

MCWILLIAMS, W.
Thioproperazine in the treatment of psychoses. *Nursing Times*, June 1, 1962, p. 706.

MADDISON, DAVID, *and others*
Psychiatric nursing, by David Maddison, Patricia Day and Bruce Leabeater. Edinburgh, Livingstone, 1963.
2nd edn., 1965.
3rd edn., 1970.

MALONEY, E.
Does the psychiatric nurse have independent functions? *The American Journal of Nursing*, June 1962, p. 61.

MANFREDA, MARGUERITE LUCY
Psychiatric nursing. 7th edn. Philadelphia, Davis, 1964.
8th edn., 1968.
[Previously by Steele, K. McLean, and Manfreda, M. L.]

MARRAM, G. D
Toward a greater understanding of mutual withdrawal in a psychiatric setting. *Journal of Psychiatric Nursing and Mental Health Services*, July/Aug. 1969, p. 160-3.

MARTIN, D. V.
Modern trends in psychiatric nursing. *Nursing Mirror*, Feb. 28, 1964, p. 483-4.

MARTIN, MORGAN
The mental ward: a personnel guidebook. Springfield, Illinois, Thomas, 1962.

MARWICK, IRIS
Psychiatric nursing in transition. Eleventh Nursing Mirror Lecture in the University of Edinburgh. *Nursing Mirror*, Mar. 7, 1969, p. 18-20; Mar. 14, 1969, p. 24-6.

MATHENEY, RUTH V., *and* TOPALIS, MARY
Psychiatric nursing. 3rd edn. St. Louis, Mosby, 1961.
4th edn., 1965.
5th edn., 1970.

MAY, A. R.
The psychiatric nurse in the community. *Nursing Mirror*, Dec. 31, 1965, p. 409-10.

MELLOW, J.
The experiential order of nursing therapy in acute schizophrenia. *Perspectives in Psychiatric Care*, Nov./Dec. 1969, p. 249-55.

MELLOW, J.
Nursing therapy. *American Journal of Nursing*, Nov. 1968, p. 2365-9.

MERENESS, DOROTHY A.
Family therapy: an evolving role for the psychiatric nurse. *Perspectives in Psychiatric Care*, Nov./Dec. 1969, p. 256-9.

MERENESS, DOROTHY A.
Psychiatric nursing. 2 vols. Dubuque, Iowa, Brown, 1966.
[Vol. 1. Developing psychiatric nursing skills; vol. 2. Understanding the nurse's role in psychiatric patient care.]

MERSKEY, H.
Electrical treatment . . . a balanced view. *Nursing Times*, Dec. 24, 1970, p. 1614-43.

MEZER, ROBERT R., *and* STANNER, SHIRLEY
Elements of psychiatry for nurses. Heinemann Medical Books, 1965.

MIDDLETON, A. B., *and* POTHIER, P. C.
The nurse in child psychiatry—an overview. *Nursing Outlook*, May 1970, p. 52-6.

MILLER, H. J. B.
Schizophrenia. *Nursing Times*, Jan. 5, 1962, p. 9-12.

MINSKI, LOUIS
A practical handbook of psychiatry for students and nurses. 5th edn. Heinemann, 1964.

MORRICE, J. K. W.
Don't step on the underdog. A personal view of the psychiatric nurse. *Nursing Times*, June 11, 1970, p. 766-7.

MORRICE, J. K. W.
Therapeutic community in the psychiatric hospital. *Nursing Mirror*, April 17, 1964, p. 59-61.

MORRIS, P. A.
The changing face of the refractory ward. *Nursing Mirror*, Jan. 18, 1963, p. viii-x.

MORRIS, WILFRED M.
Mixed psychiatric wards. *Nursing Mirror*, June 5, 1964, p. 219-20.

MORRIS, WILFRED M.
Administration of medicines to psychiatric patients. *Nursing Times*, Aug. 11, 1967, p. 1057-8.

MUNGOVAN, R.
Evolution of a therapeutic community. *Nursing Times*, Mar. 15, 1968, p. 365-6.

MUNRO, A.
Bereavement as a psychiatric emergency. *Nursing Times*, July 2, 1970, p. 841-3.

MUNRO, A.
The psychopath in a general hospital unit. *Nursing Mirror*, June 20, 1969, p. 13-4.

MURRAY, RUTH
Attitudes of professional nonpsychiatric nurses toward mental illness. *Journal of Psychiatric Nursing and Mental Health Services*, May/June 1969, p. 117-23.

NATIONAL ASSOCIATION OF CHIEF MALE NURSES
The future of mental nursing. *Nursing Mirror*, May 15, 1964, p. 147.

NATIONAL ASSOCIATION OF CHIEF AND PRINCIPAL NURSING OFFICERS
Psychiatric nurses' problems. [Report of the annual conference of the National Association of Chief and Principal Nursing Officers held in Isle of Wight, May 1969]. *British Hospital Journal and Social Service Review*, June 6, 1969, p. 1073-4.

SPECIALITIES

NEW ZEALAND NURSING JOURNAL
New ideas in psychiatric nursing. *New Zealand Nursing Journal*, Dec. 1968, p. 15-6.

NEVILLE, R., *and others*
Hysteria and its symptoms. *Nursing Mirror*, Aug. 2, 1963, p. i-iv.

NORRIS, W.
Anaesthetic care for electro-convulsive therapy. *Nursing Mirror*, June 7, 1963, p. iv-vi.

O'CONNOR, F.
A group therapy experience with regressed patients. *Journal of Psychiatric Nursing and Mental Health Services*, Sept./Oct. 1969, p. 226-9.

O'HARA, J.
Attitudes in subnormality nursing. *Nursing Mirror*, Jan. 30, 1970, p. 20-1.

PAQUETTE, A., *and* LAFAVE, H.
Halfway House. *American Journal of Nursing*, Mar. 1964, p. 121-4.

PAUL, W. K.
Research nursing in psychiatry. *The Canadian Nurse*, June 1967, p. 33-4.

PAZDUR, H.
Conflict: The nurse as therapist and researcher. *Journal of Psychiatric Nursing*, July/Aug. 1968, p. 202-7.

PECK, C.
Psychiatric nursing in Sweden. *Nursing Mirror*, Aug. 29, 1969, p. 27-30.

PEPLAU, H. E.
Interpersonal techniques: the crux of psychiatric nursing. *The American Journal of Nursing*, June 1962, p. 50.

PERCHARD, S.
Hypnosis and the pregnant woman. *Nursing Mirror*, April 7, 1967, p. i-vi.

PERCHARD, S. D.
Hypnosis in the ante-natal clinic. *Nursing Mirror*, Feb. 10, 1961, p. ii.

PERRY, M. E., *and others*
Differential attitudes of psychiatric and non-psychiatric nursing personnel. *Journal of Psychiatric Nursing*, May 1963, p. 186-97 and 232.

PERSPECTIVES IN PSYCHIATRIC CARE
Conference on hostility in the nurse-patient interaction; report. *Perspectives in Psychiatric Care*, July/Aug. 1969, p. 150-87.

PETROVICH, D. G., *and others*
Nursing apparel and psychiatric patients: a comparison of uniforms and street clothes. *Journal of Psychiatric Nursing and Mental Health Services*, Nov./Dec. 1968, p. 344-8.

PLANANSKY, K., *and* DILLMAN, E.
An experience with work therapy in the management of disturbed patients. *Nursing Research*, Spring 1962, p. 101.

POPE, J. L. W.
The changing scene of psychiatric nursing in a State Hospital. *Perspectives in Psychiatric Care*, vol. V, no. 4, 1967, p. 163-73.

RAHEJA, K. K.
The role of a nurse in a psychiatric unit. *The Nursing Journal of India*, July 1969, p. 234.

RILEY, M.
The nursing interview for psychiatric patients. *Nursing Outlook*, Oct. 1968, p. 54-7.

RITCHIE, E. A.
Administrative therapy in clinical psychiatry. *Nursing Mirror*, Oct. 9, 1970, p. 30-1.

ROBINSON, A. M.
Creativity takes courage. *Nursing Outlook*, July 1963, p. 499-501.

ROBINSON, J. T.
Rehabilitating the emotionally disabled—I. *Nursing Mirror*, April 26, 1968, p. 37-8.

ROBINSON, J. T.
Rehabilitating the emotionally disabled—II. *Nursing Mirror*, May 3, 1968, p. 37-9.

ROGERS, C. G.
The use of alienation in crisis work. *Journal of Psychiatric Nursing*, Nov./Dec. 1970, p. 7-12.

ROSE, WILLIAMINA GUNN DOULL
Management of dependence-independence factors in a nurse-patient relationship with a catatonic patient.
In
AMERICAN NURSES' ASSOCIATION
Innovations in nurse-patient relationships: nursing the patient with problems of response. New York, The Association, 1962.

ROYAL AUSTRALIAN NURSING FEDERATION
NATIONAL NURSING EDUCATION DIVISION
Bibliography on psychiatry and psychiatric nursing. Melbourne, The Federation, 1964.

ROYAL COLLEGE OF NURSING *and*
NATIONAL COUNCIL OF NURSES OF THE UNITED KINGDOM
Psychiatric nursing—today and tomorrow. [Report of a conference held by the Rcn at Caxton Hall, London, on September 26, 1969]. *Nursing Times*, Oct. 2, 1969, p. 1272-3.

ROYAL COLLEGE OF NURSES *and*
NATIONAL COUNCIL OF NURSES OF THE UNITED KINGDOM
Psychiatric nursing in Wales. *Nursing Times*, Dec. 18, 1969, p. 1628-9.

ROYAL COLLEGE OF NURSING *and*
NATIONAL COUNCIL OF NURSES OF THE UNITED KINGDOM
The role of psychiatric ward sisters and charge nurses in the rehabilitation of patients. The College, 1963.

ROYAL MEDICO-PSYCHOLOGICAL ASSOCIATION
Nurse—or educator? *Nursing Mirror*, May 1, 1970, p. 12.

SAINSBURY, M. J.
A glimpse at psychiatric nursing in New South Wales during the past fifty years. *The Lamp*, Nov. 1968, p. 16 and 19.

SAINSBURY, M. J.
A glimpse at psychiatric nursing in New South Wales during the past fifty years. Pt. 2. *The Lamp*, Dec. 1968, p. 11-3.

SANDISON, R. A., *and* HOPKIN, I.
Psychotherapy using LSD. *Nursing Times*, May 1, 1964, p. 556-7.

SAWYER, JOAN
The suicidal patient in the general ward. *Nursing Times*, Dec. 14, 1962, p. 1587.

SAWYER, JOAN
Talking with the mentally ill. *Nursing Times*, April 17, 1964, pp. 490-2.

SEAGER, C. P.
Aversion treatment in psychiatry. *Nursing Times*, Mar. 26, 1965, p. 423-4.

SHARPE, D.
The psychiatric nurse as a social visitor. *Nursing Times*, Dec. 2, 1966, p. 1578-80.

SHARROCK, R. L.
Intensive care in a psychiatric hospital. *Nursing Mirror*, Nov. 14, 1969, p. 45-7.

SHERLOCK, B. J.
Acquisition of the nursing role and the transmission of nontherapeutic orientations. *Nursing Research*, Summer 1963, p. 182-5.

SIMMONS, JANET A.
The nurse-patient relationship in psychiatric nursing. Philadelphia, Saunders, 1969.

SINGER, P., *and others*
The psychiatrist-nurse team and home care in Soviet Union and Amsterdam. *Journal of Practical Nursing and Mental Health Services*, Jan./Feb. 1970, p. 40-4.

SINKLER, G. H.
Identity and role: a nonparticipant observer discovers the importance of coherence between these two significant concepts in psychiatric nursing. *Nursing Outlook*, Oct. 1970, p. 22-4.

SMITH, E. S.
Mental illness and the district nurse. 1. Organic and neurotic reactions; 2. Depression, psychosis and mental deficiency; 3. Preventive measures. *Nursing Times*, Oct. 15, 1970, p. 1329-30; Oct. 22, 1970, p. 1363-4; Oct. 29, 1970, p. 1395-6.

SNEDDON, R.
Psychiatric geriatric assessment unit at Crichton Royal Hospital. *Nursing Mirror*, April 7, 1967, p. x-xv.

STACHYRA, M.
Nurses, psychotherapy and the law. *Perspectives in Psychiatric Care*, Sept./Oct. 1969, p. 200-13.

STAGE, T. B.
Evolution of the psychiatric nurse. *Mental Hospitals*, July 1965, p. 197-200.

STEIN, L. I., *and* JACKSON, B.
Attitudes and behavior in response to nursing staff in mufti. *Journal of Psychiatric Nursing and Mental Health Services*, Mar./April 1969, p. 82-5 and 88.

STEWART, D. R.
Psychiatric nursing in Finland and Sweden. *Nursing Times*, Feb. 12, 1970, Occasional Papers, p. 27-8.

STOKES, GERTRUDE A., *editor*
The roles of psychiatric nurses in community mental health practice: a giant step. New York, The Author, 1969.

STRONG, P. G.
Relationships in psychiatric nursing. *Nursing Mirror*, Aug. 21, 1970, p. 35-7.

SUAREZ, R.
The silent patient in group therapy. *Journal of Psychiatric Nursing*, July/Aug. 1970, p. 10-2.

SUCHINSKY, L. W.
An illustration of a behavioral therapy intervention with nursing staff in a therapeutic role. *Journal of Psychiatric Nursing*, Sept./Oct. 1970, p. 24-6.

SUGDEN, J.
Objectives in psychiatric nursing. *Nursing Times*, Oct. 8, 1970, p. 1297-8.

SULLIVAN, J. D.
Without authority. *American Journal of Nursing*, Dec. 1969, p. 2654-7.

SWEENEY, A., *and others*
Courage to change. *Journal of Psychiatric Nursing and Mental Health Services*, Mar./April 1969, p. 73-6.

SYMINGTON, A.
New in psychiatry: moditen injectable therapy and follow up care. *The Canadian Nurse*, Jan. 1970, p. 21-4.

TAUBER, I. J.
A metabolic approach to mental disorders at Hollymoor Hospital, Birmingham. *Nursing Times*, Sept. 11, 1964, p. 1172-4.

THOMAS, F. A., *and others*
A new automated psychiatric nursing report. *Perspectives in Psychiatric Care*, Sept./Oct. 1970, p. 222-9.

THOMPSON, T.
Reflections after 30 years of Psychiatric Nursing—Past, Present and Future. *Mental Health*, Summer 1961, p. 45-50.

THOMSON, C. P.
Prevention in psychiatry—1 and 2. *Nursing Times*, Nov. 19, 1965, p. 1575-6; Nov. 26, 1965, p. 1620-1.

TODD, J.
An appreciation of the mental hospital nurse. *Nursing Mirror*, July 17, 1970, p. 18-9.

TODD, J. J.
Bridging the gap. [Progressive patient care for psychiatric patients]. *District Nursing*, Dec. 1970, p. 178-9.

TRAIL, IRA DAVIS
Establishing relationships in psychiatric nursing. New York, Springer, 1966.

TRAVELBEE, JOYCE
Intervention in psychiatric nursing: process in the one-to-one relationship. Philadelphia, Davis, 1969.

TRICK, K. L. K.
The disturbed patient in a general ward. *Nursing Mirror*, Sept. 1, 1967, p. 503-5.

TRICK, K. L. K., *and* OBCARSKAS, S.
Understanding mental illness and its nursing. Pitman, 1968.

TUBBS, A.
Nursing intervention to shorten anxiety-ridden transition periods [in a child psychiatric unit]. *Nursing Outlook*, July 1970, p. 27.

TUMILTY, E. M.
Community psychiatric nursing. *Nursing Times*, Oct. 2, 1969, Occasional Papers, p. 157-60.

UJHELY, G. B.
The nurse in community psychiatry. *American Journal of Nursing*, May 1969, p. 1001-5.

UJHELY, G. B.
Nursing intervention with the acutely ill psychiatric patient. *Nursing Forum*, vol. VIII, no. 3, 1969, p. 311-325.

UNSWORTH, G. P., *and* LAWES, T.
Drug induced schizophrenia with sensory deprivation. *Nursing Mirror*, Nov. 8, 1963, p. 131-3.

URRY, N.
Behavior modification with an autistic child. *Nursing Times*, April 9, 1970, p. 456-8.

WADSWORTH, W. V.
Industrial therapy in a mental hospital. *Nursing Times*, April 7, 1961, p. 446.

WALKER, R., *and* DEMPSEY, M.
Ward behavior in schizophrenic patients ready for release and in those requiring further hospitalization. *Nursing Research*, Spring 1967, p. 174-8.

WALLACE, CLARE MARC
Electroconvulsive therapy and the nurse. *Nursing Mirror*, Jan. 31, 1969, p. 20-1.

WALLACE, CLARE MARC
Modified narcosis and the nurse. *Nursing Mirror*, Feb. 14, 1969, p. 46.

WALLACE, CLARE MARC
Portrait of a schizophrenic nurse. Hammond, Hammond, 1965.

WARD, D. J.
The central function of the mental nurse. *International Journal of Nursing Studies*, May 1967, p. 179-89.

SPECIALITIES

WARREN, W.
Psychiatric disturbance in adolescence. *Nursing Times*, July 26, 1963, p. 934-6.

WEDDELL, D.
Family centred nursing. *International Nursing Review*, vol. 8, no. 6, 1961, p. 20-5.

WEEKS, K., *and* GREENE, J.
Psychiatric nurses in the community. *Nursing Times*, Feb. 25, 1966, p. 257-8.

WERNER, J. A.
Relating group theory to nursing practice. *Perspectives in Psychiatric Care*, Nov./Dec. 1970, p. 248-61.

WHEELER, A. M.
The position of psychiatric nurses working in the occupational therapy department. *Occupational Therapy*, Apr. 1970, p. 17-21.

WHITEHEAD, J. A., *and* CORTAZZI, D., *editors*
Improving the effectiveness of hospitals and services for the mentally ill and mentally subnormal: hospital staff describe their efforts to improve patient care in and out of hospital. King Edward's Hospital Fund for London, 1968.

WHITLAM, V.
The autistic child. *Canadian Nurse*, Nov. 1970, p. 44-7.

WILKINSON, M. A.
Do-it-yourself orientation. *Nursing Outlook*, Nov. 1969, p. 53-4.

WILLIAMS, J. D.
Some social aspects of psychiatry. *Nursing Mirror*, Feb. 27, 1970, p. 22-4.

WING, J. K.
Schizophrenic patients in the community. 1. Rehabilitation and resettlement. *Nursing Mirror*, June 1, 1962, p. ii-iv.

WING, J. K.
Schizophrenic patients in the community. 2. Community care and effect of social environment. *Nursing Mirror*, June 8, 1962, p. v-vi.

WLOCH, N.
Psychiatric nursing in Scandinavia and the Netherlands. *British Hospital Journal and Social Service Review*, Dec. 29, 1967, p. 2447-9.

WOODMANSEY, A. C.
The health visitor's role in preventive psychiatry. *The Medical Officer*, June 25, 1965, p. 339-41.

WOOLLASTON, M. E. F.
Schizophrenia—a new outlook. *Nursing Mirror*, June 6, 1969, p. 33-5.

WORSLEY, J. L.
Clinical psychology in the psychiatric hospital. *Nursing Mirror*, Jan. 19, 1962, p. x.

YALOM, I. D., *and* TERRAZAS, F.
Group therapy for psychotic elderly patients. *American Journal of Nursing*, Aug. 1968, p. 1690-4.

YATES, HOWARD W.
Nursing problems in an open door hospital.
In
AMERICAN NURSES' ASSOCIATION
Culture, atmosphere and social organization: effects on nursing care of the patient. New York, The Association, 1962.

ZDERAD, LORETTA, *and* BELCHER, HELEN C.
Developing behavioral concepts in nursing: report of the regional project in teaching psychiatric nursing in baccalaureate programs. Atlanta, Ga. Southern Regional Education Board, 1968.

AFTER-CARE

BIERER, J.
Psychiatric clinics and community centres—today and tomorrow—I. *Nursing Mirror*, May 8, 1964, p. ix-x.

BIERER, J.
Psychiatric clinics and community centres—to-day and to-morrow—II. *Nursing Mirror*, May 15, 1964, p. vii and x.

BILLINGS, G. A.
The rehabilitation revolution. *Nursing Mirror*, Aug. 7, 1970, p. 38-41.

BOLTON, W. B.
Rehabilitation through education. *Nursing Times*, Oct. 5, 1962, p. 1265.

BONE, M. R.
The schizophrenic patient goes home. *Nursing Mirror*, July 10, 1964, p. 327-8.

CAMP, R. P., *and* ONNEMBO, F.
Discharged psychiatric patients' visits to a former treatment centre: a nursing dilemma. *Journal of Psychiatric Nursing*, July/Aug. 1968, p. 213-8.

CAMPBELL, W.
The Stepping Stone Club. [for ex-psychiatric patients]. *Nursing Times*, Oct. 1, 1970, p. 1273.

FAGIN, CLAIRE M.
Family-centred nursing in community psychiatry: treatment in the home. Philadelphia, Davis, 1970.

FLEMING, R., *and others*
An after-care program for patients discharged from mental hospitals. *Nursing Outlook*, Sept. 1961, p. 544.

FRAME, H. B. P., *and* BEEBY, G. J.
Conditioning the psychiatric patient for discharge. *Nursing Mirror*, Nov. 10, 1961, p. vii.

HANCOCK, C.
People who care . . . A review of voluntary organisations working with the mentally ill. *Nursing Mirror*, Dec. 20, 1968, p. 16-7.

HOGGINS, D. E.
From a psychiatric hospital to community life. *Nursing Mirror*, Sept. 13, 1970, p. 25-30.

NATIONAL ASSOCIATION FOR MENTAL HEALTH
Out of hospital—who cares? *District Nursing*, Nov. 1970, p. 153 and 156.

SHUCK, W. H.
Freedom to work [rehabilitation of chronic psychiatric patients at Middlewood Hospital, Sheffield]. *Nursing Mirror*, July 4, 1969, p. 18-21; July 11, 1969, p. 32-5.

ADMINISTRATION

ALLEN B.
Communications in the ward. *Nursing Times*, Sept. 22, 1961, p. 1230.

ALLGOOD, J.
Salmon in a psychiatric hospital group. A ward sister's view of the Salmon structure. *Nursing Mirror*, Nov. 13, 1970, p. 32-3.

AMERICAN NURSES' ASSOCIATION. RESEARCH AND STATISTICS UNIT
Survey of salaries and employment conditions in nonfederal psychiatric hospitals June 1965. New York, The Association, 1966.

ATTY, L. M.
Introducing the newcomer—the patient and the staff nurse—to a psychiatric hospital. *Perspectives in Psychiatric Care*, vol. III, no. 2, 1965, p. 25-34.

BAGGOTT, E.
Role of the hospital nurse in the wider psychiatric service. *Nursing Times*, July 28, 1967, p. 993-4.

BEUKER, KATHLEEN, *and* SAINATO, HELEN K.
A study of staffing patterns in psychiatric nursing. Washington, Saint Elizabeths Hospital, 1968.

BLACK, B.
Unit system [in psychiatric care]. The third revolution. *American Journal of Nursing*, Mar. 1970, p. 515-9.

BRAY, R. E., and BIRD, T. E.
Communication with the psychiatric patient. *Nursing Times*, April 12, 1968, p. 490-1.

BRAY, R. E., *and* BIRD, T. E.
Reception. *Nursing Times*, Mar. 18, 1966, p. 376.

BRAY, R. E., *and* BIRD, T. E.
"Relatives"—a problem in psychiatric nursing. *Nursing Times*, Mar. 6, 1969, p. 297-9.

BRAY, R. E., *and* BIRD, T. E.
Ward sister or group leader? *Nursing Mirror*, July 15, 1966, p. xiii and xvi.

CAINE, T. M., *and* WIJESINGHE, O. B.
Communication problems of student nurses in a mental hospital. *Nursing Times*, Oct. 23, 1969, Occasional Papers, p. 177-9.

CHRISTOPOULOS, A. C.
Do you read the nurses' observation notes? [A question addressed to the doctors]. *Journal of Psychiatric Nursing and Mental Health Services*, Jan./Feb. 1970, p. 24-5.

DEAN, D. J., *and others*
Patients' views of a psychiatric hospital. *Nursing Times*, July 7, 1967, p. 887-9.

DUNLAP, L., *and* MATTEOLI, R.
A team function: developing a nursing care plan in a psychiatric setting. *Journal of Psychiatric Nursing*, Sept./Oct. 1970, p. 19 and 22-3.

FLOYD, E. D.
Improving patients' clothing—and laundry services. *Nursing Times*, Jan. 27, 1967, p. 112-3 and 115.

GLANCY, J. E. MCA.
Employing communicating skills in patient care. *Nursing Mirror*, May 11, 1962, p. 109.

GORTON, JOHN V.
A guide for the evaluation of psychiatric nursing services. New York, N.L.N., 1961.

LEOPOLDT, H.
Psychiatric group homes: the economic aspects. *Nursing Mirror*, Jan. 23, 1970, p. 36-7.

LLOYD, W. A.
Integration and the principal nursing officer. *Nursing Times*, June 9, 1967, p. 774-5.

LLOYD, W. A.
Salmon in a psychiatric hospital group. The chief nursing officer's view of the Salmon structure. *Nursing Mirror*, Dec. 18, 1970, p. 36-7 and 39.

PACKARD, H.
Preparing LPNs as charge nurses and unit supervisors in a psychiatric hospital. *Journal of Practical Nursing*, Dec. 1970, p. 26-7, 31-2.

RICHARDSON, B.
Salmon in a psychiatric hospital group. The Salmon Unit in subnormality. *Nursing Mirror*, Dec. 11, 1970, p. 23-4.

YEOMANS, N. T.
The nurse's self-image and its implications. *Australian Nurses' Journal*, April 1963, p. 98-100.

EDUCATION

ACKRAL, M., *and others*
A post-registration course in child psychiatry for nurses. *Nursing Times*, April 5, 1968, Occasional Papers, p. 53-5.

ANDREWS, JOHN MICHAEL
Questions and answers on mental nursing for pupil nurses. Arnold, 1968.

ANDREWS, JOHN MICHAEL
Community therapy. Its effect on training psychiatric nurses. *Nursing Times*, Feb. 16, 1962, p. 206.

ARJE, FRANCES B., *and others, editors*
Psychiatric nursing: 1500 multiple choice questions and referenced answers, edited by Frances B. Arje, Charlotte H. Martin, Irene L. Sell. 2nd edn. New York, Medical Examination Publishing Co., 1967.
[Nursing examination review book, vol. 2.]

BADLAND, S. G.
One psychiatric register? *Nursing Times*, Feb. 12, 1965, p. 228-9.

BADLAND, S. G., *and* HULBERT, C.
Conflict—one psychiatric register? For and against. *Nursing Times*, Jan. 13, 1967, p. 56-7.

BATEY, M., *and others*
Defining graduate clinical content in psychiatric nursing. *Journal of Nursing Education*, Dec. 1962, p. 13-4 and 27-9.

BENTINCK, C., *and* MORRIS, M. L.
Teaching behavioral observation to psychiatric nursing students. *Journal of Psychiatric Nursing*, Mar./April 1968, p. 94-5 and 98-100.

BERMOSK, L. S., *and* RYKKEN, M. B.
A community approach to teaching psychiatric nursing. *Nursing Outlook*, Oct. 1962, p. 670-73.

BICKFORD, J. A. R.
Teachers in mental hospitals. *Nursing Mirror*, Sept. 22, 1967, p. x-xi.

BOORER, DAVID
Experiment at Hellingly. [In mental nurse training]. *Nursing Times*, Mar. 27, 1969, p. 401-2.

BOORER, DAVID
A code of practice [for psychiatric nurses]. *Mental Health*, Winter 1970, p. 2-4.

BUCKLES, B. V., *and others*
Learning purposeful nursing intervention. *American Journal of Nursing*, Dec. 1968, p. 2578-80.

DALTON, B. M.
Withdrawal from training of RNMS Student nurses. *Nursing Times*, Aug. 7, 1969, Occasional Papers, p. 125-8; Aug. 14, 1969, Occasional Papers, p. 129-32.

DAVIES, T. I. H.
Meeting changing needs in psychiatric nurse training. *Nursing Mirror*, Jan. 11, 1963, p. 321.

DE GRAS, L. A.
Education of the nurse for the mental health field. *Nursing Mirror*, Feb. 3, 1961, p. x.

DIERS, D., *and* JOHNSON, J. E.
How workshops prepare nurses for the therapeutic role. *Nursing Outlook*, June 1969, p. 30-4.

DONELLY, G.
Pioneering the district [The secondment of third-year psychiatric student nurses at St. Nicholas Hospital, Godforth, to the Health and Social Service Department, Newcastle upon Tyne]. *Nursing Times*, April 9, 1970, p. 472-3.

EMENS, A. E.
The clinical instructor in the psychiatric hospital. *Nursing Times*, April 28, 1967, p. 556-8.

EMERS, J.
The training of psychiatric nursing personnel in Sweden. *Journal of Psychiatric Nursing*, Sept./Oct. 1964, p. 454-9.

GELFAND, S., *and* ULLMANN, L. P.
Attitude changes associated with psychiatric affiliation. *Nursing Research*, Fall 1961, p. 200-4.

GENERAL NURSING COUNCIL FOR SCOTLAND
The training of the psychiatric nurse. Edinburgh, The Council, 1963.

SPECIALITIES

GIBSON, JOHN
Mental nursing examination questions and answers. Faber and Faber, 1964.

HALLAS, C.
Student nurse training in mental deficiency hospitals. *Nursing Times*, Aug. 9, 1968, p. 1079-80.

HALSTEAD, H.
Selecting psychiatric nurses. *Nursing Times*, Mar. 9, 1962, p. 295.

HAMM, B. H., and HARTSFIELD, S. L.
Motivation influencing students in psychiatric nursing. *Nursing Research*, Jan.-Feb. 1970, p. 79-81.

HOPKIN, I.
The first psychiatric pupil nurse assessment. *Nursing Mirror*, Aug. 25, 1967, p. 483-4.

JOHNSTONE, T., and others
A brief encounter with psychotherapy. [Attitudes of nurses seconded to the Royal Edinburgh Hospital as part of their training]. *Nursing Times*, July 3, 1969, Occasional Papers, p. 105-8.

KIRKPATRICK, W. J.
Psychiatric nurse training in British Columbia. *Nursing Times*, Feb. 2, 1965, p. 299-300.

LARSON, KENNETH H., and others
Direct care nursing: a teaching program for psychiatric nurses. New York, Macmillan, 1968.

LEWIS, GARLAND K.
An approach to education of psychiatric nursing personnel: report of Seminar Project for teachers of Psychiatric Aides; prepared by Garland K. Lewis, Marguerite J. Holmes and Fredk. Katz. New York, N.L.N., 1961. [Co-sponsored by National League for Nursing and American Psychiatric Association.]

LOGAN, D. L.
Action-oriented group therapy as a training method for psychiatric student nurses. *Journal of Psychiatric Nursing and Mental Health Services*, Sept./Oct. 1969, p. 201-6.

LOUGHLIN, T. M., and others
A comparative study of supervised and unsupervised Library periods for student nurses in psychiatric nursing. *Journal of Psychiatric Nursing*, July/Aug. 1964, p. 345-9.

McGUINNESS, A. F., and others
Psychiatric training and the development of insight. *Nursing Times*, May 1, 1969, p. 555-6.

MANFREDA, MARGUERITE LUCY
Teaching psychiatric and mental health nursing. Philadelphia, Davis, [c. 1961].

MARWICK, I.
Training psychiatric nurses in developing countries. *Journal of Psychiatric Nursing and Mental Health Services*, Mar./April 1969, p. 94-6.

MENTAL HEALTH TUTORS ASSOCIATION
Training of mental nurses. Tutors' conference views on working of the experimental syllabuses. *Hospital and Social Service Journal*, Nov. 30, 1962, p. 1341.

MORTON-MASON, S. R.
The benefits from discussion groups [in psychiatric nurse training]. *Nursing Mirror*, Mar. 25, 1966, p. v-vi.

MOULSON, F., and WHITTAKER, C. B.
Taped interviews in psychiatric nurse training. *Nursing Times*, Jan. 27, 1967, p. 106-7.

MUECKE, M. A.
Video tape recordings: a tool for psychiatric clinical supervision. *Perspectives in Psychiatric Care*, Sept./Oct. 1970, p. 200-8.

O'GORMAN, G.
Recruitment and training of mental nurses. *Nursing Times*, Aug. 3, 1962, p. 996-7.

PARKER, E. R.
RMN/SRN Training in the London Hospital Group. *Nursing Times*, May 28, 1970, p. 683-5.

PATTEMORE, W. R.
"Help! I need somebody." The value of psychiatric nursing training to the general nurse. *Nursing Times*, Mar. 18, 1966, p. 382.

PESZNECKER, BETTY L., and HEWITT, HELON E.
Psychiatric content in the nursing curriculum: a study of integration process. Seattle, University of Washington Press, 1963.

PHINNEY, R. P.
The student of nursing and the schizophrenic patient. *American Journal of Nursing*, April 1970, p. 790-2.

PILLAI, A. S.
Training of psychiatric nurses at the All India Institute of Mental Health, Bangalore. *The Nursing Journal of India*, Sept. 1967, p. 231-2.

POPKIN, D. R.
Coordination of field work experience in a course in community mental health. *Nursing Outlook*, Oct. 1969, p. 41-3.

ROBINSON, A. M.
The where of psychiatric nursing in the basic program. *Nursing Outlook*, Oct. 1963, p. 746-8.

SATA, L. S., and SHENNING, M.
Administrative implications of small group experiences. *Journal of Psychiatric Nursing and Mental Health Services*, Sept./Oct. 1968, p. 261-6.

SCHOENBERG, BERNARD, and others, editors
Teaching psychosocial aspects of patient care, edited by Bernard Schoenberg, Helen F. Pettit and Arthur C. Carr. New York, Columbia University Press, 1968.

SHEPSTONE, A.
Practical nursing with groups. *Nursing Times*, Oct. 20, 1967, p. 1413-4.

SLAVINSKY, A. T., and others
Training nursing personnel to use a rating scale. *Perspectives in Psychiatric Care*, Sept./Oct. 1969, p. 214-21.

SMITH, A. J.
A manual for the training of psychiatric nursing personnel in group psychotherapy. *Perspectives in Psychiatric Care*, May/June 1970, p. 106-26.

STRONG, P. G.
The clinical tutor in a psychiatric hospital. *Nursing Times*, Jan. 22, 1970, Occasional Papers, p. 13-6.

TAIT, J.
Educating for enlightenment. [Moorhaven Hospital, Ivybridge, S. Devon]. *Nursing Mirror*, Oct. 31, 1969, p. 20-3.

TOMSETT, V.
18 months' general nursing for mental nurses. *Nursing Mirror*, July 26, 1963, p. ii-iii.

TOOMEY, L. C., and others
Some relationships between the attitudes of nursing students toward psychiatry and success in psychiatric affiliation. *Nursing Research*, Summer 1961, p. 165-9.

VAN SANT, G. E.
Psychiatric nursing in the basic programme. *International Nursing Review*, vol. 12, no. 2, 1965, p. 30-4.

WALLACE, M. A., and MORLEY, W. E.
Teaching crisis intervention. *American Journal of Nursing*, July 1970, p. 1484-7.

WALSH, JOAN E., and TAYLOR, CECILIA MONAT
An approach to the teaching of psychiatric nursing in diploma and associate degree programs: final report on the project. New York, National League for Nursing, 1969.

WALSH, JOAN E., *and* TAYLOR, CECILIA MONAT
Integrating psychiatric-mental health nursing content in the curriculum. *Nursing Outlook*, November 1968, p. 50-3.

ZALBA, S. R., *and* ABELS, P.
Training the nurse in psychiatric group work. *Journal of Psychiatric Nursing and Mental Health Services*, Mar./April 1970, p. 7-12.

PSYCHIATRY IN THE GENERAL HOSPITAL

JOHNSON, B. S.
Psychiatric nurse consultant in a general hospital. *Nursing Outlook*, Oct. 1963, p. 728-9.

KNOX, S. J.
The nurse's role in the psychiatric unit of a general hospital. *Nursing Mirror*, Sept. 13, 1963, p. i-ii and v.

PETERSEN, S.
The psychiatric nurse specialist in a general hospital. *Nursing Outlook*, Feb. 1969, p. 56-8.

SMITH, S.
Mentally trained nurses on a general ward. *Nursing Mirror*, June 21, 1963, p. 257-8.

TUTT, N. S.
Psychiatric nurses' attitudes to treatment in a general hospital. *Nursing Times*, Sept. 17, 1970, Occasional Papers, p. 137-9.

RESEARCH

PAUL, W. K.
Research nursing in psychiatry. *The Canadian Nurse*, June 1967, p. 33-4.

PSYCHOLOGY

ALTSCHUL, A.
Aids to psychology for nurses. Bailliere, Tindall and Cox, 1962.
2nd edn., 1965.
For 1951 edn. *see* Mackenzie, Norah.

ALTSCHUL, A.
Psychology for nurses. 3rd edn. Bailliere, 1969.

BARTON, J.
The chaplain—a member of the hospital team. 1. Visiting the sick. *Nursing Mirror*, Aug. 27, 1965, p. 527-9.
Pt. II, *see* PARE, P.

BENOLIEL, J. Q.
Talking to patients about death. *Nursing Forum*, vol. IX, no. 3, 1970, p. 254-68.

BOOTH, HOWARD
Helping troubled people. *Nursing Times*, July 20, 1962, p. 933.

BOOTH, HOWARD
Spiritual healing. *Nursing Times*, Dec. 22, 1961, p. 1661.

CLARK, J. F.
The nurse's self-image and its implications. *Australian Nurses' Journal*, May 1963, p. 118-9.

COFFMAN, J. A.
Anger: its significance for nurses who work with emotionally disturbed children. *Perspectives in Psychiatric Care*, May/June 1969, p. 104-11.

COLE, J. W.
The value of psychology to the student nurse. *Nursing Times*, Aug. 10, 1962, p. 1024.

CROW, LESTER D., *and* CROW, ALICE
Human relations in practical nursing. New York, Macmillan, 1964.

CROW, LESTER D., *and* CROW, ALICE
Understanding interrelations in nursing. New York, Macmillan [1961].

DALLY, PETER, *and* FARNHAM, SUSAN
Psychology and psychiatry for nurses. English Universities Press, 1964.
2nd edn., 1967.

DENNIS, LORRAINE BRADT
Psychology of human behaviour for nurses. 2nd edn. Philadelphia, Saunders, 1962.
3rd edn., 1967.

FOX, R.
Hostility towards doctors and nurses. 1. Public and profession. 2. Face to face. *Nursing Times*, July 20, 1962, p. 918-20; July 27, 1962, p. 956.

GOLDFOGEL, L.
Working with the parent of a dying child. *American Journal of Nursing*, Aug. 1970, p. 1675-9.

GOLDSBOROUGH, J. D.
On becoming nonjudgmental. *American Journal of Nursing*, Nov. 1970, p. 2340-3.

HARMUTH, B., *and others*
The "problem" patient [By] B. Harmuth, U. Lantz, G. Oden. Newark, New Jersey, the State University College of Nursing, 1961.

HECKEL, ROBERT V., *and* JORDAN, ROSE M.
Psychology: the nurse and the patient. St. Louis, Mosby, 1963.
2nd edn., 1967.

HEIDGERKEN, LORETTA
Dynamics in group discussion. Washington, Catholic University of America Press, 1963.

JAMES, D.
The teaching of psychology. 1. Attitudes; 2. Teaching problems. *Nursing Times*, Mar. 13, 1969, p. 332-3; Mar. 20, 1969, p. 365-6.

JAMES, D. E.
Introduction to psychology for teachers, nurses and other social workers. Constable, 1968.
2nd edn., 1970.

JOHNSON, B S, *and others*
Teaching interpersonal skills to nursing students. *Nursing Outlook*, March 1964, p. 62-4.

JOHNSON, MARGARET ANNE
Developing the art of understanding: a guide for nursing students. New York, Springer, 1967.

KEMPF, FLORENCE C., *and* USEEM, RUTH HILL
Psychology: dynamics of behavior in nursing. Philadelphia, Saunders, 1964.

LAMBERTSEN, E. C.
You can't do today's nursing with yesterday's attitudes. *Modern Hospital*, Dec. 1969, p. 140.

MCGHIE, ANDREW
Psychology as applied to nursing. 2nd edn. Edinburgh, Livingstone, 1961.
3rd edn., 1963.
4th edn., 1966.
5th edn., 1969.

MCKNIGHT, E. T.
A Chaplain interprets his work. *The Canadian Nurse*, Dec. 1961, p. 1139.

MARTIN, D., *and* ALLEN, D.
A week's learning experience in the psychology of nursing. *Nursing Times*, Aug. 28, 1969, Occasional Papers, p. 137-40

MERIVALE, R. F.
The new student. *Nursing Times*, June 7, 1963, p. 704-6.

MOORE, L., *and others*
Factors influencing the behavior of students in nursing. *Nursing Research*, Spring 1962, p. 97.

MORISON, LUELLA J., *and* FARRIS, MARY AGNES
Approaches for co-workers in professional nursing. St. Louis, Mosby, 1962.

NURSES' CHRISTIAN MOVEMENT
Christianity and nursing today: the report of a working-party (1963/4) appointed by the Nurses' Christian Movement to study Christian work amongst nurses. The Epworth Press, 1964.

OAKES, J.
Pastoral care of the dying and the bereaved. *District Nursing*, Mar. 1969, p. 256-8.

O'HARA, FRANK J., *and* REITH, HERMAN R.
Psychology and the nurse. 6th edn. Philadelphia, Saunders, 1966.

PARE, P.
The chaplain—a member of the hospital team. 2. The problem of suffering. *Nursing Mirror*, Sept. 3, 1965, p. 556-7.
Pt. I, *see* BARTON, J.

PAYNE, R. L.
Psychology of racial prejudice. *Nursing Mirror*, June 17, 1966, p. i-iii.

PEARCE, EVELYN CLARE
Nurse and patient: an ethical consideration of human relations. 2nd edn. Faber, 1963.
3rd edn., 1969.

PLACHTA, SISTER MARY MIRANDA,
Spiritualize your nursing. New Jersey, Felician Sisters, 1963.

ROBISCHON, PAULETTE, *and* SCOTT, DIANE
Role theory and its application in family nursing. *Nursing Outlook*, July 1969, p. 52-7.

SANT, E. G.
Qualities of mind of a nurse. *Nursing Mirror*, April 20, 1962, p. 43.

SHAPIRO, M. B.
Behaviour therapy. *Nursing Mirror*, April 23, 1965, p. vi-vii.

SMELTZER, C. H.
Psychology for student nurses. New York, Macmillan, 1962.

THOMAS, D. HUBERT
Going into nursing. The Epworth Press, 1964.
[This book is concerned with the religious aspects of becoming a nurse.]

UJHELY, GERTRUD BERTRAND
Determinants of the nurse-patient relationship. New York, Springer, 1968.

UJHELY, GERTRUD BERTRAND
The nurse and her problem patients. New York, Springer, 1963.

VAILLOT, SISTER MADELEINE CLEMENCE,
The spiritual factors in nursing. *Journal of Practical Nursing*, Sept. 1970, p. 30-1.

WOLFSON, WILLIAM, *and* LO CASCIO, RALPH
Digit symbol performance of nursing school applicants. *Journal of Clinical Psychology*, Jan. 1961, p. 59.

WYGANT, W. E.
Dying, but not alone. *American Journal of Nursing*, Mar. 1967, p. 574-7.

PUBLIC HEALTH NURSING
GENERAL WORKS
BAILEY, D. H.
The role of the nurse in community life. *Journal of the West Australian Nurses*, June 1970, p. 18-21 and 14.

BALY, M.
Changing demands for health services—Part 1; part 2. *Nursing Times*, May 22, 1969, Occasional Papers, p. 81-4; May 29, 1969, Occasional Papers, p. 85-8.

BERGMAN, R.
Israel—team nursing in public health—pt. I. *International Journal of Nursing Studies*, Dec. 1964, p. 179-209.

BERGMAN, R.
Israel—team nursing in public health—pt. II. *International Journal of Nursing Studies*, April 1965, p. 43-71.

BERGMAN, R.
Israel—team nursing in public health—pt. III. *International Journal of Nursing Studies*, Nov. 1965, pp. 211-40.

BERGMAN, R.
Israel—team nursing in public health—pt. IV. Summary, proposals, and implications for further study. *International Journal of Nursing Studies*, Feb. 1966, p. 261-77.

BOWNS, B.
The possible dream [Co-ordination between education and service in community health nursing]. *Nursing Outlook*, Jan. 1970, p. 36-9.

BROADLEY, MARGARET E.
Nursing and community service. Longmans, 1968.

BROWN, D. E.
The nurse in the community. *District Nursing*, Oct. 1968, p. 149-50.

BULL, M. R.
Health services in Algeria: the formation of a new service for a new country. *Nursing Mirror*, Jan. 10, 1969, p. 31-3.

CANADIAN NURSES' ASSOCIATION
Statements on the recommendations of the report of the Royal Commission on Health Services. Ottawa, The Association [1965?].

CANADIAN NURSES' ASSOCIATION
Submission to the Royal Commission on Health Services. Ottawa, The Association, 1962.

CHISHOLM, A. S.
Public health nursing in Nigeria. *District Nursing*, June 1969, p. 46-7, and 49.

CHISHOLM, MARY K.
The width and depth of health education. *Nursing Mirror*, June 5, 1964, p. 211.

CLARK, G.
Parliament and public health. *Nursing Mirror*, Jan. 22, 1965, p. x-xii.

CLOUT, I. R.
New patterns of community care. *Nursing Mirror*, April 24, 1964, p. 85-6.

COLEMAN, A. M.
An introduction to community health. *Nursing Times*, Sept. 22, 1967, p. 1278-9.

CORNELIUS, D. A., *and* CONNORS, H.
The United States social security system and Medicare and Medicaid. *International Nursing Review*, vol. 17, no. 3, 1970, p. 206-23.

CUST, G.
Why health education? *District Nursing*, Oct. 1966, p. 162-4.

DAVIES, J. B. MEREDITH
Preventive medicine for nurses and social workers. English Universities Press, 1965.

DE PASS, B.
Public health nursing. *Practical Nursing*, May 1963, p. 25-6.

DESAINZ, D.
The Public Health Nurse as research interviewer. *Nursing Outlook*, Aug. 1962, p. 514-6.

BIBLIOGRAPHY OF NURSING

Dixon, P. N.
The health centre nurse. *Nursing Times*, Mar. 26, 1970, p. 399-40.

Dixon, P. N.
Work of a nurse in a health centre treatment room. *British Medical Journal*, Nov. 1, 1969, p. 292-4.

Dolton, W. D.
The health and welfare of the immigrant—1. *Nursing Mirror*, Sept. 16, 1966, p. v-vii.

Dolton, W. D.
The health and welfare of the immigrant—2. *Nursing Mirror*, Sept. 23, 1966, p. xv-xvi.

Dooley, J.
Community nursing in Zambia. *International Nursing Review*, vol. 15, no. 4, 1968, p. 359-66.

Draper, P.
Community care units. *Nursing Times*, Aug. 2, 1968, p. 1035-6.

Driscoll, B.
The changing face of public health in Gt. Britain today and the SSAFA Nursing Services. *Health Visitor*, Aug. 1970, p. 277-80.

Duffy, W.
Health education—its nature and scope—pt. I. *Nursing Mirror*, Sept. 7, 1962, p. v-vi.

Duffy, W.
Health education—its nature and scope—pt. II. *Nursing Mirror*, Sept. 14, 1962, p. xi-xii.

Dunn, M.
Haere-mai. [Public health nursing in New Zealand]. *District Nursing*, June 1969, p. 48-9.

Ellis, J. R.
Community medicine. *Nursing Mirror*, Nov. 29, 1968, p. 17-9; Dec. 6, 1968, p. 31-3.

Ennever, O. N.
An experience in community medicine for student nurses. *The Jamaican Nurse*, vol. 10, no. 1, 1970, p. 32.

Erasmus, Cora A.
Basic health problems today. *South African Nursing Journal*, Nov. 1968, p. 22-4 and 26.

Freeman, Ruth Benson
Community health nursing practice. Philadelphia, Saunders, 1970.

Freeman, Ruth Benson
Measuring the effectiveness of public health nursing service. *Nursing Outlook*, Oct. 1961, p. 605-7.

Frost, W.
Progress in public health nursing. *District Nursing*, April 1968, p. 4-6.

Gagnon, C.
The new roles of the nurse in the health team. *Canadian Nurse*, Dec. 1970, p. 20-2.

Gear, H. S., *and* Cunningham, P. J.
Modern health: a handbook for nurses and medical auxiliaries. Faber and Faber, 1965.

Gilbert, Ruth
The public health nurse and the mentally ill. *Canadian Nurse*, Oct. 1961, p. 966-8.

Glaser, W. A., *and others*
The performance of students in public health. *Nursing Research*, Spring 1965, p. 138-43.

Group, T. M.
If a nurse is to help in ghettos. *American Journal of Nursing*, Dec. 1969, p. 2635-6.

Grundy, Fred
The new public health: an introduction for midwives, health visitors and social workers. 6th edn. Luton, Leagrave Press, 1965.
7th edn. 1968.

Hansen, Ann C., *and* Levy, Judith M.
Families speak for themselves. *Nursing Outlook*, June 1961, p. 344-9.

Hansen, Ann C., *and* Levy, Judith M.
What is a public health nurse? *Nursing Research*, Spring 1961, p. 100-3.

Hansen, Ann C., *and* Thomas, D. B.
Students' disappointments in public health nursing. *Nursing Outlook*, May 1965, p. 68-72.

Harner, Ruth
Public Health nursing for male nurses. *Nursing Journal of India*, Oct. 1969, p. 361-2.

Helvie, C. O., *and others*
The setting and nursing practice. *Nursing Outlook*, Aug. 1968, p. 27-9; Sept. 1968, p. 35-8.

Highriter, M. E.
Nurse characteristics and patient progress [in public health nursing]. *Nursing Research*, Nov./Dec. 1969, p. 484-501.

Holden, D. E.
The nurse's position as a teacher in preventive medicine. *Journal of the West Australian Nurses*, April 1970, p. 4-6.

Horsley, S.
New frontiers in social medicine. *Nursing Times*, Oct. 29, 1965, p. 1473-4.

Hudson, H. H., *and* Lester, M. R.
Nurses in public health. *American Journal of Nursing*, April 1965, p. 103-7.

Huntly, Winifred L.
Aids to personal and community health. Bailliere, Tindall and Cox, 1964.
2nd edn., 1969.
[Formerly: Aids to hygiene for nurses by Edith Funnell.]

Illing, M.
Public health nursing in the USA. *Nursing Times*, Mar. 29, 1968, Occasional Papers, p. 49-51.

Immaculata, Sister M.
The sister in today's comprehensive medical center. *Hospital Progress*, April 1969, p. 78, 80, 82, 84, 88.

The Jamaican Nurse
The West Indies School of Public Health comes of age *Jamaican Nurse*, Aug./Sept. 1964, p. 19-22.

Jansen, P. W.
The social worker on the public health agency team. *Nursing Outlook*, Oct. 1968, p. 42-4.

Jeu, F., *and* Raulston, J.
A community need—nursing and medical students respond. [A medical referral service for the Negro community in Houston]. *Nursing Outlook*, Mar. 1970, p. 28-30.

Johnson, Walter L., *and* Hardin, Clara A.
Content and dynamics of home visits of public health nurses. Part I. New York, American Nurses' Foundation, [1962].
Part II, 1969.

Kallins, Ethel L.
Textbook of public health nursing. St. Louis, Mosby, 1967.

Kettle, Ellen S.
Development of rural health services in the Northern Territory. *Australian Nurses Journal*, Jan. 1969, p. 13-5.

Knopf, L.
A community gets a health centre. *American Journal of Nursing*, July 1970, p. 1498-501.

SPECIALITIES

KNUDSON, E. G.
Public health nurses' interest in occupational advancement. *Nursing Research*, July/Aug. 1968, p. 327-35.

KRISTER, J.
The community nurse as health educator. *The Australian Nurses' Journal*, Mar. 1966, p. 54-7 and 69.

KURSTEINER, P.
Public Health Services in Switzerland. *South African Nursing Journal*, Dec. 1963, p. 26-8.

LEAHY, KATHLEEN M., *and* COBB, M. MARGUERITE
Fundamentals of public health nursing. New York, McGraw-Hill, 1966.

LEWIS, I. C.
The role of the nurse in community life. *Australian Nurses Journal*, July 1970, p. 146-8, 150-1, and 154-6.

MCCORMACK, R. C., *and* CRAWFORD, R. L.
Attitudes of professional nurses toward primary care. *Nursing Research*, Nov./Dec. 1969, p. 542-4.

MAYUGA, P. N
Medical care system in the Philippines *The Philippine Journal of Nursing*, Mar /April 1965, p 76-8 and 84.

MOULTON, D. P.
A social worker's thoughts on the function of the public health nurse in relation to mental illness. *The Nursing Gazette*, Nov. 1962, p. 55.

MURDAUGH, J.
There is a difference [a social worker delineates the differences in public health nursing and social work skills]. *Nursing Outlook*, Oct. 1968, p. 45-7.

NATIONAL ASSOCIATION OF STATE ENROLLED NURSES
The State enrolled nurse in public health nursing services. [The Association, 1968].

NATIONAL LEAGUE FOR NURSING
Community nursing services. New York, National League for Nursing, 1962.

PANAYOTOVA, Z. P.
Bulgarian health services. *Nursing Mirror*, May 30, 1969, p. 28-9.

PARRY, W. H.
Health centres. *Nursing Times*, Dec. 22, 1967, p. 1728-9.

PAYNICH, MARY LOUISE, *and others*
Is there a role for the nurse clinician in public health? *Nursing Outlook*, July, 1969, p. 32-6.

PITTMAN, R., *and* KERCHNER, L.
A study of the relationship between staff attitudes and dimensions of supervisory self-actualization in public health nursing. *Nursing Research*, May/June 1970, p. 231-8.

POTTER, M. C.
The nurse as community crisis counselor. *Nursing Outlook*, Sept. 1969, p. 39-42.

RAO, K. S.
Comprehensive nursing care as practised in rural health centre today in Bagayam. *Nursing Journal of India*, Feb. 1964, p. 52-3 and 59.

ROSCHER, C. L.
The role of the public health nurse. *South African Nursing Journal*, May 1970, p. 7-9.

RUNNELS, H.
Changing patterns in public health nursing and medical social work. *Hospital Progress*, Nov. 1969, p. 106-8, and 111-3.

SAMATER, H. N.
Some health problems in the Somali Republic. *International Journal of Nursing Studies*, Mar. 1969, p. 3-14.

SANTO TOMAS NURSING JOURNAL
Issue on Public Health Nursing. *Santo Tomas Nursing Journal*, Oct. 1968.

SEARLE, CHARLOTTE, *editor*
Manual for public health nurses. Pretoria, South African Nursing Association, 1967.

SEARLE, CHARLOTTE
The role of the nursing and allied professions in health education. *South African Nursing Journal*, July 1967, p. 7-12.

SHANNON, I. R.
More nursing per square mile. *Nurisng Outlook*, April 1970, p. 42-4.

SIMON, J. R.
Nurses' ratings of patient welfare as criterion measures in the health sciences. *Occupational Psychology*, Jan. and April 1961, p. 10-22.

SIMPSON, H. M.
Research in nursing and public health nursing. *Nursing Mirror*, Jan. 19, 1968, p. 378-80.

SOBOL, EVELYN G., *and* ROBISCHON, PAULETTE
Family nursing: a study guide. St. Louis, Mosby, 1970.

SOLOMONS, G., *and* HATTON, M. L.
The public health nurse as an objective scientific observer. A new research dimension in nursing. *Nursing Outlook*, Aug. 1961, p. 486-8.

STANDARD, K.
Promoting health in the Caribbean. *The Jamaican Nurse*, Aug. 1966, p. 28-30.

STANDEVEN, M.
What the poor dislike about community health nurses. *Nursing Outlook*, Sept. 1969, p. 72-5.

SZENPETERY, K.
Community health project in West Pakistan. *District Nursing*, June 1969, p. 52-3.

TALBOT, J. A.
The teaching role of the nurse in the field of infant and maternal health. *The New Zealand Nursing Journal*, Oct. 1968, p. 15-6.

THOMAS, D. B.
Multiple discriminant analysis of public health nursing decision responses. *Nursing Research*, Mar./April 1969, p. 145-53.

THOMAS, D. B., *and* HANSEN, A. C.
Professionalization of priority decision judgments [in public health nursing]. *Nursing Research*, July/Aug. 1970, p. 343-8.

TRAINED NURSES ASSOCIATION OF INDIA
A public health manual. 2nd edn., edited by Majoo Savak Kotwal. New Delhi, the English Book Store, 1968.

UNITED STATES PUBLIC HEALTH SERVICE
Proceedings of a three-day conference on public health nursing in mental illness. Washington, Govt. Printing Office, 1961.

WALLIN, JUDITH E.
A ten-year history of the public health nurses section and school nurses branch 1952-1962. New York, American Nurses' Association (Public Health Nurses Section), 1962.

WILKIE, E. E.
Public health nursing and current social need. Tenth Nursing Mirror lecture in the University of Edinburgh. *Nursing Mirror*, Mar. 29, 1968, p. 17-20.

WILSON, A. H.
Conditions in the early health services in Rhodesia. *Rhodesian Nurse*, Sept. 1969, p. 4-7.

WILSON, M.
A guide for the public health nurse to assist elderly patients in the achievement of selected functional tasks at home. *International Journal of Nursing Studies*, Nov. 1970, p. 243-6.

WOFINDEN, R. C.
St. George Health Centre, Bristol. *Nursing Times*, July 29, 1966, p. 1004-6.

WORLD HEALTH ORGANIZATION
Aspects of public health nursing. Geneva, W.H.O., 1961. [Public Health Papers, no. 4.]

ADMINISTRATION

AMERICAN NURSES' ASSOCIATION
A guide for the utilization of personnel supportive of public health nursing services. New York, The Association, 1966.

AMERICAN NURSES' ASSOCIATION
Guidelines for the development and utilization of home health aide services in the community: a supplement to a guide for the utilization of personnel supportive of public health nursing services. New York, The Association, 1967.

BAILEY, D., *and* RAWLINSON, K.
Dictaphones in health visiting. *Nursing Times*, Oct. 16, 1969, p. 1333-4.

BELOTE, M.
Integrating a public health nursing staff. *American Journal of Nursing*, April 1965, p. 100-2.

BIRKBECK, L.
Are we meeting the needs? *Nursing Outlook*, Jan. 1961, p. 22-3.

BLACK, ISABEL
A census of nursing personnel in community health by Isabel Black and Margaret Outtier. *Canadian Journal of Public Health*, Jan. 1968, p. 1-5.

BORLICK, MARTHA M.
Guide for public health nurses working with children: from the developmental point of view. Washington, U.S. Department of Health, Education and Welfare, Children's Bureau, 1961.

BRACKETT, M. E.
The community: nursing in tomorrow's health services. *Nursing Outlook*, Sept. 1963, p. 650-3.

BROCK, M.
Public health nurse and social worker . . . no need for mutual hostility. *Canadian Hospital*, Feb. 1966, p. 49-51.

BRYANT, Z., *and* HUDSON, H. H.
The Census of Public Health Nurses. *American Journal of Nursing*, Feb. 1961, p. 94.

CANADIAN NURSES' ASSOCIATION
Continuing care: the nurse and community resources. Ottawa, Canadian Nurses' Association, 1962.

CENTRAL HEALTH SERVICES COUNCIL STANDING NURSING ADVISORY COMMITTEE
Use of ancillary help in the local authority nursing services; report of the sub-committee. . . . Ministry of Health, 1965.

CHISHOLM, M. K.
Community health builders. 1. Laying the foundations; 2. Adding the bricks. *Nursing Mirror*, Sept. 11, 1970, p. 40-1; Sept. 18, 1970, p. 38-9.

COOPER, B.
The sisters' role and responsibility toward the mother and baby, on discharge, to the health nurse in the community. *The Lamp*, Dec. 1968, p. 8-9.

CREELMAN, L.
How can nursing meet the challenge of expanding health services. *International Nursing Review*, vol. 14, no. 1, 1967, p. 21-7.

CURWEN, M., *and* BROOKES, B.
Health centres: facts and figures. *The Lancet*, Nov. 1, 1969, p. 945-8.

EVANS, M.
The community—what does it ask of the nurse? From the other side of the fence. *UNA Nursing Journal*, Mar./April 1970, p. 11-5.

EVANS, M.
A new goal for a new role. *UNA Nursing Journal*, Sept. 1968, p. 274-9.

FAIRLEY, J.
The teaching hospital and the community. *Nursing Times*, Dec. 10, 1970, p. 1592-3.

FERGUSON, MARION
How to determine nursing expenditures in small health agencies: a procedure using work units: a joint project of the Public Health Service and the National League for Nursing. Washington, Govt. Printing Office, 1962.

FERGUSON, MARION, *and* PHILLIPS, RUTH
Availability of services for nursing care of the sick at home. Washington, U.S. Public Health Service, Division of Nursing, 1964.

FREEMAN, V.
Salaries of public health nurses in selected public health nursing agencies. 1961. *Nursing Outlook*, Dec. 1961, p. 750-2.

GREAT BRITAIN. DEPARTMENT OF HEALTH AND SOCIAL SECURITY, SCOTTISH HOME AND HEALTH DEPARTMENT, *and* WELSH OFFICE
Report of working party on management structure in the local authority nursing services. Chairman E. L. Mayston. Department of Health, 1969.

HANSEN, A. C., *and* THOMAS, D. B.
Change of interest in public health nursing practice. *Nursing Research*, Summer 1966, p. 207-13.

HANSEN, A. C., *and* THOMAS, D. B.
A conceptualization of decision-making [in public health nursing]. *Nursing Research*, Sept./Oct. 1968, p. 436-43.

HARBISON, R.
Community health survey. *Journal of the West Australian Nurses*, Aug. 1970, p. 14-6.

HASLER, J. C.
The community nurse in the 70s. *District Nursing*, Dec. 1970, p. 176-7.

HATTERSLEY, F.
Co-operation with hospitals and domiciliary services. *Nursing Times*, Oct. 4, 1968, Occasional Papers, p. 153-4.

HAUGEN, I. H.
Changing role and functions of a nurse in the community. *International Journal of Nursing Studies*, Sept. 1966, p. 111-6.

HAYES, C.
Attitudes of public health nurses and social workers towards public health nursing and social work practitioners. *Nursing Research*, Sept./Oct. 1970, p. 453-6.

HENRY, A. P.
A further link between hospital and community. [A health visitor's work with patients who have undergone radiotherapy at Charing Cross Hospital, Fulham.]. *Nursing Times*, Sept. 3, 1970, p. 1127-8.

HILLER, R. B.
Communications with the local community. *Nursing Mirror*, Sept. 16, 1966, p. 587-8.

JOURNAL OF PRACTICAL NURSING
The neighborhood health center [including descriptions of five typical centers]. *Journal of Practical Nursing*, Mar. 1969, p. 24-8, 33, 42 and 44.

KOTLARSKY, C.
This nurse coordinates patient services [in hospital and community]. *The Canadian Nurse*, July 1970, p. 33-5.

SPECIALITIES

LAMB, A. M.
Community nursing development within a national health service. *International Nursing Review*, vol. 16, no. 4, 1969, p. 353-61.

LAMB, A. M.
Some aspects of nursing administration in the Local Authority Services. *International Journal of Nursing Studies*, July 1966, p. 89-95.

LINDARS, MARGARET E., *and others*
Communications and attitudes in practice: towards an integrated family health service. [An integrated scheme in Berkshire]. *International Journal of Nursing Studies*, July 1969, p. 71-9.

MCNEIL, H. J.
How to become involved in community planning. *Nursing Outlook*, Feb. 1969, p. 44-7.

MAHAR, I. R.
Where there's a will. [Interdisciplinary learning experiences for students in the public health laboratory]. *Nursing Outlook*, Oct. 1969, p. 55-7.

MARSDEN, J.
The role of the nurse in public health. *Queensland Nurses Journal*, Jan. 1969, p. 9-12.

MORRIS, M.
A new field for nursing research: preventive nursing. *Nursing Research*, Sept./Oct. 1969, p. 441-3.

NATIONAL LEAGUE FOR NURSING
DEPARTMENT OF PUBLIC HEALTH NURSING
Cost analysis for public health nursing services: Methods I and II. New York, The League, 1964.

NATIONAL LEAGUE FOR NURSING
DEPARTMENT OF PUBLIC HEALTH NURSING
Criteria for evaluating the administration of a public health nursing service. *Nursing Outlook*, Aug. 1961, p. 500-2.

O'CONNELL, P. E.
Communications in the public health team. *District Nursing*, October 1967, p. 142-4.

OHIO DEPARTMENT OF HEALTH, *and others*
Report of a study and demonstration of continuity of nursing care, directed by Doris Schwartz and Reba Birinyi. [Columbus, Ohio Department of Health], 1966.

ONTARIO DEPARTMENT OF HEALTH, RESEARCH AND PLANNING BRANCH
A census of nursing personnel employed for public health work in Ontario by position and highest academic qualifications on November 30, 1966. Toronto, The Department, 1968[?].

PETROWSKI, D. D.
How do public health nurses use the telephone? To find out whether nurses use this tool wisely, the author studied the calls of 20 nurses, over a period of five days. *Nursing Outlook*, Jan. 1965, p. 42-4.

QUEEN'S INSTITUTE OF DISTRICT NURSING
Prevention or treatment? The potential diagnostic and therapeutic range of the community health services; report of a conference organized by the Q.I.D.N. at the Royal Commonwealth Society, London, on 22 May 1964. The Institute, 1964.

REMILLET, J., *and* READING, S.
Adapting to changing community health needs [in traditional public health nursing practices]. *Nursing Outlook*, Oct. 1970, p. 47-9.

RICHARDS, I. D. G.
Planning for the community—achievements and aspirations. *Nursing Mirror*, Dec. 13, 1968, p. 9-11.

ROBERTS, DORIS E.
The staffing of public health and outpatient nursing services. Geneva, W.H.O., 1963.

ROBERTS, DORIS E., *and* HUDSON, HELEN H.
How to study patient progress. Washington, U.S. Dept. Health, Education and Welfare, 1964.

ROBERTS, DORIS E., *and others*
Census of nurses in public health. *American Journal of Nursing*, Nov. 1970, p. 2394-9.

ROYAL COLLEGE OF NURSING *and*
NATIONAL COUNCIL OF NURSES OF THE UNITED KINGDOM
Administering the local authority nursing service. Rcn, 1968.

ROYAL COLLEGE OF NURSING *and*
NATIONAL COUNCIL OF NURSES OF THE UNITED KINGDOM
The future of public health nursing in relation to the needs of the community. Rcn, 1969.

ROYAL SOCIETY OF HEALTH CONGRESS 1970
Teamwork of community care. Report of RSH Congress opening session. *Nursing Mirror*, May 8, 1970, p. 11-4.

RUNNELS, H.
Changing patterns in public health nursing and medical social work. *Hospital Progress*, Nov. 1969, p. 106-8, and 111-3.

SHAPIRO, S. G., *and* DILLON, A.
The changing emphasis in public health nursing programs. *Nursing Outlook*, June 1965, p. 62-5.

SIMMONDS, E. H.
Placement of staff by administrative nursing officers. *Health Visitor*, Oct. 1970, p. 325-6.

SOLOMONS, G., *and* HATTON, M. L.
The public health nurse as an objective scientific observer. A new research dimension in nursing. *Nursing Outlook*, Aug. 1961, p. 486-8.

SUBHADRA, V., *and* SUJATA BASU
An evaluation of public health nursing services at an Urban Health Centre [in India]. *International Journal of Nursing Studies*, Nov. 1970, p. 257-65.

SWEENEY, B. T.
Family-centered care in public health nursing. *Nursing Forum*, vol. IX, no. 2, 1970, p. 169-75.

UNITED STATES PUBLIC HEALTH SERVICE,
DIVISION OF NURSING
Class specifications for nursing positions: a guide for state and local public health agencies. Washington, U.S. Public Health Service, 1964.

UNITED STATES PUBLIC HEALTH SERVICE,
DIVISION OF NURSING
Community planning for nurses in the District of Columbia Metropolitan Area: source book for planning. Arlington, Virginia, U.S. Department of Health, Education and Welfare, [1967].

UNITED STATES PUBLIC HEALTH SERVICE,
DIVISION OF NURSING
Services available for nursing care of the sick at home, Jan. 1966. Arlington, Virginia, Department of Health, Education and Welfare, 1967.

VREELAND, E. M.
The Government's interest in public health research. *Nursing Research*, Fall 1966, p. 323-9.

VREELAND, E. M.
Nursing research programs of the public health service. *Nursing Research*, Spring, 1964, p. 148-58.

WALKER, C., *and* DEUBLE, H.
A scheme for analysis of accident prevention activities in public health nurses' records. *Nursing Research*, Sept./Oct. 1968, p. 408-14.

WALKER, D.
The future public health nurse and her team. *District Nursing*, Nov. 1965, p. 200-3.

DISTRICT NURSING
General Works

BENNETT, B. A.
The changing pattern of nursing and its effect on the work of the district nurse. *Nursing Mirror*, July 17, 1964, p. x-xii.

BODDY, F. A.
General practitioner's view of the home nursing service [in Scotland]. *British Medical Journal*, May 17, 1969, p. 438-41.

BOORER, D.
Home nursing in Birmingham. *Nursing Times*, June 11, 1970, p. 741-3.

BRYANT, ZELLA
Report on nursing care of the sick at home in incorporated U.S. cities with population of 25,000 and over. Washington, U.S. Public Health Service, 1962.

CARR, A. J.
The district nurse in our society. *Nursing Times*, Jan. 28, 1966, p. 109-10.

CARSTAIRS, VERA
Home nursing in Scotland, report of an enquiry into the local authority domiciliary services. Edinburgh, Scottish Home and Health Department, 1966.

FRY, J.
What the family doctor asks of the district nurse. *Nursing Times*, May 3, 1963, p. 551-2.

GALLAHAR, E., and others
A study of health visiting and district nursing in Bolton. *The Medical Officer*, Mar. 27, 1970, p. 161-7.

GANDER, D. R.
Psychiatric domiciliary visiting. *Nursing Times*, Jan. 26, 1968, p. 109-10.

HOCKEY, LISBETH.
District nursing sister attached to hospital surgical department. An experiment to show use of district nurse in after care of surgical patient and early discharge from hospital. *British Medical Journal*, April 18, 1970, p. 169-71.

HOCKEY, LISBETH
Feeling the pulse: a survey of district nursing in six areas. Queen's Institute of District Nursing, 1966.

HUGO, C. M.
The need for the expansion of district nursing services in South Africa. *South African Nursing Journal*, Aug. 1966, p. 25-6.

IRVEN, I. D.
District nurse in Kenya. *Nursing Mirror*, Feb. 7, 1969, p. 42-3.

KENNEDY, ELTA M.
Expanding home nursing in rural Kansas. *American Journal of Nursing*, April 1967, p. 763-6.

KING, V. M.
Night nursing service in Hertfordshire. *Nursing Mirror*, April 19, 1963, p. viii-ix.

KING EDWARD'S HOSPITAL FUND FOR LONDON HOSPITAL CENTRE
Continued nursing care: ward sisters and district nurses confer. *Nursing Times*, Oct. 11, 1968, p. 1384-5.

MACARA, A. W.
A forward look at district nursing. *Nursing Mirror*, Mar. 5, 1965, p. 535-6; Mar. 12, 1965, p. 563-4.

MAZZARELLA, M. C.
Banding together for rural home care. *American Journal of Nursing*, Dec. 1969, p. 2658-60.

MORRIS, I. H.
The S.E.N. and the home nursing service [in Birmingham]. *Nursing Mirror*, May 30, 1969, p. 10-1.

NEEDLE, A.
Queen's Nurse in an Indian village. *Nursing Mirror*, Jan. 25, 1963, p. 365-6.

QUEEN'S INSTITUTE OF DISTRICT NURSING
Nursing in the community. The Institute, 1970.

QUEEN'S INSTITUTE OF DISTRICT NURSING
State enrolled nurses on the district. The Institute, [1967].

REID, M., and WADDICOR, P. E. E.
Continuity of patient care. *Nursing Times*, June 18, 1970, p. 786-8.

SMITH, B. L.
The district nurse in the team. *District Nursing*, Oct. 1970, p. 133-4.

SMITH, E. S.
Mental illness and the district nurse. 1. Organic and neurotic reactions; 2. Depression, psychosis and mental deficiency; 3. Preventive measures. *Nursing Times*, Oct. 15, 1970, p. 1329-30; Oct. 22, 1970, p. 1363-4; Oct. 29, 1970, p. 1395-6.

SPRIGGS, C.
A night nursing service. *District Nursing*, Oct. 1969, p. 128-30.

TRASLER, B. J.
The district nurse and the health services. *Nursing Times*, Dec. 21, 1962, p. 1604-6.

VERRILL, M. T.
Introduction to rural district nursing. *District Nursing*, Sept. 1963, p. 137.

WENBORN, J. K.
The community health nurse. *The Medical Officer*, Mar. 11, 1966, p. 131-2.

WENBORN, J. K.
The community health nurse. *Nursing Times*, April 22, 1966, p. 535-6.

WILKIE, E. E.
Changing values in community nursing. *District Nursing*, Jan. 1969, p. 209 and 214.

WILSON, ALBERTA B.
Long-term nursing care in rural Minnesota. *Nursing Outlook*, Oct. 1964, p. 68-70.

WRIGHT-WARREN, P.
Image of a district nurse. A survey on recruitment and publicity to discover what lies behind the shortage of district nurses. *District Nursing*, Mar. 1963, p. 273-6.

Administration

BANKS, A. LESLIE
Role of the district nurse in the community. *Nursing Mirror*, Mar. 8, 1963, p. iii-v.

CANADIAN RED CROSS SOCIETY, NATIONAL NURSING COMMITTEE
Report of the pilot project on nursing and related services in the home. Toronto, The Society, 1964.

DISTRICT NURSING
Management structure in the local authority nursing services. *District Nursing*, Feb. 1970, p. 229-31.

FORMAN, J. A. S.
What the G.P. expects of the district nurse and the midwife. *District Nursing*, July 1963, p. 74-5.

FORMAN, J. A. S.
What the G.P. expects of the district nurse and the midwife. II. *District Nursing*, Aug. 1963, p. 102-4.

GILLIE, A.
A pattern of integration. *District Nursing*, Jan. 1969, p. 208 and 223.

SPECIALITIES

HASLER, J. C., and others
Development of the nursing section of the community health team. *Nursing Times*, Feb. 13, 1969, Occasional Papers, p. 28; Feb. 20, 1969, Occasional Papers, p. 32.

HOCKEY, L.
The place of research in district nursing. *Nursing Mirror*, Mar. 18, 1966, p. 685-6.

LAMB, A. M.
The changing pattern within the domiciliary field. *Nursing Mirror*, Jan. 17, 1969, p. 20-3.

LUNT, J.
Bridging the gap in continuity of care. *Nursing Times*, Mar. 19, 1970, p. 372.

LYON, W. M.
A report on the first International Congress on Domiciliary Nursing. *New Zealand Nursing Journal*, May 1970, p. 24-5.

RIDDELL, J.
An enquiry into domiciliary nursing. Comparisons in Midlothian and Peeblesshire between 1958-61 and 1962-65. *The Medical Officer*, Feb. 23, 1967, p. 105-7.

ROWLAND, A. J., and others
Evaluation of home nurse attachment in Bristol. *British Medical Journal*, Nov. 18, 1970, p. 545-7.

TODD, J. J.
Bridging the gap [Mentally trained district nurses help psychiatric patients in the community]. *District Nursing*, Dec. 1970, p. 178-9.

WALKER, D.
The hospital plan and the domiciliary nursing service. *Nursing Times*, June 21, 1963, p. 766-8.

Education

BYATT, J.
Practical work instructors' course for district nurses. *Nursing Mirror*, Dec. 18, 1970, p. 28-9.

CAMPBELL, I., and KENNEDY, E. A.
The role of the practical work instructor in district nurse training. *Nursing Times*, July 31, 1969, Occasional Papers, p. 121.

EVANS, M.
Preparation of the nurse for domiciliary nursing. *Queensland Nurses Journal*, Feb. 1969, p. 5, 6 and 8.

GEORGE, V. M.
Principles of examining as applied to district nursing. *Nursing Times*, Nov. 8, 1968, Occasional Papers, p. 173-4.

HOCKEY, L.
Survey of district nurse training, 1962/63. Queen's Institute of District Nursing, 1964.

JENKINSON, V.
William Rathbone Staff College: The three month course. *District Nursing*, July 1965, p. 88-91.

KEYWOOD, O.
Modern aims in district nurse training. *Nursing Mirror*, Jan. 23, 1970, p. 17-9.

LAMB, A. M.
The work of the Panel of Assessors and the Training of District Nurses. *Nursing Times*, Sept. 24, 1970, p. 1246-7.

LINDARS, M. E.
What is required of district nurse training? *District Nursing*, Sept. 1967, p. 129-30.

LINDARS, M. E., and THOMAS, D. J.
A successful venture: learning community care. [District nurse training for third-year students in Reading.]. *Nursing Times*, June 5, 1969, Occasional Papers, p. 89-92.

QUEEN'S INSTITUTE OF DISTRICT NURSING
General principles of district nursing practice. 2nd edn. The Institute, 1966.

ROYAL COLLEGE OF NURSING and
NATIONAL COUNCIL OF NURSES OF THE UNITED KINGDOM
The future of district nurse training. *Nursing Times*, Mar. 20, 1969, Occasional Papers, p. 45-8.

HEALTH VISITING
General Works

AKESTER, JOYCE M., and MACPHAIL, ANGUS N.
Health visiting in the sixties, based on a survey carried out in the City of Leeds. Macmillan (for the *Nursing Times*), 1963.

AMERICAN NURSES' ASSOCIATION
Exploring progress in public health nursing practice. New York, The Association, 1966.

AMERICAN NURSES' FOUNDATION
Home visits by public health nurses. Focus of study by Foundation. *Nursing Research Report*, Sept. 1969, p. 1, and 5-8.

ARNSTEIN, MARGARET G.
Research in public health nursing.
See
WALTER REED ARMY INSTITUTE OF RESEARCH
Report on nursing research conference, 1959. Washington, The Institute, 1961.

BAVIN, J.
Mental handicap—the role of the health visitor. *Midwife and Health Visitor*, July 1970, p. 248-51.

BLISS, S. G.
Health visiting—time for a new look? *Nursing Times*, Dec. 23, 1966, p. 1679-81.

BLODGETT, F. M., and WESSELL, M. A.
When the medical student visits with a visiting nurse. *Nursing Outlook*, Aug. 1961, p. 475-6.

BRITISH TUBERCULOSIS ASSOCIATION
JOINT TUBERCULOSIS COMMITTEE
Health visitors and chest diseases. *The Medical Officer*, Oct. 28, 1966, p. 237-9.

BROOKS, C.
Group work with mothers in a health visiting service. *Nursing Times*, June 1, 1962, p. 710-3.

BROOKS, C.
Tomorrow's health visitor. *District Nursing*, July 1964, p. 84.

BURTON, P. M.
The South African Nursing Association Seventh biennial congress for white members. The growth and development of public health nursing. *South African Nursing Journal*, Dec. 1970, p. 22-3 and 26-7.

CAMPBELL, K., and SPALDING, W. J.
The male health visitor. *Nursing Mirror*, Jan. 26, 1968, p. 35-6.

CHISHOLM, MARY K.
Health visitors and the elderly. *Midwife and Health Visitor*, Jan. 1970, p. 28-30.

CHISHOLM, MARY K.
An insight into health visiting. Bailliere, 1970.

CHISHOLM, MARY K.
"This is my work—my life". *Nursing Mirror*, June 11, 1965, p. 263-4.

CORCORAN, LUCILLE E., and CORRIGAN, MARJORIE J., editors
Knowledge for the practice of public health nursing. Washington, Catholic University of America Press, 1962.

CUNNINGHAM, P. J., editor
The principles of health visiting. Faber and Faber, 1967.

DARRAH, WINONA E.
Public health nursing interventions in changing patterning of fear in an ex-state hospital patient.
In
AMERICAN NURSES' ASSOCIATION
Effects of continuity in nursing scare on patient welfare. New York, The Association, 1962.

DOWNEY, D.
Public health nurses' attitudes toward patients with a psychiatric diagnosis. *Nursing Research*, May/June 1969, p. 244-50.

FRANKS, J., *and others*
Health visiting in the seventies. *Nursing Times*, Sept. 4, 1969, p. 1149-50.

FREEMAN, RUTH B.
Public health nursing practice. 3rd edn. Philadelphia, Saunders, 1963.

GLASER, W. A., *and* MCVEY, F. A.
Evaluation of performance in public health nursing. *Nursing Research*, Winter, 1961, p. 32-7.

GORRIE, M. G.
The expanding role of health visiting. *Public Health*, Jan. 1962, p. 69-82.

GRAHAM, A. A.
Future of the health visitor. *Nursing Times*, Dec. 1, 1961, p. 1574-6.

GRAHAM, J. A. G.
A health visitor work study. *The Medical Officer*, Dec. 30, 1966, p. 360-1.

GREENING, P.
Health visitors and hospitals. Paper given at the 69th Congress of The Royal Society of Health held at Scarborough 9th-13th April, 1962. *The Royal Society of Health 69th Congress Papers*, 1962, p. 135.

HALE, ROSEMARY, *and others*
The principles and practice of health visiting by Rosemary Hale, Marion K. Loveland, Grace M. Owen. Oxford, Pergamon Press, 1968.

HALL, I.
Health visiting in a county borough [Hartlepool]. *Nursing Mirror*, Aug. 30, 1968, p. 25-7.

HEALTH VISITORS' ASSOCIATION
Health visiting: a manifesto. The Association, [1970].

KANE, A. H.
Health visiting in an immigrant area. *Nursing Mirror*, Oct. 14, 1966, p. xi-xiii and xvi.

KELLEY, A. J.
Colorado's visiting nurse services program. *Hospitals*, Aug. 1, 1963, p. 53-5.

KEMP, I. W.
Health visiting in Scotland. *Health Bulletin*, April 1969, p. 21-9.

LAMONT, D. J.
Men in health visiting. 2. The preparation. *Nursing Times*, Aug. 26, 1966, p. 1129-30.

LAMONT, D. J., *and* MACQUEEN, I. A. G.
Male health visitors. *Nursing Times*, Jan. 10, 1964, p. 46-8.

THE LANCET
Health visitors of the future. *The Lancet*, Feb. 15, 1969, p. 356.

LANGTON, B. M.
Auxiliaries in health visiting. *Nursing Times*, Sept. 22, 1961, p. 1220-2.

LANGTON, B. M.
Early health visiting. *Nursing Times*, Oct. 4, 1963, p. 1247-8.

LEMIN, B.
What is a male health visiting officer? *Nursing Mirror*, Nov. 28, 1969, p. 37-9.

LINDSEY, E. M.
Towards a comprehensive health visiting service. *Nursing Mirror*, May 5, 1961, p. v-vii.

LINES, M. B.
The health visitor and the care of the elderly. *Nursing Times*, Sept. 24, 1970, p. 1242-3.

MCEWAN, MARGARET
Health visiting: a textbook for health visitor students. 4th edn. Faber, 1962.

MACLEOD, H. M.
Tuberculosis and the health visitor. *Nursing Mirror*, May 26, 1961, p. vi-vii and xvi.

MCMILLAN, E. B. B.
Men in health visiting. 3. The work. *Nursing Times*, Aug. 26, 1966, p. 1131.

MACQUEEN, I. A. G.
Attitudes of health visitors to possible developments. *The Medical Officer*, April 1, 1966, p. 177-9.

MACQUEEN, I. A. G.
The emergence of the male health visitor. *Public Health*, January 1962, p. 89-94.

MACQUEEN, I. A. G.
Health visiting developments in a city. *Health Bulletin*, Oct. 1966, p. 102-4.

MACQUEEN, I. A. G.
Male health visitors—the present position. *Medical Officer*, Oct. 21, 1966, p. 223-4.

MACQUEEN, I. A. G.
Men in health visiting. 1. The need. *Nursing Times*, Aug. 26, 1966, p. 1128-9.

MARSHALL, E. H.
The health visitor—her role in the future. *Nursing Mirror*, April 12, 1963, p. 37-8.

MARSHALL, E. H.
The health visitor—widening the scope. *Nursing Mirror*, April 19, 1963, p. 57-8.

MASON, E. M.
Health visiting in France. *Nursing Mirror*, Oct. 19, 1962, p. 53.

MASON, R., *and* MAJOR, K.
Health visitors with a medical research unit. *Nursing Times*, Aug. 24, 1962, p. 1081-3.

MAY, L.
New HVs and students: their difficulties. *Nursing Times*, May 29, 1969, p. 692-4.

MEDICAL OFFICER
Men in health visiting. *The Medical Officer*, April 23, 1965, p. 227-8.

MUMFORD, D.
Some aspects of health visiting. *International Journal of Nursing Studies*, Sept. 1968, p. 195-201.

NAIRN, M.
Developments in health visiting [in Aberdeen]. *Mother and Child*, Sept./Oct. 1969, p. 6-8.

NATION, M. B.
The creed of the health visitor. *Nursing Mirror*, Feb. 4, 1966, p. 536-7.

NEWINGTON, D. K.
The birth of rural health visiting. *Nursing Mirror*, July 6, 1962, p. iv-vii.

NURSING MIRROR
Scotland's health visitor story. *Nursing Mirror*, May 25, 1962, p. xii-xiii.

SPECIALITIES

NURSING MIRROR
Scotland's health visitor story—2. *Nursing Mirror*, June 1, 1962, p. xi-xii.

NURSING MIRROR
Scotland's health visitor story (conclusion). *Nursing Mirror*, June 8, 1962, p. 185-6.

NURSING TIMES
Health visiting: the past, the present and the future. *Nursing Times*, June 29, 1962, p. 847-8.

NURSING TIMES
Specialist health visiting for Brighton's old people. *Nursing Times*, May 12, 1961, p. 601-2.

O'CONNELL, P. E.
Health visiting at the crossroads. *Nursing Times*, Oct. 23, 1964, p. 1409.

OPARINDE, S. O.
A male health visiting officer's training experiences. *Mother and Child*, Jan./Feb. 1969, p. 17-9.

OWEN, G. M.
The health visitor in the social context—I. *Midwife and Health Visitor*, Oct. 1970, p. 373-5.

OWEN, G. M.
The health visitor in the social context—II. *Midwife and Health Visitor*, Nov. 1970, p. 413-6.

PREECE, S.
Problems of health visiting—1. "Know then thyself." *Nursing Times*, Jan. 4, 1963, p. 6-8.

PREECE, S.
Problems of health visiting—2. Dangerous generalizations! *Nursing Times*, Jan. 11, 1963, p. 45-7.

PREECE, S.
Problems of health visiting—3. Problem to whom? *Nursing Times*, Jan. 18, 1963, p. 72-4.

PREECE, S.
Problems of health visiting—4. A day in the life of ... *Nursing Times*, Jan. 25, 1963, p. 110-3.

PRINCE, G. S.
Mental health and the health visitor. *Nursing Mirror*, Sept. 20, 1963, p. ii-iv; Sept. 27, 1963, p. xiv-xvi.

REID, J. J. A.
The health visitor and the hospital. *British Hospital Journal and Social Service Review*, May 19, 1967, p. 913-4.

ROBERTS, I.
Health visiting: a view of the future. *Nursing Times*, Mar. 1, 1968, Occasional papers, p. 33-5.

ROBINSON, E.
The public health nurse. *Nursing Mirror*, June 22, 1962, p. 221-3.

ROYAL COLLEGE OF NURSING (PUBLIC HEALTH DEPT.) *and* HEALTH VISITORS' ASSOCIATION
Centenary of health visiting 1862-1962: addresses given at commemorative meeting and exhibition, 18th and 19th June 1962. The College and the Association, 1962.

SAUNDERS, MARY
Health visiting practice. Oxford, Pergamon Press, 1968.

SCOTT, J.
Health visiting—lets face it. *Health Visitor*, July 1970, p. 255-6.

SHEEN, E. M., *and* DUNCAN, E. H. L.
The health visitor's work among the chronic sick and aged. *Nursing Times*, Aug. 18, 1961, p. 1057-9.

SIMPSON, H. M.
Research and health visiting. *Health Visitor*, May 1970, p. 174-5, and 177

STRUTHERS, J. E., *and* MAGUIRE, R. E.
Health visitors and nurses in community medicine. [The Authors, 1966?].
[*Note:* Report of Council of Europe Medical Fellowship, 1966.]

THORPE, E., *and* THORPE, A.
Is sociology relevant for the health visitor? *Health Visitor*, Oct. 1970, p. 321-4.

WILKIE, E. E.
Health visiting. *Women's Employment*, Dec. 4, 1964, p. 355-6.

WOODWARD, P.
Health visitors' attitudes towards family planning. *Health Visitor*, Nov. 1970, p. 360-1.

Administration

BILTON, K.
Health visitors, social work and Seebohm. *Health Visitor*, Jan. 1970, p. 13-4.

DAVIES, J. B. M.
Health visitors and social workers—is there a place for both? *Nursing Mirror*, Oct. 22, 1965, p. 191-2.

DOWNS, B.
Some problems of health visiting in Central London. *International Journal of Nursing Studies*, July 1966, p. 97-102.

DRAPER, P., *and others*
The health visitor after Seebohm—1. *Nursing Times*, Jan. 9, 1969, p. 40-1.

DRAPER, P., *and others*
The health visitor after Seebohm—2. *Nursing Times*, Jan. 16, 1969, p. 82-3.

DRAPER, P., *and others*
The health visitor after Seebohm—3. *Nursing Times*, Jan. 23, 1969, p. 114-5.

GALLAHER, E., *and others*
A study of health visiting and district nursing in Bolton. *The Medical Officer*, Mar. 27, 1970, p. 161-7.

RYAN, T. M.
A note on health visiting statistics for England and Wales, 1953-62. *The Medical Officer*, Sept. 25, 1964, p. 190-2.

SANGSTER, J. O.
Recently qualified health visitors—1. An employment survey. *Nursing Times*, Dec. 23, 1966, p. 1691-3.

SANGSTER, J. O.
Recently qualified health visitors—2. Health visiting and health visiting combined with district nursing and/or midwifery. *Nursing Times*, Dec. 30, 1966, p. 1726-7.

SANGSTER, J. O.
Employment of recently qualified health visitors—a survey carried out through standing conference of representatives of health visitor training centres. *International Journal of Nursing Studies*, Feb. 1967, p. 47-54.

TORRIE, A.
The health visitor and the new Mental Health Act. *Nursing Mirror*, Feb. 9, 1962, p. 367-9.

WEAKLEY, L. R., *and* HAINS, C. K.
Use of health visitor potential. *South African Nursing Journal*, Jan. 1969, p. 10-1 and 38-9; Feb. 1969, p. 26-9.

Education

AKESTER, J. M.
Nursing training of the health visitor. *Nursing Times*, Mar. 17, 1961, p. 335-7.

BARNARD, D.
Family planning seminars for health visitors. *Health Visitor*, Mar. 1970, p. 81-3.

BAUMGART, A. J.
Preparation for health team practice. *The Canadian Nurse*, Sept. 1968, p. 42-3.

BEATTIE, I. E.
In-service mental health training for health visitors. *Nursing Times*, Feb. 24, 1961, p. 242-4.

BORLICK, MARTHA M., *and others, editors*
Community health nursing: 1600 multiple choice questions and referenced answers: edited by Martha M. Borlick, Beverly Henry Bowns, Velena Boyd and Carolyn Feher Waltz. New York, Medical Examination Publishing Co., 1969.
[Nursing examination review book, vol. 9.]

BYRNE, M.
Modern teaching methods in a developing country. *Nursing Mirror*, Aug. 18, 1967, p. x-xiii.

BYRNE, M. W.
This I believe ... about the baccalaureate graduate in a VNA. *Nursing Outlook*, July 1970, p. 28-31.

CHIVERS, T. S.
Sociology for health visitors—1 and 2. *Nursing Times*, Jan. 23, 1969, Occasional Papers, p. 13-5; Jan. 30, 1969, Occasional Papers, p. 17-20.

COHN, HELEN, *and others*
Manual for nurses in family and community health, by Helen Cohn, Joann Eckels, Betty Ford, Ann Lord, Joyce Tingle. Boston, Little, Brown, 1969.

COUNCIL FOR THE TRAINING OF HEALTH VISITORS
First report 1962-64 [in progress].

COUNCIL FOR THE TRAINING OF HEALTH VISITORS
The health visitor: her function and its implications for training. The Council, 1970.

DANCER, M. E. G.
Community nurse tutor. *District Nursing*, Dec. 1970, p. 170-1.

GOODACRE, R.
For public health nurses. A description of in-service education in a provincial public health nursing service. *The Canadian Nurse*, May 1962, p. 422-3.

GREAT BRITAIN. PARLIAMENT
Health visiting and social work (training) act, 1962. H.M.S.O., 1962.

ILLING, M.
Fieldwork instruction. *Nursing Times*, Dec. 6, 1968, Occasional Papers, p. 189-90.

LINDBERG, H. G.
Mental health concepts in in-service education. *Nursing Outlook*, April 1969, p. 34-5.

LINDSAY, D. W.
An experiment in teaching student health visitors. *Nursing Times*, May 26, 1967, p. 693-4.

LOUGHLIN, B. W.
Aide training reaches the Navajo Reservation. *American Journal of Nursing*, July 1963, p. 106-9.

MENCEL, Z.
Poland's students learn to teach health education. *American Journal of Nursing*, Jan. 1963, p. 98-9.

POWELL, M. B.
Recent advances in training public health nurses. *Royal Society of Health Journal*, Jan./Feb. 1964, p. 36-7 and 41.

REMILLET, J. G.
Using community resources to teach public health nursing: a design. *Nursing Forum*, vol. IV, no. 1, 1965, p. 73-93.

SMITH, S. B., *and others*
The new health visitor training. 1. From a tutor's point of view, by S. B. Smith; 2. A field work instructor's point of view, by Florence Matthews; 3. From a recent student's point of view, by June Clark. *Mother and Child*, April 1968, p. 9-14.

SOTEJO, J. V.
Preparing the nurse for first level position in public health nursing in the basic nursing curriculum. *International Journal of Nursing Studies*, June 1968, p. 89-102.

WILKIE, E. E.
A course in community nursing. Royal Society of Health, 1963.
[Paper read before the Health Congress of R.S.H. at Eastbourne, 29 April to 3 May 1963.]

WILKIE, E. E.
Training health visitors. *Nursing Times*, Nov. 12, 1965, p. 1558-60.

WILLIAMS, HEATHER M.
The integrated nurse/health visitor course: a report of the first five years of the experimental course organized by the University of Southampton and the Nightingale School St. Thomas' Hospital. [Southampton University], 1962.

WILLIAMS, I. D.
Twenty-five years of public health refresher courses in Manchester. *Nursing Times*, April 23, 1965, p. 565.

Health Visiting and General Practice

AKESTER, J. M., *and* MACPHAIL, A. N.
Health visiting and general practice. *The Lancet*, Aug. 22, 1964, p. 405-8.

AKESTER, J. M., *and* MACPHAIL, A. M.
Health visiting and general practice. *Nursing Mirror*, Feb. 5, 1965, p. 423-4, and 436.

ALLEN, W. H., *and* KING, V. M.
A study of health visitor attachment to general practitioners in Hertfordshire. *Nursing Times*, Nov. 15, 1968, Occasional Papers, p. 177-9.

AMBLER, M., *and others*
The attachment of local health authority staff to general practices. *The Medical Officer*, May 31, 1968, p. 295-9; *Nursing Times*, Aug. 23, 1968, Occasional Papers, p. 129-32.

ANDERSON, J. A. D.
Attachment of community nurses to general practices. A follow-up study. *British Medical Journal*, Oct. 10, 1970, p. 103-5.

ANDERSON, J. A. D., *and others*
The attachment of local authority staff to general practices. *Medical Officer*, Nov. 17, 1967, p. 249-51.

BAKER, C. D.
The extent in England of health visitor attachment to general practices. *The Journal of The College of General Practitioners*, Sept. 1964, p. 171-8.

BATES, B.
Nurse-physician teamwork. *Medical Care*, April/June 1966, p. 69-80.

BOORER, D.
Nurses in a group practice. *Nursing Times*, July 2, 1965, p. 903-5.

BREWIN, P. H.
Contact between general practitioners and public health nursing staff in the West Riding. *The Medical Officer*, Mar. 29, 1968, p. 171-2.

BUTTERWORTH, J.
The general practitioner and the health visitor. *Nursing Mirror*, Jan. 8, 1965, p. 337-9.

BUTTERWORTH, J., *and* MCDONAGH, V. P.
General practitioner and health visitor. *The Lancet*, Mar. 7, 1964, p. 549-50.

CARTWRIGHT, A., *and* SCOTT, R.
The work of a nurse employed in a general practice. *British Medical Journal*, Mar. 18, 1961, p. 807-8, and 809-13.

SPECIALITIES

Clow, J. T.
Attachment of health visitors to general practitioners. *The Medical Officer*, Mar. 29, 1968, p. 173-6.

Flack, G.
Work of the health visitor in relation to the general practitioner. *International Journal of Nursing Studies*, Feb. 1966, p. 297-304.

Fletcher, W. B.
A district nurse/GP attachment. *The Medical Officer*, Mar. 31, 1967, p. 169-71.

Forbes, F. A.
A health visitor attached to a general practice. *Health Bulletin*, Jan. 1964, p. 20-2.

Francis, H. W. S.
The family doctor, the health visitor and the computer. *Nursing Times*, Feb. 23, 1968, p. 252-4.

Fry, J.
Should midwives, health visitors and nurses be attached to general practice? *Maternal and Child Care*, June 1965, p. 47-9.

Fry, J., *and others*
The evolution of a health team: a successful general practitioner-health visitor association. *British Medical Journal*, Jan. 16, 1965, p. 181-3.

Gebbie, K. M., *and others*
Levels of utilization: nursing specialists in community mental health. *Journal of Psychiatric Nursing and Mental Health Service*, Jan./Feb. 1970, p. 37-9.

Gettings, B.
Health visiting needs in general practice. *Health Visitor*, Feb. 1970, p. 43-6.

Gilmore, M.
A pilot study of the work of a nursing team in general practice. *The Medical Officer*, Oct. 30, 1970, p. 238-43.

Great Britain. Department of Health and Social Security, Social Science Research Unit
Nursing attachments to general practice: staff implications of scheme for attachment of local authority staff (health visitors and home nurses) to general practice, by R. Ann Abel. H.M.S.O., 1969.

Gunn, A. D. G.
The nurse and the family doctor. *Nursing Times*, Oct. 7, 1966, p. 1311-2; Oct. 14, 1966, p. 1370-2; Oct. 21, 1966, p. 1388-90; Oct. 28, 1966, p. 1429-30.

Hall, T.
Experiment in cooperation. An account of health-visitor/general practitioner liaison. *The Lancet*, June 19, 1965, p. 1325-7.

Hardy, S.
Primary care in general practice. *Nursing Mirror*, Nov. 6, 1970, p. 14-5.

Hattersley, F. G.
Health visitor attachment. *Nursing Times*, May 24, 1968, p. 695-6.

Hayes, K. J.
Health visitor in general practice. *Nursing Times*, Jan. 6, 1961, p. 14-5.

Hockey, Lisbeth
Care in the balance: a study of collaboration between hospital and community services. Queen's Institute of District Nursing, 1968.

Hockey, Lisbeth, *and* Buttimore, Anne
Co-operation in patient care: studies of district nurses attached to hospital and general medical practices. Queen's Institute of District Nursing, 1970.

Howard, A. L.
Twelve months' attachment: from the local authority [in Birmingham]. *Nursing Times*, Oct. 29, 1970, p. 1390-1.

Hunter, D. A.
Doctors and nurses in Brent—1. A study in group attachment; 2. A study in group attachment. *Nursing Times*, May 1, 1969, p. 560-3; May 8, 1969, p. 594-5.

Hutchinson, D. A., *and* Mumby, D. M.
Public health nurses work with family physicians. *The Canadian Nurse*, Jan. 1970, p. 28-31.

Jones, P. E.
The public health nurse and general practice. *The Canadian Nurse*, July 1968, p. 43-4.

Jones, P. E., *and* Bondy, D. M.
Family health service: the PHN and the GP. *Canadian Nurse*, Sept. 1969, p. 38-40.

Kuenssberg, E. V.
The nurse—a luxury or a necessity in general practice.
In
Royal College of General Practitioners
Report of a symposium on the management of staff in general practice. . . .

Lamb, A. M.
Development of attachment schemes. *The Medical Officer*, July 24, 1970, p. 61-3.

Lewis, T. D.
The health visitor and the family doctor. *Journal of the Royal College of General Practitioners*, April 1968, p. 241-3.

Lord, W. J. H.
The general practitioner, the social worker and the health visitor. *The Journal of the College of General Practitioners*, Nov. 1965, p. 247-56.

McGregor, Angus
Total attachment of community nurses to general practices [in Southampton]. *British Medical Journal*, Aug. 2, 1969, p. 291-3; *Nursing Times*, April 9, 1970, p. 465-8.

McNabola, E. K. A., *and* Alexander, I. R. W.
The Restairig group attachment. *Nursing Mirror*, Dec. 15, 1967, p. 264-6.

Mansbridge, I.
Attachment of district nurses to a group practice. *Nursing Times*, July 23, 1965, p. 1013-4.

Marsh, G. N.
Group practice nurse: an analysis and comment on six months' work. *British Medical Journal*, Feb. 25, 1967, p. 489-91.

"A Medical Officer of Health"
The general practitioner and the health visitor. *Mother and Child*, Sept. 1964, p. 7 and 14.

Mottram, E.
Extended use of nursing services in general practice. *Nursing Mirror*, June 21, 1968, p. 20-3.

Parish, P. A.
Health visitor attachment in general practice. *Nursing Times*, Feb. 23, 1968, p. 256-9.

Parry, W. H., *and* Lunn, J. E.
A "pre-attachment" study of the attitudes of nurses in the city of Nottingham. *The Medical Officer*, Aug. 28, 1970, p. 119-20.

Pickworth, K. H., *and others*
Nurses in general practice. *Nursing Times*, Feb. 23, 1968, p. 247-8.

Pinsent, R. J. F. H.
A nurse attachment study. *Journal of the Royal College of General Practitioners*, May 1968, p. 402-8.

Pinsent, R. J. F. H., *and others*
The health visitor in a general practice. *British Medical Journal Supplement*, April 8, 1961, p. 123-7.

PLAYER, D. A.
Attachment of health visitors and district nurse/midwives to G.P. in Dumfries. *Health Bulletin*, Jan. 1969, p. 6-12.

RAWLINSON, K.
Impressions of a field work instructor in group practice. *Health Visitor*, Dec. 1970, p. 386-9.

RIDDELL, D. M.
Liaison between health visitors and hospital staff in Edinburgh. *Health Bulletin*, July 1968, p. 41-2.

ROYAL COLLEGE OF GENERAL PRACTITIONERS
The practice nurse: further development of her role in general practice and its effects on the doctor's work. The College, 1968.

ROYAL COLLEGE OF GENERAL PRACTITIONERS
Report of a symposium on the management of staff in general practice, held at the New Medical Lecture Theatre, the Radcliffe Infirmary, University of Oxford, 20th April 1969. *Journal of the Royal College of General Practitioners* [Supplement no. 3, vol. 19 (no. 95)].

RYAN, M.
The district nursing team in a group practice. *District Nursing*, April 1969, p. 6-7.

SARGEAUNT, B. Z.
The health visitor in the team. *District Nursing*, Oct. 1970, p. 132-4.

SMITH, J. WESTON, and MOTTRAM, E. M.
Extended use of nursing services in general practice. *British Medical Journal*, Dec. 16, 1967, p. 672-4.

SOCIETY OF MEDICAL OFFICERS OF HEALTH, and others
JOINT WORKING PARTY ON GROUP ATTACHMENT
Attachment of nursing services in general practice. Report of the Joint Working Party ... set up by the Society of Medical Officers of Health, Royal College of Nursing, Health Visitors Association, Queen's Institute of District Nursing, Royal College of Midwives, Association of Supervisors of Midwives and Royal College of General Practitioners. Educare, 1970.
[Chairman: D. E. Cullingtton.]

SWIFT, G., and MACDOUGALL, I. A.
The family doctor and the family nurse. *British Medical Journal*, June 27, 1964, p. 1697-9.

WALKER, J. H., and MCCLURE, L. M.
Community nurses' view of general practice attachment. *British Medical Journal*, Sept. 6, 1969, p. 584-7.

WARIN, J. F.
General practitioners and nursing staff: a complete attachment scheme in retrospect and prospect. *British Medical Journal*, April 6, 1968, p. 41-5.

WATERS, N. W.
Reflections after two and a half years of general practice attachment. *Health Visitor*, Oct. 1970, p. 326-7.

SCHOOL NURSING

AMERICAN NURSES' ASSOCIATION
A rationale for school nurse certification. New York, The Association, 1966.

AMERICAN NURSES' ASSOCIATION
Functions and qualifications for school nurses. New York, The Association, 1966.

AMERICAN NURSES' ASSOCIATION,
PUBLIC HEALTH NURSES' SECTION
School nursing practice: a guide for evaluating, implementing, and improving the functions of school nurses, prepared by the Committee on Functions, Standards and Qualifications for Practice, School Nurses Branch, Helen G. Ennis, Chairman. N.Y., A.N.A., 1961.

BASCO, D.
Evaluation of school nursing activities. *Nursing Research*, Fall 1963, p. 212-21.

BRIGG, M.
School nursing in the good old days (in South Africa). *South African Nursing Journal*, Oct. 1963, p. 30-1.

BRUEGGEN, STELLA L.
The role of the school nurse in a program for the partially seeing.
In
AMERICAN NURSES' ASSOCIATION
Nursing of patients with loss of perceptions. New York, The Association, 1962.

CAUFFMAN, J. G.
The nurse and health care of school children. *Nursing Research*, Sept./Oct. 1969, p. 412-7.

COAKLEY, J. M., and PARKER, J. M.
Education of nurses for school nursing. *American Journal of Nursing*, Nov. 1965, p. 84-7.

CROMWELL, GERTRUDE E.
The nurse in the school health program. Philadelphia, Saunders, 1963.

DITHRIDGE, E. H.
Administration of school health services: a review. *Nursing Outlook*, May 1966, p. 50-3.

FLORENTINE, HELEN GOODALE
The preparation and the role of nurses in school health programs. New York, National League for Nursing, 1962.

HENDERSON, P.
The health visitor in the school health service. *Midwife and Health Visitor*, June 1965, p. 54-6.

KING, J. S.
A school nurse in Bolivia. *Nursing Outlook*, Nov. 1968, p. 37-9.

LUNN, J. E.
School health service work in the ordinary day schools—Parts I and II. *Nursing Times*, April 26, 1968, Occasional Papers, p. 65-8; May 3, 1968, Occasional Papers, p. 69-72.

MCCULLOUGH, L.
School health services. *Australian Nurses' Journal*, Dec. 1964, p. 293-7.

NEMIR, ALMA
The school health program: a textbook for teachers, school nurses, school administrators and others who are concerned with the health of school-age youth. 2nd edn. Philadelphia, Saunders, 1965.

O'BRIEN, MARGARET J.
Team nursing in school health [In New York City]. *Nursing Outlook*, July 1969, p. 28-30.

RUTLEDGE, F.
Health education in schools. *Health Visitor*, Sept. 1970, p. 281-3.

SMITH, P.
The health visitor and the school. *Health Visitor*, Sept. 1970, p. 286.

STOBO, ELIZABETH C., and others
Report of the nurse in the elementary school: promotion of mental health, by Elizabeth C. Stobo, Dorothy Shoobs, Rosemary McKevitt and Grace Matsunage. New York, Teachers College, Columbia University, 1968.

TROOP, E. H.
Sixty years of school nurse preparation. *Nursing Outlook*, May 1963, p. 364-6.

WAYNE, DORA
School nursing and team teaching. *Nursing Outlook*, July 1969, p. 37.

WHITELEY, J.
School nurse in Uganda. *Nursing Mirror*, Feb. 27, 1970, p. 44-5.

SPECIALITIES

RESPIRATORY SYSTEMS

ADRIANI, J.
Hyperventilation: effects on acid-base balance and circulation during anaesthesia. *Journal of American Association of Nurse Anesthetists*, Feb. 1969, p. 41-8.

BEDSIDE NURSE
Rehabilitation of emphysema and chronic bronchitis patients. *Bedside Nurse*, Mar./April 1969, p. 23-7.

BLACKSTOCK, C. R.
Artificial respiration. *The Canadian Nurse*, May 1962, p. 411.

BLOCH, V. C.
Helping the patient to ventilate. *Nursing Outlook*, Oct. 1969, p. 31-3.

BROWN, C.
Breathlessness. *Nursing Times*, Sept. 20, 1968, p. 1258-9.

BROWN, C.
Breathlessness—2. *Nursing Times*, Sept. 27, 1968, p. 1300-2.

CHEST AND HEART ASSOCIATION
The "chesty" child: report of a meeting for doctors, nurses, health visitors, social workers, voluntary care committee members and parents held at the Guildhall, London, 2nd June 1965. The Association, 1965.

CLAYTON, J. I., *and* LAMBRECHTS, W.
Modern methods of artificial respiration including expired air resuscitation. *Nursing Mirror*, Jan. 13, 1961, p. 1333.

CROPPER, C. G. J.
Heart-lung resuscitation. "When seconds count". *Nursing Times*, Aug. 28, 1969, p. 1095-7.

DEAKIN, HARRY G., *and* RANN, SUSAN E.
Artificial ventilation. *Nursing Times*, Mar. 27, 1969, Occasional Papers, p. 49-52.

ELLIS, C. R.
Fundamental breathing exercises. *Nursing Mirror*, Feb. 20, 1970, p. 34-5.

ELWOOD, EVELYN
The battle of breathlessness: a study of the nursing care of the patient with chronic, obstructive pulmonary emphysema.
In
AMERICAN NURSES' ASSOCIATION
Nursing care of the disoriented patient. New York, The Association, 1962.

FELL, A. V.
The Bird respirator in cardiothoracic surgery. *Nursing Times*, May 22, 1964, p. 652-3.

GUMBLEY, C. N.
"Farmer's lung", one of the more uncommon pneumoconioses. *Nursing Mirror*, July 21, 1961, p. 1383.

HARRISON, G. G.
Respiratory nursing care. *Nursing Mirror*, May 31, 1963, p. i-iii and vi.

JACOBY, N. M.
Steroid treatment of asthmatic children. *Nursing Times*, June 16, 1967, p. 789-90.

JONES, M. C.
Acute viral respiratory diseases. *Nursing Times*, Jan. 15, 1970, p. 82-4.

KEARNS, B.
Tracheotomy suctioning technique. *The Canadian Nurse*, Feb. 1970, p. 44-8.

KELLEHER, W. H.
Iron lungs and their use. Development of an entirely new pattern. *Nursing Mirror*, Nov. 30, 1962, p. vii-x.

KNIGHT, R. K.
Spontaneous pneumothorax. *Nursing Times*, Nov. 3, 1967, p. 1470-2.

KRAMER, H.
Chest pain. *American Association of Industrial Nurses Journal*, Feb. 1963, p. 16-8.

MACBETH, R.
Chronic paranasal sinusitis. *Nursing Mirror*, June 20, 1969, p. 33-5.

MCCLELLAND, R. M. A.
Mechanical means of artificial respiration. *Nursing Times*, May 3, 1963, p. 541-3.

MALCOMSON, K. G.
Upper respiratory infections. *Nursing Mirror*, April 10, 1970, p. 29-32.

MILLER, I. C.
Respiratory problems in an intensive care unit. *Journal of the West Australian Nurses*, Jan. 1969, p. 8, and 10-2.

NETT, L. M., *and* PETTY, T. L.
Why emphysema patients are the way they are. *American Journal of Nursing*, June 1970, p. 1251-3.

NORMAN, A. P.
Asthma in childhood. *Nursing Mirror*, May 19, 1961, p. 633.

PAULLEY, J. W.
Asthma. *Nursing Times*, April 12, 1963, p. 466-8.

QUARRELL, E. J.
Artificial ventilation—1. Normal respiratory mechanism and function; 2. Indications and techniques for artificial ventilation; 3. Nursing care. *Nursing Times*, Oct. 8, 1970, p. 1289-91; Oct. 15, 1970, p. 1323-5; Oct. 22, 1970, p. 1360-2.

ROBINSON, F. N.
Nursing care of the patient with pulmonary emphysema. *American Journal of Nursing*, September 1963, p. 92-6.

SCHWAID, M. C.
The impact of emphysema. *American Journal of Nursing*, June 1970, p. 1247-50.

SCOTT, M. E.
The asthmatic child in a residential school—1. *Nursing Times*, Nov. 20, 1969, p. 1492-3.

SCOTT, M. E.
The asthmatic child in a residential school—2. Individual case histories. *Nursing Times*, Nov. 27, 1969, p. 1525-6.

SECOR, JANE
Patient care in respiratory problems. Philadelphia, Saunders, 1969.

SEMPLE, S. J. G., *and* SPENCER, G. T.
The treatment of emphysema. *Nursing Times*, June 15, 1962, p. 762-6.

SITZMAN, J.
Respiratory problems and the nurse's changing responsibilities. *Cardio-Vascular Nursing*, May/June 1970, p. 41-5.

STUNT, C. L.
An automatic alarm system: for use in the management of respiratory ventilation. *Nursing Times*, Oct. 15, 1970, p. 1321-2.

VAUGHAN, V. C.
The place of drug therapy in childhood asthma. *American Journal of Nursing*, May 1966, p. 1049-52.

WALLACE, C. A.
Resuscitation: open airway and rescue breathing. *Journal of American Association of Nurse Anesthetists*, Aug. 1968, p. 267-73.

WILLIAMS, M. H.
Pulmonary emphysema. *American Journal of Nursing*, Sept. 1963, p. 88-91.

WILSON, FRANK
Tracheostomy for the nurse. Edward Arnold, 1970.

SOCIAL PROBLEMS AND NURSING
GENERAL WORKS

ABDELLAH, F. G.
Approaches to protecting the rights of human subjects. *Nursing Research*, Fall, 1967, p. 316-20.

GUNN, A. D. G.
Vulnerable Groups—The underprivileged and underpaid. *Nursing Times*, April 26, 1968, p. 563-4.

KARVONEN, M. J.
Woman and work: the two roles of woman. *District Nursing*, Oct. 1966, p. 174-5.

MACQUEEN, I. A. G.
Social work in Scotland. *District Nursing*, May 1970, p. 37-8.

SPICER, C. C.
Vital statistics and the nurse. *Nursing Mirror*, Mar. 1, 1963, p. 472-4.

ABORTION

BAILEY, M.
The unmarried pregnant teenager. *Bedside Nurse*, July/Aug. 1968, p. 13-6.

CHESSER, E.
Termination of pregnancy. *Nursing Mirror*, Sept. 20, 1963, p. 535-6.

GUNN, A. D. G.
The legal termination of pregnancy—and the lessons to be learnt from a year's experience. *Nursing Times*, Sept. 4, 1969, p. 1130-2.

HAZER, A., and others
Legalized abortion: what do nurses think? *Hospital Topics*, Nov. 1966, p. 109-11.

LILEY, A. W.
Execution without trial (Abortion). *New Zealand Nursing Journal*, Dec. 1970, p. 6-7.

NURSING TIMES
Effects of Abortion Act: some observations. *Nursing Times*, July 12, 1968, p. 931-2.

SCOTT, J. S.
Implications of abortion law reform. *Nursing Times*, Nov. 11, 1966, p. 1478-80.

SIMMS, M.
Abortion Act in operation. *Nursing Mirror*, Feb. 7, 1969, p. 21.

UNIVERSITY OF COLORADO SCHOOL OF NURSING
Abortion. *American Journal of Nursing*, Sept. 1970, p. 1919-25.

ALCOHOLISM

ARMSTRONG, J. D.
Alcoholism as a disease. *The Canadian Nurse*, Aug. 1965, p. 614-7.

BAGENSTOSE, M.
How can the public health nurse help the alcoholic? *Pennsylvania Nurse*, Jan. 1969, p. 4-9.

BUTT, J.
Hospital treatment of alcoholism. *Nursing Times*, Dec. 28, 1962, p. 1639-43.

EDWARDS, G.
Alcoholism is a disease. *Nursing Times*, Aug. 9, 1963, p. 991-3.

EPP, M. L.
Nursing the alcoholic. *The Canadian Nurse*, Aug. 1965, p. 618-20.

FELSTEIN, I.
The nurse and the alcoholic. *Hospital World*, Oct. 1970, p. 5.

FREED, EARL X.
The dilemma of the alcoholic patient in a psychiatric hospital. *Journal of Psychiatric Nursing and Mental Health Services*, May/June 1969, p. 113-6.

GILLESPIE, C.
Nurses help combat alcoholism. *American Journal of Nursing*, Sept. 1969, p. 1938-41.

GRIFFITHS, S. H.
Video recordings [in the treatment of alcohol and drug dependency]. *Nursing Times*, Sept. 17, 1970, p. 1208-9.

HEINEMANN, E., and RHODES, R. J.
How nurses view the tuberculous alcoholic patient. *Nursing Research*, Fall 1967, p. 361-5.

HUGHES, J. P. W.
Education on alcoholism. *Occupational Health*, May/June, 1969, p. 143-6.

HUNTER, C. B., and others
"Project alcoholism". *Nursing Mirror*, Aug. 8, 1969, p. 17-21.

KING EDWARDS HOSPITAL FUND FOR LONDON
HOSPITAL CENTRE
Meeting of nurses from alcoholic units. *Nursing Times*, Jan. 23, 1969, p. 120.

MOORE, M.
An account of a nurse's role and functions in an alcoholic treatment program. *Journal of Psychiatric Nursing and Mental Health Services*, May/June 1970, p. 21, and 24-7.

RITSON, E. B., and COLLIE, A. W.
The treatment of alcoholism in a specialised unit. *Nursing Mirror*, Nov. 4, 1966, p. i-iv.

DRUG ADDICTION

ASSOCIATION FOR THE PREVENTION OF DRUG ADDICTION
Heroin addiction. A case history. *Nursing Times*, Jan. 19, 1968, p. 79-81.

CASKEY, K. K., and others
The school nurse and drug abusers. *Nursing Outlook*, Dec. 1970, p. 27-30.

CHILDRESS, G.
The role of the nurse with the drug abuser and addict. *Journal of Psychiatric Nursing and Mental Health Services*, Mar./April 1970, p. 21-3, and 26.

EPP, M. L.
Care of patients addicted to non-narcotic drugs. *The Canadian Nurse*, Mar. 1967, p. 42-4.

FREEDMAN, A. M.
Drug addiction. Action research in a treatment center. *American Journal of Nursing*, July 1963, p. 57-60.

GARDNER, R.
Amphetamine dependence and misuse. *Nursing Mirror*, Mar. 6, 1970, p. 22-5.

GELBER, I.
Drug addiction. The addict and his drugs. *American Journal of Nursing*, July 1963, p. 53-6.

GLATT, M. M.
Group therapy with young drug addicts—the addicts' point of view. *Nursing Times*, April 21, 1967, p. 519-20.

HALLIDAY, R.
Use of narcotics in addict therapy. *The Canadian Nurse*, Mar. 1967, p. 39-41.

HEATON, D.
Drug dependence. *Nursing Mirror*, Mar. 1, 1968, p. 36-8.

SPECIALITIES

HINE, C. H.
The role of the industrial nurse in the detection and prevention of drug abuse. *Occupational Health Nursing*, April 1969, p. 15-7.

HINE, C. H., *and* WRIGHT, J. A.
A program for control of drug abuse in industry. *Occupational Health Nursing*, April 1970, p. 17-8, and 41.

HOLDEN, H. M.
Social considerations of drug taking. *Nursing Times*, April 14, 1967, p. 476-8.

JONES, K., *and others*
A comparison of the nursing role in units for alcohol and drug dependence. *Nursing Times*, Nov. 8, 1968, p. 1535-6.

KING EDWARD'S HOSPITAL FUND FOR LONDON
HOSPITAL CENTRE
Alcoholic and drug addiction units. *Nursing Times*, Jan. 26, 1968, p. 111.

KING EDWARD'S HOSPITAL FUND FOR LONDON
HOSPITAL CENTRE
The nurse and the drug addict. *Nursing Times*, Feb. 20, 1969, p. 249.

MCDERMOTT, R.
Maintaining the methadone patient. *Nursing Outlook*, Dec. 1970, p. 22-6.

MCGUINNESS, J. P.
Drug dependence. *Nursing Times*, Oct. 2, 1969, p. 1255-7.

MERRY, J.
Heroin addiction: some of its problems. *Nursing Times*, Jan. 19, 1968, p. 77-8.

OWENS, J., *and others*
Nursing the drug addict. *Nursing Times*, May 3, 1968, p. 584-5.

POLAR, J. F.
Characteristics of nurse addicts. *American Journal of Nursing*, Jan. 1969, p. 117-9.

PRACTICAL APPROACHES TO NURSING SERVICE
ADMINISTRATION
Participation of the nursing service department in programs related to drug habituation. *Practical Approaches to Nursing Service Administration*, Fall 1970, p. 1-4.

ROHDE, I. M.
Drug addiction. The addict as an inpatient. *American Journal of Nursing*, July 1963, p. 61-6.

RUSSAW, E. H.
Nursing in a narcotic-detoxification unit. *American Journal of Nursing*, Aug. 1970, p. 1720-3.

SOHN, D., *and others*
Drug screening in industrial nursing. *Occupational Health Nursing*, Aug. 1970, p. 7-10.

TARRY, C.
Addicts in a therapeutic community. *Nursing Mirror*, Sept. 11, 1970, p. 32-4.

WILLIS, J. H.
Drug dependency. *Nursing Times*, April 14, 1967, p. 474-6.

FAMILY PLANNING

ABRAHAM, A.
Perception and attitude of nursing personnel towards family planning. *Nursing Journal of India*, Oct. 1967, p. 258-63.

BARNARD, D.
Family planning seminars for health visitors. *Health Visitor*, March 1970, p. 81-3.

BARNARD, D.
Health visitors and the Family Planning Act. *Nursing Mirror*, Dec. 13, 1968, p. 34-5.

DAVID, H. P.
Psychosocial studies in family planning behavior in Central and Eastern Europe: a preliminary report of a developing program. *Journal of Psychiatric Nursing*, Sept./Oct. 1970, p. 28-33.

ELDER, M. S.
Nurse counseling on sexuality. *Nursing Outlook*, Nov. 1970, p. 38-40.

FEROZE, R. M.
Advantages and the disadvantages of the contraceptive pill. *Nursing Mirror*, Sept. 27, 1968, p. 20-1.

FOX, THEODORE
Family planning. *Nursing Mirror*, Feb. 23, 1968, p. 17-21.

HERZIG, N.
Nurse's role in family planning at a municipal hospital. *Hospital Topics*, Feb. 1970, p. 101 and 104.

HILL, H.
The challenge of family planning. *Nursing Mirror*, Aug. 21, 1970, p. 27-32.

KAMALAMMA, S.
The role of a public health nurse in family planning programme. *Nursing Journal of India*, Dec. 1968, p. 392-3 and 397.

LOUDON, N.
Training of nurses in family planning. *Nursing Mirror*, July 24, 1970, p. 28-9.

MIZER, H. E.
Curriculum should include fertility regulation. *Nursing Outlook*, Nov. 1970, p. 42-3.

NURSING TIMES
Marriage guidance: the student nurses, by a Student Nurse; Marriage guidance: the tutors by a Principal Tutor; Marriage guidance: who are the Counsellors? by an official of the National Marriage Guidance Council. *Nursing Times*, Feb. 9, 1968, p. 195-8.

POLE, K. F.
Family planning and the Catholic nurse. *Nursing Times*, April 26, 1968, p. 569-71.

SMITH, E.
Family planning coordinator in a City Hospital. *American Journal of Nursing*, Nov. 1970, p. 2363-5.

SWYER, G. I. M.
The pill. *Nursing Mirror*, June 19, 1970, p. 19-21; June 26, 1970, p. 34-6.

WOODWARD, P.
Health visitors' attitudes towards family planning. *Health Visitor*, Nov. 1970, p. 360-1.

PROBLEM FAMILIES

HUNT, J. E.
Problem families. *District Nursing*, July 1963, p. 78-80.

LITTLE, K.
Integration of immigrant families in Britain. *Midwife and Health Visitor*, June 1966, p. 231-4.

WELLER, M. F.
Immigrants. Some problems of integration. *Health Visitor*, April 1970, p. 115-7.

WORGAN, M.
The care of special families in Bristol. *Health Visitor*, Nov. 1970, p. 358-60.

SURGERY

GENERAL WORK

BAILEY, HAMILTON
Demonstrations of operative surgery for nurses. 3rd edn. Edinburgh, Livingstone, 1967.

BAILEY, HAMILTON, *and* LOVE, R. J. MCNEILL
Surgery for nurses. 9th edn. Lewis, 1964.

BAIN, WILLIAM H., *and* WATT, J. KENNEDY
Cardio-vascular surgery for nurses and students. Edinburgh, Livingstone, 1970.

BOURNE, J. G.
Post-operative fainting: brain damage in patients propped up after operation. *Nursing Times*, Aug. 3, 1962, p. 984-6.

BRADBY, M. B.
Prosthetic valves in cardiac surgery—1. *Nursing Times*, July 19, 1963, p. 901-2.

BRADBY, M. B.
Prosthetic valves in cardiac surgery—2. Valvular surgery. *Nursing Times*, July 26, 1963, p. 926-7.

BRICKER, D. L.
Progress in cardiac surgery. *AORN Journal*, April 1970, p. 44-9.

CAIRNEY, JOHN
Surgery for students of nursing. 5th edn. Christchurch, N.Z., Peryer, 1969.

CLARK, J. A
Leucotomy—yesterday and today. 1. Pre-frontal leucotomy—its development and procedure. *Nursing Mirror*, Mar. 23, 1962, p. 490-2.
Pt. 2, *see* FERNIE, W. W.

CLARKSON, G.
Stereotactic tractotomy theatre routine. *Nursing Times*, May 8, 1969, p. 587-9.

COLEMAN, D.
Surgical alleviation of coronary artery disease. *American Journal of Nursing*, April 1968, p. 763-6.

CONNELL, A.
Plastic surgical drapes. An evaluation. *American Journal of Nursing*, March 1970, p. 512-4.

DAVIDSON, J. S.
Surgery of the oesophagus. *Nursing Mirror*, Aug. 26, 1966, p. iv-ix.

DEVANE, D. J.
The hazards of the operating theatre. *Irish Nurses' Journal*, July 1969, p. 10-2.

DOUGLAS, E.
Introduction to recovery room. *Barbados Nursing Journal*, April/May 1968, p. 14-5.

EDINBURGH ROYAL INFIRMARY
Theatre work without drudgery. The Edinburgh pre-set tray system. *Nursing Times*, Mar. 1, 1963, p. 254-5.

FELL, A. V.
The Bird Respirator in cardiothoracic surgery. *Nursing Times*, May 22, 1964, p. 652-3.

FERNIE, W. W.
Leucotomy—yesterday and today. 2. Psychological and nursing care of the patient. *Nursing Mirror*, Mar. 30, 1962, p. 508-10.
Pt. 1, *see* CLARK, J. A.

FIEBER, W. W.
Massive fluid therapy. *Journal of American Association of Nurse Anesthetists*, Dec. 1968, p. 426-32.

FRASER, J., *and* GILL, W.
Cryosurgery. 1. Controlled cooling as a therapeutic agent. *Nursing Times*, Dec. 4, 1969, p. 1543-5.

FRASER, J., *and* GILL, W.
Cryosurgery. 2. The special fields in which cryosurgery is being used. *Nursing Times*, Dec. 11, 1969, p. 1587-9.

GRONDIN, P., *and* MEERE, C.
Recent advances in heart surgery. *The Canadian Nurse*, Jan. 1967, p. 32-5.

HAMILTON, D. I.
Cardiac surgery. The changing horizon. *Nursing Times*, Feb. 27, 1969, p. 263-4.

HAMILTON, G. L., *and* HATCHER, C. R.
Surgery for complications of myocardial infarction. *AORN Journal*, Oct. 1969, p. 44-9.

HARDMAN, F. G.
Oral surgery for nurses. Bristol, Wright, 1962.

HARLOW, F. WILSON, *editor*
Modern surgery for nurses. 5th edn. Heinemann, 1961.
6th edn., 1963.
7th edn., 1965.
8th edn., 1968.

HARRISON, D. F. N.
Surgical repair after pharyngolaryngectomy. *Nursing Times*, July 7, 1967, p. 895-7.

HEALY, K. M.
A pre-operative patient teaching program. *AORN Journal*, Oct. 1969, p. 37-43.

HOLT, P. J. L.
Surgery in rheumatoid arthritis—1 and 2. *Nursing Times*, Oct. 30, 1969, p. 1393-6; Nov. 6, 1969, p. 1417-8.

JACKSON, H.
Advances in cataract surgery. *Nursing Mirror*, Aug. 22, 1969, p. 14-7.

KIMBALL, C. P.
Psychological responses to open heart surgery. *AORN Journal*, Feb. 1970, p. 73-83.

KIRKWOOD, E. C.
The management of intercostal drainage tubes. *Nursing Mirror*, April 21, 1961, p. iv-vi.

KNIGHT, G.
Chronic depression and drug addiction treated by stereotactic surgery. *Nursing Times*, May 8, 1969, p. 583-6.

LARGEY, LILLIE B.
Knowledge, understanding and skill necessary to meet the nursing needs of the adult patient who has undergone open-heart surgery.
In
AMERICAN NURSES' ASSOCIATION
Technical innovations in health care: nursing implications. New York, The Association, 1962.

LLOYD, J. W.
Chest injuries and their management. *Nursing Mirror*, Sept. 8, 1967, p. iv-vi.

LUCK, M.
Management of surgery and operating theatres. *NATNews*, Autumn 1969, p. 19-21, 23 and 25.

MCKENZIE, W.
Stapes surgery. *Nursing Mirror*, Feb. 10, 1967, p. i-iii.

MCMILLAN, I. K. R.
Cardiothoracic surgery. *Nursing Times*, Nov. 6, 1964, p. 1454-5; Nov. 13, 1964, p. 1499-500.

MICHIE, W.
The complications of thyroidectomy for thyrotoxicosis. *Nursing Times*, Dec. 13, 1968, p. 1689-92.

MIDDLETON, M. D.
Gastrectomy. *Nursing Times*, Sept. 6, 1968, p. 1190-2.

MILLER, A.
Nephrectomy. *Nursing Times*, Aug. 31, 1962, p. 1096-9.

MORONEY, JAMES
Surgery for nurses. 7th edn. Edinburgh, Livingstone, 1961.
8th edn., 1962.
9th edn., 1964.
10th edn., 1966.
11th edn., 1967.

SPECIALITIES

Morse, R. M., *and* Litin, E. M.
Postoperative delirium: a study of etiologic factors. *AORN Journal*, Nov. 1969, p. 85-92.

Muirhead, I. E.
Theatre routine for cardiac bypass. *Nursing Times*, Aug. 9, 1963, p. 984-6.

Mullard, K., *and others*
Surgical treatment of post-cricoid carcinoma. *Nursing Times*, Jan. 16, 1969, p. 69-72.

Parsons, H. M.
Surgery for diseases of the mastoid process. *Nursing Times*, July 23, 1970, p. 942-5.

Polley, M.
Rectal surgery. *Nursing Mirror*, Mar. 1, 1968, p. 17-20.

Rains, A. J. Harding
Arterial surgery for nurses. Macmillan (for *Nursing Times*), 1965.

Rains, A. J. Harding
Arterial surgery for nurses—1. Historical introduction and types of arterial disease. *Nursing Times*, Feb. 26, 1965, p. 276-8.

Rains, A. J. Harding
Arterial surgery for nurses—2. Intermittent claudication rest, pain and gangrene, the ischaemic limb. *Nursing Times*, Mar. 5, 1965, p. 313-5.

Rains, A. J. Harding
Arterial surgery for nurses—3. Observations, investigations and indications for operation. *Nursing Times*, Mar. 12, 1965, p. 353-6.

Rains, A. J. Harding
Arterial surgery for nurses—4. Operations on arteries—1. *Nursing Times*, Mar. 19, 1965, p. 387-90.

Rains, A. J. Harding
Arterial surgery for nurses—5. Operations on arteries—2. Treatment of the various conditions. *Nursing Times*, Mar. 26, 1965, p. 418-22.

Rains, A. J. Harding
Arterial surgery for nurses—6. Care after arterial operations. *Nursing Times*, April 2, 1965, p. 454-6.

Rains, A. J. Harding
Arterial surgery for nurses—7. Palliative procedures, out-patient conservative measures, amputations. *Nursing Times*, April 9, 1965, p. 489-92.

Ring, P. A.
Chest injuries. *Nursing Times*, June 28, 1963, p. 796-9.

Ross, J. K.
Reconstructive surgery of the heart. *Nursing Mirror*, Oct. 10, 1969, p. 55-6.

Rothnie, N. G.
Sutureless skin closure. *Nursing Mirror*, April 10, 1964, p. v-vii and xiii.

Savage, C. R.
Direct arterial surgery. *Nursing Times*, Aug. 11, 1967, p. 1052-3.

Schurr, P. H.
Cerebral Surgery—1. Some modern treatment in the neurosurgical field. *Nursing Mirror*, Jan. 27, 1961, p. v-vii.

Schurr, P. H.
Cerebral Surgery. *Nursing Mirror*, Feb. 3, 1961, p. v-vi.

Schweisheimer, W.
Cryogenics in surgery. *Nursing Mirror*, June 3, 1966, p. viii-x.

Stanley, P. H.
Open heart surgery. *The Canadian Nurse*, Mar. 1964, p. 249-57.

Sugden, B.
Instrument shadow boards. *Nursing Mirror*, Feb. 3, 1967, p. v-vii.

Swinney, J.
Conservative surgery of the kidney. *Nursing Mirror*, Feb. 9, 1968, p. 33-7.

Tagart, R. E. B.
A handbook of general surgery for nurses. Pitman, 1968.

Townsend, N.
Major day case surgery. *District Nursing*, Dec. 1970, p. 173 and 188.

Trimble, A. S.
Advances in surgery for coronary artery disease. *Canadian Nurse*, Jan. 1969, p. 32-4.

Viljoen, J. F.
Myocardial revascularization procedures: anesthetic technic. *Journal American Association of Nurse Anesthetists*, Aug. 1968, p. 261-6.

Vineberg, Arthur
The value of revascularization surgery. *Canadian Nurse*, Jan. 1969, p. 28-31.

Wakeley, J.
The changing face of surgery in a provincial hospital. *Nursing Mirror*, Sept. 18, 1970, p. 23-5.

Warltier, A. W.
New approach to dressing raw surfaces. *Nursing Times*, Dec. 9, 1966, p. 1608-9.

Williams, M. M.
An investigation into surgical dressing techniques. *Journal for Industrial Nurses*, Jan./Feb. 1961, p. 11-4.

Wolfer, J. A., *and* Davis, C. E.
Assessment of surgical patients' preoperative emotional condition and postoperative welfare. *Nursing Research*, Sept./Oct. 1970, p. 402-14.

ACCIDENTS, BURNS

Akey, D. T.
The employee with critical burns. *American Association of Industrial Nurses Journal*, Oct. 1968, p. 17-9.

American Nurses' Association
Nursing care of the burned patient. N.Y., A.N.A., 1962.

Archambeault, C. A.
Maintaining the burn nursing team. *AORN Journal*, Feb. 1970, p. 60-5.

Armitage, S.
Hospital mobile accident units. *Nursing Times*, Nov. 10, 1967, p. 1514-5.

Bell, H. S.
Nursing service in the emergency department. *Nursing Outlook*, June 1962, p. 392-3.

Bennett, H. J.
Burns first aid and emergency care. *American Journal of Nursing*, Oct. 1962, p. 96.

Bennett, J. P.
Skin grafting and the treatment of burns. *Nursing Times*, Dec. 10, 1970, p. 1584-7.

Broomfield Hospital, Chelmsford
Crush injuries of the chest. *Nursing Times*, April 7, 1967, p. 451-8.

Cason, J. S.
The treatment of burned patients. *Nursing Times*, Jan. 8, 1970, p. 40-2.

Cheetham, J.
Treatment of burns with compressed air. *Nursing Times*, Feb. 10, 1961, p. 170.

CHUTZ, ADRIAN
The development of a nursing categorization of burn patients and a burn patient nursing care index. New York, National League for Nursing, 1969.

COLLINS, J. A.
The early care of accident victims: contrasting approaches. *AORN Journal*, July 1969, p. 35-9.

DOWLING, J. J.
"Whiplash" injuries. *American Association of Industrial Nurses Journal*, May 1964, p. 12-5 and 34-5.

ERRERA, D. W.
Care and treatment of the burn patient. *Hospital Topics*, June 1969, p. 101-8.

FAHEY, PAULINE M.
Nursing care of a child with extensive burns.
In
AMERICAN NURSES' ASSOCIATION
Nursing care of the burned patient. New York, The Association, 1962.

FARROW, RAYMOND
The nursing of accidents. English Universities Press, 1964.

FISHER, LUCILLE C.
Discussion—with emphasis on variations of nursing care in flame and radiation burns sustained in disaster.
In
AMERICAN NURSES' ASSOCIATION
Nursing care of the burned patient. New York, The Association, 1962.

FITZPATRICK, K.
Nursing care of severely burned patients. *Nursing Times*, Dec. 10, 1970, p. 1588-91.

HENLEY, N. L.
Sulfamylon for burns. *American Journal of Nursing*, Oct. 1969, p. 2122-3.

JOHNS, L. A.
Nursing care of the burned patient. *American Association of Industrial Nurses Journal*, May 1963, p. 16-9.

LAING, J. ELLSWORTH, and HARVEY, JOYCE
The management and nursing of burns. English Universities Press, 1967.

LAMBERTON, C. J.
A guide to the care of the injured patient. *Nursing Times*, Mar. 12, 1970, p. 335-7; Mar. 19, 1970, p. 368-71; Mar. 26, 1970, p. 402-4.

LARSON, D., and GASTON, R.
Current trends in the care of burned patients. *American Journal of Nursing*, Feb. 1967, p. 319-27.

LIN, P. M.
Management of head injuries. *American Association of Industrial Nurses Journal*, Feb. 1963, p. 22-4.

LONDON, P. S.
Nursing emergencies. Oxford, Blackwell, 1967.

LOWERY, M., and DOBBIE, K.
Suspected diathermy burns. *NATNews*, Winter 1968, p. 17-9.

LYNCH, M. D.
Nursing care of a badly burned child. *Nursing Mirror*, June 26, 1970, p. 28-31.

MACLENNAN, W. D.
Severe facial injuries—emergency hospital care. *NATNews*, Summer, 1970, p. 15-7.

MANN, T. S., and others
Accident surgery for nurses, by T. S. Mann in collaboration with Wm. Henry Reid, A. B. M. Telfer and Robert Tym. Edinburgh, Livingstone, 1969.

MEEHAN, A. R.
Accident prevention in a geriatric setting. *Journal of Psychiatric Nursing*, May 1963, p. 214-9.

MINCKLEY, B. B.
Expert nursing care for burned patients. *American Journal of Nursing*, Sept. 1970, p. 1888-93.

MORRISTON-DAVIES, M.
Nursing a patient with 40 per cent burns. *Nursing Mirror*, April 11, 1969, p. 40-3.

NAISH, B.
Accidents in the home. *Nursing Times*, June 23, 1961, p. 805-7.

NURSING CLINICS OF NORTH AMERICA
Symposium on the patient with trauma. *Nursing Clinics of North America*, Dec. 1970, p. 549-630.

NURSING MIRROR
Transport dressing for burns. *Nursing Mirror*, Aug. 12, 1966, p. 450-1.

OSMOND, J. D.
The role of the nurse in acute accident cases. *South African Nursing Journal*, Feb. 1970, p. 11-4.

PEARSON, R. J. C.
Accident and emergency departments. Sisters' views. *Nursing Times*, June 16, 1967, p. 796-8.

PRICE, W. R., and WOOD, M.
Operating room care of burned patients treated with silver nitrate. *American Journal of Nursing*, Aug. 1968, p. 1705-7.

RAINS, A. J. H.
Injuries to arteries and veins. *Nursing Mirror*, Nov. 13, 1970, p. 25-7 and 31.

SLATER, R. R.
Triage nurse in the emergency department. *American Journal of Nursing*, Jan. 1970, p. 127-9.

SMITH, JACQULYN M.
Discussion—with emphasis on variations of nursing care of the adult burn patient.
In
AMERICAN NURSES' ASSOCIATION
Nursing care of the burned patient. New York, The Association, 1962.

WALKER, K.
Accidents in hospitals. *Nursing Mirror*, Nov. 13, 1970, p. 38-9.

WATSON, J.
Treatment and nursing of the severely burned patient. *Nursing Mirror*, Jan. 30, 1970, p. 13-5.

ORTHOPAEDICS

ARNOLD, H. M.
Elderly diabetic amputees. *American Journal of Nursing*, Dec. 1969, p. 2646-9.

BAME, K. B.
Halo traction. *American Journal of Nursing*, Sept. 1969, p. 1933-7.

BARLOW, T. G.
Congenital dislocation of the hip. *Nursing Times*, July 19, 1968, p. 967-8.

BETTS, G. A.
An adjustable plastozote splint—for the hand or arm. *Nursing Times*, Dec. 3, 1970, p. 1556-7.

BRADLEY, D.
Fractures of the upper end of the femur—1. Clinical features; 2. Treatment. *Nursing Times*, Nov. 26, 1970, p. 1523-5; Dec. 3, 1970, p. 1552-5.

BRIGDEN, R. J.
Metric measurement for orthopaedic implants. *Nursing Times*, Sept. 6, 1963, p. 1122-5.

BURGESS, D. M.
Alvik Traction—a new technique. *Nursing Times*, July 16, 1970, p. 908-10.

SPECIALITIES

CALDERWOOD, CARMELITA
Orthopedic nursing; revised by Carroll B. Larson and Marjorie Gould. 5th edn. St. Louis, Mosby, 1961.
7th edn., 1970.
[For earlier editions of this work *see* Funsten and Calderwood, "Orthopedic nursing".]

CHOLMELEY, J. A.
The history of orthopaedic nurse training. *Nursing Times*, Sept. 4, 1969, p. 1144-5.

DURBIN, F. C.
Frozen shoulder. *Nursing Times*, June 3, 1966, p. 743-5.

ELSON, REGINALD
Practical management of spinal injuries for nurses. Edinburgh, Livingstone, 1965.

GILCHRIST, M. I.
Posterior ilio-psoas transplants. *Nursing Times*, Dec. 11, 1969, p. 1575-8.

GOWDA, S. BASAVE
Nurses' role on a patient with fractured neck of the femur. *The Nursing Journal of India*, July 1969, p. 231, 236.

KERR, AVICE
Orthopedic nursing procedures. 2nd edn. New York, Springer, 1969.

LAM, S. J.
Arthroplasty. *Nursing Times*, May 8, 1964, p. 586-8.

LAM, S. J.
Fractures—1. *Nursing Times*, Mar. 25, 1966, p. 410-2.

LAM, S. J.
Fractures—2. General principles. *Nursing Times*, April 1, 1966, p. 446-7.

LAMB, D. W.
Amputation surgery and rehabilitation. *Nursing Mirror*, Jan. 3, 1969, p. 26-31.

LOWRY, M. F.
Congenital dislocation of the hip. *Nursing Times*, Jan. 15, 1970, p. 72-4.

MCCARRICK, H.
Orthopaedic uses for Plastozote. *Nursing Times*, May 15, 1969, p. 618-9.

MCFARLAND, B.
Osteoarthritis of the hip. *Nursing Times*, July 13, 1962, p. 890-3.

MCKEE, G. K.
Replacement hip surgery. *Nursing Times*, July 28, 1967, p. 984-7.

MCKIBBIN, B.
Sources of error in early recognition of congenital dislocation of the hip. *Nursing Mirror*, April 24, 1970, p. 23-5.

MONCRIEFF, M. J.
Problems, principles and practices in the care of patients in plasters. *The Canadian Nurse*, Nov. 1963, p. 1040-52.

MONCUR, S. D.
Rehabilitation of a lower limb amputee. *Nursing Times*, Mar. 20, 1969, p. 372-4.

NAYLOR, ARTHUR
Fractures and orthopaedic surgery for nurses and masseuses. 5th edn. Edinburgh, Livingstone, 1964.
6th edn., 1968.

NEW ZEALAND DEPARTMENT OF HEALTH, RESEARCH AND PLANNING UNIT
Patient-nurse dependency: orthopaedic surgery; an analysis of survey data from three public hospitals in Christchurch 1962. Wellington, Owen, 1965.

NEWCOMBE, J.
Through-knee amputation. *Nursing Times*, July 10, 1969, p. 871-4.

NICOLL, K.
Understanding traction—I, II, III, IV, V, VI, VII and VIII. *Nursing Times*, Sept. 13, 1963, p. 1142-5; Sept. 20, 1963, p. 1170-2; Sept. 27, 1963, p. 1203-5; Oct. 4, 1963, p. 1239-42; Oct. 11, 1963, p. 1284-6; Oct. 18, 1963, p. 1326-9; Oct. 25, 1963, p. 1359-61; Nov. 1, 1963, p. 1389-91.

NICOLL, K.
Understanding traction—IX. *Nursing Times*, Nov. 8, 1963, p. 1412-5.

NURSING MIRROR
Safe splint for broken limbs. Pre-hospital first-aid. *Nursing Mirror*, Aug. 29, 1969, p. 39.

NURSING MIRROR
To replace human bones. New material developed in the U.S. *Nursing Mirror*, Mar. 11, 1966, p. 673.

PENROSE, J. H.
Upper femoral osteotomy in children. *NATNews*, Winter 1969, p. 12-6.

PFALTZGRAFF, R. E.
Developing a prosthesis for amputees. *Nursing Mirror*, June 21, 1963, p. v-vii.

PLAISTED, L. M., and FRIZ, B. R.
The nurse on the amputee clinic team. *Nursing Outlook*, October 1968, p. 34-7.

POWELL, MARY
Orthopaedic nursing. 4th edn. Edinburgh, Livingstone, 1969.
5th edn., 1965.
6th edn., 1968.

RANGREJI, D. S.
Modern trends in orthopedic nursing. *Nursing Journal of India*, July 1970, p. 222 and 236.

ROAF, ROBERT
Perthes' Disease. *Nursing Times*, May 24, 1963, p. 642-3.

ROAF, ROBERT
Spinal Injuries—1. *Nursing Times*, Nov. 3, 1961, p. 1422-4.

ROAF, ROBERT
Spinal injuries—2. *Nursing Times*, Nov. 10, 1961, p. 1467-9.

ROAF, ROBERT, and HODKINSON, LEONARD J., *editors*
The Oswestry textbook for orthopaedic nurses. Pitman Medical, 1962.

SHEWCHUK, M., and YOUNG, Z.
The amputee and immediate prosthesis. *Canadian Nurse*, May 1969, p. 47-9.

STEELE, S.
Children with amputations. *Nursing Forum*, vol. VII, no. 4, 1968, p. 411-23.

STONE, R. M.
The changing concepts of orthopaedic nursing. *International Journal of Nursing Studies*, vol. 2, no. 3, 1965, p. 247-50.

TILL, K., and MURRIE, E.
Spinal dysraphism: hidden congenital malformations. *Nursing Times*, April 16, 1970, p. 488-90.

TWOMEY, SISTER M. REDEMPTA
Halo pelvic traction. *Nursing Times*, Sept. 24, 1970, p. 1225-8.

WIEBE, ANNE M.
Orthopedics in nursing. Philadelphia, Saunders, 1961.

WINSTON, M. E.
Total prosthetic replacement in hip surgery. *Nursing Times*, Nov. 22, 1968, p. 1588-9.

SURGICAL NURSING

ALEXANDER, EDYTHE LOUISE, *and others*
The care of the patient in surgery, including techniques 4th edn. St. Louis, Mosby, 1967.

ALODIA, SISTER MARY
Cardiovascular surgical intensive care unit. Roslyn, New York, St. Francis Hospital, 1968.

AMERICAN COLLEGE OF SURGEONS
Surgical nurses' observation vital to patient's recovery. *Hospital Topics*, May 1962, p. 78-80.

ANDERSON, BARBARA L.
Nursing care of the patient with the cardiac pace-maker monitor.
In
AMERICAN NURSES' ASSOCIATION
Technical innovations in health care: nursing implications. New York, The Association, 1962.

ASSOCIATION OF OPERATING ROOM NURSES
STATEMENT COMMITTEE
Definition and objective for clinical practice of professional operating room nursing. *AORN Journal*, Nov. 1969, p. 43-8.

ARMSTRONG, KATHERINE F.
Aids to surgical nursing. 7th edn. Bailliere, Tindall and Cox, 1961.
8th edn., 1969.

AUDETTE, A.
Nursing care in cardiovascular surgery. *Canadian Nurse*, Mar. 1964, p. 259-70.

BAKER, SISTER M. EUGENE
Operating room technicians. *Nursing Outlook*, Nov. 1963, p. 807-8.

BALL, B. M.
Hospital-trained surgical technicians lighten nursing load. *Hospitals*, June 1, 1967, p. 87-90.

BAYNHAM, J. E., and others
Advances in nursing care of thoracic surgical patients. *AORN Journal*, Aug. 1969, p. 56-60.

BEAL, JOHN M., and ECKENHOFF, JAMES E.
Intensive and recovery room care. Collier-Macmillan, 1969.

BEER, G. E.
Postoperative pain relief: report of a cooperative study. *Journal of American Association of Nurse Anesthetists*, Oct. 1970, p. 379-84.

BERNADETTE POIRIER, REV. SISTER
Changing role of the O.R. nurse. *Hospital Administration in Canada*, April 1970, p. 62, 64 and 66.

BERRY, D. M., and MICHAEL, M. G.
Professional nurse on the operating room team. *AORN Journal*, Feb. 1970, p. 41-4.

BETSCHMAN, LUCILLE I.
Handbook of recovery room nursing. Philadelphia, Davis, 1967.

BORDICKS, KATHERINE J.
Nursing care of patients having chest surgery. New York, Macmillan, 1962.

BRAMBILLA, MARY A.
A teaching plan for cardiac surgical patients. *Cardiovascular Nursing*, Jan./Feb. 1969, p. 1-4.

BRESLAU, R. C.
Intensive care following vascular surgery. *American Journal of Nursing*, Aug. 1968, p. 1670-6.

BRIGDEN, RAYMOND J.
Operating theatre technique: a textbook for nurses, technicians, medical students, house surgeons and others associated with the operating theatre. Edinburgh, Livingstone, 1962. 2nd edn., 1969.

BRIGGS, LOUISE
Nursing care—a specialty—as related to the patient with a prosthetic heart valve.
In
AMERICAN NURSES' ASSOCIATION
Technical innovations in health care: nursing implications. New York, The Association, 1962.

BRITTAIN, G. J. C.
The post-operative recovery ward. *Nursing Mirror*, Feb. 17, 1961, p. i.

BROCK, RUSSELL CLAUD
The importance of nursing care in cardiac surgery. *Nursing Mirror*, Oct. 14, 1966, p. 33-5.

BROOME, W. E.
Dressing technique—a cause of confusion. *Nursing Mirror*, July 25, 1969, p. 9-10.

BROOME, W. E.
Recording levels of consciousness. *Nursing Mirror*, Feb. 8, 1963, p. 415-6.

BRUNNER, LILLIAN SHOLTIS, and others
Textbook of medical-surgical nursing by Lillian Sholtis Brunner, Charles Phillips Emerson, L. Kraeer Ferguson and Doris Smith Suddarth. Philadelphia, Lippincott, 1964. 2nd edn., 1970.

CENTRAL HEALTH SERVICES COUNCIL
JOINT SUB-COMMITTEE OF THE STANDING MEDICAL AND STANDING NURSING ADVISORY COMMITTEES
The organisation and staffing of operating departments. H.M.S.O., 1970.

CHARTER, D.
Is the operating room nurse part of a vanishing breed? *Canadian Hospital*, Nov 1970, p 56-7

CHILDS, PETER
Nurses guide to surgery Bristol, John Wright, 1962.

CHOW, RITA
Postoperative cardiac nursing research: a method for identifying and categorizing nursing action. *Nursing Research*, Jan./Feb. 1969, p. 4-13.

CLARKE, M. K.
Illustrated guide to theatre instruments. Butterworths, 1966.

CLEMONS, B.
The OR nurse in the patient care circuit. *American Journal of Nursing*, Oct. 1968, p. 2141-5.

COOKE, R. GORDON
The nurse's guide to common surgical operations. Faber and Faber, 1967.

DAVIDSON, A.
No nurses in operating theatres? Report of Institute of Operating Theatre Technicians Congress, held at Eastbourne, May 21-23, 1970. *NATNews*, Summer 1970, p. 12.

DAVIS, R. W.
Post-operative care of the craniotomy patient. *Bedside Nurse*, May/June 1969, p. 23-8.

DE GUTIERREZ-MAHONEY, C. G., and CARINI, ESTA
Neurological and neurosurgical nursing. 4th edn. St. Louis, Mosby, 1965.
5th edn. by Carini and Guy Owens, 1970.

EDWARDS, M.
Post-registration theatre course [at United Manchester Hospitals]. *NATNews*, Summer 1969, p. 19.

ELAINE, REV. SISTER MARY
The OR nurse of the future. *Hospital Administration in Canada*, Feb. 1970, p. 38, 40, 42 and 44.

FORDHAM, MARY E.
Cardiovascular surgical nursing. New York, Macmillan, 1962.

FRASER, J. R.
Some aspects of trainee nurses' evaluation of their term of operating theatre nursing duties. *Australian Nurses' Journal*, Jan. 1969, p. 16-21.

GINSBERG, FRANCES, and others
A manual of operating room technology, by Frances Ginsberg, Lillian Sholtis Brunner and Vernita L. Cantlin. Philadelphia, Lippincott, 1966.

SPECIALITIES

GLIEDMAN, M. L.
ORN—conservation of the species. *AORN Journal*, June 1970, p. 60-4.

GOWIN, J.
Staff development in the operating room. *American Journal of Nursing*, May 1965, p. 117-9.

GRUENDEMANN, B. J.
Social structure of hospital operating rooms. *AORN Journal*, May 1970, p. 43-8.

GRUENDEMANN, B. J., *and others*
Operating room nursing in the basic curriculum: an opinion. *Nursing Outlook*, Jan. 1970, p. 44-5.

HARVEY, R. H.
Nursing care in direct arterial surgery. *Nursing Times*, Aug. 11, 1967, p. 1055-6.

HEALY, K. M.
A pre-operative patient teaching program. *AORN Journal*, Oct. 1969, p. 37-43.

HEIMLICH, HENRY J.
Postoperative care in thoracic surgery: a manual of practical information for internes, residents and nurses. Springfield, Thomas, 1962.

HOOPER, REGINALD
Neurosurgical nursing. Springfield, Thomas, 1964.

HOPKIN, D. A. BUXTON
Anaesthesia, recovery and intensive care. English Universities Press, 1970.

HOUGHTON, MARJORIE, *and* HUDD, JEAN
Aids to theatre technique. 3rd edn. Bailliere, Tindall and Cox, 1961.
4th edn., 1967.

HURT, R. L.
Nursing care after lung resection. *Nursing Times*, July 26, 1963, p. 920-3.

JACKSON, F. E., *and* SMITH, M. E.
Increasing nursing skills and responsibilities in neurosurgical nursing. *Nursing Times*, Sept. 6, 1968, p. 1206-7.

JARVIS, D.
Open heart surgery: patients' perceptions of care. *American Journal of Nursing*, Dec. 1970, p. 2591-3.

JOHNSON, B. A., *and others*
Research in nursing practice. *Nursing Research*, July/Aug. 1970, p. 337-42.

JOHNSON, J. E., *and others*
Psychosocial factors in the welfare of surgical patients. *Nursing Research*, Jan./Feb. 1970, p. 18-29.

LANGAN, E.
Nursing care of neurosurgical patients—admission and discharge. *Nursing Times*, Jan. 20, 1967, p. 77.

LANGAN, E.
Nursing care of neurosurgical patients. Post-operative care. *Nursing Times*, Jan. 27, 1967, p. 111.

LEMAITRE, GEORGE D., *and* FINNEGAN, JANET A.
The patient in surgery: a guide for nurses. Philadelphia, Saunders, 1965.
2nd edn., 1970.

LEUNG, J. S. M.
A discussion on some problems in the post-operative management after open heart surgery. *The Hong Kong Nursing Journal*, Nov. 1970, p. 63-8.

LEVINE, D. C., *and* FIEDLER, J. P.
Fears, facts and fantasies about pre- and post-operation care. *Nursing Outlook*, Feb. 1970, p. 26-8.

LOUISE, SISTER MARY,
The operating room technician. St. Louis, Mosby, 1965.

MCGRATH, MARION E., *and* MOORE, BETTY
Correlating operating room nursing with the total nursing curriculum. *Journal of Nursing Education*, Nov. 1967, p. 13-5, 17 and 32-3.

MARTIN, M. A.
The ABC of the recovery room. *Nursing Times*, Dec. 21, 1962, p. 1621-2.

MATTHIAS, A. MARJORIE, *and others*
Illustrated guide for theatre nurses, by A. Marjorie Matthias, Margaret J. Penfold, and Susan Fry. Butterworths, 1961.

MEMORIAL HOSPITAL FOR CANCER AND ALLIED DISEASES
NURSING DIVISION
Home care for the patient after urological surgery. New York, The Hospital, 1966.

MEYER, SEYMOUR W.
Functional bandaging, including splints and protective dressings. New York, American Elsevier Publishing Co., 1967.

MEZZANOTTE, E. J.
Group instruction [of patients] in preparation for surgery. *American Journal of Nursing*, Jan. 1970, p. 89-91.

MILLER, J.
Planning effective in-service program for O.R. nurses and technicians. *Hospital Topics*, Nov. 1970, p. 73-7 and 80.

MINCKLEY, BARBARA B.
OR nursing research—1. and 2. *AORN Journal*, Nov. 1969, p. 65-6; Dec. 1969, p. 47-9.

MORAN, SISTER ANN,
A new nurse becomes a patient-centered nurse practitioner in the operating room. *AORN Journal*, Feb. 1970, p. 49-54.

MORRIS, R. P.
Training student nurses in theatre. *NATNews*, Summer 1970, p. 21.

NASH, D. F. ELLISON
The principles and practice of surgical nursing. 2nd edn. Arnold, 1961.
3rd edn., 1965.
4th edn., 1969.

NATIONAL ASSOCIATION OF THEATRE NURSES
WEST RIDING BRANCH
Theatrician—a new profession. *NATNews*, Winter 1970, p. 17, and 20.

NEW ZEALAND DEPARTMENT OF HEALTH,
RESEARCH AND PLANNING UNIT
Patient-nurse dependency: general surgery an analysis of survey data from three public hospitals in Christchurch 1962. Wellington, Owen, 1964.

O'CONNOR, V.
Theatrician—a name for the future? *Nursing Mirror*, Oct. 23, 1970, p. 28.

PARKER, D. J.
Intensive therapy after cardiac surgery. *Nursing Times*, Mar. 13, 1969, p. 341-2.

PEARCE, EVELYN
Instruments, appliances and theatre technique. 4th edn. Faber, 1962.
5th edn., 1967.

PENFOLD, MARGARET J.
Instruments without tears. Macmillan (for *Nursing Times*), 1964.

PENFOLD, MARGARET J., *and* MOUSLEY, J. S.
The theatre nurse and emergency surgery. Macmillan (for *Nursing Times*), 1965.

PHILIPP, ELLIOT E., *and* GEARING, K. L.
The student nurse in the operating theatre, Edinburgh, Livingstone, 1964.

POPIEL, E. S.
The operating room nurse and continuing education. *AORN Journal*, Feb. 1970, p. 35-7.

POTTER, J. M.
Nursing observation of patients with head injuries. *Nursing Times*, Oct. 19, 1962, p. 1310.

POWERS, MARYANN, *and* STORLIE, FRANCES
The cardiac surgical patient: pathophysiologic considerations and nursing care. New York, Macmillan, 1969.

PRENTICE, G. M.
Nursing care in oesophageal surgery. 1. Pre-operative care. *Nursing Times*, Jan. 4, 1963, p. 4-5.

PRENTICE, G. M.
Nursing care in oesophageal surgery. 2. Post-operative care. *Nursing Times*, Jan. 11, 1963, p. 39-49.

PRENTICE, G. M.
Nursing care in oesophageal surgery. 3. Post-operative care. *Nursing Times*, Jan. 18, 1963, p. 80-1.

PRENTICE, G. M.
Nursing care in oesophageal surgery. 4. Palliative and therapeutic procedures. *Nursing Times*, Jan. 25, 1963, p. 99-101.

RAINS, A. J. HARDING
Care after arterial operations. *Nursing Times*, April 2, 1965, p. 454-6.

RAY, RUTH M.
Independent and dependent judgements of the nurse in the care of selected surgical patients.
In
AMERICAN NURSES' ASSOCIATION
The nurse-patient-doctor triadic relationships: effects on nursing care of the patient. New York, The Association, 1962.

RHODES, IONE B.
Discussion—nursing care for open-heart surgery.
In
AMERICAN NURSES' ASSOCIATION
Technical innovations in health care: nursing implications. New York, The Association, 1962.

SAUNDERS, H. B.
Colostomy. The nurse's contribution to the patient's welfare. *Nursing Times*, April 26, 1963, p. 504-6.

SCHROEDER, H. G.
Post-operative respiratory intensive care. *NATNews*, Autumn 1969, p. 13-6.

SCOTT, DONALD F., *and* DODD, BARBARA
Neurological and neurosurgical nursing: an introduction. Oxford, Pergamon, 1966.

SIMONDS, A.
Two methods of teaching in the OR. *Nursing Outlook*, Feb. 1970, p. 29-31.

SOLOSKO, A.
Nursing care of the gallbladder patient. *Bedside Nurse*, Mar./April 1968, p. 11-5.

TARSITANO, JOHN J., *and others*
Nursing care after oral surgery. *American Journal of Nursing*, July 1969, p. 1493-6.

TAYLOR, SELWYN, *and* WORRALL, OLGA
Principles of surgery and surgical nursing. English Universities Press, 1961.
2nd edn., 1969.

TEWINKLE, M. B.
Care of the patient with chest surgery. *Journal of Practical Nursing*, Feb. 1970, p. 24-5, 36-8, 40, 42-4 and 46-7.

TROUTEN, F.
Are changes in nursing education removing students from operating room experience? *Hospital Administration in Canada*, Aug. 1968, p. 64-6.

TYRRELL, B.
Extra-corporeal circulation. Nursing after-care. *Nursing Times*, April 24, 1964, p. 518-20.

UNITED STATES PUBLIC HEALTH SERVICE
DIVISION OF NURSING
Closed drainage of the chest: a programed course for nurses. Washington, U.S. Dept of Health, Education and Welfare, 1965.

WASS, JUDITH R.
Nursing the patient after heart surgery. *Canadian Nurse*, Jan. 1969, p. 35-7.

WELLS, P.
Interrelated surgical patient care. The need to communicate. *AORN Journal*, Aug. 1969, p. 35-46.

WHITESIDE, J. E.
Surgical nursing. Sydney, Angus & Robertson, 1967.

WILLINGHAM, JACQUELINE
Logic of operating room nursing. New York, Springer, 1962.
2nd edn., 1967.

WILSON, FRANK
Nursing care of the anaesthetized patient. Oxford, Blackwell, 1962.

WULFSOHN, N. L.
Aids to pre- and post-operative nursing. 2nd edn. Bailliere, Tindall and Cassell, 1963.

CENTRAL STERILE SUPPLY DEPTS.
Sterilization, Infection, Cross-infection

ALDER, V. G.
Low-temperature steam disinfection of wool blankets. *Nursing Times*, Oct. 4, 1963, p. 1234-6.

AYLIFFE, G. A. J.
Control of infection in domiciliary practice. *District Nursing*, Jan. 1970, p. 197-8 and 200.

BETHUNE, S.
Pseudomonas Aeruginosa: the role of the nurse/research assistant in a study of the spread of clinical infection. *Nursing Times*, Nov. 8, 1968, p. 1517-8.

BRIGDEN, R. J.
Macintoshes *can* be sterilized by autoclaving. *Nursing Times*, Nov. 2, 1962, p. 1410.

BROOME, W. E.
Isolation techniques. *Nursing Times*, May 10, 1963, p. 574-5.

BURKE, J. F.
Environmental sanitation. Bacteria-free nursing unit—a new approach to isolation procedures. *Hospitals*, Jan. 16, 1969, p. 86-9.

CHRISTIE, J. E.
Why nurses should run central service. *Modern Hospital*, July 1968, p. 120.

CLEAVELY, K. B.
Decrease in ward hygiene. *Nursing Mirror*, Sept. 4, 1970, p. 10.

COCKER, P., *and* WHITE, D. K.
Doing without ward boilers and drums. *Nursing Mirror*, Jan. 17, 1964, p. 347-9.

COLUMBIA UNIVERSITY, TEACHERS COLLEGE
Introduction to asepsis: a programed unit in fundamentals of nursing, by Marie M. Seedor. New York, Columbia University Teachers College Bureau of Publications, 1963.

EDGEWORTH, D.
Nursing and asepsis in the modern hospital. *Nursing Outlook*, June 1965, p. 54-6.

SPECIALITIES

FLICK, J. A.
Sterilization techniques. *American Association of Industrial Nurses Journal*, Feb. 1963, p. 14-5.

GERMAINE, A.
Centralization of supplies: what it means to the nursing department. *Hospital Administration in Canada*, vol. 11, no. 8, Aug. 1969, p. 30-2 and 34.

GILLESPIE, W. A.
Staphylococcal cross-infection. *Nursing Mirror*, Sept. 9, 1962, p. 473-4, and 476.

GINSBERG, F.
Private scrub nurses can be blessing—or a curse. *The Modern Hospital*, Feb. 1967, p. 129 and 132.

GREENE, V. W.
Microbiological contamination control in hospitals. Role of nursing service. *Hospitals*, Nov. 16, 1969, p. 71-5 and 78.

HANKIN, E., *and* LEMIN, B.
Pre-sterilized dressing service for district nurses. *Nursing Times*, Sept. 8, 1967, p. 1216-7.

HOPE, T.
Autoclaving does not sterilize macintoshes. *Nursing Times*, Oct. 19, 1962, p. 1335-6.

HOPE, T.
Boiler or autoclave? The sterilization of bowls and instruments. *Nursing Times*, June 8, 1962, p. 744-5.

HUGHES, E.
Central sterilization of equipment for domiciliary midwives and district nurses. *The Medical Officer*, Dec. 14, 1962, p. 371-3.

HUGHES, T. A.
Planning and equipping a CSSD for a new hospital. *Nursing Times*, Mar. 19, 1965, p. 399-400.

IRVINE, M. B., *and* GOOD, E. R.
An alternative scheme for central sterile department. *Nursing Mirror*, April 28, 1961, p. ii-iv.

JAMES, D.
The CSD unit. *South African Nursing Journal*, vol. 36, no. 6, June 1970, p. 18-22.

JENKINS, M. M.
CSSD and the nurse—1. 2. 3. Packs for catheterization: bladder irrigation: clean procedure sets. 4. Packs for specific medical and surgical procedures. 5 & 6. Procedure packs for the specialised units. 7 & 8. Procedure packs for the specialised units. 9. The way ahead. *Nursing Times*, April 23, 1970, p. 517-20; April 30, 1970, p. 557-61; May 7, 1970, p. 593-6; May 14, 1970, p. 619-23; May 21, 1970, p. 650-3; May 28, 1970, p. 688-92; June 4, 1970, p. 722-4; June 11, 1970, p. 744-8; June 18, 1970, p. 777-9.

JOHNSON, A.
Aseptic techniques. 1. Using sterile packs. 2. Methods of distribution. 3. A pack for use in operating theatres. 4. Packs issued to district nurses and midwives. *Nursing Times*, Feb. 24, 1967, p. 254-9.

JOHNSON, A.
Principles and practice of sterilization. 1 & 2. Sterilization by steam. 3. Quality control in the CSSD. *Nursing Times*, Oct. 6, 1967, p. 1344-5; Oct. 13, 1967, p. 1391-2; Oct. 20, 1967, p. 1427-8.

KING, M. J.
Theatre service centre, The Royal Infirmary of Edinburgh. *International Journal of Nursing Studies*, Nov. 1969, p. 225-35.

LIBRACH, I. M.
Barrier nursing and cross-infection. *Hospital and Social Service Journal*, April 13, 1962, p. 423.

LOWBURY, E. J. L., *and* PATH, F. C.
Research on control of hospital infection by air-conditioned isolation wards. *Nursing Mirror*, Sept. 17, 1965, p. vii-viii.

MAGUIRE, J. M.
The sterile pack system. As used in the operating room suite at Grey's Hospital, Pietermaritzburg. *South African Nursing Journal*, March 1962, p. 15.

MELLINGS, M.
Prevention of staphylococcal infection in surgical wards. *Nursing Times*, Nov. 22, 1963, p. 1484-6.

NURSING CLINICS OF NORTH AMERICA
Symposium on infection and the nurse. *Nursing Clinics of North America*, Mar. 1970, p. 85-174.

PARNELL, J. W.
C.S.S.D. scheme between hospital and local authority. *Nursing Mirror*, Feb. 18, 1966, p. 591-2.

PARRY, W. H.
Hospital infection. *Nursing Times*, Sept. 24, 1965, p. 1305-7.

PEQUEGNAT, D.
Infections in the hospital. *The Canadian Nurse*, Mar. 1969, p. 27-9.

QUEEN'S INSTITUTE OF DISTRICT NURSING
Safer sterilising of equipment: a study of traditional methods of sterilisation in current district nursing practice in selected areas, and of the provision of pre-sterilised supplies for the domiciliary health team by local authorities throughout England and Wales. The Institute, 1965.

RIDLEY, M.
Barrier nursing. *Nursing Times*, Mar. 16, 1962, p. 340.

ROCKWELL, V. T.
Surgical hand scrubbing. *American Journal of Nursing*, June 1963, p. 75-81.

SMITH, B. J.
Disinfectants in hospitals. *Nursing Times*, May 22, 1969, p. 647-9.

SMITH, S.
New suture dispensing system. *NATNews*, Spring 1969, p. 11 and 26.

SPEERS, R., *and others*
Contamination of nurses' uniforms with staphylococcus aureus. *The Lancet*, Aug. 2, 1969, p. 233-5.

WELCH, J. D.
Central sterile supply to wards. *Nursing Mirror*, Mar. 1, 1963, p. vii-ix.

WHYTE, B. BRYSSON
The human element (in Central Sterile Supply). *Nursing Times*, June 5, 1964, p. 720-3.

Infection Control Sister

BRADBEER, T. L., *and others*
Duties and status of an infection control sister in the Exeter Hospital Group. *Monthly Bulletin of the Ministry of Health and the Public Health Laboratory Service*, Nov. 1966, p. 269-76.

BRADBEER, T. L., *and others*
The infection control sister. *Nursing Times*, May 26, 1967, p. 698-700.

COOPER, R. G.
An infection control sister in a children's hospital. *South Australian Journal of Nursing*, Sept. 1968, p. 17-20.

CRAWFORD, M.
Infection control in the OR. *AORN Journal*, May 1970, p. 54-61.

DAVIS, N. C., *and others*
The infection control sister. Her role in a large hospital. *The Lancet*, Dec. 21, 1963, p. 1321-2.

DAY, V. M.
Infection control sister. *Nursing Mirror*, June 9, 1967, p. 224-6.

FORMAN, A.
Infection control sister. *Nursing Times*, Feb. 8, 1963, p. 158-61.

GARDNER, A. M. N., *and others*
The infection control sister. *The Lancet*, Oct. 6, 1962, p. 710-1.

GINSBERG, F.
Control nurse is needed to keep infection committee in action. *Modern Hospital*, Oct. 1969, p. 122.

GRANT, M. L.
Infection control sister. *Nursing Times*, May 21, 1970, p. 659-60.

MOORE, B.
Control of infection: the employment of a senior member of the nursing staff as a member of the control of infection team in general hospitals. [Bristol, South Western Regional Hospital Board,] 1961.

MOORE, B.
The infection control sister in British hospitals. *International Nursing Review*, vol. 17, no. 1, 1970, p. 84-91.

NAHMIAS, A. J.
Infections associated with hospitals. To combat this problem, the addition of a full-time infection control nurse to the hospital staff has been proposed. *Nursing Outlook*, June 1963, p. 450-3.

Transplants, Skin Grafts, Plastic Surgery

ALSOP, J. A.
Augmentation mammaplasty. *Nursing Times*, Dec. 17, 1970, p. 1617-20.

ARGAMASO, R. V.
Skin grafts and the care of the grafted patient. *Bedside Nurse*, Nov./Dec. 1968, p. 11-4.

BIGUE, C., *and* PAPLAUSKAS-MACDONALD, R.
Heart transplants in Canada. *The Canadian Nurse*, Oct. 1968, p. 34-9.

BOIS, M. S., *and others*
Nursing care of patients having kidney transplants. *American Journal of Nursing*, June 1968, p. 1238-9, and 1242-7.

CARNEY, L., *and* CONROY, M. D.
The transplant nurse. *AORN Journal*, Dec. 1969, p. 43-4.

COOLEY, D. A.
Cardiac transplantation and the OR nurse. *AORN Journal*, Dec. 1969, p. 35-41.

DOSSETOR, J. B.
Present status of renal transplantation. *The Canadian Nurse*, Oct. 1967, p. 32-4.

FRANCIS, P. C.
Renal transplantation in Australia. *The Lamp*, Dec. 1970, p. 17-39.

HALL, G. C.
The first human heart transplantation. Groote Schuur Hospital. Ward case history. *South African Nursing Journal*, Mar. 1968, p. 27-32.

HAYTER, J.
Organ transplants—a new type of nursing? *Canadian Nurse*, Nov. 1968, p. 49-53.

HOPKINS, S. J.
Role of drugs in tissue grafting. *Nursing Mirror*, Aug. 7, 1970, p. 24.

ILLINGWORTH, CHARLES
Organ transplantation. *Nursing Times*, May 31, 1968, p. 743-4.

JENKINS, MAIR M.
Plastic surgery nursing. Macmillan, 1964.

JORDAAN, P.
The first human heart transplant. *Nursing Times*, July 19, 1968, p. 956-8.

LUNDE, D. T.
Psychiatric complications of heart transplants. *AORN Journal*, Dec. 1969, p. 86-91.

MCGREGOR, IAN A., *and* REID, WM. HENRY
Plastic surgery for nurses. Edinburgh, Livingstone, 1966.

MACLEAN, D. M., *and* FOWLER, E. A.
Heart transplant. Early postoperative care. *American Journal of Nursing*, Oct. 1968, p. 2124-7.

MAGINN, R. R.
Renal transplantation logistics and the operating room nurse. *AORN Journal*, Sept. 1969, p. 40-5.

MAGUIRE, J. M.
Natal's first heart transplant operation. An outline of the nursing service organization. *South African Nursing Journal*, July 1969, p. 7-9, 11 and 13-5.

MARTIN, A. J.
Renal transplantation: surgical technique and complications. *American Journal of Nursing*, June 1968, p. 1240-1.

MORLEY, G. H.
Plastic surgery and accidents. *Nursing Mirror*, May 5, 1967, p. i-iii.

NOLAN, B.
Transplantation of the kidney. *Nursing Mirror*, Mar. 22, 1963, p. i-iii.

RATCHFORD, P.
The first human heart transplant operation at Groote Schuur Hospital, Cape Town. *South African Nursing Journal*, Mar. 1968, p. 24-6.

STICKEL, D. L.
The law and organ transplants. *Journal of Practical Nursing*, Sept. 1970, p. 28-9, 40 and 42.

TYMAN, B. M.
The role of the nurse in renal transplantation. *AORN Journal*, Sept. 1969, p. 35-9.

WHITE, H. J. O.
Liver transplantation. *Nursing Times*, June 21, 1968, p. 820-1.

WILLIAMS, G.
Transplantation. 1. Introduction. 2. Kidney transplantation, (a) The donor. 3. Kidney transplantation, (b) The recipient. 4. Other tissues and organs. 5. Problems. *Nursing Times*, June 5, 1969, p. 711-2; June 12, 1969, p. 753-4; June 19, 1969, p. 778-81; June 26, 1969, p. 818-20; July 3, 1969, p. 849-50.

WOOD-SMITH, DONALD, *and* POROWSKI, PAULINE C., *editors*
Nursing care of the plastic surgery patient. St. Louis, Mosby, 1967.

THERAPEUTICS

ANAESTHETICS

ADRIANI, J.
Complications of anesthesia due to adjunctive drugs. *The Journal of the American Nurse Anesthetists*, Aug. 1967, p. 265-72.

ADRIANI, J.
Hyperventilation: effects on acid-base balance and circulation during anesthesia. *Journal of American Association of Nurse Anesthetists*, Feb. 1969, p. 41-8.

BELTON, M. K.
Nurse anesthetists in Canada? *The Canadian Nurse*, Jan. 1966, p. 36-7.

BERRY, M.
Anesthetist's view of the traumatized patient. *Canadian Nurse*, Nov. 1968, p. 38-41.

SPECIALITIES

BLOCH, M.
Hypothermia and its clinical considerations—1. *Nursing Mirror*, Sept. 21, 1962, p. iv.

BLOCH, M.
Hypothermia and its clinical considerations—2a. *Nursing Mirror*, Sept. 28, 1962, p. ii.

BLOCH, M.
Hypothermia and its clinical considerations—2b. *Nursing Mirror*, Oct. 5, 1962, p. xi.

BRECKENRIDGE, FLORA J., *and* BRUNO, PAULINE
Nursing care of the anesthetized patient. *American Journal of Nursing*, July 1962, p. 74-8.

BUTLER, R. O.
Induced hypothermia in cardiac surgery. *Nursing Times*, Mar. 6, 1964, p. 296-8.

CAMPBELL, M. B., *and* CLEVERDON, J.
Notes on pediatric anesthesia. *Journal of the American Association of Nurse Anesthetists*, June 1969, p. 183-96.

CARRIER, P. J., *and others*
Notes on geriatric anesthesia. *Journal of the American Association of Nurse Anesthetists*, Aug. 1969, p. 273-83.

DORNETTE, W. H. L.
Monitoring the anesthetized patient: practical aspects and legal connotations. *Journal of American Association of Nurse Anesthetists*, Dec. 1968, p. 420-5.

DURRANT, C. W.
The power of suggestion on the unconscious patient. *The Canadian Nurse*, Oct. 1968, p. 46-8.

ELLIS, M.
Cold sprays for the relief of pain. *Nursing Mirror*, June 1, 1962, p. v-vi.

FIGUEROA, MIGUEL
Anesthesia and you. *AORN Journal*, Nov. 1969, p. 49-51.

GILSTON, A.
Return to nursing. Recent advances in anaesthesia. *Nursing Mirror*, May 23, 1969, p. 29-33.

GUNN, I. P.
Current nursing issues and their implications for the preparation of nurse anesthetists. *Journal of American Association of Nurse Anesthetists*, Dec. 1968, p. 413-9.

HEHRE, F. W.
Obstetrical anesthesia: some physiological responses and common problems. *Journal of the American Association of Nurse Anesthetists*, Dec. 1970, p. 459-64.

HICKEY, MARY CATHERINE
Nursing care for patients in hypothermia.
In
AMERICAN NURSES' ASSOCIATION
Technical innovations in health care: nursing implications. New York, The Association, 1962.

HOLDERNESS, M. C.
Anaesthesia for gynaecological surgery. *Nursing Times*, Sept. 8, 1967, p. 1195-7.

JACOBSON, J.
The management of patients taking drugs prior to anesthesia. *Journal of American Association of Nurse Anesthetists*, Dec. 1968, p. 433-42.

JOHNSON, BRIAN D.
The nurse and the anaesthetic. *Nursing Times*, 1961.

KUZUCU, E. Y.
Anesthesia for obstetrics and resuscitation of the newborn. *Journal of the American Association of Nurse Anesthetists*, June 1969, p. 212-9.

LUCAS, B. G. B.
Medication before and after operation. *Nursing Times*, Sept. 17, 1965, p. 1270-2.

LUNDGAARD, M. J.
Educational programs in nursing anesthesia and related services in Minnesota Hospitals: 1955-April 1968. *Journal of American Association of Nurse Anesthetists*, Oct. 1968, p. 358-65.

LUNDY, J. S.
From this point in time: some memories of my part in the history of anesthesia. *The Journal of the American Association of Nurse Anesthetists*, April 1966, p. 95-102.

MCQUILLEN, F. A.
Nurse anesthetists in the United States. *The Canadian Nurse*, January 1966, p. 34-5.

MARROW, N.
The care of the anaesthetised patient. *Nursing Times*, Aug. 21, 1969, Occasional Papers, p. 133-5.

MINCKLEY, B. B.
Physiologic hazards of position changes in the anesthetized patient. *American Journal of Nursing*, Dec. 1969, p. 2606-11.

NORRIS, W., *and* CAMPBELL, D.
A nurse's guide to anaesthetics, resuscitation and intensive care. Edinburgh, Livingstone, 1964.
2nd edn., 1965.
3rd edn., 1967.
4th edn., 1969.

PAYNE, J. P.
Modern trends in anaesthesia. 1. Training and range of anaesthetic practice. *Nursing Mirror*, June 16, 1961, p. ii-iv.

PAYNE, J. P.
Modern trends in anaesthesia. 2. Pain Clinics, Hypnosis and Research. *Nursing Mirror*, June 23, 1961, p. vi-vii.

PESCHIN, A.
Clinical and electronic monitoring for the nurse anesthetist. *Journal of American Association of Nurse Anesthetists*, Oct. 1969, p. 371-6.

RICKS, M. J.
The explosion of knowledge and the nurse anesthetist. *Journal of American Association of Nurse Anesthetists*, Feb. 1969, p. 33-6.

ROBSON, J. G.
The newer anaesthetics. *Nursing Mirror*, Feb. 18, 1966, p. 583-5.

RUBIN, A. P.
Present value of epidural anaesthesia in obstetrics. *Midwife and Health Visitor*, Jan. 1970, p. 11-5.

RUSSELL, J. T.
Modern anaesthesia—protecting the patient. *South African Nursing Journal*, Dec. 1963, p. 7-9.

SEYMOUR, C. A.
Anaesthetics for the student nurse. *Nursing Times*, July 2, 1970, p. 844-6.

SIMMONS, P. H.
Anaesthesia for nurses. Heinemann, 1966.

SORBIE, C.
Intravenous regional anaesthesia. *Nursing Mirror*, Dec. 2, 1966, p. i-iv.

SPHIRE, R. D.
Anesthesia for neurosurgery—a challenge. *Journal of the American Association of Nurse Anesthetists*, Oct. 1970, p. 385-92.

STEPHEN, C. R.
Pediatric anesthesia. *Journal of the American Association of Nurse Anesthetists*, Dec. 1970, p. 441-7.

WALTERS, E.
Dental office anesthesia: pre-induction precautions. *Journal of the American Association of Nurse Anesthetists*, Aug. 1969, p. 285-96.

WILLIAMS, J. E.
Treatment by hypothermia in Australia. *Nursing Mirror*, Feb. 10, 1968, p. 33-41.

ZUCK, DAVID
The principles of anaesthesia for nurses. Pitman, 1969.

ZUCK, DAVID
Post-operative epidural analgesia. *Nursing Times*, Aug. 11, 1967, p. 1059-62.

DIETETICS AND NUTRITION

BAKER, AUDREY Z.
Dietetics and nutrition: a textbook for nurses and dietitians. Faber and Faber, 1964.

BECK, MARY E.
Nutrition and dietetics for nurses. Edinburgh, Livingstone, 1962.
2nd edn., 1965.

BROWN, ANN M.
Practical nutrition for nurses. Heinemann, 1966.

CABOT, E. E.
If nurses talk to dietitians food service will get better. *Modern Hospital*, Dec. 1969, p. 146.

CAREY, M. E.
Diet therapy and the nurse: dietitian's viewpoint. *Nursing Times*, April 21, 1961, p 486-9.

ERLANDER, D.
Dietetics—a look at the profession. *American Journal of Nursing*, Nov. 1970, p. 2402-5.

ENSING, E. C.
Bon appétit. A new centralised method of distributing and serving food in hospital, which enables the patients to receive their meals while hot and appetising. *Nursing Mirror*, June 28, 1963, p. x-xii.

HARRIS, C. F.
Teaching nutrition and dietetics to nurses. *Nutrition*, Winter 1963, p. 147-8.

HOWE, PHYLLIS S.
Nutrition for practical nurses. 3rd edn. Philadelphia, Saunders, 1963.
4th edn., 1967.

JENSEN, MARY, *and others*
Nursing: fundamentals of nutrition. Subject matter specifications by Mary Jensen, Doris Moses and Jeannette Poindexter; programing by Mirian Sierra-Franco. 2 vols. Michigan, Educational Systems Development, 1967.

KLUGMAN, H. B.
Nutrition in the aged. *South African Nursing Journal*, Mar. 1964, p. 7-9.

MERKEL, R., *and* BROWN, C. M.
Evaluating feeding activities in a CCU. *American Journal of Nursing*, Nov. 1970, p. 2348-50.

MIRENDA, ROSE, *and others, editors*
Nutrition and diet therapy: 1500 multiple choice questions and referenced answers, edited by Rose Mirenda, Antoinette V. Grundy and Esther K. Plotner. New York, Medical Examination Publishing Co., 1969.
[Nursing examination review book, vol. 8.]

MOWRY, LILLIAN
Basic nutrition and diet therapy for nurses. 2nd edn. St. Louis, Mosby, 1962.
3rd edn., 1966.
4th edn., 1970, by L. Mowry and S. R. Williams.

ROBINSON, CORINNE H.
Basic nutrition and diet therapy. New York, Macmillan, 1965.

RYNBERGEN, HENDERIKA J.
Teaching nutrition in nursing. 5th edn. Philadelphia, Lippincott, 1963.

SALTER, R. H.
Diet and alimentary disease—is it really "goodbye to all this"? *Nursing Times*, July 31, 1969, p. 970-1.

SHACKELTON, ALBERTA DENT
Practical nurse nutrition education. 2nd edn. Philadelphia, Saunders, 1966.

SPIKANTIA, S. G.
Nutrition of mother and child. *Nursing Journal of India*, Sept. 1970, p. 291-2 and 308.

WALIKE, B. C.
Studies of eating behavior. *Nursing Research*, Mar./April 1969, p. 108-13.

WILSON, C. T.
Speaking of food. . . . *Nursing Times*, Dec. 13, 1968, Occasional Papers, p. 195-6.

MUSIC AND ART THERAPY

BEAVERS, S. V.
Music therapy. *American Journal of Nursing*, Jan. 1969, p. 89-92.

BURWELL, D. M.
Psychodrama. *Canadian Nurse*, May 1969, p. 44-6.

FELL, J. H.
Drama and the subnormal patient. *Nursing Mirror*, Oct. 2, 1970, p. 36-7.

FORREST, C.
Music in psychiatry. *Nursing Mirror*, Dec. 13, 1968, p. 22-3.

FORSYTH, B., *and* KRATTER, F.
Music therapy. *Nursing Times*, May 19, 1967, p. 668-9.

HURLEY, H. P.
Art therapy. *Nursing Times*, Nov. 15, 1968, p. 1555-8.

NEWNHAM, W. H.
Music therapy in a neurosis centre. *Nursing Times*, Feb. 3, 1967, p. 146 and 148.

ROLLIN, H. R.
Music therapy in a mental hospital. *Nursing Times*, Sept. 18, 1964, p. 1219-22.

TAIT, E. A.
Art appreciation and the nurse. *Journal of Nursing Education*, April 1970, p. 29-33.

WALL, B. A.
Music in the mental hospital. *Nursing Times*, April 12, 1963, p. 450-1.

OXYGEN THERAPY

ADAMS, J. G.
Hyperbaric oxygen therapy. *American Journal of Nursing*, June 1964, p. 76-9.

AUGENSTEIN, D.
Hyperbaric oxygen radiation therapy. *Nursing Forum*, vol. VII, no. 3, 1968, p. 324-35.

BULTERIJS, A.
Application of oxygen under high atmospheric pressure. *International Nursing Review*, vol. 12, no. 1, 1965, p. 20-2.

CAMPBELL, D.
Oxygen therapy at home. *Nursing Mirror*, Feb. 3, 1967, p. xii-xv.

CATTERALL, M.
Oxygen therapy. *Nursing Mirror*, June 30, 1967, p. v-viii.

COCKERILL, G., *and* O'CONNOR, R.
Hyperbaric oxygenation—a new field opened for nurses. *Nursing Times*, Feb. 17, 1967, p. 216-8.

COTES, J. E.
Oxygen therapy. *Nursing Times*, Sept. 15, 1967, p. 1237-41.

SPECIALITIES

FEGAN, F. J.
Hyperbaric oxygen therapy centers. *Nursing Forum*, vol. III, no. 2, 1964, p. 90-101.

FISCHER, B. H.
Topical hyperbaric oxygen. Treatment of pressure sores and certain skin ulcerations. *Nursing Times*, May 14, 1970, p. 613-6.

FLATTER, P. A.
Hazards of oxygen therapy. *American Journal of Nursing*, Jan. 1968, p. 80-4.

GRIFFITHS, J. C.
Oxygen therapy in a high pressure environment. Recent advance in treatment. *Nursing Mirror*, Nov. 23, 1962, p. 171-3.

GUNTER, V.
Gas gangrene treated by hyperbaric oxygen. *Nursing Times*, April 24, 1969, p. 526-8.

HANSON, G. C.
Hyperbaric oxygenation. *Nursing Times*, Feb. 17, 1967, p. 213-6.

LEDINGHAM, I. McA.
High pressure oxygen. *Nursing Times*, Feb. 7, 1964, p. 171-3.

MARKS, A. E.
Hyperbaric medicine. *Journal of Practical Nursing*, Oct. 1969, p. 24-6.

MATHESON, J. G., *and* THOMSON, C. W.
Nursing severe head injuries in oxygen tents. *The Lancet*, Mar. 12, 1966, p. 591-4.

MAUDSLEY, R. H., *and others*
Experience with a hyperbaric oxygen unit. *Nursing Mirror*, Sept. 9, 1966, p. x-xii.

NEELON, V. J.
Hyperbaric oxygenation benefits and hazards. *American Journal of Nursing*, Oct. 1964, p. 73-8.

SOUTH AFRICAN NURSING JOURNAL
Hyperbaric oxygenation. *South African Nursing Journal*, Aug. 1967, p. 24-7.

SYKES, M. K.
Oxygen therapy. *Nursing Times*, Mar. 9, 1962, p. 300-2.

THURSTON, J. C. B.
Hyperbaric oxygen. *Nursing Times*, Oct. 1, 1970, p. 1271-2.

VENGER, M. J., *and* JACOBSON, J. H.
Hyperbaric oxygenation. A nursing challenge. *International Nursing Review*, vol. 12, no. 1, 1965, p. 17-9.

VENGER, M. J., *and* JACOBSON, J. H.
Nursing plans for a hyperbaric unit. *American Journal of Nursing*, Oct. 1964, p. 79-81.

ZILM, GLENNIS
Hyperbaric oxygen units—high pressure nursing. *Canadian Nurse*, Feb. 1969, p. 37-40.

PHARMACOLOGY

AMERICAN NURSING HOME ASSOCIATION
Pharmaceutical services in the nursing home. Washington, The Association, 1963.

ASHER, P.
Drugs—their administration, action and uses. *Nursing Mirror*, Jan. 3, 1964, p. 303-5.

ASPERHEIM, MARY KAYE
The pharmacologic basis of patient care. Philadelphia, Saunders, 1968.

ASPERHEIM, MARY KAYE
Pharmacology for practical nurses. 2nd edn. Philadelphia, Saunders, 1967.

AYD, F. J.
Chemical assault on mental illness—The minor tranquilizers. *American Journal of Nursing*, May 1965, p. 89-96.

BAILEY, R. E.
Aids to pharmacology for nurses. Bailliere, Tindall and Cox, 1964.
2nd edn., 1967.

BIDDLE, HARRY C., *and* SITLER, DISA W.
The mathematics of drugs and solutions: a workbook designed to supplement textbooks on drugs and solutions for schools of nursing. 7th edn. Philadelphia, Davis, 1961.

BINGLE, J.
Current antibiotics. *Nursing Times*, Oct. 15, 1965, p. 1396-9.

BLUME, DOROTHY M.
Dosages and solutions. Philadelphia, Davis, 1969.

BOYLE, JAMES A.
Lecture notes in pharmacology and therapeutics for nurses. Edinburgh, Livingstone, 1967.

CAIE, H. B.
Prescribing and administering drugs. *Nursing Times*, May 7, 1965, p. 621-3.

CASSELL, M.
A nurse views the trends in pharmaceutical dispensing practices. *Hospital Management*, June 1963, p. 80, 82 and 84.

CONWAY, B., *and others*
The seventh right [administering drugs to children]. *American Journal of Nursing*, May 1970, p. 1040-3.

COOK, ALICE C., *and* MACAW, KATHERINE D.
A mathematical guide to dosage and solutions. 2nd edn. Philadelphia, Saunders, 1962.

DAWSON, W. B.
Chemotherapy of malignant disease. *Nursing Times*, Dec. 1, 1961, p. 1563-5.

DIXON, N.
Measurement of drugs and dilution of lotions. *Nursing Times*, June 2, 1961, p. 692-4.

DOLL, R.
Recognition of unwanted drug effects—1 and 2. *Nursing Times*, Oct. 16, 1969, p. 1328-30; Oct. 23, 1969, p. 1363-5.

DOUGLAS, FRANCES N.
Essentials of pharmacology in clinical nursing. Butterworths, 1970.

EDWARDS, L. G., *and* BARKER, K. N.
Pharmacy notes for nurses. *American Journal of Nursing*, Oct. 1962, p. 68-9.

ELLIS, S.
Drug rounds in small hospitals. *Nursing Times*, Aug. 20, 1970, p. 1069-71.

EMMANUEL, S.
The clinical pharmacist and his relationship to nursing practice. *Hospital Management*, May 1970, p. 44-6, 48 and 53.

FALCONER, MARY W., *and* NORMAN, MABELCLAIRE RALSTON
The drug, the nurse, the patient. 2nd edn. Philadelphia Saunders, 1962.
2nd edn., 1962. Includes "Current drug handbook 1962-4", by Mary W. Falconer and H. R. Patterson.
4th edn., 1970.

FEINSTEIN, MAURICE B., *and* LEVINE, HARRIET, *editors*
Pharmacology: 1500 multiple choice questions and referenced answers. New York, Medical Examination Publishing Co. 1966.
[Nursing examination review book, vol. 6.]

FOGG, J.
Patients, drugs and nurses. *Nursing Times*, April 8, 1966, p. 473-5.

GARB, SOLOMON, *and* CRIM, BETTY JEAN
Pharmacology and patient care. New York, Springer, 1962.

GIBSON, JOHN
The nurse's materia medica. Oxford, Blackwell, 1965.
2nd edn., 1970.

GOODLAND, N. L.
A confusion of drugs. *Nursing Times*, Oct. 5, 1962, p. 1268-9.

GOUGH, M. A.
Teaching the care of drugs. *Nursing Times*, Mar. 5, 1965, p. 310-2.

GOVONI, LAURA E., *and others*
Drugs and nursing implications, by Laura E. Govoni, Faye Clark Berzon and Marilyn Bellini Fall. New York, Appleton-Century-Crofts, 1965.

HART, LAURA K.
The arithmetic of dosages and solutions a programmed presentation. 2nd edn. St. Louis, Mosby, 1969.

HECHT, A. B.
Self-medication inaccuracy and what can be done. *Nursing Outlook*, April 1970, p. 30-1.

HOCKEY, L.
Three Ds. Drugs—danger—disposal. *District Nursing*, Nov. 1963, p. 176-7.

HOLLIDAY, C. B.
Rebirth of folk medicine. *Nursing Mirror*, Mar. 8, 1968, p. 17.

HOPKINS, S. J.
Drugs and pharmacology for nurses. Edinburgh, Livingstone, 1963.
2nd edn., 1965.
3rd edn., 1966.
4th edn., 1968.

HOPKINS, S. J.
Psychotrophic Drugs. 1. A signpost through the maze. 2. Towards a unifying concept. *Nursing Times*, June 21, 1968, p. 837-8; June 28, 1968, p. 880-1.

HOPKINS, S. J.
Role of drugs in tissue grafting. *Nursing Mirror*, Aug. 7, 1970, p. 24.

HOPKINS, S. J.
The storage of drugs. *Nursing Times*, April 10, 1969, p. 459-61.

HYMOVICH, D. P., *and* JOHNS, M. P.
Whither pharmacology in the curriculum? *Nursing Outlook* Aug. 1968, p. 58-60.

JAMES, D. G.
The operative umbrella of drugs. *Nursing Times*, May 7, 1970, p. 587-8; May 14, 1970, p. 624-6.

JAMISON, SARA
Solutions and dosage. 4th edn. New York, McGraw Hill, 1962.

JONES, B. R.
Getting with the metric system [in the administration of drugs]. *Nursing Mirror*, Mar. 7, 1969, p. 23-5.

KEANE, CLAIRE B., *and* FLETCHER, SYBIL M.
Drugs and solutions: a programed introduction for nurses. Philadelphia, Saunders, 1965.
2nd edn., 1970.

KENNA, F. REGIS
Orienting the registered nurse: pharmacy procedures. *Hospital Topics*, July 1968, p. 39-41.

KNUDSEN, E. T.
The semi-synthetic penicillins. 2 parts. *Nursing Mirror*, Nov. 9, 1962, p. 119-22; Nov. 16, 1962, p. 147-8.

KRUG, ELSIE E., *and* McGUIGAN, HUGH ALISTER
Pharmacology in nursing. 9th edn. St. Louis, Mosby, 1963.
10th edn., 1966, by Betty Berkerson and Elsie Krug.

LEVINE, M. E.
Breaking through the medications mystique. *American Journal of Nursing*, April 1970, p. 799-803.

LEWIS, B. J.
Prescribing and handling drugs in hospital. *Nursing Mirror*, Oct. 16, 1970, p. 24-7.

MORAVEC, D. F.
A review of pharmacy for nurses. *Hospital Management*, Jan. 1968, p. 46-9; Feb. 1968, p. 68 and 70; Mar. 1968, p. 72, 75, 76.

MURPHREE, H. B.
The use of potent analgesics. *American Journal of Nursing*, Sept. 1963, p. 104-9.

NAPKE, E.
Drug adverse reaction program—and the nurse's role. *Canadian Nurse*, Dec. 1969, p. 40-3.

NAST, MINETTE
Simplified drugs and solutions for nurses; including arithmetic. 3rd edn. St. Louis, Mosby, 1964.
4th edn., 1968, by M. Nast and Norma Dison.

NIGHTINGALE, C. H.
The effect on nursing of the changing role of the pharmacist. *Nursing Forum*, vol. IX, no. 4, 1970, p. 400-7.

PARE, C. M. B.
Psychotrophic drugs and their use—1. *Nursing Mirror*, Dec. 28, 1962, p. 271-4.

PARE, C. M. B.
Psychotropic drugs and their use—2. *Nursing Mirror*, Jan. 4, 1963, p. 295-6.

PARRY, DOROTHY WALTON
Mathematics of drugs and solutions. 3rd edn. New York, Putnam, 1961.

PEEL, J. S.
Materia medica and pharmacology for nurses. 4th edn. Christchurch, New Zealand, Peryer, 1962.
5th edn., 1964.
6th edn., 1967.
7th edn., 1969.

PLEIN, JOY B., *and* PLEIN, ELMER M.
Fundamentals of medications: a text-workbook of dosages, solutions, mathematics and introductory pharmacology. Philadelphia, Lippincott, 1967.

RIDDELL, A. G.
New techniques in chemotherapy for malignant disease. *Nursing Mirror*, April 3, 1964, p. 7-8.

RIDLEY, M.
The age of antibacterial chemotherapy. *Nursing Times*, Jan. 15, 1970, p. 77-9; Jan. 22, 1970, p. 103-4; Jan. 29, 1970, p. 146-8.

ROBSON, J. M.
Drugs and placental function. *Midwife and Health Visitor*, Feb. 1970, p. 68-70.

RODMAN, MORTON J., *and* SMITH, DOROTHY W.
Pharmacology and drug therapy in nursing. Philadelphia, Lippincott, 1968.

ROSENBERG, J. M.
The team approach to collecting adverse reactions to drugs. *AORN Journal*, Oct. 1969, p. 71-6.

SAPEIKA, N.
The common tranquillisers. *Nursing Mirror*, May 13, 1966, p. 133-4.

SAXTON, DOLORES F., *and* WALTER, JOHN F.
Programmed instruction in arithmetic, dosages and solutions. St. Louis, Mosby, 1966.

SPECIALITIES

Sears, W. Gordon
  Materia medica for nurses: a textbook of drugs and therapeutics. 5th edn. Arnold, 1962.
  6th edn., 1966.

Smith, S. E.
  Drugs and hypertension. *Nursing Times*, Jan. 3, 1964, p. 21-3.

Squire, Jessie E.
  Basic pharmacology for nurses. 2nd edn. St. Louis, Mosby, 1961.
  3rd edn., 1965.
  4th edn., 1969.

Suzanne Marie, Sister
  Pharmacology for practical nurses. Philadelphia, Saunders, 1963.

Taverner, D.
  Drugs and their drawbacks. *Nursing Mirror*, Sept. 2, 1966, p. 535-6.

Tewari, S. N., *and* Blenkiron, C. H.
  A comparison of non-barbiturate sedatives in elderly patients. *Nursing Times*, Feb. 5, 1970, p. 178-80.

Thomas, S.
  Medication errors *can* be prevented. *Canadian Nurse*, May 1969, p. 50-1.

Timoney, R. F.
  Drugs: the nurse's responsibility. *Irish Nurses' Journal*, May 1969, p. 10-2.

Tonkin, Richard D.
  Nurses handbook of current drugs. Heinemann, 1961.
  2nd edn., 1967, by R. D. Tonkin and F. B. Gibberd.

Trounce, J. R.
  Pharmacology for nurses; with a chapter on anaesthetic drugs, by J. M. Hall. 2nd edn. Churchill, 1961.
  3rd edn., 1964.
  4th edn., 1967.
  5th edn., 1970.

Whittow, M.
  Problems of ward prescribing. *Nursing Times*, Dec. 1, 1967, p. 1620-2.

Worley, Eloise
  Pharmacology and medications for vocational nurses. Philadelphia, Davis, 1967.

PHYSICAL MEDICINE

Alexander, D. M., *and* Simon, G.
  Cerebral angiography. *Nursing Times*, Jan. 27, 1961, p. 116-7.

Andrews, J. T., *and* Pope, R. A.
  Radio-isotopes in medicine. *Nursing Mirror*, Feb. 16, 1968, p. 23-6.

Booth, C.
  Radiotherapy nursing. *Nursing Times*, Mar. 8, 1963, p. 290-3.

Chesney, D. N.
  Diagnostic radiology and the nurse—1. X-rays and contrast agents. *Nursing Times*, April 30, 1965, p. 580-2.

Chesney, D. N.
  Diagnostic radiology and the nurse—2. Preparing patients for radiography. *Nursing Times*, May 7, 1965, p. 624-6.

Chesney, D. N.
  Radiography of gastro-intestinal tract—1. The barium meal. 2. The barium enema. *Nursing Times*, May 14, 1965, p. 666-8; May 21, 1965, p. 704-6.

Croft, D. N.
  Radioisotopes in clinical medicine—1. The physics; thyroid function and treatment. *Nursing Times*, Oct. 18, 1968, p. 1416-8.

Croft, D. N.
  Radioisotopes in clinical medicine—2. Non-thyroid function tests. *Nursing Times*, Oct. 25, 1968, p. 1443-6.

Cullinan, J.
  Radioisotopes in medical diagnosis and investigation. *Nursing Times*, Mar. 1, 1968, p. 287-9.

Deeley, T. J., *and others*
  A guide to radiotherapy nursing, by T. J. Deeley, Joan Hart, Eliner Clarke, Joyce M. Charters and Mary McCarthy. Edinburgh, Livingstone, 1970.

Easson, Eric
  Radiation therapy. *Nursing Times*, April 17, 1964, p. 499-500.

Flatman, G. E.
  Lymphography and its adaptation for endolymphatic radiotherapy. *Nursing Times*, Oct. 18, 1968, p. 1400-2.

Goldman, Myer
  Focus on the X-ray department: emergencies. *Nursing Mirror*, Mar. 31, 1967, p. x-xiii.

Goldman, Myer
  A nurse's guide to the X-ray department. Edinburgh, Livingstone, 1967.

Goldman, Myer
  75 years of X-rays. *Nursing Mirror*, Nov. 6, 1970, p. 32-5.

Goldman, Myer
  Return to nursing. Recent advances in radiology. *Nursing Mirror*, Apr. 4, 1969, p. 36-8.

Graveling, B.
  Physiotherapy for replacement of arthritic hip. *Nursing Times*, Sept. 27, 1968, p. 1297-9.

Haines, J.
  Cold therapy used by physiotherapists. *Nursing Times*, July 12, 1968, p. 925-6.

McIntyre, P. H.
  Total body irradiation. *American Journal of Nursing*, Sept. 1961, p. 62.

Macvicar, J.
  Exercises before and after thoracic surgery. *American Journal of Nursing*, Jan. 1962, p. 61-3.

Memorial Hospital for Cancer and Allied Diseases, Nursing Division
  A handbook on radiation for nurses. New York, The Hospital [196?].

Nursing Times
  Physiotherapy helps nursing. Nursing Times, 1963.

Parker, B.
  Nursing in a radiotherapy unit. *Nursing Times*, April 17, 1964, p. 500-2.

Rees, S.
  Radiological examination of the heart. *Nursing Times*, Oct. 25, 1968, p. 1450-2.

Rummerfield, P. S., *and* Rummerfield, M. K.
  What you should know about radiation hazards. *American Journal of Nursing*, April 1970, p. 781-6.

Rusell, J. G. B.
  The place of radiology in modern obstetrics—1. *Midwife and Health Visitor*, Oct. 1969, p. 401-3.

Rusell, J. G. B.
  The place of radiology in modern obstetrics—2. *Midwife and Health Visitor*, Nov. 1969, p. 441-3.

Thomson, W.
  Protection from radiation. *Nursing Times*, June 4, 1970, p. 720-1.

Wares, E.
  Cathetron. A new word in the field of medicine. *Nursing Times*, Nov. 22, 1968, p. 1585-7.

WILD, A. A.
The nurse and the X-ray department. *Nursing Times*, Jan. 16, 1969, p. 76-7.

REHABILITATION

ALLGIRE, MILDRED J., *and* DENNEY, RUTH R.
Nurses can give and teach rehabilitation: a manual. 2nd edn. New York, Springer, 1968.

BLUNDY, M. G.
Rehabilitation day centre. *Nursing Times*, Mar. 3, 1967, p. 274-6.

BOORER, D.
Steps to independence. Industrial rehabilitation at St. John's Hospital, Lincoln. *Nursing Times*, April 22, 1966, p. 537-40.

BRAY, R. E., *and* BIRD, T. E.
Rehabilitation and resettlement—they're different. *Nursing Times*, Mar. 3, 1967, p. 280-2.

BROMPTON, A. W.
Rehabilitation in the patient's home. *Nursing Times*, Feb. 5, 1970, p. 174-7.

CAMERON, F., *and* NICOLL, S.
Industrial and social therapy. An account of the Bristol experiment in the rehabilitation of the mental patient. *Nursing Times*, Feb. 3, 1961, p. 144-6.

COOK, D. W.
The nursing contribution to rehabilitation. *Occupational Health*, May/June 1963, p. 125-32.

COOMBES, D. B., *and* ROGERS, W. H.
The way back. A resettlement unit in a mental hospital. *Nursing Times*, Mar. 16, 1962, p. 334-7.

ENGBERG, E.
Family flats with a nursing annexe; a Danish experiment for the disabled. *Lancet*, May 20, 1961, p. 1106.

FUHRER, M. J., *and others*
The nursing attendant's role in a rehabilitation setting: conceptions and attitudinal correlates. *Nursing Research*, July/Aug. 1968, p. 343-8.

GREEN, W. M., *and* COULDREY, B. M.
Rehabilitation nursing. *District Nursing*, April 1966, p. 7-9.

GROVE, E.
Occupational therapy and the nurse. *Nursing Times*, Nov. 6, 1969, p. 1423-5; Nov. 13, 1969, p. 1452-4.

HALL, LYDIA E.
The Loeb Center for nursing and rehabilitation, Montefiore Hospital and Medical Center, Bronx, New York. *International Journal of Nursing Studies*, July 1969, p. 81-95.

HALL, M. E.
Training and rehabilitation of the disabled at St. Loyes College, Devon. *Nursing Mirror*, Sept. 29, 1967, p. vii-xi.

HOWARTH, W.
Living as a totally disabled person—I. *Nursing Mirror*, Oct. 27, 1967, p. i-v.

HOWARTH, W.
Living as a totally disabled person—II. *Nursing Mirror*, Nov. 3, 1967, p. vi-ix.

JENSEN, DEBORAH MACLURG, *editor*
Principles and technics of rehabilitation nursing; by Florence Jones Terry, Gladys S. Benz, Dorothy Mereness, Frank R. Kleffner; Deborah MacLurg Jensen, editor. 2nd edn. St. Louis, Mosby, 1961.

LEOPOLDT, L.
Rehabilitation 1965 - 1967. *Nursing Mirror*, Oct. 25, 1968, p. 20-1.

LITTLE, DONNA
Nursing and the patient's motivation toward rehabilitation.
In
AMERICAN NURSES' ASSOCIATION
Nursing and the patient's motivations. New York, The Association, 1962.

LOCKHART, P.
Sheltered work centre for victims of head injury. *Nursing Times*, Dec. 8, 1967, p. 1667.

LOCKHART, P.
Social rehabilitation following severe head injuries. *Nursing Mirror*, April 17, 1964, p. 48-50.

LUNN, A. G. M.
Beauty treatment and its place in hospital. *Nursing Times*, Sept. 20, 1968, p. 1268-70.

MCNICHOLLS, J.
Back to work. The Ministry of Labour and the employment of the disabled. *Nursing Times*, Feb. 26, 1965, p. 291-2.

MARTIN, N.
The rehabilitation process. A challenge to nursing. *Occupational Health Nursing*, Nov. 1970, p. 13-6.

MARTIN, N., *and others*
The nurse therapist in a rehabilitation setting. *American Journal of Nursing*, Aug. 1970, p. 1694-7.

MAULE, H. G.
Rehabilitation of the long-term patient—1. Patients in hospital. *Nursing Mirror*, Feb. 1, 1963, p. x-xii.

MAULE, H. G.
Rehabilitation of the long-term patient—2. Accident patients. *Nursing Mirror*, Feb. 8, 1963, p. vi-vii.

MOUNTFORD, S. W.
Modern concepts of occupational therapy. *International Journal of Nursing Studies*, Nov. 1969, p. 205-14.

MYERS, E. N.
Rehabilitation after radical surgery of the tongue. *AORN Journal*, Feb. 1970, p. 55-9.

NATIONAL LEAGUE FOR NURSING,
RESEARCH AND STUDIES SERVICE
Rehabilitative aspects of nursing; a programed instruction series. Part 1. Physical therapeutic nursing measures. Unit 1. Concepts and goals. New York, The League, 1966

PAGE, S. C.
Made to order [Rehabilitation of patients at Clifton Hospital, York]. *Nursing Mirror*, Oct. 3, 1969, p. 24-5.

PLAISTED, L. M.
The clinical specialist in rehabilitation nursing. *American Journal of Nursing*, Mar. 1969, p. 562-4.

ROTHBERG, J. S.
The challenges for rehabilitative nursing. *Nursing Outlook*, Nov. 1969, p. 37-9.

RUDD, T. N.
The background to rehabilitation—1. Analysing the problem; 2. Clothes rehabilitation; 3. Rehabilitation through the mind. *Nursing Mirror*, July 9, 1965, p. 345-6; July 16, 1965, p. 373-4; July 23, 1965, p. 411-2.

RUDD, T. N.
The nurse's role in physiotherapy. *Nursing Mirror*, July 14, 1967, p. i-iii.

SABEL, M. E.
Using aids for the disabled particularly in the home. *International Journal of Nursing Studies*, Sept. 1966, p. 145-55.

SIMPSON, J.
The nurse in rehabilitation medicine. *Nursing Times*, April 23, 1965, p. 566-7.

SPECIALITIES

TENNEY, D. A.
Patients' progress—one step forward. *Nursing Outlook*, Nov. 1967, p. 30-3.

TIBBS, T.
Rehabilitating laryngectomees. *American Association of Industrial Nurses' Journal*, Feb. 1968, p. 23-6.

TIMOTHY, SISTER M.
Interdepartmental planning among nurses for rehabilitative care.
In
AMERICAN NURSES' ASSOCIATION
Effects of continuity in nursing care on patient welfare. New York, The Association, 1962.

UNITED STATES PUBLIC HEALTH SERVICE
DIVISION OF NURSING
Elementary rehabilitation nursing care. Washington, U.S. Govt. Printing Office, 1966.

WEST, W. L.
Occupational therapy philosophy and perspective. *American Journal of Nursing*, Aug. 1968, p. 1708-11.

WHEELER, A. M.
The position of psychiatric nurses working in the occupational therapy department. *Occupational Therapy*, April 1970, p. 17-21.

WHEELER, R. H.
"Nursed" factory work—a form of industrial therapy. *Nursing Times*, Feb. 18, 1966, p. 222-4.

WILKINSON, M.
Rehabilitation of patients with neurological deficit. *Nursing Times*, Mar. 3, 1967, p. 289-91.

WILLIAMS, W.
A course in rehabilitative nursing at the Devonshire Royal Hospital, Buxton. *Nursing Times*, July 23, 1965, p. 1007-10.

WILMSHURST, M. K.
"Strengthen the things which remain..." *Nursing Times*, Jan. 20, 1961, p. 75-7.

WILSON, A. B. K.
Power-driven artificial limbs. *Nursing Times*, Feb. 22, 1963, p. 233-6.

TUBERCULOSIS NURSING

ALLEN, JAMES CONSTANCE
A psychodynamic approach of the nurse in combating denial of the disease—tuberculosis.
In
AMERICAN NURSES' ASSOCIATION
Nursing approaches to denial of illness. New York, The Association, 1962.

AMROLIWALLA, F. K.
Tuberculosis today. *Nursing Times*, Sept. 6, 1968, p. 1196-8.

CADY, LOUISE LINCOLN
Nursing in tuberculosis. 2nd edn. Philadelphia, Saunders, 1961.

DAMHACHER, E., *and others*
Critique of the study: nurse specialist effect on tuberculosis. *Nursing Research*, Fall, 1967, p. 327-32.

DEWOLFE, A. S., *and* GOVERNALE, C. N.
Fear of tuberculosis and prior psychiatric experience. *Nursing Research*, Summer 1963, p. 175-80.

DRUMMOND, E. E.
Patient-centered and task-centered tuberculosis nursing. *Nursing Research*, Winter 1964. p. 56-62.

FAGERHAUGH, S. Y.
Mental illness and the tuberculosis patient. *Nursing Outlook*, Aug. 1970, p. 38-41.

FIELDER, J.
Rehabilitation of tuberculosis patients in Poland. *Nursing Mirror*, Sept. 6, 1968, p. 36-7.

FRENAY, M. A. C.
Drugs in tuberculosis control. *American Journal of Nursing*, April 1961, p. 82-5.

GRIMWOOD, J. M.
Tuberculosis control amongst the Bantu. *District Nursing*, June 1969, p. 50-1 and 54.

HLOHINEC, E. M.
Hospital care for the tuberculous child. *American Journal of Nursing*, Sept. 1968, p. 1913-5.

HOPKINS, S. J.
New treatment for tuberculosis. *Nursing Mirror*, Dec. 12, 1969, p. 30-1.

LITTLE, D. E., *and* CARNEVALI, D.
Nurse specialist effect on tuberculosis. *Nursing Research*, Fall 1967, p. 321-6.

LUNTZ, G. R. W. N.
Tuberculosis—the changing picture. *Nursing Times*, June 16, 1961, p. 756-8.

NATIONAL TUBERCULOSIS ASSOCIATION,
NURSING ADVISORY SERVICE ON TUBERCULOSIS AND OTHER
RESPIRATORY DISEASES *and* NATIONAL LEAGUE FOR NURSING
Annual nursing advisory service seminar, May 21, 1966. New York, N.L.N., 1966.

NATIONAL TUBERCULOSIS ASSOCIATION. NURSING ADVISORY
SERVICE ON TUBERCULOSIS AND OTHER RESPIRATORY DISEASES
and NATIONAL LEAGUE FOR NURSING
Nursing and the task force report to the Surgeon General and keys to improved patient care. New York, National League for Nursing, 1965.

QUARRELL, EDWARD J.
Pulmonary tuberculosis—1. *Nursing Times*, Jan. 30, 1969, p. 144-5.

QUARRELL, EDWARD J.
Pulmonary tuberculosis—2. The mycobacterium tuberculosis. *Nursing Times*, Feb. 6, 1969, p. 178-80.

QUARRELL, EDWARD J.
Pulmonary tuberculosis—3. The pathology of tuberculosis. *Nursing Times*, Feb. 13, 1969, p. 210-1.

QUARRELL, EDWARD J.
Pulmonary tuberculosis—4. Signs and symptoms of pulmonary tuberculosis. *Nursing Times*, Feb. 20, 1969, p. 242-5.

QUARRELL, EDWARD J.
Pulmonary tuberculosis—5. Nursing care of patients suffering from pulmonary tuberculosis. *Nursing Times*, Feb. 27, 1969, p. 267-8.

QUARRELL, EDWARD J.
Pulmonary tuberculosis—6. Surgical treatment for pulmonary tuberculosis. *Nursing Times*, Mar. 6, 1969, p. 309-10.

QUARRELL, EDWARD J.
Pulmonary tuberculosis—7. Community aspects of tuberculosis—1 and 2. *Nursing Times*, Mar. 13, 1969, p. 338-40; Mar. 20, 1969, p. 367-8.

STOCK, F. E.
Anterior spinal fusion—1. *Nursing Times*, April 24, 1969, p. 532-4.

STOCK, F. E.
Anterior spinal fusion—2. A radical approach to the treatment of tuberculosis of the spine. *Nursing Times*, May 1, 1969, p. 564-6.

VENEREAL DISEASE NURSING

CATTERALL, R. D.
Venereology for nurses: a textbook of the sexually transmitted diseases. English Universities Press, 1964.

HALLIS, N. O. J.
Venereology and the sexually transmitted diseases in Denmark, Sweden and Holland. *Nursing Times*, July 23, 1970, Occasional Papers, p. 105-8; July 30, 1970, Occasional Papers, p. 109-12.

MORTON, R. S.
Health education and venereal diseases. *Nursing Times*, July 21, 1967, p. 957-8.

OBAYAN, M. N.
Has the nurse any responsibility in the control of venereal disease in the Nigerian community? *Nigerian Nurse*, July 1970, p. 17-8.

SCHWARTZ, BENJAMIN
Clinical venereology for nurses and students. Oxford, Pergamon, 1966.

HOSPITALS

GENERAL WORKS

ABEL-SMITH, BRIAN
The hospitals, 1800-1948: a study in social administration in England and Wales. Heinemann, 1964.

BIRMINGHAM REGIONAL HOSPITAL BOARD
The balanced hospital community. A new concept of patient care. *Nursing Mirror*, June 9, 1961, p. 929-30.

BOLITHO, H.
Hospitals—from the patient's point of view. *Nursing Times*, July 12, 1963, p. 860-1.

CARTWRIGHT, ANN
Human relations and hospital care. Routledge and Kegan Paul, 1964.

CONSULTATIVE COUNCIL ON THE GENERAL HOSPITAL SERVICE
Nurses and our hospitals, as envisaged in the report of the Consultative Council on the General Hospital Service. *Irish Nurses' Journal*, Feb. 1969, p. 5-6 and 8.

COWAN, P.
Some observations concerning the increase of hospital provision in London between 1850 and 1960. *Medical History*, Jan. 1970, p. 42-52.

CRAIG, J. B.
King Edward's Hospital Fund for London: The Hospital Centre. *International Journal of Nursing Studies*, Dec. 1968, p. 255-64.

CRICHTON, ANNE, and CRAWFORD, MARION P.
Disappointed expectations? Report on a survey of professional and technical staff in the hospital service in Wales, 1963. Cardiff, Welsh Hospital Board, 1963.

DRAPER, P.
The functions of the district general hospital. *Nursing Times*, Jan. 8, 1970, p. 58-9.

GREAT BRITAIN—MINISTRY OF HEALTH
Abstracts of efficiency studies in the hospital service—50. Nursing: patient/nurse talk-back system; 51. Nursing: ward telephone calls. H.M.S.O., 1961.

GREAT BRITAIN—MINISTRY OF HEALTH
Abstracts of efficiency studies in the hospital service—96. Nursing: work in wards—the most time-consuming activities. H.M.S.O., 1961.

GREAT BRITAIN—MINISTRY OF HEALTH
Abstracts of efficiency studies in the hospital service—136. Nursing: Relieving nurses of non-nursing duties. H.M.S.O., 1961.

KING EDWARD'S HOSPITAL FUND FOR LONDON
HOSPITAL CENTRE
Hospital internal communications—1. The community general hospital. *Nursing Times*, Aug. 20, 1965, p. 1137-8.

KING EDWARD'S HOSPITAL FUND FOR LONDON
HOSPITAL CENTRE
Hospital internal communications—2. The community general hospital. *Nursing Times*, Aug. 27, 1965, p. 1185-6.

PINKER, ROBERT
English hospital statistics 1861-1938. Heinemann, 1966. [This book is a companion volume to Brian Abel-Smith, *Hospitals* 1800-1948.]

POWELL, ENOCH
Human relations in hospital service. An address given to the 1961 Annual General Meeting of the Association of Hospital Matrons. *Nursing Mirror*, June 23, 1961, p. 1125-6.

RYDER, M.
The community hospital—a pilot project. *District Nursing*, Dec. 1970, p. 174, 175 and 177.

THOMSON, W.
Modern trends in hospital practice. *Nursing Times*, Feb. 5, 1970, Occasional Papers, p. 21-4.

ADMINISTRATION

ALEXANDER, F. M., and ZIX, L. G.
Streamlining nurses' reports. *Hospitals*, Jan. 1, 1963, p. 48-9.

AMERICAN HOSPITAL ASSOCIATION
Administrative records in the department of nursing. *Practical Approaches to Nursing Service Administration*, vol. 9, no. 1, Winter 1970, p. 1-4.

BOGUSLAWSKI, M., and others
Tape-recording patient interviews: a minimester project. *Nursing Outlook*, May 1969, p. 41-5.

BOORER, D.
The new administration—1. United Oxford Hospitals. *Nursing Times*, Jan. 28, 1966, p. 115-6.

BOORER, D.
The new administration—2. United Liverpool Hospitals. *Nursing Times*, April 22, 1966, p. 544-5.

BOURNE, M. W.
Network analysis and commissioning the nursing services of a new hospital. *Nursing Times*, Aug. 6, 1965, p. 1070-3.

CARRIKER, D.
Automated nursing notes. *Journal of Practical Nursing*, Feb. 1970, p. 26-9.

CENTRAL HEALTH SERVICES COUNCIL,
STANDING NURSING ADVISORY COMMITTEE
Relieving nurses of non-nursing duties in general and maternity hospitals: a report by the sub-committee. H.M.S.O., 1968.

CHRISTIE, L. S.
Is hospital management all it could be? *Nursing Times*, Feb. 12, 1970, p. 218-9.

CHRISTOPOULOS, A. C.
Do you read the nurses' observation notes? [A question addressed to the doctors]. *Journal of Psychiatric Nursing and Mental Health Services*, Jan./Feb. 1970, p. 24-5.

COLLIER, C.
Domestic work in hospitals—1. Is it a problem? *Nursing Times*, Mar. 3, 1962, p. 289-92.

COLLIER, C.
Domestic work in hospitals—2. How is it managed? *Nursing Times*, Mar. 16, 1962, p. 327-30.

COLLIER, C.
Domestic work in hospitals—3. Contract cleaning? *Nursing Times*, Mar. 23, 1962, p. 369-72.

COLLIER, C.
Domestic work in hospitals—4. What can be done? *Nursing Times*, Mar. 30, 1962, p. 405 and 411-2.

DELAHANTY, M. B.
Staff-line conflict in hospitals. *The Canadian Nurse*, Nov. 1969, p. 35-7.

DONOVAN, H. M.
Principles of administration applied to the small hospital. *Nursing Outlook*, Aug. 1963, p. 568-70.

FLOYD, E. D.
Improving patients' clothing—and laundry services. *Nursing Times*, Jan. 27, 1967, p. 112-3 and 115.

GLOSTER CRUSADER VENDING LIMITED
Attitudes of nurses and others at St. Bartholomew's Hospital towards catering. Research study conducted for Gloster Crusader Vending Ltd., by Market and Opinion International. 1970.

GREENWOOD, G. A.
Multi-disciplinary management course. *Nursing Mirror*, Aug. 23, 1968, p. 32-3.

HILL, S. G.
The myth of tripartite administration. *Nursing Times*, Jan. 28, 1966, p. 103-5.

KING EDWARD'S HOSPITAL FUND FOR LONDON
HOSPITAL CENTRE
The hospital and its relationships. [Report of a conference]. *Nursing Times*, Jan. 22, 1970, p. 127.

KING EDWARD'S HOSPITAL FUND FOR LONDON
HOSPITAL CENTRE
Information services for a management by objectives programme in a psychiatric hospital [St. James' Hospital, Portsmouth]. *Nursing Times*, May 1, 1969, p. 569.

KING EDWARD'S HOSIPTAL FUND FOR LONDON
HOSPITAL CENTRE
Staff participation in management [Report of a conference] *Nursing Times*, Mar. 20, 1969, p. 357.

KITCHIN, C. H.
Who's managing whom? *Nursing Mirror*, Aug. 11, 1967, p. 447-8.

KNIGHT, J. E., and STREETER, J.
The computer as an aid to nursing records. *Nursing Times*, Feb. 19, 1970, p. 233-5.

KRIEGEL, J.
Cost control at the nurse's station. *Hospitals*, Nov. 16, 1961, p. 64 and 66-7.

McCORMICK, W.
Labour relations in hospitals. *American Journal of Nursing*, Dec. 1970, p. 2606-9.

MACRAE, A. K.
Do hospitals need an inspectorate? *Nursing Mirror*, Mar. 15, 1968, p. 11-3.

MADSEN, INGER MARGRETHE
Report on procedures on discharge of patients from hospital. Royal College of Nursing and National Council of Nurses of the U.K., 1965.

MAILLÉ, PAULINE
The philosophy of hospital administration. *Canadian Nurse*, Aug. 1963, pp. 719-22.

OLSSON, D. E.
Automating nurses' notes—first step in a computerized record system. *Hospitals*, June 16, 1967, p. 64-9.

PANTALL, J., and COND, R.
The use of job descriptions in hospital management. *Nursing Times*, July 12, 1968, Occasional Papers, p. 105-8.

PEDELTY, K. M.
The ward sister and medical records. *The Medical Record*, Nov. 1962, p. 593-5.

ROSENBERG, M., and CARRIKER, D.
Automating nurses' notes. *American Journal of Nursing*, May 1966, p. 1021-3.

ROSENBERG, M., and others
Comparison of automated nursing notes as recorded by psychiatrists and nursing service personnel. *Nursing Research*, July/Aug. 1969, p. 350-4.

ROYAL COLLEGE OF NURSING
Central supply services. Report of a conference held by the Royal College of Nursing in London, March 1962. *Nursing Times*, Mar. 16, 1962, p. 351-2.

RUSSELL, C. H.
Survey shows how doctors, nurses and hospitals agree and disagree on health care issues and outlook. *Modern Hospital*, Nov. 1970, p. 88-93 and 136.

STEIN, R. F.
An exploratory study in the development and use of automated nursing reports. *Nursing Research*, Jan./Feb. 1969, p. 14-21.

WALKER, V. H., and SELMANOFF, E. D.
A study of the nature and uses of nurses' notes. *Nursing Research*, Spring 1964, p. 113-21.

WATKIN, B.
Training nurses for top management. *International Nursing Review*, vol. 15, no. 3, 1968, p. 215-22.

WEBB, J.
The nurse and the medical records office. *Nursing Mirror*, July 27, 1962, p. 319-20.

WESTBROOK, G. M.
The nursing profession and the medical record. *The Medical Record*, May 1966, p. 253-7.

ZIMMER, J. G., and GROOMES, E. W.
An observer reliability study of physicians' and nurses' decisions in utilization review of chronic-care facilities. *Medical Care*, Jan./Feb. 1969, p. 14-20.

STAFF

BOORER, D.
The domestic administrator. *Nursing Times*, Jan. 22, 1970, p. 122-4.

GREAT BRITAIN—MINISTRY OF HEALTH
Abstracts of efficiency studies in the hospital service—42. Nursing: recording sickness of nursing staff. H.M.S.O., 1961.

GREAT BRITAIN—MINISTRY OF HEALTH
Abstracts of efficiency studies in the hospital service—69. Nursing: nurses health records. H.M.S.O., 1961.

GREAT BRITAIN—MINISTRY OF HEALTH
Abstracts of efficiency studies in the hospital service—117. Nursing: Work in out-patient departments—the allocation of duties between trained staff, auxiliary nurses and domestic staff. H.M.S.O., 1961.

GREAT BRITAIN—MINISTRY OF HEALTH
Abstracts of efficiency studies in the hospital service—138. Nursing: Ward and departmental staffing list. H.M.S.O., 1961.

KING EDWARD'S HOSPITAL FUND FOR LONDON
HOSPITAL CENTRE
Aspects of hospital management. Establishing a personnel department [Report of a conference]. *Nursing Times*, Mar. 6, 1969, p. 313.

NURSING TIMES
Volunteer service. *Nursing Times*, Jan. 14, 1966, p. 40-1.

PEPPERELL, E. M.
Staff relations in hospitals—1. Staff management. *Nursing Mirror*, July 28, 1961, p. 1405-6.

PEPPERELL, E. M.
Staff relations in hospitals—2. Recruiting and selecting staff. *Nursing Mirror*, Aug. 4, 1961, p. 1433-4.

PEPPERELL, E. M.
Staff relations in hospitals—3. The art of interviewing. *Nursing Mirror*, Aug. 11, 1961, p. 1455-6.

PEPPERELL, E. M.
Staff relations in hospitals—4. The democratic approach. *Nursing Mirror*, Aug. 18, 1961, p. 1475-6.

PEPPERELL, E. M.
Staff relations in hospitals—5. Creating high morale. *Nursing Mirror*, Aug. 25, 1961, p. 1491-2.

HOSPITALS

PEPPERELL, E. M.
Staff relations in hospitals—6. Where responsibility lies. *Nursing Mirror*, Sept. 1, 1961, p. xi-xii.

ROSENBAUM, M. J.
College students as a source of attendant help. *Perspectives in Psychiatric Care*, Sept./Oct. 1969, p. 228-34.

TURNER, W. J.
Volunteers in health and extended facilities: their role and function in the nursing home. *Bedside Nursing*, Nov. 1970, p. 24-31.

WEST CUMBERLAND HOSPITAL
Ward staffing at the West Cumberland Hospital. *British Hospital Journal and Social Service Review*, Aug. 27, 1965, p. 1640-2.

WILLCOCKS, A. J.
Filling the gap—voluntary work in the N.H.S. *Nursing Mirror*, Dec. 15, 1967, p. i-iii.

WARD CLERKS—HOTEL SERVICES

ASSOCIATION OF HOSPITAL AND WELFARE ADMINISTRATORS
Right roads and wrong ones. All administrative and clerical duties should be carried out by staff trained to perform those duties and nursing staff allowed to get on with the work for which they trained. *British Hospital Journal and Social Service Review*, June 3, 1966, p. 1022-4.

COOKE, M.
Adopting the housekeeper in the psychiatric hospital. *Nursing Times*, June 3, 1966, p. 736-8.

CRAIG, J. B.
Ward housekeepers. *Nursing Times*, May 6, 1966, p. 607-8.

CRAIG, J. B.
Ward housekeeping. *Hospital Management*, Mar./April 1970, p. 150-1.

DALY, O. M.
Ward housekeeping experiment. *Nursing Times*, July 5, 1963, p. 837-9.

ELLIOTT, F.
Ward clerks *do* help [Royal Victoria Hospital, Belfast]. *Nursing Times*, Sept. 7, 1962, p. 1138-40.

HANNIGAN, E.
How housekeeping can aid nursing. At St. John's Hospital, Hamilton, Ontario. *Canadian Hospital*, May 1961, p. 64.

HOLDER, S.
Hostesses of Harlow. *Nursing Times*, Jan. 7, 1966, p. 15-8.

JOLLY, C. R.
Hotel services for the patients. *Nursing Mirror*, July 21, 1961, p. viii-x.

KING EDWARD'S HOSPITAL FUND FOR LONDON
HOSPITAL CENTRE
Non-nursing duties in wards. *Nursing Times*, Jan. 28, 1966, p. 121-2.

KING EDWARD'S HOSPITAL FUND FOR LONDON
HOSPITAL CENTRE
Ward housekeepers. *Nursing Times*, Nov. 17, 1967, p. 1547-9.

LEICESTER ROYAL INFIRMARY
Ward assistants. *Nursing Times*, May 18, 1962, p. 637-40.

OXFORD REGIONAL HOSPITAL BOARD
Ward housekeepers: report of a study carried out at the Miller General Wing Greenwich District Hospital, Greenwich and Deptford H.M.C. Oxford, The Board, 1966.

ROBINSON, W.
A waitress service at Burton-on-Trent. *Nursing Times*, Oct. 29, 1965, p. 1481-3.

STRYKER, RUTH PERIN
The hospital ward clerk. St. Louis, Mosby, 1970.

WARREN, D. DE M.
Ward housekeepers. *Nursing Times*, Nov. 20, 1964, p. 1527-9.

WEST CUMBERLAND HOSPITAL
"As many nurses as we can afford" [deals with employment of ward clerks and waitresses]. *Nursing Times*, Nov. 26, 1965, p. 1622-4.

WILLIAMS, W.
Ward clerks at the Royal Free Hospital, London. *Nursing Times*, April 9, 1965, p. 493-5.

PLANNING

ALLEN, R. W.
Designed for nursing. *American Journal of Nursing*, Feb. 1964, p. 91-3.

ALTNAGELVIN HOSPITAL, LONDONDERRY
Matron's assessment of a new hospital. *Nursing Mirror*, Nov. 22, 1963, p. iv-v.

ASHWORTH, P. M.
Intensive care ward. Broadgreen Hospital, Liverpool. *Nursing Times*, July 3, 1964, p. 867-9.

BREGANDE, B. J.
Role of the director of nursing in planning new hospital facilities. *Nursing Forum*, vol VII, no. 4, 1968, p. 398-410.

CRAFT, N. B., and BOBROW, M. L.
New design enhances nursing efficiency. *Hospital Progress*, Oct. 1969, p. 42-4.

CRAIG, J. S.
Group corridor plan nursing units. *Canadian Hospital*, Aug. 1963, p. 43-4 and 92.

CUSDIN, S. E. T.
Hospital plans and the nurse. *Nursing Times*, Mar. 6, 1964, p. 313-4.

GREAT BRITAIN—MINISTRY OF HEALTH
Training school for nurses. H.M.S.O., 1961.
[Hospital Building Note No. 14. Includes Appendix E.]
[Reprinted with amendments, 1964.]

GREAT BRITAIN—MINISTRY OF HEALTH
Ward units. H.M.S.O., 1961.
[Hospital Building Note No. 4. Rev. edn., 1968.]

GRIFFIN, H.
Falkirk Ward: nurses' impressions. *Nursing Times*, Oct. 18, 1968, p. 1406-10.

HECTOR, W.
Called on to plan? *Nursing Times*, July 30, 1965, p. 1037-8 and 1048.

HEYWARD, J.
The nurse and hospital planning—1. The nurse's contribution to planning and design. *Nursing Mirror*, Jan. 20, 1961, p. 1430-2.
See also HUDDLESTON, R. G., and PALLISTER, R. K.

HIGH PLAINS BAPTIST HOSPITAL, AMARILLO, TEXAS
Hospital built for nurses works well for everyone. High Plains Baptist Hospital, Amarillo, Texas. *Modern Hospital*, Nov. 1970, p. 94-7.

HUDDLESTON, R. G.
The nurse and hospital planning—2. How to read a plan. *Nursing Mirror*, Jan. 27, 1961, p. 1525-7.
See also HEYWARD, J., and PALLISTER, R. K.

KAMINKER, B.
Planning the nursing unit. *Hospital and Health Management*, July 1964, p. 503.

KING EDWARD'S HOSPITAL FUND FOR LONDON
HOSPITAL CENTRE
"A crucible of humanity". Hospital planning procedures for nurses. *Nursing Times*, Jan. 17, 1964, p. 93-4 and 97.

KING EDWARD'S HOSPITAL FUND FOR LONDON
HOSPITAL CENTRE
Design of intensive care units. Report of a conference held at the Centre, July 29th, 1965. *Nursing Times*, Aug. 13, 1965, p. 116-7.

KING EDWARD'S HOSPITAL FUND FOR LONDON
HOSPITAL CENTRE
Office accommodation for nursing administration. *Nursing Times*, Oct. 4, 1968, Occasional Papers, p. 155-6.

KING EDWARD'S HOSPITAL FUND FOR LONDON
HOSPITAL CENTRE
Planning of training schools. *Nursing Times*, Mar. 4, 1966, p. 305-6.

KING EDWARD'S HOSPITAL FUND FOR LONDON
HOSPITAL CENTRE
The ward of the future. Report of a conference held at the Hospital Centre, London, December 1965. *Nursing Times*, Dec. 24, 1965, p. 1771.

LETOURNEAU, C. U.
Tandem nursing units provide flexibility of service. *Hospital Management*, Dec. 1965, p. 42-3.

MCLAUGHLIN, H.
Systems study supports triangular shapes [triangular nursing units]. *Modern Hospital*, May 1969, p. 105-9.

MCLAUGHLIN, H.
What shape is best for nursing units. *The Modern Hospital*, Dec. 1964, p. 84-9.

MOUNTFORD, P. A.
Ward plan for a new hospital. *Nursing Times*, Sept. 17, 1965, p. 1276-9.

NORTHWICK PARK HOSPITAL
The Northwick Park Project. *Nursing Times*, Mar. 18, 1966, p. 367-9.

NURSING MIRROR
The "cloverleaf" hospital. New concept in hospital design. *Nursing Mirror*, Dec. 20, 1963, p. xiii.

PALLISTER, L. K.
The nurse and hospital planning—3. Future trends in ward design. *Nursing Mirror*, Feb. 3, 1961, p. 1617-20; Feb. 10, 1961, p. 1718-20.
See also
HEYWARD, J., *and* HUDDLESTONE, R. G.

PECKHAM, A. H.
Nurses must play an active role on the hospital planning team. *Hospital Administration in Canada*, Nov. 1968, p. 61.

PETRIE, P.
Operating department planning in the United Kingdom. *International Nursing Review*, vol. 17, no. 1, 1970, p. 53-65.

QUIGLEY, C. J. P., *and* BARNES, A. L.
The importance of ward design in the socialisation of subnormal patients. *Nursing Times*, May 14, 1970, Occasional Papers, p. 67-8.

ROYAL COLLEGE OF NURSING *and*
NATIONAL COUNCIL OF NURSES OF THE UNITED KINGDOM
Hospital planning—the nurse's contribution. *British Hospital and Social Services Journal*, Dec. 11, 1964, p. 1802-3.

SCOTTISH HOME AND HEALTH DEPARTMENT
Ward design. Edinburgh, H.M.S.O., 1963.

SCOTTISH HOSPITAL CENTRE
The importance of detail. Report of a conference held at the Scottish Hospital Centre on 23rd June 1967. *Nursing Times*, Sept. 1, 1967, p. 1170.

SCOTTISH HOSPITAL CENTRE
Upgrading of wards. Edinburgh, The Centre, 1967.

SHEE, W. A.
The ward of the future. *Nursing Times*, Mar. 4, 1966, p. 288-9.

SOUTH EAST METROPOLITAN REGION, GREENWICH AND DEPTFORD HOSPITAL MANAGEMENT COMMITTEE
Greenwich district hospital: staff residential accommodation. [Greenwich, The Hospital, 1966.].

STRACHAN, D. W.
Colour in hospitals. *Nursing Times*, May 7, 1965, p. 627-9.

THOMPSON, J. D.
Efficiency and design in the hospital outpatient unit. *International Nursing Review*, vol. 10, no. 5, 1963, p. 45-9.

UNITED STATES PUBLIC HEALTH SERVICE,
DIVISION OF HOSPITAL AND MEDICAL FACILITIES
General standards of construction and equipment for nurses' residence, school of nursing, public health centers, state public health laboratories and diagnostic or treatment centers. Washington, U.S. Dept. of Health, Education and Welfare, Public Health Service, 1962.

WYLIE, N. A.
Hospital design is a nursing affair [McMaster University Health Sciences Centre]. *Canadian Nurse*, Oct. 1969, p. 42-4.

EQUIPMENT

ACTON HOSPITAL, LONDON
"Experiment disposable." Report of important trials being conducted at Acton Hospital, London. *Nursing Mirror*, Jan. 10, 1964, p .330-2.

AGNEW, K.
Medicine trolley design—report of a recent study. *Nursing Mirror*, Nov. 8, 1963, p. 137-8.

BOGASH, R. C.
The effect of disposables on the roles of the pharmacist and the nurse. *Hospital Topics*, Sept. 1965, p. 85-9.

ENSING, E. C.
The scope and value of disposables in hospital. *Nursing Mirror*, Nov. 16, 1962, p. 157-60 and 162-3.

GREEN, M. D., *and* BENNETT, M. H.
How to use disposable giving sets. *Nursing Times*, Mar. 1, 1963, p. 263-6.

HARGEST, T. S.
A new concept in patient care: the air-fluidized bed. *AORN Journal*, Sept. 1969, p. 50-3.

INTERNATIONAL WOOL SECRETARIAT
Nursing sheepskins. The Secretariat, [196?].

KING EDWARD'S HOSPITAL FUND FOR LONDON
HOSPITAL CENTRE
Design of hospital beds. *Nursing Times*, May 13, 1966, p. 632-4.

LEHR, L. W.
Disposables? *AORN Journal*, Oct. 1969, p. 88-92.

MARSH, V. W.
Nursing personnel show preference for carpeting. *Hospitals*, Nov. 16, 1969, p. 83-5.

MEADE, D. M.
Disposable bedpans. The Vernaid system. *Nursing Times*, Oct. 18, 1963, p. 1320-1.

NORTON, DOREEN
By accident or design: a study of equipment development in relation to basic nursing problems. Edinburgh, Livingstone, 1970.

NURSING MIRROR
Disposable products for hospital use. *Nursing Mirror*, May 31, 1968, p. 43-8.

NURSING MIRROR
Nurse inventor solves ward problem [a feeding table for subnormal patients]. *Nursing Mirror*, July 31, 1970, p. 30.

OXFORD REGIONAL HOSPITAL BOARD
Report of the Working Party on ward nursing facilities for long-stay patients. 3rd edn. The Board, 1968.

SCHWABACHER, H.
Disposable bedpans. *Nursing Times*, Jan. 31, 1964, p. 145-7.

SIMON, P. L.
Pilot scheme on use of disposable dressings. *Nursing Mirror*, Sept. 9, 1968, p. 19-23.

SOUTH EASTERN REGIONAL HOSPITAL BOARD, SCOTLAND
Disposable procedure pack service. *Nursing Mirror*, Sept. 19, 1969, p. 10-3.

WILMARTH, M. G.
Disposables—panacea or problem? *AORN Journal*, May 1970, p. 49-53.

WILSON, L.
A nurse's view of disposables. *Canadian Hospital*, Oct. 1970, p. 63.

HISTORY OF HOSPITALS

GENERAL WORKS

DAINTON, COURTNEY
The story of England's hospitals. Museum Press, 1961.

NADARAJAH, I.
A brief early history of the hospital services, Singapore. *Berita Jururawat*, Nov. 1968, p. 33-41.

POYNTER, F. N. L.
The evolution of hospitals in Britain. Pitman, 1964.

RISLEY, MARY
The house of healing: the story of the hospital. Hale, 1962.

SIMPSON, H. MARJORIE
The influence of professional nursing on the development of the modern hospital.
In
POYNTER, F. N. L.
The evolution of hospitals in Britain. Pitman, 1966.

HISTORY OF INDIVIDUAL HOSPITALS

ARCHER MEMORIAL HOSPITAL OF LAMONT
The Lamp is golden: Lamont and its nurses, 1912-1962. Lamont, Archer Memorial Hospital, 1962.

BLACKBURN AND EAST LANCASHIRE ROYAL INFIRMARY
A history of the Blackburn and East Lancashire Royal Infirmary, 1865-1965, by the Blackburn and District Hospital Management Committee. [Blackburn], The Committee, 1965.

BOURTON-ON-THE-WATER COTTAGE HOSPITAL
Centenary of the Bourton-on-the-Water Cottage Hospital, 1861-1961. Bourton-on-the-Water House Committee, [1961].

BRISTOL. UNITED BRISTOL HOSPITALS
A history of the United Bristol Hospitals. Bristol, the Board of Governors of the United Bristol Hospitals, 1965.

BROMLEY HOSPITAL, KENT
Centenary of Bromley Hospital, 1869 to 1969. A commemorative record compiled for the Bromley Hospital Management Committee by Sydney W. Collett. Farnborough, Kent, The Committee, 1969.

CHARING CROSS HOSPITAL
The two pillars of Charing Cross: the story of a famous hospital, by R. J. Minney. Cassell, 1967.

CLATTERBRIDGE HOSPITALS
A short history of Clatterbridge Hospitals, by the Central Wirral Hospital Management Committee. Wirral, the H.M.C., 1966.

DINGLETON HOSPITAL, MELROSE
The past, the present and the future. [Galashiels, Meigle Printers, 1969].

EAST LONDON HOSPITAL
East London Hospital for Children, Shadwell, 1868-1963. Queen Elizabeth Hospital for Children, Shadwell by V. A. J. Swain and L. Woodall. *British Medical Journal*, Dec. 14, 1968, p. 694-9.

ELIZABETH GARRETT ANDERSON HOSPITAL
Elizabeth Garrett Anderson Hospital Centenary, by Janet Aitken. *British Medical Journal*, Aug. 6, 1966, p. 354-5.

EVELINA HOSPITAL
The Evelina: the story of a London children's hospital, 1869-1969, by H. E. Priestley. Guy's Hospital, 1969.

KINGSTON PUBLIC HOSPITAL, JAMAICA
History of Kingston Public Hospital. *The Jamaican Nurse*, April 1966, p. 19 and 22.

LANCASTER MOOR HOSPITAL
Lancaster Moor Hospital 150th anniversary, 1816-1966 by the North Lancashire and South Westmorland Hospital Management Committee. Lancaster, The Committee, [1966].

LAWN HOSPITAL, LINCOLN.
One hundred and fifty years at the Lawn, by B. L. Melton [The Author, 1969?].

LEEDS GENERAL INFIRMARY
The General Infirmary at Leeds. Vol. I: the first hundred years, 1767-1869, by S. T. Anning. Livingstone, 1963.
Vol. II: the second hundred years, 1869-1965. 1966.

LONDON HOSPITAL
The London: a study in the voluntary hospital system by A. E. Clark-Kennedy. Pitman, 1962-63.
Vol. I: the first hundred years, 1740-1840. 1962.
Vol. II: the second hundred years, 1840-1948. 1963.

NEWCASTLE GENERAL HOSPITAL
The history of Newcastle General Hospital, [1870-1966], by George Hurrell, assisted by George P. Harlan. Newcastle upon Tyne, Newcastle upon Tyne Hospital Management Committee, [1967].

NEW PLYMOUTH PUBLIC HOSPITAL, NEW ZEALAND
New Plymouth Public Hospital Centenary, by K. A. Hood. *New Zealand Nursing Journal*, Mar. 1967, p. 11-12.

PRINCE OF WALES'S GENERAL HOSPITAL, TOTTENHAM
The Prince of Wales's General Hospital, Tottenham: a centenary history by Brian Watkin. Tottenham Group H.M.C., 1967.

QUEEN VICTORIA HOSPITAL, EAST GRINSTEAD
Celebrating a centenary, by M. A. Duncombe. *International Nursing Review*, vol. 10, no. 3, 1963, p. 38-42.

QUEEN'S HOME AND THE QUEEN VICTORIA MATERNITY HOSPITAL, ADELAIDE, SOUTH AUSTRALIA
A brief history of the Queen's Home and the Queen Victoria Maternity Hospital, Adelaide, South Australia. *The South Australian Journal of Nursing*, Dec. 1966, p. 8-10.

RADCLIFFE INFIRMARY, OXFORD
A short history of the Radcliffe Infirmary, by A. H. T. Robb-Smith. Oxford, Church Army Press for United Oxford Hospitals, 1970.

THE RETREAT, YORK
A history of The Retreat at York—I., by M. R. Glover. *Nursing Mirror*, Aug. 7, 1964, p. 413-4.

THE RETREAT, YORK
A history of The Retreat at York—II. by M. R. Glover. *Nursing Mirror*, Aug. 14, 1964, p. 442-4.

THE RETREAT, YORK
A history of The Retreat at York—III, by M. R. Glover. *Nursing Mirror*, Aug. 21, 1964, p. 462-4.

ST. JOHN'S HOSPITAL FOR DISEASES OF THE SKIN
St. John's Hospital for Diseases of the Skin, 1863-1963, edited by Brian Russell. Edinburgh, Livingstone, 1963.

St. Leonard's Hospital, Shoreditch
St. Leonard's Hospital, 1863-1963: a short history by D. A. Brassett. Priv. print., 1963.

St. Thomas' Hospital
St. Thomas' Hospital, by E. M. McInnes. Allen & Unwin, 1963.

Salisbury General Hospital
Salisbury 200: the bi-centenary of Salisbury Infirmary, 1766-1966, by members of the hospital staff. Salisbury, The Hospital, 1967.

Vancouver General Hospital
Annual report, 1962. (Diamond jubilee issue, including the history of the hospital from 1902). Vancouver General Hospital, 1962.

Victoria Hospital For Children, London
The Victoria Hospital for Children, a short commemorative history, 1866-1964, by George Edwards. St. George's Hospital, 1964.

Victoria Infirmary, Glasgow
The Victoria Infirmary of Glasgow: history of a voluntary hospital 1890-1948, by Ian Murray. Glasgow, C. L. Wright, 1967.

Westminster Hospital
Westminster Hospital, 1716-1966, by J. G. Humble and Peter Hansell. Pitman, 1966.

Worcester State Hospital, Massachusetts
The state and the mentally ill: a history of Worcester State Hospital in Massachusetts, 1830-1920, by Gerald N. Grob. Chapel Hill, University of North Carolina Press, 1966.

Yeatman Hospital, Sherbourne
A century of service: the story of the Yeatman Hospital [Sherborne], 1866-1966, by Elizabeth O. Cockburn and J. Elise Gordon. Sherborne, The Friends of the Yeatman Hospital, 1966.

SPECIAL DEPARTMENTS AND UNITS

Arrowsmith, Ron
Geriatric welfare institutions management; nursing administration. Ottawa, 1967.

Central Health Services Council
Standing Nursing Advisory Committee
Duties of nurses in out-patient departments. H.M.S.O., 1965.

Confederation of Health Service Employees
Survey of nursing services of certain general psychiatric and mentally subnormal hospitals for the purpose of establishing the necessity for a Royal Commission in accordance with the resolution adopted by the T.U.C. September 1962. The Confederation, 1963.

Great Britain—Ministry of Health
Abstracts of efficiency studies in the hospital service—97. Nursing: work in out-patient departments—the most time-consuming activities. H.M.S.O., 1961.

James, F. R.
Family-centred nursing at the Cassel Hospital. *Nursing Times*, Aug. 4, 1961, p. 999-1002.

Lee, J. M.
Outpatients departments—1. How to run an outpatient clinic; 2. The medical clinic; 3. The surgical clinic; 4. The *Nursing Times*, Sept. 9, 1966, p. 1183-4; Sept. 16, 1966, p. 1233-4; Sept. 23, 1966, p. 1267-8; Sept. 30, 1966, p. 1292-4.

Mauksch, Ingelborg Grosser, *project director*
A community-wide approach to the study of nursing activities in hospital outpatient departments. Chicago, Council on Community Nursing, 1963.

Norton, Doreen
Hospitals of the long-stay patient: a study of their practical nursing problems and solutions. Oxford, Pergamon, 1967.

Pearson, R. J. C.
Outpatient nursing: sisters' views. *Nursing Times*, June 23, 1967, p. 834-5.

Rayner, Claire
Essentials of outpatient nursing. Arlington Books, 1967.

Schulz, Esther D., *and* Rudick, Eleanor
Nursing in ambulatory units. Dubuque, Iowa, Brown, 1966.

INDEX 1859-1960

a, after page number denotes the left hand column of the page
b, after page number denotes the right hand column of the page

Abbott, M. E. S., 1a, 15b
Abbott, R. D., 115a
Abdellah, F. G., 58a, 62a, 64b, 69b, 79b, 82a
Abel-Smith, B., 2b
Aberg, H. L., 79b
Abraham, S., 87b
Ackner, B., 107b
Acland, Sir H. W., 91a
Adams, A. O., 27b, 44b, 58a, 68b, 70a
Adams, A. R. D., 95a
Adams, G. K., 11b
Adams, H., 107a
Adams, M. L., 103b
Adams, M. M., 103b
Adams, R., 8a, 72b
Adams, W. S., 88b
Adamson, F. K., 104a
Adelson, D., 122b
Adranvala, T. K., 39a
Afleck, J. W., 116a
Agate, M. A., 49a
Agnew, G. H., 82a
Agnew, L. R. C., 15b
Ahla, A. M. M., 110b
Ahla, M., 56a
Aikenhead, M. A., 130b
Aikens, C. A., 49a, 60a, 92b, 126b
Aikin, R. C., 108b
Aird, E., 95a
Aitken, R. S., 126a
Aitkenhead, M., 11b
Aitken-Swan, J., 87a
Akester, J., 89b
Akester, J. M., 33a, 39a, 112a, 116a
Alabama University. Committee on Human Relations, 63b
Alcott, L. M., 8b
Aldis, M., 15b
Alexander, E. L., 118a
Alexander, J., 118b
Alford, B. L., 31a
Alger, G. W., 19a
Alinquist, 39a
Alkin, E., 11b
Allan Memorial Institute of Psychiatry. McGill University, 104a
Allemang, M., 79b
Allen, D. E., 3b, 52a
Allen, M., 22a, 58b
Allgire, M. J., 124a
Alline, A. L., 54a
Allwood-Paredes, J., 110a
Alma, Sister, 92b
Almack, J. C., 117b
Aloysia, Sister, 48a
Aloysius, Sister M., 8b
Alphonsa, Mother (R. H. Lathrop), 14b
Alsop, H. A., 11b
Altschul, A., 28a, 51a, 104a, 107b
Amadeus, Sister, 79a
Amberg, E., 2b
American Association of Industrial Nurses, 98a, 98b, 100a, 100b
American Association of Industrial Nurses. Committee on Education, 100a
American Association of Industrial Nurses. Management Advisory Council, 100a
American Association of Medical Social Workers, 39a
American Association of Nurse Anaesthetists, 32b

American Brake Shoe Company. Medical Department, 98b
American Cancer Society, 87a
American College of Nurse-Midwifery, 96b
American Conference of Governmental Industrial Hygienists, 100a
American Dietetic Association. Professional Education Committee, 122a
American Hospital Association, 34b, 36a, 66a, 68b, 70a, 72b, 73a, 118b
American Hospital Association. Division of Nursing, 68b
American Journal of Nursing, 28a, 31a
American Library Association. Joint Committee on Standards for Hospital Libraries, 51a
American Medical Association, 39a
American Medical Association. Council on Industrial Health, 32b, 98b
American National Red Cross Society, 7b
American Nurses' Association, 26a, 28a, 34b, 36b, 60a, 64b, 70a, 71a, 72a, 83a, 110a, 112b
American Nurses' Association. Industrial Nurses' Section, 98b
American Nurses' Association. Public Health Nurses' Section, 112b
American Nurses' Association. Research and Statistics Unit, 58a
American Nurses' Foundation, 39a, 58a
American Nurses' Foundation. International Nursing Project, 28a
American Public Health Association, 124b
American Red Cross Society, 116b
American School of Home Economics, Chicago, 94a
American Society of Superintendents of Training Schools for Nurses, 28a
Amidon, B., 26a
Amieriro, M., 127b
Amor, A. J., 100b
Anderson, A., 98b
Anderson, B. E., 26a, 32b, 33a, 48b
Anderson, C. E., 2a
Anderson, G., 5b
Anderson, G. W., 91a
Anderson, J., 92b
Anderson, J. W., 38b
Anderson, L., 57a
Anderson, L. C., 58a, 66a
Anderson, M., 11b
Anderson, M. C., 23a
Anderson, M. E., 109a
Anderson, R., 48a
Anderson, T., 89a
Andrell, M., 64b
Andrewes, F. W., 34b
Andrews, —, 5b
Andrews, C. T., 15b
Andrews, H. R., 96b
Andrews, M. R. S., 15b
Andrews, M. S., 119b
Annis, J. W., 79b
Anon, 23b
Apley, J., 101b
Appleyard, M. L., 11b
Archard, T., 8b
Archer, P., 27b
Archibald, —, 1a
Ardley, D. G., 123a
Arkansas State Nurses' Association, 67b

Arkle, A., 4b
Arlitt, A. H., 101b
Armiger, B., 39a, 68b
Armitage, C. P., 112b
Armstrong, I. L., 101b
Armstrong, K. F., 49b, 75b, 86a, 93b, 119b
Arnold, V., 20a
Arnstein, M., 39a
Arnstein, M. G., 15b, 41b, 58a, 60a, 67b, 68b, 69a, 70a, 91a, 112b
Arthritis and Rheumatism Foundation, 92b
Ashby, I. M., 13a
Ashby, L. E., 35b, 112b
Ashdown, A. M., 73a, 85a
Asher, P., 93a, 117b
Ashford, M. E., 95b
Associated Hospital Service of New York, 110b
Association of Collegiate Schools of Nursing, 46b
Association of Hospital Matrons, 66a
Association of Women Science Teachers, 48b
Atherton, W. H., 15a
Athlone, Earl of, 25a
Atkins, H. J. B., 119b
Atkinson, W. J., 119b
Atlee, H. B., 39a
Atteberry, M., 66a
Aubuchon, M., 13a
Auckland Psychiatric Hospital, 128b
Auerbach, A. B., 96b
Aufhauser, T., 49a, 101b
Austen, A., 33b
Austen, K., 11b
Austin, A. L., 1a, 56b, 58a
Austin, C. L., 89b
Australian Army Nursing Service, 4b
Australian Nurses' Association, 28a
Aveling, J. H., 96b
Averill, L. A., 109a
Avery, L. M., 22b
Aydelotte, M. K., 80a
Aylett, S., 119b
Ayllon, T., 104a
Aynes, E. A., 12a, 39a

Baarslag, C. A. La B., 23b
Bacala, J. C., 20a
Baggallay, O, 20a, 57a
Bagot, R. A., 73a
Bahirathi, 101b
Bailey, E. C., 100a
Bailey, H., 93a, 104a, 118a
Bailey, J. T., 58a
Bailey, M. E., 66a
Baker, N. B., 12a
Baker, R., 17b
Baker, S. M., 64b
Baker, T. J., 119a
Bakst, H. J., 110b
Baldwin, J. C., 101b
Ball, F. E., 36b
Ball, R. M., 33b
Balme, H., 39a
Bancroft, M. C., 101b
Banfield, M., 11b
Banfill, B. J., 22b
Barbee, G. C., 32b
Barckley, V., 87a, 104a
Barclay, J., 36b
Barclay, M. K., 73a

Barfield, K. A., 98b
Bark, E., 7b
Barnett, E. A., 65b, 77a
Barnett, R. P., 2b
Barnowe, T. J., 69a
Barr, A., 34b, 35a, 39a
Barrett, J., 66a
Barrington, B. G., 112b
Barrington, S. E., 131a
Barrus, C., 104a
Barschak, E., 98b
Barth, R. S., 15b
Bartlett, H. C., 29a
Barton, C., 7b, 11b
Barton, E. C., 6b, 11b, 65b, 72a
Barton, G., 8b
Barton, J., 80a
Barton, P. H., 103b
Barton, W., 11b
Barwell, R., 73a
Batchelor, R. C. L., 125b
Bateman, F. J. A., 73a
Baumberger, T. S., 38a
B.C.H., 64b
Beachcroft, C. M., 12a
Beal, J. M., 79a
Beams, R., 127b
Beard, M., 110a
Beard, R. O., 50b
Beardsley, J. M., 119b
Beasley, F. A., 95b
Beatrice, Sister, 12a
Beattie, I. T., 112b
Beatty, M. M., 66a
Beatty, W. K., 31a, 51a
Beauchamp, P., 8b
Beauclair, R. R., 81b
Beaudin, N. R., 33b
Beaumont, W., 124a
Beccle, H. C., 104a
Beck, F., 41b
Beck, M. B., 60a
Beckett, J. D. H., 67b
Beckett, J. S., 73a
Beeby, N. V., 31a
Befers, E. C., 126a
Behrer, M. R., 92b
Beith, J. H., 4b
Belcher, C. D., 80a
Belcher, H. C., 39a, 43a
Belcher, J. R., 118a
Belilios, A. D., 73a
Belknap, E. L., 98b
Bell, A. T., 116a
Bell, C., 92a
Bell, D., 35a
Bell, H. G., 39a
Bell, J., 119b
Bell, L. M., 56b
Bellevue Hospital, New York, 56a, 128b
Bellevue Hospital, New York.
   Training School for Nurses, 56a, 73a
Benedict, J., 130a
Bennallack, F. M., 80a
Benne, K. D., 20a, 46b
Bennett, A., 123b
Bennett, A. E., 104b
Bennett, B. A., 3a, 24b, 36b, 39a, 48a, 73a, 85a
Bennett, S. V., 36b
Bennis, W., 20a
Bentley, R. S., 20a
Benz, E. G., 58a, 69a
Benz, G. S., 101b
Berg, M. J., 66a
Berke, M., 70b
Berkeley, C., 24b, 90a
Berkowitz, J. E., 39a
Berkowitz, N. H., 39a
Berman, P., 73a
Bernadette de Lourdes, Sister, 89b
Bernard, J., 62a
Bernstein, E., 67b
Berry, E. C., 118a
Berry, F. D., 16a
Berthiaume, A. B., 39a

Bertozzi, E., 58a
Bertrande, Sister, 39b
Best, S. H., 7b
Bethlehem Hospital, 128b
Bett, W. R., 1a
Bevington, S. M., 24b
Bews, D. C., 100a
Beyerl, M. C., 38a
Bickerdyke, M. A., 12a
Bickerton, —, 12a
Bickford, E., 118a
Bicknell, E. P., 7b
Biddle, H. C., 87b, 122b
Bien, R. V., 73a, 122a
Bietsch, E. M., 80a
Billington, M. F., 7b, 16a
Billroth, C. A. T., 73a
Birch, C. A., 93a
Bird, A. H. K., 36b
Bird, B., 62a, 120a
Bird, E. P., 73a
Birdwood, G. T., 96b
Birmingham and Midland Eye Hospital, 128b
Birmingham Children's Hospital, 103a
Birmingham General Hospital, 128b
Birmingham Regional Hospital Board.
   Mental Health Services Committee, 107a, 107b, 127a, 127b
Bishop, T. H., 11b, 18b
Bishop, W. J., 16a, 20a
Bixler, G. K., 20a, 45a, 52a
Bixler, R. W., 20a, 45a
Bjornstad, E. M., 129b
Black, A., 50b, 112a
Black, C. V., 18a
Black, I., 110a
Black, K., 46b, 104b
Blacker, H., 108a
Blacklock, C., 62a
Blackwood, B., 47a
Blackwood, M. D., 110b
Blair, D., 13a, 104b
Blair, J., 60a
Blair, L. B., 73a
Blair-Fish, H. M., 27b
Blake, E. L., 58a
Blake, F. G., 66a, 101b
Blanchfield, F. A., 12a
Bleakley, E., 2b
Bleazby, E., 85a
Bliss, A. R., 104a
Block, L., 45b
Blocker, T. G., 119a
Blockley Hospital, Philadelphia, 128b
Blomfield, J., 131b
Bluestone, E. M., 80a
Blumberg, A., 63b
Blumenthal, A., 123a
Boak, E., 98b
Boardman, M. T., 7b
Bocock, E. J., 85a, 86a
Bodine, W., 80a
Bodley, —, 6b
Bodley, A. M. E., 12a
Boek, W. E., 116a
Bogardus, E. S., 62a
Böge, E., 65b, 110b
Bogie, H., 104b
Bojar, S., 80a
Bolduan, C. F., 86a
Bolduan, N. W., 86a
Bolliger, W., 70b
Bomford, M. K., 127b
Bond, D. H., 31a
Bone, A. I. C., 39b
Bonell, P. R., 120a
Bonham-Carter, H., 2b
Bookmiller, M. M., 96b
Booth, S., 87a
Borcherds, M. G., 31b
Boshowers, H., 67b
Bosquet, M. M., 94a
Boston Children's Hospital, 128b
Boston Children's Hospital. School of Nursing, 56a

Boston Floating Hospital, 128b
Boston University School of Nursing, 69a
Botts, W. H., 70b
Bourne, A. W., 96b
Bourne, P. J., 80a
Bowden, J., 8b
Bowditch, N. I., 130a
Bowe, A. B., 80a
Bowe, E. J., 2a, 22b
Bower, A. G., 91a
Bowers, H. G., 110a
Bowers, L., 63b
Bowlby, A. A., 130b
Bowser, T., 8b
Box, K., 26a, 38a
Boyd, D. D., 79b
Boyd, H., 60a
Boyd, L. C., 3b, 50b
Boyer, V. S., 70b
Boyle, R. E., 58b, 62a
Boyles, E. R., 82b
Boylston, H. D., 11b
Boynton, R., 90b
Bracker, M., 130a
Brackett, M. E., 39b, 52a
Bradley, E. M., 12a
Bradshaw, A. F., 14b
Bradshaw, M. C., 117a
Brady, K., 110b
Bragdon, J. S., 49a, 120a
Brainard, A. M., 5b, 115a
Brand, M., 98b
Brandon, A. N., 51b
Branson, H. K., 35a
Brantl, V. M., 119a
Brass, R., 104b
Braun, A. E., 46a
Breay, M., 2b, 29a, 30a, 35a, 56b, 72a, 96b, 110b, 128a, 129a, 131b, 132a
Brech, E. F. L., 66a
Breckenridge, S. D., 121a
Breckinridge, M., 3b
Bredenberg, V. C., 48a, 58b, 66a, 69a
Bredow, M., 93a
Breen, G. E., 91a
Bregg, E. A., 49a
Bresnahan, D., 70b
Bressler, M., 26a
Brethorst, A. B., 49a, 62a
Brewerton, H., 12a
Bridge, B. C., 52a
Bridge, H. L., 73b
Bridges, D. C., 20a, 48a, 64b, 73b, 80a
Bridgman, M., 39b, 46a
Bridson, —, 12a
Briess, L., 49a
Briggs, G. G. B., 7b
Briggs, S. L., 94a
Brigh, M., 79a
Bright, P., 24b
Brinton, M. W., 12a
Bristol Eye Hospital, 128b
Bristol Royal Infirmary, 118a, 128b
Bristowe, L. S., 30a
British Hospitals Association, 25b, 55b
British Journal of Nursing, 3a
British Medical Association, 3a, 94a
British Medical Journal, 8b, 38a
British Nurses' Association, 3a, 28a
   (See also: Royal British Nurses' Association)
British Red Cross Society, 7b
Britten, J. D., 73b
Broadhurst, J., 28a, 86b
Broadwell, L., 74b
Brockbank, W., 130a
Brodie, E. P., 123b
Brodie, J., 36a
Brodman, E., 58b
Brodrick, A. L., 4b
Brody, W., 112b, 115a
Broe, E., 39b, 41b
Broer, M. R., 39a
Brogan, J. M., 60a
Broglie, Prince E. de, 14b

Brompton Hospital, 129a
Brookes, H. S., 120a
Brooklyn Hospital. Orthopaedic Dispensary and Training School for Nurses, 51a
Brooks, L., 116b
Brooks, S. M., 49a
Brooksbank, M., 128a
Brotherston, J. H. F., 20a
Browder, J. J., 101b
Brower, J. V., 91a
Brown, A. F., 38a, 46b, 49a, 51a, 58b, 73b, 93a
Brown, B. J., 49a, 119a
Brown, C. A., 39b, 73b
Brown, E. L., 26a, 80a, 112b
Brown, F. J., 62a, 89b
Brown, G. L., 96b
Brown, J. P., 87b
Brown, J. R., 89b
Brown, L. G., 127b
Brown, M. L., 35a, 98b, 100a, 100b, 117b, 122a
Brown, M. M., 104b
Brown, S., 119a
Browne, O. T. D., 96b, 131a
Browne, S., 4b, 65b
Brownell, K. O., 73b
Bruen, E., 73b
Bryan, E. S., 112b
Bryan, M. de G., 35b
Bryant, A., 70b
Bryant, R. D., 98a
Bryant, V., 90b
Buch, F. S., 125b
Buchanan, M. E., 73b
Buchanan, S. H., 124b, 125a
Buckingham, M. A., 12a
Buckinghamshire County Council. North Bucks Technical Education Committee, 5b
Buckley, A. C., 96a
Buckoke, L., 24b
Budd, E., 118a
Buechel, J. F. M., 45a
Buffham, A. H., 131a
Bulkley, L. D., 88a
Bull, T., 96b
Bullock, R. P., 26b
Bullough, J., 92a
Bulman, M. W., 96b, 118a
Bundy, E. R., 85a
Bunford, A. M., 5b
Bunge, H. L., 40a, 58b
Burbridge, D. H. D., 83a
Burden, J., 24b
Burdett, H. C., 24b, 35a, 126b, 127b
Burdon, I. M., 85a
Burgess, E. C., 12a
Burgess, M. A., 34b, 54a
Burke, C., 107b
Burkett, J. E., 116a
Burleigh, A. L., 12a
Burleigh, K. L., 12a
Burling, T., 64a, 126b
Burns, M. G., 36b
Burr, A. M., 103a
Burr, M., 39b, 45a
Burton, D. E., 71a
Burton, G., 62a
Busche, M. J., 63b
Bush, C. K., 69a
Bushby, A. M., 12a
Butler, G., 70b
Butterley Company. Medical Department, 100b
Butterworth, Lady, 129a
Button, D., 86a
Buxton, O. V., 125a
Byrne, A., 112b

Cable, J. V., 93a
Cabot, H., 120a
Cabot, R. C., 73b
Cadbury, M. C., 12a

Cadmus, R. R., 82a
Cadogan, W., 101b
Cady, L. L., 125a
Cafferty, K. W., 50b
Cairney, J., 85a, 85b, 90a, 118a
Cairns, E., 54a
Calabro, A. M., 98b
Calder, J. M., 1a
Calderwood, C., 119a
California State. Department of Public Health, 103b
California State Nurses' Association, 67b
Callahan, J., 37b
Callaway, C. S., 95b
Calvet, J., 19a
Calvey, Sister M. E., 63a
Camara, A., 23b
Cambray, P. G., 7b
Cambridge School of Nursing, Mass., 56a
Cameron, C. M., Jr., 110a
Cameron, D., 100b
Cameron, H., 12a
Cameron, H. C., 129b
Campbell, A. D., 90a
Campbell, D., 105b
Campbell, F., 94a
Campbell, J., 103b
Campbell, M., 52a, 116a, 130a
Campbell, M. F., 56b
Campbell, P. E., 83a
Campion, F. L., 92a
Canada. Department of National Health. Civil Service Health Division, 100b
Canada. Dominion Bureau of Statistics, 110b
Canadian Nurses' Association, 22b, 28a, 47a, 58b, 66a, 67b
Candland, L., 99a
Canfield, S. A. M., 54a
Cantlin, V. L., 120a
Capes, M., 103a
Caplan, H., 101b
Caraman, E., 12a
Card, W. I., 20a
Cardew, E. C., 49a
Cardew, E. M., 47a
Carey, H. W., 86b
Carey, M., 91b
Carini, E., 120a
Carling, E. R., 126a
Carlisle, B., 82b
Carlson, H. E., 89a
Carmichael, F. A., 104b
Carmon, M. C., 97a
Carpenter, H. M., 64b, 112b
Carroll, M. F., 31a
Carse, J., 95b
Carson-Rae, A., 12b
Carter, D., 112b
Carter, G. B., 24b, 47a, 58b
Carter, G. M. M., 125a
Cartrell, M., 22b
Carvisiglia, F. F., 119b
Cascio, J., 132a
Case Western Reserve University. Frances Payne Bolton School of Nursing. See Frances Payne Bolton School of Nursing
Caseley, D. J., 73b, 93a
Cassie, E., 103b
Cassinari, E., 14a
Catchings, M. W., 116b
Cates, J. E., 88b
Cathcart, H. R., 39b
Catherine de Jesus Christ, 60b
Catherine of Sienna, Saint, 12b
Catholic University of America, 46a, 49a, 58b, 69a
Catto, I. M., 112b
Caufield, W. B., 73b
Cavaglieri, N., 62b, 87a
Cavell, E., 12b
Cavers, A. S., 58a

Cavey, M., 107b
Caws, A. G., 52a
Central Committee for the State Registration of Nurses, 3a
Central Council for District Nursing in London, 5b, 28a
Central Council for Health Education, 62a
Central Hanover Bank & Trust Co., New York, 112b
Central Health Services Council, 62a, 103a
Central Health Services Council. Standing Nursing Advisory Committee, 8a, 71a
Central Midwives' Board, 97b
Chadwick, M., 104b, 109a
Chagas, A. W., 31b
Chalke, H. D., 116b
Chaloner, L., 110b
Chamberlain, E. N., 93a
Chamberlain, R., 20a
Chambers, L., 80a
Champion, R., 119a
Chandler, E. M., 87a, 124a
Chang, R. K., 91b
Chant, O., 64b
Chapanis, A., 59b
Chapman, —., 104b
Chapman, J., 104b
Chapman, M. P., 54b
Chard, S. D., 99a
Charing Cross Hospital, London, 56a
Charles, E., 49a, 90b
Charles Marie, Sister, 39b
Charleton, J. W., 52a
Charley, I. H., 6b, 99a
Charlotte, Sister, 70b
Chase, J. A., 12a
Chase, R. H., 107b
Chayer, M. E., 26b, 116b
C.H.C., 73b
Chester Royal Infirmary, 129a
Chetwynd, C. A., 73b
Chiga, D. E., 80a
Child, L. M., 94a
Chittick, R., 2a, 22a, 52a, 58b
Christ, E. A., 3b, 64a, 65a, 68a
Christian, H.R.H. Princess, 30a
Christman, L., 82b
Church Home and Hospital, Baltimore, 56a
Churchill, S., 94a
City of London Hospital for Diseases of the Heart and Lungs, 129a
Civil Service Chronicle, New York, 39b
Clancey, I. L., 108a
Clare, Saint, 5a
Claridge, S. A., 12b
Clark, E. I., 86b
Clark, F. Le Gros, 101b
Clark, H. E., 39b
Clark-Kennedy, A. E., 62a, 93a
Clarke, E. A., 125b
Clarke, E. K., 95b
Clarke, E. M., 94a
Clarke, F., 39b
Clarke, M. A., 12b
Clarkson, P., 119a
Clay, M. J. H., 49a
Clay, R. M., 128a
Claybury Hospital, 129a
Claye, A. M., 129b
Clemence, M., 39b
Cleveland, A. J., 130b
Clewes, E. S., 73b
Clifford, S. C. A., 36b
Cline, D. S., 39b
Clint, M. B., 8b
Clyne, D. G. W., 39b, 90a, 97a
Cobb, B., 64a
Cobbe, F. P., 6b
Coburn, E. P., 112b
Cochrane, M. S., 24b
Cockayne, E., 24b, 39b, 66a
Cocker, D. E., 95a

185

Coggan, N. E., 60b
Cohen, J., 37b
Coladarci, A. P., 39b
Colburn, E. W., 51a
Cole, G. E., 101a
Cole, M., 11a
College of Nursing, 3a, 28a, 30a, 30b, 33a
 (*See also:* Royal College of Nursing)
Coletti, A. C., 66a
Collins, W. J. T., 131a
Collis, J. L., 118a
Colonial, *pseud.*, 22b
Colonial Hospital, Port-of-Spain, Trinidad, 56a, 129a
Colored Home and Hospital, New York City, 129a
Colp, R., 120a
Colquhoun, D. R., 80a
Coltman, G., 73b
Columbia University. Department of Nursing, Faculty of Medicine, 40a
Columbia University Teachers' College, 40a, 52a, 56a
Columbia University Teachers' College. Division of Nursing Education, 68a, 82b, 116a
Colvin, S. T., 12b
Committee for the Study of Nursing Education, 40a
Committee on the Function of Nursing, 26b
Committee on the Grading of Nursing Schools, 26b, 34b, 54a
Committee on the Structure of National Nursing Organizations, 26b
Community Council of Greater New York. Research Department, 34b
Compton, D. E., 103a
Conference on State Registration of Nurses, 3a
Connecticut State Department of Health. Bureau of Industrial Hygiene, 99a
Connecticut State Nurse Association, 28b
Connecticut Training School for Nurses, 56b, 94a
Connolly, E. C., 125a
Connolly, M. G., 80a
Conta, A. L., 33a
Cooch, J. W., 83a
Cook, E., 16a
Cook, J. B., 73b
Cooke, G., 12b
Cooke, H. J., 130a
Cooke, J. B., 97a
Cooke, R. G., 93a
Cooke, R. V., 87b
Coombe, M. E., 80a
Cooper, C., 49a
Cooper, M., 108a
Cooper, P., 128b
Cooper, P. S., 36b
Cooper, Y. V., 90b
Cope, Z., 3a, 5b, 13a, 16a, 57b, 64b, 66a, 110b, 126a, 127b, 131b
Copeman, W. S. C., 132a
Corbin, H., 97a
Corbin, M., 45a
Corcoran, J., 51b
Corey, B. W., 105a
Cork, R. M., 117b
Corley, C., 90a
Cornell University. New York Hospital, 129a, 130b
Cornell University, New York Hospital School of Nursing, 56b, 57a, 80a
Corry, S., 73b
Costello, C. G., 104b, 109a
Coston, H. M., 49a
Couey, E. D., 72a
Coultas, R., 88a
Coulter, E. B., 117b
Coulter, P. P., 49a, 110a
Counihan, H. E., 35a

Courtney, M. E., 49b
Cousens, H. M., 40a, 99a
Couzins, E. M., 91b
Coville, W., 47a
Cowan, F. P., 47a
Cowan, M. C., 90a
Coward, R., 83a
Cowen, E. D. H., 35a
Cowles, E., 80a
Cowlin, G., 40a
Cox, B. R., 58b
Cox-Davies, R., 18b
Crabbe, V. E., 65b, 103b
Cragg, M. J., 99a
Craig, M., 103b
Craig, W. S., 101b
Crain, C., 12b
Crandall, E. P., 112b
Craven, D., 110b
Craven, M. E., 60b
Crawford, A. L., 108a
Crawford, A. M., 123a
Crawford, J. A., 3a
Crawford, M. E., 124a
Creelman, L., 20a, 113a
Creighton, H., 32b, 60b
Crew, F. A. E., 5a, 113a
Crews, E. R., 119a
Crick, H. A., 131a
Critchley, M., 130b
Crombie, D. L., 116b
Cromwell, G. E., 116b
Crosby, J. W., 128b
Cross, K. W., 36b, 116b
Cross, W. H., 30a
Crossen, H. S., 90a
Crossen, R. J., 90a
Crossey, B., 58b
Crow, L. D., 109a
Croy, Princess M. De, 8b
Cruickshank, W. H., 95b
Crumpsall Hospital, 51a
Cruze, W. W., 109a
Cuff, H. E., 78b, 93a
Cullingworth, C. J., 73b, 97a
Cullwick, H. R., 88a
Culver, V. M., 26b
Cumming, E., 108a
Cumming, J., 108a
Cumming, K., 8b
Cummings, G. O., 130a
Cunningham, B. V., 15b, 109a
Cunningham, E. V., 52a
Cunningham, M. R., 40a
Cunningham, P. J., 40a, 77b, 123a
Cunningham, R., 23a
Cureton, M. N., 12b
Curran, J. A., 20a, 40a
Curran, W. M., 74a
Cutbush, E., 4b
Cutbush, R. E., 40a
Cuthbert, T. M., 36b, 48b
Cutler, B., 12b
Cutler, B. I., 101b
Cutler, G. E., 94a

D'Abreu, A. L., 118a
Dafoe, C. A., 120b
Dagsland, H., 58b
Daikos, G. K., 36a
Dakin, F., 74a
Dale, B., 109a
Daley, A., 80b
Dally, J. F. H., 87b
Dalrymple-Smith, M., 74a
Dalzell-Ward, A. J., 20a, 95b, 110b
Damart, L. M., 99a
Dan Mason Nursing Research Committee, 65a
Dancey, T. E., 35a
Daniel, M. P., 64a
Daniells, N. C., 113a
Daniels, D. W., 118a
Daniels, M. L., 105b
Danto, J. L., 35b

Darche, L., 12b, 54a
Darcy, R., 91b
Darley, V. E., 36b
Darling, H. C. R., 90b, 120a
Darmady, E. M., 74a
Darnell, L. M., 25a
Daughters of Charity of St. Vincent de Paul, Los Angeles, 4a
Davidson, M., 129a
Davies, D. M., 36a
Davies, D. V., 85a
Davies, H. V., 90b
Davies, J. B. M., 85a
Davies, J. O., 35a
Davies, J. W., 12b
Davies, M., 74a, 94a
Davies, M. E., 33b
Davies, M. E., 113a, 115a
Davies, R. L., 127b
Davies, W. T., 119b
Davis, D., 89a
Davis, E., 12b
Davis, E. K., 113a
Davis, E. P., 97a
Davis, J. A., 103b
Davis, J. H., 119a
Davis, M. B., 12a
Davis, M. E., 97a
Davison, E. H., 113a
Dawson, J. B., 97b
Dawson, P. M., 85a
Dax, E. C., 104b
Day, M. A. C., 74a
Day, P. E., 67a
Deakin, B. M., 124a
Deans, A. G., 56b
Dearmer, M., 8b
DeBacker, D., 79a
De Camp General Hospital, 126b
Decary, M., 58b, 82b
Deegan, D., 122a
De Gutierrez-Mahoney, C. G., 120a
Delacato, C. H., 49b
Delano, J. A., 12b
Delavan, D. B., 130b
De Lee, J. B., 97a
Delehanty, M. E., 99a
Deleuran, H., 47a
Deming, D., 26b, 74a, 125a
Denham, M., 87b
Denison, A. H., 88b
Denney, R. R., 124a
Dennis, L. B., 109a
Denny, F. P., 47a
Densford, K. J., 64a
De Paul, Sister, 48a
De Pelchin, K. P., 13a
De Pledge, J. L., 20a
Derham, R. F., 80b
Derryberry, M., 113a
Desjardins, M., 102a
Despres, L. M., 32b
Deutsch, A., 7a
Deutscher, I., 26b, 36b, 40a
Devereux, G., 26b, 33a
De Witt, K., 72a
DeYoung, L., 43b
Diamond, L. K., 36b, 40b
Dick, E. C., 97a
Dickie, H. M., 74a
Dickinson, D. M., 90a
Dicks, R. L., 60b, 73b
Diehl, H. S., 90b
Dietz, L. D., 64a
Diller, D., 118b
Dillner, E., 2b
Dimock, H. G., 101b, 103a
Disbrow, M., 103b
District Nursing Association of Northern Westchester County (N.Y.), 28b
Ditchfield, A. L., 47a
Dix, D. L., 13a
Dobson, J., 4b
Dock, L. L., 1a, 1b, 7b, 13a, 20a, 24a, 26b, 54a, 74a, 125b, 126b

Dr. Steevens' Hospital, Dublin, 129a
Dodds, G. H., 90a
Dodge, B. S., 1a
Dodge, J. S., 36b, 62a, 68a, 80b
Dodsworth, E., 73a
Doggart, J. H., 101a
Dohahoe, M. F., 74a
Doherty, B., 130a
Doherty, M. K., 74a
Doman, G. J., 49b
Domville, E. J., 74a
Donnelly, P. R., 36b
Donovan, A. C., 82a
Donovan, H. M., 48a, 66a
Dooley, M. S., 123a
Dopson, L., 131b
Dora, Sister, 13a
Dorffeld, M. E., 38a
Dormer, E. W., 131a
Dorsey, N. L., 28b
Dougherty, E., 13a
Douglas, G. M., 94a
Douglas, J., 47a
Dowding, M. K., 70b
Dowling, G. B., 88a
Downey, E., 125a
Dowson-Weisskopf, A. B., 99a
Doyle, A., 5a
Doyon, R., 113a
Drakard, M., 65b, 91b
Drake, E. M., 60b
Drake, M. F., 124a
Drew, M., 94a
Druckman-Frankenstein, R., 23b
Drummond, E. E., 40a
Drummond, W. B., 94a
Dryborough-Smith, E., 25a
Dublin Metropolitan Technical
 School for Nurses, 56b
Duchess of York Hospital for Babies,
 Manchester, 103b
Duder, R., 74a
Duff-Grant, L., 40a
Duffus, R. L., 19a
Dufton, L., 57a
Du Gas, B. W., 47a
Duggan, M. G., 99a
Dukes, C. E., 86b, 131b
Dulles, R. F., 7b
Dunant, J. H., 7b
Dunbar, C., 113a
Dunbar, V. M., 57b
Duncan, A., 95a
Duncan, E. H. L., 114b
Duncan, S., 24a
Duncan-Johnstone, D., 73a
Duncanson, B., 58a
Dundas, G. H. G., 91b
Dundee Royal Infirmary, 129a
Dunn, M. A., 118a
Dunstan, E. M., 83a
Dunton, W. R., 124a
Dunwiddie, M., 29a
Durrant, M. M., 74a
D'Ursel, L., 22b
Dusseault, R., 120a
Dutch Nurses' Association, 28b
Dutton, G., 89a
Dwyer, M. T., 109a
Dwyer, S. M., 89a
D'Yonville, M., 13a

Eager, R., 104b
Earp, K. A., 112b
Eason, H., 126a
Easter, E. M., 116a
Eastman, N. J., 98a
Eastwood, C. G., 5b
Eaton, J., 54a
Eaton, L. K., 128a
Ebaugh, F. G., 104b
Eccles, W. M., 85a
Eddleson, R. B., 69a
Eddy, J. P., 32a
Eden, A. J., 104a

Edgell, B., 60b
Edgeworth, D. R., 86b
Edinburgh Royal Infirmary, 129a
Edinburgh University, 52a
Edman, H., 111a
Edmonds, S. E. E., 8b
Edge, G., 8b, 10a
Edwards, A. D., 116b
Edwards, M. A. F., 83a
Edwards, M. M., 80b
Edwards, M. P., 115a
Edwards, R., 101a
Edwards, W., 74a
Efron, H. Y., 35b
Egloff, F. R. L., 55b
Egstrom, L., 36b
Elder, A. T., 111a, 113a
Eldred, S. H., 62a
Eldridge, R. W., 113a
Eliason, E. L., 74a, 120a
Elizabeth of Hungary, 13a
Elkins, W. H., 52a
Ellenberg, M., 35a
Ellenbogen, B. L., 90a
Elles, G. W., 104b
Elliman, V. B., 7b, 83a
Elliott, F. E., 20b, 29a, 47a, 49b, 52a,
 54b
Elliott, J. E., 21a
Elliott, J. T., 88a
Elliott, S. M., 94a
Elliott, V., 99a
Ellis, M., 119a
Ellsworth, R., 70b
Elms, J., 101a
Emblem, R. G., 112a
Emerson, C. P., 93a
Emory, F. H. M., 113a
Emory University Hospital, 129a
Enarson, H. L., 40a
Engells, A. M., 97a
Engle, B., 104b
Englefield, A. M., 124a
Enriques, B., 40a
Fnsworth, H., 91b
Epler, P. H., 11b
Epstein, B. W., 19b
Epstein, C., 100b
Erickson, F., 103a
Erickson, M. E., 52a
Erne, M. J., 96a
Eron, L. D., 58b
Erwin, G. S., 125a
Erxleben, M. C., 102a
Esau, M. C., 74b
Eshleman, F., 125a
Essex-Cater, A. J., 111a
Evans, A. D., 128a
Evans, B. L., 104b
Evans, P. J., 101a
Evans, S. J. H., 32a
Evanston School of Nursing, Illinois,
 56b
Evatt, G. J. H., 4b
Eve, E., 113a
Evelyn, G. P., 8b
Everett, M. L., 64a
Ewell, T., 97a
Eyre, J. G., 125a
Eyre, M. B., 109a

Faber, G., 17a
Fabiola, Saint, 13a
Faddis, M. O., 49b, 62b, 74b, 93b, 123a
Fagan, E. A., 40b
Fair, E., 38a
Fair, E. W., 80b
Falck, H. S., 68a
Falconer, M. W., 123a
Falk, H. C., 120a
Falkiner, N. M., 23a
Falls, F. H., 90a, 97a
Falther, A. R., 116b
Farfor, U. C. M., 101a
Faris, M., 110b

Farnol, R. T., 78b
Farnworth, M., 74b
Farquarson, M. D., 13a, 47a
Farr, M., 99a
Farrell, M., 35a
Farrow, R., 102a
Fash, B., 92b
Faughnan, J. E., 103a
Favreau, C., 54b
Fawkes, B. N., 52a
Faxon, N. W., 130a
Fedden, M., 8b
Federated Superannuation Scheme for
 Nurses and Hospital Officers
 (Contributory), 33b
Feeney, E., 49b
Fegan, A. C., 1b
Feiling, A., 129b
Felter, R. K., 120b
Felton, B. L., 82a
Felton, J. S., 100b
Fenwick, B., 117b
Fenwick, E. G., 3a, 13a, 20b, 23b,
 28b, 29a, 30a, 65a
Ferguson, E. S., 123a
Ferguson, I. L., 123a
Ferguson, L. E., 99a
Ferguson, L. K., 120a
Ferguson, M., 66a, 87a, 113a, 115a
Ferguson, R. G., 36a
Ferrand Training School for Nurses,
 Detroit, Michigan, 56b
Ferris, E. A., 86b
Fey, L. H., 66a
Fidler, F. G., 62a
Fidler, N. D., 31b, 52a, 59a
Field, M., 80b, 82b
Fieldhouse, A. E., 40b
Filimore, A., 29b
Filson, M., 76b
Finer, H., 66b, 72a
Finette, F., 45a
Fink, L. G., 60b
Fink, S. L., 124b
Finlay, R. B., 30a
Finnie, W. J., 121b
Fisher, A., 13a, 79a
Fisher, A. M., 86b
Fisher, E., 74b, 93b
Fisher, J. W., 104b, 109a
Fisher, M., 116b
Fisher, W., 59a
Fisk, J. E., 120b
Fitzgerald, —, 8b
Fitzgerald, C. E., 85a
Fitzpatrick, E., 98a
Fitzroy, Y., 9a
Fitzsimmons, L. W., 108a
Fiumara, N. J., 116a
Flanagan, E. C., 96a, 120b, 127b
Fletcher, H. E., 113a
Fletcher, N. C., 7b
Fliedner Institute, Kaiserswerth,
 Germany, 56b, 72a
Flikke, J. O., 4b
Flitter, H. H., 59a, 85b, 104a
Florence, M., 66b
Florence Nightingale International
 Foundation, 28b, 41b, 52b, 54b
Florentine, H. G., 38a
Flores, F., 29a, 64a
Flynn, C. W., 56a
Foggo-Thompson, H., 72b
Folck, M. M., 40b
Foley, E. L., 111a
Foley, M. M., 40b, 49b, 54a, 54b
Follmann, J. F., Jr., 115a
Foote, J., 40b
Foote, R. R., 88a
Foran, J. K., 15a
Forbes, R., 32a
Ford, B. M., 51a
Ford, L. C., 82a
Ford, T. R., 63b, 71a
Fordham, M. E., 87b
Forest Gate Hospital, 129a

Forman, D. H., 66b
Forman, J. A., 116b
Forrer, G. R., 104b
Forrest, C., 13a
Fortescue-Brickdale, J. M., 74b, 123a
Fortin, D., 80b
Fortman, A. G., 127a
Foster, J. B., 101a
Foster, L. M., 102a
Foster, M. L., 95b
Fowler, D., 87a
Fowler, G. R., 104b
Fowler, K. A. B., 25a
Fox, A. M., 13a
Fox, D. J., 36b, 40b
Fox, E. M., 3a, 13a, 60b, 65a, 65b, 66b, 74b
Fox, J., 80b
Fox, V., 80b
Frances Payne Bolton School of Nursing, 52a
Frances Xavier, Sister, 51a
Francis, C. C., 85b
Francis, H. W. S., 111a
Francis, S. G. M., 128a
Francoise de Chantal, Sister, 66b
Franghiadi, M., 13a
Frank, Sister C. M., 1a, 20b
Frankel, H. M., 80b
Frankland, A. W., 85a
Fraser, E. G., 57b
Fraser, R. D., 107b
Frasier, E. S., 100a
Fream, W. C., 86a
Frederick, H. K., 74b
Freedman, M. G., 74b
Freeman, E., 74b
Freeman, R. B., 46b, 52a, 62a, 62b, 66b, 113a, 115a
French, C. N., 131b
French, M., 97a
French, M. A., 104b, 111a
French, T., 108b
Frey, L. M., 104b
Frey, M., 68a, 82b
Frey, T. E., 60a
Friedman, G. A., 32a
Friedman, T. T., 107b
Friend, C. P., 49b
Fritz, E. L., 80a
Frobisher, M., 86b
Frodsham, W., 52b
Frost, H., 20b
Frumkin, R. M., 26b
Fry, E., 13a, 13b
Fry, V., 59a
Fuerst, E. V., 40b, 74b
Fujikura, Y. Y., 113a
Fullagar, C., 13b
Fullerton, A. M., 90a, 97a
Fulmer, H., 5b
Fulton, J. T., 88a
Funnell, E. M., 90b
Funsten, R. V., 119a
Furfey, P. H., 63b
Furguson, K., 94b

Gabig, M. G., 40b
Gabriel, Sister J., 49b, 60b, 62b
Gage, E. B., 105b
Gailani, D. M., 74a
Gaines, M. J., 51a
Galpine, J. F., 36a
Gamester, E. R., 129a
Gant, F. J., 25a
Gardiner, L. A., 83a
Gardner, B., 98a
Gardner, C., 4a
Gardner, K. E., 80b
Gardner, M., 13b, 33a
Gardner, M. S., 13b, 113a
Garesché, E. F., 60b
Garland, G. W., 90a, 97a
Garland, P., 101a
Garmon, B. L., 83b

Garnsey, C. E., 123a
Garside, A. H., 117a
Garside, R. F., 38a
Gass, F., 82b
Gates, K. H., 83b
Gaved-Wills, L., 13b
Gazaway, R., 62b
Gazdar, E. J., 104b
Geddes, A. K., 103b
Geddes, J. D. C., 49b
Geffen, D., 89b
Geister, J. M., 20b, 28b, 69b, 120b, 121b
Gelber, I., 107b
Gelinas, A., 26b, 40b
General Nursing Council for England and Wales, 25a, 28b, 29a, 37b, 40b, 48b, 54b, 97b
George, F. L., 80b
George, G. R., 62b
Gerber, W., 84a
Gerds, G., 65a
Germain, L. D., 66b
German Nurses' Federation, 90a
Gerstenburger, H. J., 115a
Gibbon, J. M., 2a, 30b
Gibbons, Cardinal, 72a
Gibbs, P., 9a
Gibson, A. G., 130b
Gibson, H. J., 129a
Gibson, J., 85b, 90b, 108b
Gibson, M., 74b
Gibson, R. M., 111a
Gibson, R. W., 62b
Giddings, L., 82a, 82b
Gidseg, L., 94b
Gilbert, A. J., 123a
Gilbert, J., 113a
Gilbert, J. G., 109a
Gilbert, N. S., 94b
Gilbert, R., 113b
Gilbertson, H. C., 72b
Giles, D., 56a
Giles, M. D., 120a
Gilhooly, M. A. N., 29a, 54b
Gill, H. Z., 78a
Gillan, R. I., 23b, 67b
Gillet, J. A., 103b, 111a
Gillis, L., 108a, 120b
Gilmour, M., 57a
Gilpin, F., 13b
Gilson, M., 102a
Gipe, F. M., 66b
Gips, C. D., 52b
Girard, A., 66b
Gittins, E. A., 13b
Giunti, I. di T., 2b
Given, L. I., 32b, 54b, 86b
Gladstein, S., 66b
Gladwin, M. E., 7b, 60b
Glague, E., 34b
Glasgow City Corporation, 116a
Glasgow Royal Infirmary, 40b, 41a, 129a
Glassman, J. A., 120b
Gleeson, I., 104b
Gliddon, P., 60b
Gloucester Infirmary, 129a
Gloucestershire Royal Hospital, 129a
Godbout, R. A., 59a
Goddard, H. A., 69a
Goddard, L., 7a
Godden, G. M., 25a, 41a
Godfrey, A. E., 103a
Godwin, E., 121b
Goik, M. C., 95b
Gold, R. L., 71a
Golder, C., 1a
Golder, G. M., 117b
Goldfinch, D. A., 35b, 128a
Goldman, L., 88a
Goldmann, F., 80b, 89b
Goldmark, J., 40a
Goldowsky, S. J., 129b
Goldring, D., 92b
Goldsmith, M., 16a
Goldstein, R. L., 26b

Goller, G., 96b
Gooch, M., 45a
Goodale, R., 104a
Goodman, M., 9a
Goodnow, M., 1a, 74b, 83b, 104a
Goodrich, A. W., 13b, 41a, 54b, 60b
Goodrich, F. W., 97b
Goodsell, W., 17a
Goodwin, D., 56b
Goodyear, K., 48b
Goostray, S., 13b, 15b, 17a, 56a, 68b, 73a, 123a
Gordon, A. K., 41a, 91b
Gordon, Br., 51b
Gordon, E. M., 100b, 110a
Gordon, P., 46b, 69a
Gordon, R. E., 59a
Gorham, D. R., 108b
Gorman, M. R., 23b
Gorsky, J. A., 32a
Got, A., 12b
Gotten, N., 96a
Gould, —, 62b
Gould, E. M., 23b
Gould, M. E., 57a
Goulding, F. A., 74b
Gow, W. J., 97b
Gowing, T., 9a
Gowland, W. P., 85b
Graf, C. N., 59b
Graffam, S., 120b
Graham, —, 102a
Graham, A. A., 117a
Graham, J. C., 99a
Grand, D. E., 101a
Grand Forks Deaconess Hospital, 129a
Grant, A. H., 113b
Grant, I. W. B., 118a
Grant, J., 25a
Grant-Smith, R., 105a
Gration, H. M., 74b, 90a
Graves, L. M., 87b
Gray, A. M. H., 126a
Gray, C. E., 97a
Gray, J., 57a
Gray, J. I. L., 83b
Gray, K. G., 31b
Grazier, G. M., 111a
Great Britain. Board of Control, 107b
Great Britain. Central Health Services Council. See: Central Health Services Council
Great Britain. Colonial Office, 41a
Great Britain. Interdepartmental Committee on Nursing Services, 25a, 69a, 107b
Great Britain. Ministry of Education, 116a
Great Britain. Ministry of Health, 37a, 37b, 52b, 76b, 85a, 88a, 112a, 126a
Great Britain. Ministry of Health. Nurses' Salaries Committee, 34a
Great Britain. Ministry of Health. Working Party on the Field of Work, Training and Recruitment of Health Visitors, 114a
Great Britain. Ministry of Labour, 34a
Great Britain. Parliament, 32a, 32b, 97b
Great Britain. Parliament. Select Committee on the G.N.C., 25a
Great Britain. Scotland. Department of Health. See: Scotland. Department of Health
Great Britain. Scottish Health Services Council. See: Scottish Health Services Council
Great Britain. War Office. See: War Office
Great Ormond Street Hospital for Sick Children, 41a, 102a, 129b
Green, D., 36a
Green, E., 57b
Greenberg, A. J., 36a
Greenbie, M. B., 7b
Greenblatt, M., 59a
Greene, J. C., 122a

Greene, J. M., 122a
Greenhough-Smith, M., 41a
Greenlaw, B. L., 13b
Greenwood, F. J. L., 6a
Greenwood, L. L., 91b, 109a
Gregg, A. L., 95a
Gregory, A. S., 13b
Greig, D. S., 18a
Greisheimer, E. M., 85b
Gremp, Z. Von, 74b
Gretter, E. L., 60b
Greville, T., 99a
Grey, E., 12b
Grey, M. E., 25a
Grey's Hospital, Pietermaritzburg, 129a
Griffin, A. E., 120b
Griffith, J. Q., 94b
Griffith, O. F., 33a, 105a
Gring, A. C., 116a
Grisell, J. L., 104b
Grivest, M. T., 68a
Grobbelaar, A., 24a
Gross, S. D., 41a
Grossman, J., 117a
Grosvenor, A. G., 125a
Group for the Advancement of Psychiatry. Committee on Hospitals, 105a
Group for the Advancement of Psychiatry. Committee on Psychiatric Nursing, 105a
Grouse, G., 89b
Grove, L., 51b
Grover, E. P., 124b
Groves, E. W. H., 74b
Gruener, J. R., 80b
Grundy, F., 110a
Grygier, P., 38a
Guinee, K. K., 36b
Gullan, M. A., 75a
Gumpert, M., 7b
Gurel, L., 70b
Guthrie, D., 1a, 131a
Guy, J., 90b
Guy's Hospital, 56b, 129b
Guy's Hospital Nurses' League, 52b
Guy's Hospital Training School, 57b

Habel, M. L., 72b, 113b
Habenstein, R. W., 65a
Haber, M. E., 96a
Hackney Group Hospital Management Committee, 128a
Hadley, E. C., 41a
Haggart, A., 83b
Haines, R. W., 85a
Haldane, E., 3b, 7a, 25a
Haldeman, J. C., 82a
Hale, T., 37a
Hall, B. H., 49b, 105a, 108a
Hall, D. L. A., 36b
Hall, E. D., 120b
Hall, E. F., 16a
Hall, G. M., 59a
Hall, J. B., 113b
Hall, M. N., 115b
Hall, W., 20b
Hallas, C. H., 108b
Hallock, G. T., 16a
Hallowes, R. M., 13a, 13b, 14a, 14b, 17b, 18b, 19b
Halpin, J., 89b
Hamby, W. B., 120b
Hamilton, A., 23a
Hamilton, D. I. W., 41a
Hamilton General Hospital School of Nursing, 56b
Hamilton, T. S., 20b, 54b
Hamilton-Paterson, J. L., 85b
Hamley, H. R., 28b
Hammarlund, M., 9a
Hammersley, D. P., 118b
Hampton, I. A., 1a, 6a, 7a, 41a, 41b, 54a, 56b, 57b, 64b, 72a, 75a, 98a, 110b, 112a

Hanbury, —, 75a
Hanisch, V. K., 87a
Hanlon, M. R., 69a
Hannan, J., 74b
Hansen, H. F., 64a, 75a
Hanson, L. M., 87b
Hardaway, R. M., 79b
Hardin, C. A., 59a
Harding, A., 60b
Harding, G., 60b
Harding, W., 91b
Hardman, E., 33b
Hardy, C. H., 65a
Hardy, G. M., 13b, 25a, 75a, 92a
Harlan, H. R., 88a
Harlow, F. W., 118a
Harlow, M. J., 36a
Harmer, B., 49b, 75a
Harriman, P. L., 109a
Harrington, G. M., 71a
Harris, C. F., 122a
Harris, P., 105a
Harrison, A., 9a
Harrison, E., 94b
Harrison, G., 32b, 60b, 64a
Harrison, L., 13b
Hart, B. C., 50b
Hart, B. H., 49b
Hart, B. L., 80b
Hart, M. H., 3b
Harvey, D., 77b
Harvey, J. E., 118a
Harvey, S., 41a
Hasenjaeger, E., 91b
Hassard, A. R., 83b
Hassard, E. M., 83b
Hassenplug, L. W., 41a, 50b, 52b, 70b, 122a
Hathaway, J. S., 35a
Hattersley, A. F., 129a
Haug, C. H., 82b
Hauge, C. H., 83b
Haughey, R., 124a
Haver, H. T., 132b
Haward, L. R. C., 38b
Haward, W., 65a
Hawes, A. T., 75a
Hawkins, C., 55a
Hawkins, D. M., 9a
Hawkins, K. L., 124a
Hawkins, N. G., 47a
Hawkins-Ambler, G. A., 25a, 90b, 94b
Hawkins-Dempster, H., 41a, 75a
Hay, M. E. D., 65b, 71a
Hayden, M. L., 124a
Haydon, M. O., 65b, 97b
Hayes, E. J., 60b
Hayes, W., 62b
Hayman, C. R., 80b
Hayman, J. M., 74b, 93b
Haynes, I., 83b
Haynes, W. G., 120b
Hayt, E., 32b
Hayt, L. R., 32b
Head, P., 65b, 105a
Headlee, R., 105a
Healy, Sister F., 45a
Heather-Bigg, M., 13b
Heaton, H. M., 41a
Hecker, H., 35a
Hector, W., 75a, 90b
Headman, L. L., 107b
Heely, P. I., 116a
Heidgerken, L. E., 20b, 41a, 45a, 48a, 49b, 52b, 59a
Heil, L. M., 62b, 87a
Heim, E. M., 43b
Heinemann, E., 125a
Hellier, J. B., 90b
Hellyer, E. M., 121a
Hely, A. E., 13b
Henderson, L., 75a, 94b
Henderson, L. M., 119a, 120b
Henderson, V., 13b, 59a, 75a
Henke, H. F., 82b
Henrietta, Sister, 9a

Henriksen, H. L., 46a, 99a, 101a
Henry, J. N., 93b
Henry, M., 28a, 29a
Hentsch, Y., 49a
Herdan, I. M., 96a, 120b
Hereford General Hospital, 129b
Herz-Haber, Z. G., 24a
Heslin, H. L., 80b
Heslin, L., 69a
Hess, J. H., 103b
Hetherington, H. W., 125a
Hewer, C. L., 121b
Hewer, J. L., 102a
Hewitt, G. K., 131a
Heyse, M. F., 47a
Hezlett, E., 13b
Hickey, F. C., 88a
Hickey, N. M., 48a
Hickman, W. H., 20b
Hicks, W. J., 35a
Higgins, A. C., 109a
Higgins, T. T., 129b
Higham, A. R., 131b
Highley, B. L., 109a
Hilbert, H., 59a
Hilkemeyer, R., 87a
Hill, D. D., 75a
Hill, E., 65a
Hill, W. T., 12b
Hilliard, L. T., 108b
Hillman, O. S., 118a
Hindes, G., 123a
Hiner, B., 48a
Hines, M., 50b
Hinson, J. A., 120b
Hird, N. G., 105a
Hirsh, J., 130a
Hislop, R., 87a
Hitch, M., 75b, 78a, 93b
Hoban, L., 70b
Hobson, E. C., 4a
Hobson, J. M., 128a
Hochbaum, G. M., 59a
Hodgkinson, S., 127b
Hodgson, V. H., 99a, 115b, 125a
Hodson, J., 26b
Hoehling, A. A., 12b
Hoffmann, J., 57a
Hofling, C. K., 105a
Hogarth, M., 111b
Holgate, W., 83b
Holland, D. L., 49b, 90a
Holland, D. S., 25a
Holland, M. A. G., 9a
Holland, S., 3b, 14b, 33a, 60b
Hollander, B., 105a
Hollender, A. R., 88b
Holliday, J., 27b
Holloway, S. W., 5b
Holm, E. M., 13b
Holman, M. C., 131b
Holman, P., 109a
Holmes, G., 130a
Holmes, J., 72b
Holmes, K. M., 6b
Holmes, M. J., 62b
Holmes, T. M., 113b
Hone, E., 65a
Hood, D. W. C., 93b
Hope, G. H., 94b
Hope, M. E., 13b, 22b
Hopkins, S. J., 123a
Horder, Lord, 25b
Hormuth, R. P., 113b
Horner, C. M., 111a
Horner, H. H., 41a
Hospital, 32a, 45a
Hospital and Health Management, 37a
Hospital Association, London, 25a
Hospital for Joint Diseases, New York City, 129b
Hospital for Sick Children, Great Ormond Street, 41a, 102a, 129b
Hospital for Women, Leeds, 129b
Hospital of St. John and St. Elizabeth, 129b

A Hospital Secretary, 127a
Hospitals Association. Joint Sectional Committee of Registration, 3b
L'Hotel Dieu, Paris, 129b
Houghton, L. E., 125a
Houghton, M., 75b, 118b
Houle, E. L., 122a
Houliston, M., 105a
Houston, J. C., 93b
Houts, D. C., 62b
Howard, J., 128b
Howard, L. G. R., 128a
Howard, R., 120b
Howe, P. S., 122a
Howell, C., 120b
Howell, L. N., 83b
Howell, S. K., 62b
Howell, T. H., 89b
Howells, G., 35b, 85a
Howkins, J., 90b
Howson, J. S., 5b
Hoxie, G. H., 93b
Hubble, D., 16a, 17a
Hudd, J., 118b
Hueston, R. M., 82a
Huffman, V. M., 100b
Hughes, A., 6a, 14a, 97b, 111a
Hughes, A. A., 128a
Hughes, E. C., 27a
Hughes, F., 14a
Hughes, J. M., 119a
Hughes, L. W., 72b
Hughes, M. F., 1b
Hull, E., 75b, 93b
Hull, E. J., 47a
Hull Royal Infirmary, 129b
Hume, R. F., 16a
Hume, W. E., 130b
Humfrey, M., 6b, 30a, 97b
Humphry, L., 75b
Hungate, T. L., 45a
Hunt, A., 14a
Hunt, A. M., 122a
Hunt, H. C., 130b
Hunt, J., 93b
Hunter, J. B., 126a
Hunter, R. A., 7a
Hunter, R. M., 128b
Hunter, T. G., 29a, 115b
Hurd, A. W., 109a
Hurd, H. M., 16a, 54b
Hureblatt, E., 14a
Hurry, J. B., 112a
Hurst, E. H., 132b
Hurst, I., 54b
Hurwitz, I., 59a
Hutton, I. E., 9a
Hutton, M., 94b
Huxley, M., 14a
Hyde, R. W., 60b, 105a

Ibadan University College School of Nursing, 56b
Iffert, R. E., 27a, 38b
Ilgenfritz, H. C., 118b
Illing, M., 112a
Illinois State Nurses' Association, 29a
Illinois Training School for Nurses, 56b
Incorporated Society for Promoting the Higher Education and Training of Nurses, 29a
India. Ministry of Health. Committee to Review Conditions of Service, Emoluments, etc. of the Nursing Profession, 33b
Indiana State Board of Health, 80b
Indiana University Medical Center, 80b
Ingles, T., 20b, 21a, 41a, 41b, 49b, 62b, 75b, 82b
Inglis, K. S., 131a
Ingmere, A. E., 49b
Ingram, J. T., 88a
Ingram, M. E., 105a
Interdepartmental Committee on Nursing Services, 25a, 69a
Interdepartmental Committee on Nursing Services. Sub-Committee on Mental Nursing and the Nursing of the Mentally Defective, 105a
International Congress of Charities, Correction and Philanthropy, Chicago, 27a
International Council of Nurses, 20b, 29a, 33a, 35a, 59a, 61a, 108b
International Council of Nurses. Economic Welfare Committee, 33a
International Council of Nurses. Education Committee, 41b, 52b
International Council of Nurses. Eleventh Quadrennial Congress, 38b
International Council of Nurses. Florence Nightingale International Foundation, 28b, 41b, 52b, 54b
International Hospital Federation, 80b
International Labour Organization, 33a
Iowa Methodist Hospital, 129b
Iowa State Association of Registered Nurses, 29a
Irish Nuses' Association, 29a
Irvin, I. D., 111b
Isaacs, B., 47a
Israel, J., 41b
Israel. Ministry of Health, 23b
Ives, A. G. L., 128b
Iwamoto, S., 70b
Iyi Enu Hospital, Nigeria, 129b
Izycka, J., 41b
Izzard, W. P., 105a

Jacks, L. V., 15a
Jackson, A. M., 49b
Jackson, J. A., 22b
Jackson, J. C., 75b
Jackson, M. L., 120b
Jackson, Q. M., 102a
Jackson, R., 129b
Jackson, W. L., 6a
Jacob, F. H., 130b
Jacobsen, M., 32b
Jacobson, F. N., 62b
Jacques, —, 23b
Jacques, M., 111a
Jamaica Hospital, New York, 129b
James, C. F., 103a
James, H. M., 103a
James, J. T., 20b
Jameson, A. B., 5b
Jameson, Sir W., 114a
Jamieson, E. B., 85b
Jamieson, E. M., 1b
Jamison, S., 123a
Jamme, A. C., 75b
Jane, M. A., 51b
Jarrett, R. F., 37a, 108b
Jarvi, K., 2a
Jaton, R., 20b
Jeanne, Sister M., 95b
Jeans, P. C., 102a
Jeffrey, B., 9a
Jellett, H., 97b
Jenkins, B., 69b
Jenkins, P., 66b
Jenkins, S. B., 105a
Jenkinson, V. M., 80b, 83a
Jennings, L. A., 50b
Jensen, A. C., 59a
Jensen, D. M., 1b, 50a, 62a, 66b, 75b, 80b, 93b, 124a
Jensen, F. T., 66b, 70b
Jensen, J., 93b
Jensen, K., 85b
Jephcott, P., 37a
Jessee, R. W., 41b, 86a
Jeune, M., 30a
Jewesbury, E. C. O., 131a
Johannesen, L., 123b
John Gabriel, Sister, 64a
Johns, E., 28a, 56b, 58a, 65a
Johns, R., 12b

Johns Hopkins Hospital, Baltimore. Alumnae Association of Nurses, 61a
Johns Hopkins Hospital, Baltimore. School of Nursing, 56b
Johnson, B. D., 61a
Johnson, D. E., 20b
Johnson, M., 72a
Johnson, M. L., 125a
Johnson, M. M., 21a
Johnson, P. V., 83b
Johnson, R. W., 75b, 94b
Johnson, S. C., 95a
Johnston, M. E., 8b
Johnston, R. V., 41b
Johnstone, F., 91b
Joint Committee of Nursing Service and Nursing Education, 35a
Joint Orthopaedic Nursing Advisory Service, 119a
Joint Tuberculosis Council, 36a
Jolly, J. D., 120b
Jones, A., 14a
Jones, A. T., 126b
Jones, B. R., 86a
Jones, G. C., 69a
Jones, H., 21a
Jones, J. A., 59a
Jones, K., 7b
Jones, M., 105a
Jones, R. A., 108a
Jones, R. M., 83a
Jones, S. E., 113b
Jones, T. B., 131a
Jones, W. B., 27a, 38b
Jordan, C. H., 46b
Jordan, H. J., 56b, 129a
Jorden, E., 9a
Jordheim, A., 113b
Jorgensen, J., 12b
Joseph, R. R., 76a
Joseph Ovide, Sister, 109a
Josie, G. H., 68a
Joule, J. W., 93b
Jourard, S. M., 62b
Joy, E. M., 14a
Jubilee Congress of District Nursing, Liverpool, 1909, 6a
Judson, H., 12b
Julian, E. E., 7a
Jurkowitz, M., 132b

Kaariainen, H., 111a
Kaback, G. R., 46b
Kahl, F. R., 100a
Kaiserswerth Institute, 56b, 72a
Kakosh, M., 37a, 68a
Kalkman, M. E., 105b
Kandel, P. M., 66b, 127a
Kane, H. H., 94b
Kane, J. J., 21a
Kansas State Nurses' Association, 29a
Kansas State Nurses' Association. Nursing Functions Committee, 65a
Kaplan, S. M., 105b
Karim, R. B., 24a
Karll, A., 14a, 23b
Karnosh, L. J., 105b
Kassler, R., 108b
Kathleen Mary, Sister, 62b
Keane, V. R., 63a, 97b
Keefe, A. E., 41b
Keele, K. D., 94b
Keevil, J. J., 11b
Keezer, D. M., 37a
Keith, H., 68a
Kelber, M., 52b
Kelleher, R. P., 52b
Keller, M. W., 57b, 120a
Kelley, H. W., 117a
Kellogg, F. S., 12a
Kellogg, W., 115b
Kellog Foundation, 71a
Kelly, B. M., 14a
Kelly, C. W., 8a, 71a

Kelly, I. V., 76a
Kelly, P. W., 37a
Kelman, R. J., 83a
Kelsall, M. T., 131a
Kemble, J., 118b
Kempf, F. C., 64a, 109a
Kenealy, A., 2a, 27a
Kenealy, H., 30a
Kennaway, E., 80b
Kenneally, C. M., 4a
Kennedy, D. A., 102a
Kennedy, J., 46b
Kennedy, M. E., 107b
Kennedy, M. V., 103a
Kennedy, P. E., 92b
Kennedy, R. B., 82a
Kenny, E., 14a, 92a
Kent, B., 72b
Kent, K., 13b
Kent County Mental Hospital, 129b
Keogh, I. C., 14a
Kephart, W., 26a
Kernodle, P. B., 8a
Kerr, A., 119b
Kerrigan, Sister M. R., 62b
Kershaw, J. D., 113b
Kessel, I., 102a
Kilander, V. C., 108a
Killby, M. M., 28b
Kilmer, E. W., 99a
Kimball, L., 108a
Kimber, W. J. T., 109a
Kimerer, N. S., 31a
Kinch, A., 83b
Kindbom, H., 14a
King, E., Bishop of Lincoln, 61a
King, E. J., 8a
King, V. G., 33b
King Edward VII's Hospital for Officers, 129b
King Edward's Hospital Fund for London, 35a, 37b, 54b, 62b, 69b, 127b
King Edward's Hospital Fund for London. Nursing Recruitment Service, 37a
Kingcade, M. E., 95b
King's College Hospital, London, 48b, 129b
Kingsbury, V., 48a
Kinney, D. H., 14a
Kirk, T. E., 89b
Kirk, V., 109b
Kirkcaldie, R. A., 9a
Kirkconnell, N. E., 51a
Kirkpatrick, T. P. C., 61a, 129a
Kirwin, T. J., 89a
Kitchin, J. B., 68a
Kitching, R. L., 111a
Klein, H. R., 106b
Klemme, R. M., 120b
Klingelhoffer, A., 59a
Klosz, W. H., 23b
Klump, O. M., 68a
Klutas, E. M., 47b, 100b
Knapp, L., 41b
Knapp, M., 87a
Knepler, H. W., 50a
Knight, G., 14a
Knighton, P. H., 128a
Knocke, F. J., 119b
Knocke, L. S., 119b
Knott, L. K., 45a
Knowles, L. N., 8a, 62b
Knowlton, G. C., 85b
Koch, H. B., 13b
Kohn, M. L., 118a
Kohn, R., 115b
Kollen, Dr., 41b
Koontz, A. R., 21a, 62b
Koos, E. L., 81a
Kopf, E. W., 16a
Korkis, F. B., 88b
Kough, A. M., 14a
Kovacs, R., 124a
Kozma, W. A., 70b

Krafft, C., 24b, 56b
Krakower, H., 41b
Kranock, A., 62b, 81a
Krause, M. V., 122a
Kreuter, F. R., 82b
Kristal, H. F., 116a
Kroeger, L. J., 67b
Krog, G., 24b
Krueger, E., 81b
Krug, E. E., 123b
Krush, T. P., 108a
Kuehn, R. P., 80b
Kullmann, G., 38b
Kulp, D. H., 62b
Kurtz, G., 68a

Labour Party, 25a
Laboure, C., 14a
La Croix, M. A., 41b
A Lady, pseud., 7a, 9a
Lage, L. C., 51b
Laird, D. A., 109b
Laird, S. L., 105b
Lake, V. M., 41b
Lakeland, K., 85b
Lamb, J. T., 105b
Lamb, M. C. N., 41b, 83a
Lamb, R. J., 79b
Lambersten, E. C., 41b, 52b, 68a, 82b
Lambeth Hospital, 129b
Lambie, M. I., 2b, 14a
Lammond, D., 16a
Lamont, D. J., 113b, 116a
Lamont, M., 14b
Lancaster, A., 61a
Lancet, 3b, 31b, 35a, 36a, 64a, 81a, 82a, 105b
Lancet Commission on Nursing, 37a
Lancet Sanitary Commission for Investigating the State of the Infirmaries of Workhouses, 7a
Landale, E. J. R., 7a, 41b, 66b
Landles, H. G., 14b
Landon, D. M., 14b
Lane, H. C., 124b
Lane, R. E., 101a
Langdon-Davies, J., 132a
Langley, G., 95ı, 99a
Langton, B. M., 113b
Larkin, C. M., 46a
Lartio, M., 111a
Lasky, J. J., 68a
La Source School of Nursing, Lausanne, 56b
Lathrop, R. H. (Mother Alphonsa), 14b
Lattimore, J. G., 4b
Laughlin, H. D., 48a
Launceston General Hospital, Launceston, Tasmania, 47a
Laurence, E. C., 3b, 14b, 76a
Lawrence, B., 105b
Lawrence, C., 78a
Lawrence, I., 14b
Lawrence, R. D., 88b
Lawson, M., 14b
Lawson, M. G., 14b, 21a
Leach, M. M., 102a
League of Red Cross Societies, 8a
League of St. Bartholomew's Nurses, 29a
League of School Nurses, 29a
Leahy, K. M., 38b, 54b, 56a, 116a
Leake, M. J., 76a
Learmont, D., 113b
Leask, J., 113b
Leavell, L. C., 117b
Lebecki, G., 35a
Lee, A. N., 70b
Lee, E., 57b
Lee, J. T., 104a
Lee, M. M., 87a
Lee, P. F., 59a
Lee, S. S., 132b
Lee, T., 38b

Lee, V. T., 63a
Lee, W. R., 99a
Leeds, H., 12b
Leeds General Infirmary, 129b
Lees, F. S., 14b, 66b, 111a
Lefebvre, D., 54b
Leicester Royal Infirmary, 50a
Leininger, M. M., 105a
Leipoldt, C. L., 117a
Lembright, K. A., 99b
Lemkau, P. V., 105b
Lennon, M. I., 50a, 63a, 64a
Lentz, E. M., 59a
Leone, L. P., 21a, 37a, 59b, 65a, 66b, 71b, 81a
Leopold, A. K., 34b
Leopold, I. H., 132a
Lersner, O. Von, 52b
Lesnick, M. J., 32b
Lesparre, M., 54b
Lesser, M. S., 63a, 97b
Lesson, G., 6a, 111a
Lester, M. R., 28a, 77b, 91b
Letourneau, C., 61a, 122a
Lett, H., 126a
Levin, D., 35a
Levine, E., 53a, 62b, 69b, 70a, 79b
Levison, H., 88a
Levy, L. 35a
Lewin P., 119b
Lewin, W., 121a
Lewis, E. K., 120a
Lewis, E. P., 18a
Lewis, G. G., 101a
Lewis, G. K., 46b, 70b
Lewis, I., 33b
Lewis, J. A., 117b
Lewis, L. Z., 86b
Lewis, P. G., 76a
Lightwood, R., 103b
Lilly, H. A., 118b
Lilly, J. L., 76b
Lindberg, S. M., 37a, 45a
Lindsay, J., 81a
Lindsay, W. F., 121a
Linklater, G. J. I., 90b
Lipeles, J. C., 42a, 117a
Lippott, L. C., 94b
Lipsett, G. E. A., 22b
Lipton, M. B., 35b
Liston, M. F., 63a, 105b, 115b
Littlewood, C. M., 85b
Liu, J. K. C., 1b
Livermore, M. A., 9a
Liverpool Nurses' Training School, 43a, 56b
Liverpool University. Department of Social Science, 64a, 66b, 107b
Livingston, M. C., 30b, 92b
Livingstone, H. M., 124a
Loane, M., 38b, 111a, 122a
Lobban, M., 2b
Local Government Board, 7a
Loch, C. G., 4b, 14b
Locke, E. I. J., 9a
Lockerby, F. K., 8a, 41a, 63a
Locket, S., 93b
Lockitt, M. A., 14b
Lockwood, C. D., 121a
Lockwood, H. J., 82a, 82b
Lodge, P. M., 85b
Lofthouse, E. M., 87a
Logan, J. S., 48b
Logsdon, A., 28a, 66b
London Biblewomen and Nurses Mission, 6a
London County Council, 111b, 128b
Long, J., 42a, 76a
Long, L. M., 48a
Longhurst, G. M., 125a
Longmore, T., 9a
Longshore, J. S., 76a
Lonie, T. C., 42a
Lonni, L. J., 82a
Lonsdale, M., 17b
Lord, A. R., 42a

Lorentz, M., 37a
Los Angeles. County Superintendent of Schools, 117a
Loucks, P. M., 42a
Loughran, H. A., 18b
Louise de Marillac, Saint, 14b
Louisiana State Nurses' Association, 29a
Lovat, Lady, 14b
Love, R. J. M., 118a
Lovell General Hospital, Portsmouth Grove, Rhode Island, 129b
Lovely, E. M., 102a
Low, R. B., 128a
Lowbury, E. J. L., 118b
Lowry, E. B., 94b
Lowsley, O. S., 89a
Lowson, K. J., 129b
Luard, K. E., 9a
Lub, A., 119a
Lucal, M. W., 6b
Luckes, E. C. E., 14b, 66b, 76a
Lucow, W. H., 42a
Ludlam, R., 65a
Lueth, H. G., 83b
Lundblad, E., 91b
Lundeen, E. C., 103b
Lynch, T. I., 91b
Lyon, H. F., 47a
Lyon, R. A., 102a
Lyons, G., 14b
Lyons-Bergman, R., 24a

Mabbit, L. E., 118a
Mabry, J. H., 81a
McAllister, J. B., 61a
MacAndrew, C., 21a, 33a
McArthur, A. C., 83a
MacArthur, C., 124b
McArthur, H. G., 22b
Macaulay, E. L., 108a
McBride, E. D., 103a, 119b
McBride, M., 27a
McCabe, G. S., 59b, 108a
McCain, R. F., 51a
Maccalman, D. R., 105b
McCarthy, V., 103a
McCaul, E., 9a
McClain, M. E., 76a, 86a
McClure, C. R., 103b
McCombs, R. S., 102a
McConnell, R. A., 21a
McCorkle, M. D., 47a
McCormick, V., 28a
McCoull, G., 48b
McCracken, M. C., 46b
McCrae, A., 15a, 76a
McCullough, W., 76a
McCune, H. L., 50a
Macdermot, H. E., 15a, 57a
McDermott, A. T., 110b
McDermott, V. V., 110b
Macdonald, I., 3b, 11b
Macdonald, J. M., 105b
MacDonald, M. G., 99b
MacDonald, S., 85a, 99b
Macdonald, V. M., 95b, 113b
MacDonald, W. J., 59b
MacDougall, A. A., 105b
McDowell, E. M., 51a, 53a
McEwan, M., 14b, 113b
McFadden, G. M., 54b
McFarland, J., 64a
McFee, W. F., 120a
MacFie, M., 113b
McGabe, G. S., 81a
McGaffin, C. G., 130b
McGahey, S. B., 22b
McGahey, S. M., 15a
McGhie, A., 105b, 109b
McGill University, 106a
McGill University. Allan Memorial Institute of Psychiatry, 104a
McGill University. School for Graduate Nurses, 11a

McGirr, P. O. M., 71b, 99b
McGlothlin, W. J., 53a
McGolrick, B., 70b, 76a
McGrath, B. J., 99b
McGregor, E. M., 105b
MacGregor, F. C., 42a, 81a
MacGregor, J. E., 22b
McGuigan, H. A., 123b
McGuire, M., 120b
Macintyre, K. V., 15a
McIntyre, M. J., 88a
McIntyre, P. H., 50a
McIsaac, I., 15a, 61a, 76a, 90b
McIver, P., 27a, 65b, 114a
Mack Training School, St. Catherine's Hospital, Ontario, 56b
Mackay, P. M. M., 125a
McKechnie, M. W., 47a
McKenna, F. M., 27a
Mackenzie, E., 15a
Mackenzie, M. A., 15a
Mackenzie, N., 25a, 53a, 109b
Mackenzie, T., 131a
Mackie, T. T., 95a
McKinney, J. C., 21a
Mackintosh, J. M., 83b
MacLaggan, K., 42a
McLaren, B., 9b
McLaren, E. S., 128b
McLaughlin, A. I. G., 87b
McLaughlin, C. R., 118b
McLaughlin, J. R., 90a, 97a
McLaughlin, M., 115a
Maclean, H., 2b, 15a
Maclehose, O., 15a
MacLeod, A. I., 21a, 51b
MacLeod, C., 70b, 111b
MacMahon, R. P., 54b
Macmanus, E. E. P., 9b, 15a, 83b, 127a
McManus, R. L., 21a, 27a, 42a, 52a, 54b
McMenemey, H., 132a
McMillan, M. H., 53a
MacNab, G. H., 102a
McNaught, E., 50a
McNealy, R. W., 120b
McPartland, T. S., 26a, 39a
MacPhail, H., 42a
McQuarrie, F., 42a, 54b
McQuater, F., 92b
McQueen, E. U., 53a
Macqueen, I. A. G., 53a, 113b, 114a
MacQueen, K. S., 15a
Macrae, A. D., 36a
McRae, C., 22b
MacRea, M. C., 48a
McWatt, F., 111b
Maddin, S., 35b
Maddox, H., 105b
Maegraith, B. G., 95a
Magee, R. B., 79b
Magnussen, A. K., 83b
Magnussen, E., 38b
Maguire, Sister M. A., 54b
Maher, M. A., 116a
Maher, M. H., 119a
Mahood, N. P., 118b
Maida Vale Hospital, 129b
Maine General Hospital, 130a
Malachowski, L. T., 115b
Malecka, A. B., 123b
Mallory, E., 21a, 42a
Maloney, E. M., 123b
Mance, J., 15a
Manchester Northern Hospital, 130a
Manchester Regional Hospital Board, 51a, 69b, 106a, 107b, 127b
Manchester Royal Infirmary, 130a
Manchester University, 51a, 106a
Mandelbrote, B., 106a
Manfreda, M. L., 107a
Mann, T. P., 74b
Mannin, E., 110a
Manning, A. R., 76a
Mannino, S. F., 124b
Manoch, H., 51b

Mansell, E. M., 111b
Mansfield, E. O., 55a
Mansfield, L., 53a
Manzer, H. G., 63a
Marchant, E. P., 48b
Marchesini, E. H., 106a
Margaret Vincent, Sister, 69a
Marianne, Mother, 15a
Marie Curie Memorial, 87a
Marie Edgar, Sister, 121a
Marin, A., 64b
Markowitz, A., 88a
Markus, F. E., 35b
Marple, C. D., 88a
Marriner, —, 15a
Marsh, E. L., 81a
Marsh, H. N., 29a
Marshall, J., 96a
Marshall, M. L., 11a
Marshall, R., 131a, 131b
Marshall, S., 86b, 89a
Martin, A. M., 4a
Martin, D. V., 61a, 106a
Martin, H. W., 21a, 42a, 106a
Martin, J., 53a
Martin, M. F., 87a
Martin, M. M., 88b
Martin, S. E., 64a
Martineau, H., 76a
Martinez, R. E., 103a
Martin-Scott, I., 35b
Marwick, I. I., 106a
Mary, Sister, 50a
Mary Agnes, Sister, 48b
Mary Albert, Sister, 48b
Mary Carolyn, Sister, 42a
Mary Crown of Thorns, Sister, 81a
Mary Emil, Sister, 53a
Mary Felicitas, Sister, 42a
Mary Fletcher Hospital, Burlington, Vermont, 130a
Mary Louise, Sister, 66b
Mary Margarella, Sister, 67a
Mary Maurita, Sister, 69a
Mary Stephen, Sister, 37a
Maryland State Nurses' Association, 29a
Maryo, J. S., 68a
Mason, M. A., 93b
Massachusetts General Hospital, 130a
Massachusetts General Hospital. School of Nursing, 57a
Masachusetts Memorial Hospital, 29a
Massachusetts State Nurses' Association, 29b
Masterman, C., 33a
Masters, R. E., 99a
Maternity Centre Association, New York, 6b
Matheney, R. V., 106a
Matheson, A., 16a
Matheson, V., 23a
Mathews, B., 53b
Mathewson, M. S., 2a
Matrons' Council, 4b, 29b
Matson, D. D., 102a
Matthews, A., 15a
Matthews, F., 76a
Matthews, H. J., 13a
Matthews, M. L. W., 15a
Matthews, O., 63a
Mattick, —, 15a
Mattingley, C. B., 87b
Mauksch, H. O., 81a
Maule, H. G., 81a
Maunders, S. H., 99b
Maxwell, A. C., 76a
Mayes, M., 97b
Maynard, E. L., 110a
Maynard, T., 19a
Meachen, G. N., 86b, 88b, 125a
Mead, M., 21a
Medical Officer, *pseud.*, 117a
Medico-Psychological Association of Great Britain and Ireland, 108a. *See also:* Royal Medico-Psychological Association

Medill, —, 15a
Meigs, J. W., 35a, 98b
Meir, E., 53a, 106a
Melanie, M., 81a
Mellor, M. D., 35b
Mellow, J., 108b
Mendoza, R., 59b
Mental Hospital and Institutional Workers' Union, 29b
Menzies, I. E. P., 69b
Mercier, C. A., 21a, 61a
Merrick, E., 11b, 27a
Merrill, B. E., 4a
Merrill, M. G., 57b
Merritt, W., 34a
Merrow, S., 35a
Merry, E. J., 48b, 111b
Merton, R. K., 21a
Methuen, D., 50a
Metropolitan and National Association for Providing Trained Nurses for the Sick Poor, 6a
Metropolitan Asylums Board, 37a
Metropolitan Life Insurance Company, 122a
Metzger, M. E., 42a
Metzner, C. A., 81b
Meyer, B., 68a, 82a
Meyer, G. R., 59b, 61a
Meyer, R. T., 50a
Meyers, M. E., 15a
Michael, J., 104a
Michaels, R., 8a
Michaels, R. G., 59a
Michal-Smith, H., 108b
Michigan Department of Health, 117a
Michigan University. School of Public Health, 87a
Mickey, J. E., 81a
Middlesex Hospital, 41a, 130a
Middleton, A. B., 66a, 107b
Midgley, R. L., 76b
Midland Doctor, *pseud.*, 25a
Mildmay Mission Hospital, 130a
Miles, H., 116a
Miles, H. B., 53a
Mill, C. R., 15a, 81a
Millard, S., 9b
Miller, D., 97b
Miller, H., 42a
Miller, H. A., 54b
Miller, J. D., 9b
Miller, J. D., Jr., 79b
Miller, L. B., 51b
Miller, M. A., 48b
Miller, M. C., 57b
Miller, N. F., 90b
Miller Hospital and Royal Kent Dispensary, 130a
Mills, A. C., 97b
Mills, C. K., 106a
Mills, H. C., 45a
Mills, K. A., 70b
Milne, J. H., 15b
Milton, H. D., 72b, 113b
Mindess, H., 38b
Miner, L., 110a
Ministry of Education. *See:* Great Britain. Ministry of Education
Ministry of Health. *See:* Great Britain. Ministry of Health
Ministry of Labour. *See:* Great Britain. Ministry of Labour
Minks, M., 15b
Minnesota Board of Nursing, 27a
Minnesota Nurses' Association, 27a
Minnesota University. Center for Continuation Study, 100b
Minnesota University. School of Nursing, 53a, 57a, 76b
Minski, L., 106a
Minter, S., 121a
Mishler, E. G., 107b
Missouri University, 57a
Mrs. H., 9b
Mitchell, A. G., 102a

Mitchell, I. A., 122b
Mitchell, R. J., 42a
Mitchell, S. D., 106a
Mitchell, S. W., 27a, 61a
Mitchiner, P. H., 9b, 83b
Mitchison, E. L., 23b
Mitman, M., 91b
M.M.W., 131a
Moak, F. L., 37b
Modell, W., 87b, 123b
Modern Hospital, 82a, 128a
Moersch, F. P., 96a
Mohan, T., 50a
Mohs, E. L., 94b
Moles, C. L., 25a, 94b
Molgren, R., 37b
Molleson, A., 122a
Mollett, M., 7a, 15b, 21a, 42a, 61a, 64a
Mollett, N., 51b
Monahan, S., 69b
Moncrieff, A., 25a, 102b
Mongrain, L., 69b
Monkhouse, M., 65b, 114a
Montag, M. L., 42b, 46b, 70b, 76b
Montalembert, Count, 13a
Montefiore Hospital, New York, 130a
Monteith, J. W., 22b
Montgomerie, H. L., 15b
Montreal General Hospital, 57a
Montreal Royal Victoria Hospital, 106a
Moody, S., 123a
Moore, F., 9b
Moore, L., 71b
Moore, N., 131b
Mooreland, M., 119a
Moorhaven Hospital, 130a
Morgan, J., 81a
Morgan, K., 27a
Morgan, M. M., 70b
Morgan, M. P., 59b
Morgan, W., 41a
Moriarty, H. R., 42b
Morimoto, F. R., 63a
Morland, V., 68a
Morley, H., 94b
Moroney, J., 118b
Morrell, M. A., 61a
Morris, E., 122a
Morris, E. E., 22b
Morris, E. H., 125b
Morris, I. H., 111a
Morris, J. M., 22b
Morrison, L. J., 1b, 27a, 106a
Morrison, R. M., 50a
Morrissey, A. B., 124b
Morrissey, M., 51b
Morrow, J. T., 111b
Morse, E. C., 87b
Morse, M. E., 86b
Morson, C., 131b
Morten, H., 1b, 15b, 25a
Morton, A. L., 123b
Morton, T. G., 130b
Morwyn, J., 25b
Mosby, C. V., 16a
Mosby's Comprehensive Review of Nursing, 27a
Mosenthall, W. T., 79b
Moses, E. B., 27a, 72b
Mount Sinai Hospital, New York, 130a
Mount Vernon Hospital, Northwood, 130a
Mowla, K., 24a
Mowry, L., 122b
Mudge, J., 53a
Mullane, M. K., 21a, 45a, 69b
Mullaney, G., 114a
Muller, T., 50a
Muller, T. G., 106a, 109b
Mulvany, M. F., 15b
Mumford, E. M., 129a
Mumford, E. W., 99b
Munro, A., 27a, 76b
Munro, E., 97b
Munson, H. W., 28b
Muntyan, B., 46b

Murphy, D. G., 1b
Murphy, M., 116a
Murphy, R. J., 61a
Murray, J. G., 53a
Murray, M., 37b
Murray, R., 42b
Murrell, M., 125b
Murrell, T. W., 81a
Murrey, N., 90b
Musallam, A., 24a
Muse, M. B., 15b, 42b, 109b
Musgrove, J., 127a
Mussallem, H. K., 55a
Musselman, G., 53a
Musson, E. M., 15b, 35b, 53a
Myers, G. W., 130a
Myers, J. A., 125b
Myers, R. S., 71a, 81a
Myles, M. F., 97b

Nabbe, F. C., 83b
Nahm, H., 21a, 42b, 55a, 108b
Nash, D. F. E., 121a
Nash, R., 16a, 16b
Nast, M., 123b
Nathan, H., 61b
National Association for Practical Nurse Education, 71b
National Association of Local Government Officers, 25b-
National Association of State Enrolled Assistant Nurses, 71b
National Committee for the Improvement of Nursing Services. Sub-Committee on School Data Analysis, 55a
National Council of Nurses for Great Britain and Ireland, 29b
National Council of Trained Nurses of Finland, 76b
National Council of Trained Nurses of Great Britain and Ireland, 5a
National Council of Women of Great Britain and Ireland, 34a
National Federation of Belgian Nurses, 76b
National Heart Hospital, London, 130a
National Hospital for Nervous Diseases, London, 130a, 130b
National League for Nursing, 29b, 38b, 42b, 45b, 46a, 51b, 59b, 67a, 83b, 100b
National League for Nursing. Committee on Careers, 27a, 27b, 37b, 42b
National League for Nursing. Committee on the Future, 27b
National League for Nursing. Department of Baccalaureate and Higher Degree Programs, 42b, 53a
National League for Nursing. Department of Diploma and Associate Degree Programs, 47b
National League for Nursing. Department of Hospital Nursing, 67a, 81a, 118b
National League for Nursing. Department of Public Health Nursing, 81a, 110a, 111b, 114a, 115b, 116a, 117a
National League for Nursing. Division of Nursing Education, 42b, 53a, 55a
National League for Nursing. Tuberculosis Nursing Advisory Service, 36a, 125b
National League of Certificated Nurses of Great Britain and Ireland, 29b
National League of Nursing Education, 11a, 27a, 29b, 37b, 38b, 42b, 43a, 45a, 46a, 47b, 53a, 55a, 64b, 65b, 66a, 68b, 73a, 108a, 119b
National League of Nursing Education. Committee on Curriculum, 55a
National League of Nursing Education. Committee on Vocational Guidance, 55a

National League of Nursing Education. Committee to Study Administration in Schools of Nursing, 55a
National League of Nursing Education. Department of Studies, 34b, 65b
National League of Nursing Education. Joint Orthopaedic Nursing Advisory Service, 92a
National Nursing Council, 55a
National Nursing Council. History Committee, 29b
National Nursing Council for War Service, 46b
National Organization for Public Health Nursing, 92a, 95b, 110a, 111b, 114a, 115b, 116a
National Organization for Public Health Nursing. Committee on Nursing in Medical Care Plans, 110a
National Organization for Public Health Nursing. Committee on Parti-Time Nursing Service to Industry, 99b
National Organization for Public Health Nursing. School Nursing Section, 117a
National Organization of Hospital Schools of Nursing, 55b
National Pension Fund, 29b
National Society for the Prevention of Blindness, 101a
National Union of Trained Nurses, 29b
Nattestad, L., 101a
Navran, L., 59b
Nayer, D. D., 43a
Naylor, A., 119b
Neal, M. V., 84a
Neal, R. E., 87b
Nebraska State Nurses' Association, 29b
Needham, C. E., 67b
Neef, F. E., 121a
Neil, C. A., 92b
Neil, J. H., 89a
Neil, T. H., 89a
Nelson, J., 26b
Nelson, K. L. J., 59b, 124a
Nelson, R. C., 21a
Nelson, S. C., 15b
Neter, E., 86b
Netherlands Consulting Centre for Hospital Planning, 33b
New, P. K., 37b, 69b, 70a
New Brunswick University, 43a, 57a
New South Wales Assembly, 33b
New South Wales Trained Nurses' Association, 29b
New York City Children's Hospital, Randall's Island, New York, 130b
New York City. Department of Health, 116a
New York City. Department of Hospitals. Committee on Nursing Standards, 77a
New York City. Manhattan Eye, Ear and Throat Hospital, 89a
New York City. Mayor's Committee of Women on National Defence, Standing Committee on Nursing, 84a
New York City Training School for Nurses, 57a
New York Hospital, 129a, 130b
New York Hospital School of Nursing, 56b, 57a, 80a
New York Postgraduate Medical School and Hospital, 57a
New York State, 4a
New York State. Department of Health, 87a, 114a
New York State. Department of Health. Nutrition Bureau, 122b
New York State. Departmental Health Council, 43a
New York State University. State Education Department, 43a
New York University. Department of Nurse Education, 68a

New Zealand. Department of Health, 2b
New Zealand, Parliament, 31b
Newcastle Regional Hospital Board, 8a
Newcastle-upon-Tyne Infirmary, 130b
Newcomb, D. P., 83a
Newcomb, E., 9b
Newell, H., 29b
Newington, D. K., 114a
Newman, C., 51a
Newman, Sir G., 16b
Newman, L., 15b
Newsholme, H. P., 63a
Newsome, E., 76b
Newstead, W. K., 29b
Newton Hospital, Massachusetts, 57a
Newton, K., 89b
Newton, M. E., 16b, 51a, 67a, 121a, 122b, 127b
Newton, M. G., 115b
Nicholson, E., 15b
Nicholson, N. G., 116b
Nickolls, —, 102b
Nicole, J. E., 109b
Nie, P. J., 40b
Nightingale, F., 14a, 15b, 16a, 16b, 17a, 21a, 21b, 25b, 43a, 56b, 61a, 77a, 91a, 97b, 111b, 128a
Nightingale, G. S., 131b
Nightingale School of Nursing, Toronto, 58a
Nightingale Training School, London, 57a, 57b
Nite, G., 37b, 50a, 70a
Nixon, J. A., 74b
Norbury, F., 34a
Nordmark, M. T., 43a, 77a
Norfolk and Norwich Hospital, 130b
Norman, L. G., 119a
Norman, M. R., 123a
Norrie, C., 23a
Norris, C. M., 50a, 109a
Norris, C. N., 81a
Norris, S., 68a
North, F. H., 56a
North Carolina Baptist Hospital, 130b
North Carolina State, 4a
North Carolina University. Institute for Research in Social Science, 106a
Northcroft, G. B., 121a
Northern Ireland. Parliament, 32a, 34a
Norton, D., 89b, 121a
Norton, F., 67a, 77a, 85b, 90b
Norton, I., 84a
Norwalk Hospital, 130b
Norwegian Nurses' Association, 121a
Notter, L., 116b
Nottingham General Hospital, 130b
Noyes, A. P., 106a
Nuesse, C. J., 1b
Nuffield Provincial Hospitals Trust, 37b, 68a, 77a
Nuffield Provincial Hospitals Trust. Scottish Advisory Medical Committee, 127b
Nunez, M., 23a
Nurses' Associated Alumnae of the United States and Canada, 29b
Nurses' Association of China, 29b
Nurses' Association of China. Education Committee. 47b
Nurses' House Inc., 35b
Nursing Directory, 25b
Nursing Mirror, 6b, 8a, 37b, 61a, 63a, 77a, 84a
Nursing Mirror. Committee on Overtaxed Nurses, 35b
Nursing Outlook, 21b, 27b, 43a, 53b, 71b
Nursing Record, 2b, 3b, 6b, 45a, 51b, 55b, 106b
Nursing Research, 59b
Nursing Times, 5a, 8a, 33b, 53b, 61b, 65a, 65b, 71a, 71b, 72a, 91b, 97b, 103b, 105a, 106a, 110b, 114a, 117a, 125b
Nutini, S., 53b

Nuttall, P., 25b
Nutting, M. A., 1b, 17a, 43a, 45a, 55b

Oakes, L., 90b, 94b, 123b
Oberteuffer, D., 117a
O'Boyle, M., 68b
O'Connell, P. E., 48b, 51a, 116b
O'Connor, M. E., 17a
Oddie, W. A., 13a
Odier, L., 5a
Odlum, D., 109b
O'Donoghue, E. G., 128b
O'Driscoll, B. J., 85a
Ogg, E., 42b
Ogle, W., 17a
O'Hara, F. J., 109b
Ohlson, A., 29a
Oklahoma State Nurses' Association, 29b
Old Internationals' Association, 61b
An Old Woman, pseud., 21b
Oleksyn, E. E., 120b
Olive, A. H., 104a
Olnhausen, M. P., 9b
Olsen, B. M., 50b
Olson, A. F., 67b
Olson, J. F., 55b
Olson, L. M., 77a
Olson, M. E., 59b, 70a
O'Malley, I. B., 16b
O'Malley, M., 81a
O'Neill, H. C., 65b, 77a
Ontario. Department of Health. Division of Venereal Disease Control, 125b
Ophthalmic Nursing Board, 101a, 101b
Oppenheim, A. N., 108a
Orange Training School for Nurses, Orange, New Jersey, 57b
Orbison, K. T., 77a
Order of St. John of Jerusalem, 7b
Ordiz, R. A., 38b
Orem, D. E., 71b
Orme, S. E., 53b
Orn, E., 24a
O'Roarke, E. M., 52b
Orr, J. M., 17a
Osborne, S. G., 9b
Osgood, G. A., 69b
Osler, W., 21b, 93b
Osmond, H., 22a
Ostenso, M., 14a
Ottley, L. J., 81a
Ouellet, F. M., 102b
Ouimet, J., 58b, 121a
Our Lady's Hospice, Dublin, 130b
Ouseley, M. H., 50a, 59b
Overlock, M. G., 95a
Ovington, L. H., 95a
Owen, M. C., 116b
Owen, M. R., 43a
Oxford, M. N., 77a
Oxford Regional Hospital Board, 35b, 43a

Pacific Coast Journal of Nursing, 11a
Packard, J. H., 43a
Padwick, C. E., 11a
Paget, R., 17a
Paine, L. H. W., 63a
Palmer, M. E., 53b, 96a
Palmer, S. F., 17a
Parent, A., 121a
Park, A., 17a
Park, P. M., 27b
Parker, C., 100b
Parker, E. M., 121a
Parker, N. A., 121b
Parker, S., 17b, 63a
Parkinson, R. H., 89a
Parloff, M. B., 109b
Parmet, M., 95b
Parrish, H. M., 81b, 127a
Parson, J. S., 17b

Parsons, F. G., 131b
Parsons, H. F., 128a
Parsons, L. G., 126a
Parsons, S. E., 21b, 57a, 61b
Pasanen, U., 23a, 57b
Patmore, E., 37b, 50a, 83a
Patrick, J., 129a
Patrick, M., 125a
Patriot Daughters of Lancaster, 9b
Patterson, M. G., 64a
Patterson, T. K., 53b
Pattison, D. W., 17b
Pavey, A., 1b, 91a, 93b, 122b, 127a
Peabody, F. W., 77a
Pearce, D., 61b
Pearce, E. C., 24b, 63a, 77a, 85b, 91a, 91b, 119b, 121a
Pearn, O. P. N., 106b, 108b
Pearse, H. L., 17b, 43a, 110a, 117a
Pearson, E., 8a
Peebles, A., 110b
Peel, J. S., 123b
Pegg, F. G., 17b
Pemberton, D. A., 99b
Pennant, A., 15b
Penney, M., 15a
Pennock, M. R., 11a
Pennsylvania Hospital, 130b
Pennsylvania State Nurses' Association, 72b
Peplau, H. E., 50a, 63a, 106b
Percival, F. H., 88b
Percy, D. M., 115b
Perkins, D. T., 100b
Perkins, E. W., 121a
Perkins, L. D., 80b
Perkins, R. A., 102b
Perrodin, C. M., 70a, 75b, 93b
Perry, A., 77b
Perry, C. B., 93b
Perry, H., 35b
Perry, I., 127a
Perry, S. E., 107b
Peter, P. W., 17b
Peters, F. N., 87b
Peters, G. A., 29a
Peterson, R. I., 124b
Pether, G. C., 99b
Petrie, A., 38b
Petry, L., 45b
Petty, R., 117a
Peyton, A. B., 122b
Pfefferkorn, B., 50a, 56b, 65a, 66a
Philadelphia Episcopal Hospital, 130b
Phillips, E. C., 124b
Phillips, F. L. M., 67a
Phillips, M., 113b
Phillips, M. G., 57b
Philpott, N., 114b
Phinney, M., Baroness Von Genhausen, 17b
Pickens, M. E., 68b, 115b
Pickett, S. E., 8a
Picture Facts Associates, 65b
Pierce, B., 106b
Pierce, E., 101b
Pierre, Sister, 131b
Pilkington, F., 130a
Piette, E. C., 86b
Pike, C. F., 99b
Pilant, E. P., 91a
Pillers, M. E., 1b
Pillsbury, M. E., 92a
Pinanski, V. R., 71a
Pinchard, S. T. B., 17b
Pines, A., 85a
Piper, P. M., 77b
Pittman, H., 47b
Place, D. J., 123b
Plass, F. G., 98a
Platt, E., 6a
Plogsted, H., 50a, 105b
Plum, W., 17b
Pochin, E. E., 124a
Pohowalla, J. N., 102b
Poland, R., 130a

Polden, S. E., 17b
Pollard, E. F., 16b
Pollard, J. C., 106b
Poole, D., 43b, 84a
Poole, E., 4a, 6a
Poole, H., 3b
Poorman, A., 65b
Pope, A. E., 76a, 77b, 94a
Pope, F. M., 64b
Pope, G., 9b, 98a
Porter, E., 109b
Porter, E. K., 51b
Porter, M. F., 109b
Portland Hospital, 130b
Potter, G. W., 30b
Potter, H. G., 5b
Potter, H. W., 106b
Potter, M., 17b, 114b
Potter, R., 57a
Potter, R. M., 53b, 70a
Poulos, E. S., 59b
Powell, M., 119b
Powell, M. B., 38b, 60b, 127a
Powell, N. W., 77b, 123b
Powers, R. A., 53b
Prabhu, M. B., 102b
Practitioner, 111b
Prangley, R. R., 43b
Pratt, D. L., 68b
Preher, Sister L. M., 63a
Presbyterian Hospital, New York, 130b
Presbyterian Hospital, New York. School of Nursing, 57b
Pressland, D., 17b
Preston, A., 77b
Price, A. L., 77b
Price, E. D., 71b
Price, T. W., 31b
Priest, M. A., 91a
Pringle, A. L., 17b, 21b, 25b
Prior, P. L., 77b
Pritchard, E., 102b
Professional Union of Trained Nurses, 30a
Proudfit, F. T., 122b
Pugh, W. T. G., 77b
Pumroy, S. S., 72b
Purdy, K. E., 64b

Queen Alexandra's Imperial Military Nursing Service, 5a, 9b
Queen Alexandra's Royal Naval Nursing Service, 6b
Queen Alexandra's Royal Naval Nursing Service Reserve, 6b
Queen Charlotte's Lying-in Hospital, 130b
Queen Victoria's Jubilee Institute for Nurses, 6a
Queen's Institute of District Nursing, 6a, 87a, 111b, 112a
Queensland. Parliament, 31a
Quine, A. E., 126a
Quiros, A., 117b
Quixley, J. M. E., 90a, 97a

Rabin, C. B., 104a
Rabo, M., 47b
Radcliffe Infirmary, Oxford, 130b
Radwanski, D. M., 99b
Radzialowski, R., 67a
Raeburn, H. A., 85b
Raeburn, J. K., 85b, 86a
Raisig, L. M., 85b
Rakich, J. H., 77b
Ramos, L. F., 114b
Randall, M., 67a
Randall, M. G., 115b
Randall, O. A., 89b
Randle, B. B., 117a
Randle, J., 125b
Rappaport, J., 123a
Rappaport, M. B., 117a
Rathbone, W., 6a

Rattner, H., 88b
Rauth, J. E., 109b
Raven, R. W., 87a
Ravitz, M. J., 21b
Ray, M. E., 17b
Ray, T. S., 38a
Rayner, C. B., 37b
Rayner, J. F., 84a
Reader, G., 81b
Recicar, C., 9b
Red Crescent School of Nursing, Istanbul, 57b
Redman, P. W., 81b
Redmond, J., 9b
Redmond, M. M., 48b, 77b
Reed, C. A. L., 21b
Reed, C. B., 98a
Reed, W. H., 9b
Rees, M. I. H., 96a
Rees, T. P., 106b
Reese, D. E., 43b
Regan, W. A., 32b, 49a, 82a, 122a
Regardie, V. H., 121a
Registered Nurses' Parliamentary Council, 30a
Reid, A. E., 28a, 50a
Reid, E. G., 16b
Reid, E. P., 77b
Reid, J. P., 37b
Reid, L. D., 37b
Reid, M., 68b, 111b
Reijnvaan, J. P., 17b
Reilly, C. E., 65b
Reimann, C., 70a
Reinhardt, J. M., 27b, 63a
Reinhart, A., 5b
Reissman, L., 69b
Render, H. W., 63a, 106b
Renton, B. H., 125b
The Retreat, York, 130b
Reuell, C. H., 53b
Revans, R. W., 37b, 68b, 127a
Rexford-Welch, S. C., 4b
Reynolds, J., 81b
Reynolds, W. M., 75b
Rezler, A., 115b
Rhode Island Hospital, 57b
Rhode Island Training School for Nursing, 77b
Rhodes, V. A., 119b
Rhodes, W. C., 95b
Rice, F. F., 21b, 65b
Rice, G. U., Jr., 114b
Rich, F. R., 54b
Richards, E. L., 106b
Richards, L., 17b, 55b, 57b
Richardson, D. C., 92a
Richardson, G., 24a
Richardson, H. B., 81b
Richardson, T. E., 9b
Richardson, W. L., 72b
Richie, J., 114b, 125b
Richmond, K. E., 17b
Richomme, A., 14b
Richwagen, L. E., 67a
Riddell, M. S., 43b, 77b, 78a
Ridding, L., 98a
Riddle, M. M., 55b, 67a
Ridley, M., 17b
Riley, F., 36a
Riley, F. G., 129b
Riley, T. P., 96a
Rippington, A. E., 37b
Ritchie, G., 102b
Ritchie, J. A., 70a
Robb, I. H., 4a, 18a, 30a, 43b, 61b
Roberts, D. I., 63a, 111b
Roberts, G. W., 78a
Roberts, J. G., 89a
Roberts, K., 65b
Roberts, L., 111b, 114b
Roberts, M. M., 4a, 5a, 13a, 13b, 18a, 19b
Roberts, R. L., 78a, 91a
Roberts, T., 108a
Roberts, W., 81b
Robertson, E., 71a

BIBLIOGRAPHY OF NURSING

Robertson, G. M., 106b
Robertson, J. D., 112a
Robins, D., 18a
Robins, R. A., 86a
Robinson, A. M., 106b, 108b
Robinson, E. S., 109b
Robinson, G. C., 81b
Robinson, J., 56a
Robinson, J. M., 5b
Robinson, M., 34a
Robinson, M. G., 95b
Robinson, P., 102b
Robinson, V., 1b
Robson, P. L., 8a
Roche, A. E., 89b
Rochester General Hospital, New York, 131a
Rochester Regional Hospital Council, 81b
Rockberger, H., 35b
Rockefeller Foundation, 43b
Rodabaugh, J. H., 4a
Rodabaugh, M. J., 4a
Rodeman, C. R., 106b
Rogan, J., 5a
Rogers, D. L. M., 107b
Rogers, G. A., 18a
Rogers, H., 86b
Rogers, L. L., 117a
Rohrer, J. H., 69b
Rohweder, A. E., 43a, 77a
Rohweder, A. W., 50b, 80b
Rolfe, P. J., 107b
Roosevelt Hospital, New York. School of Nursing, 57b
Rose, D. E., 55b
Rosemont, V. L., 71a
Rosenberg, A., 129b
Roseveare, M. P., 129b
Ross, A., 102b
Ross, A. D., 21b
Ross, C. F., 71b, 83a
Ross, I., 11b
Ross, J. S., 78a
Ross, J. W., 5a
Ross, M., 18a
Ross, R. I., 21b
Rossitter, E., 33b
Rossman, I. J., 95a
Roth, A., 29b
Rotherham County Borough Council, 103a, 103b
Rothweiler, E. L., 78a
Rotter, K., 89a
Rottman, M., 50a
Rotunda Hospital, Dublin, 131a
Rourke, A. J., 81b
Routhier, A. M., 89b
Rouvray, F. G., 129a
Rovetta, C. A., 66a
The Roving Englishman, *pseud.*, 9b
Rowbotham, G. F., 118b
Rowe, H. R., 85b
Rowe, J. W., 86a
Rowe, P. R. M., 108a
Rowland, M. A., 65b
Rowley, M., 84a
Royal Berkshire Hospital, 131a
Royal British Nurses' Association, 30a
(*See also:* British Nurses' Association)
Royal College of Nursing, 25b, 37b, 48b, 51b, 53b, 55b, 69a, 69b, 71b
(*See also:* College of Nursing)
Royal College of Nursing. Education Department, 50b, 53b
Royal College of Nursing. Occupational Health Section, 99b
Royal College of Nursing. Public Health Section, 34a, 115a
Royal College of Nursing. Sister Tutor Section, 51b
Royal College of Nursing. Ward and Departmental Sisters Section, 106b
Royal College of Physicians of London. Paediatric Committee, 103a

Royal Edinburgh Hospital for Sick Children, 131a
Royal Eye Hospital, London, 131a
Royal Gwent Hospital, 131a
Royal Hospital, Haslar, 131a
Royal Medico-Psychological Association, 106b, 108a, 108b
(*See also:* Medico-Psychological Association, etc.)
Royal Melbourne Hospital, 131a
Royal National Hospital for Rheumatic Diseases, Bath, 131a
Royal National Pension Fund for Nurses, 30b
Royal Northern Hospital, London, 131a
Royal Northern Infirmary, Inverness, 131a
Royal United Hospital, Bath, 131a
Royal Victoria Hospital, Belfast, 131a
Royal West Sussex Hospital, 131a
Rubery Hill and Hollymoor Hospitals, 131a
Rubin, C., 96a
Rudd, T. N., 89b, 90a
Rue, C. B., 114b
Rumball, M., 18a
Rundall, F. B. A., 16b
Rundle, H., 9b
Rundle, M. S., 18a, 47b
Runell, E. S., 21b, 67a
Rushcliffe, Lord, 34a
Rushton, J. G., 96a
Russell, C. H., 43b
Russell, C. M., 84a
Russell, E. K., 21b, 43a, 43b, 82b
Russell, S. M., 27b
Russell, V. D., 130b
Russell, W. H., 9b
Russell, W. L., 106b
Rutan, E. L., 48b
Ryan, T., 130b
Ryer, I., 99a
Rykken, M. B., 96a
Ryle, A. E., 67a
Ryle-Horwood, E. M., 125b
Rynbergen, H. J., 122b

Sabshin, M., 63a
Sachs, E., 121a
Sachs, G., 91b
Sackheim, G. I., 104a
Sadler, S., 92b
Sadler, W. S., 106b
Safford, B. J., 82b
Safren, M. A., 59b
Sage, V., 58a
St. Alfege's Hospital, Greenwich, 131a
St. Bartholomew's Hospital, London, 131a, 131b
St. George's Hospital, London, 131b
St. John, C. F., 16b
St. John, M., 72a
St. Joseph Hospital School of Nursing, 57b
St. Joseph's Hospital, Woodside, 131b
St. Louis City Hospital. Training School for Nurses, 57b
St. Luke's Hospital, Woodside, 131b
St. Luke's Hospital School of Nursing, 57b
St. Luke's Hospital Training School for Nurses, New York, 57b
St. Mary's Hospital, Paddington, 57b, 103b, 131b
St. Mary's Hospital, Rochester, Minnesota, 118b, 131b
St. Mary's School of Nursing, Milwaukee, Wisconsin. Guidance Committee, 46b
St. Paul's Hospital, London, 131b
St. Peter's Hospital for Stone, London, 131b
St. Thomas's Hospital, London, 128a, 131b

St. Thomas's Hospital, London. Nightingale Training School, 57a, 57b
St. Vincent's Hospital, Dublin, 131b
Salisbury, P. F., 79b
Salter, K., 88a
Salvador, A., 72b
Samaritan Free Hospital, 131b
Samson, H. P., 63b
Sand, O., 43b, 47b
Sandbach, B., 10a
Sanders, B. H., 21b
Sanders, E. K., 19a
Sanders, G. J., 78a
Sands, I. J., 96b
Sanford, T. H., 59b
Santos, E. H., 7b
Sara, D., 94b
Sargent, E. G., 90a
Sarwer-Foner, G. J., 35a
Satchwell, —, 106b
Satchwell, E., 18a
Sauer, L. W., 102b
Saunders, H. St. G., 130a
Saunders, L., 21b
Savage, W. G., 126a
Sawers, J., 38b
Sayer, J., 89b
Saynajarvi, R., 101a
Scales, M., 67a
Schade, J. A., 132b
Schafer, M. K., 70a, 84a
Scheffel, C., 33a
Schiff, S., 102b
Schlotfeldt, R. M., 59b, 82b
Schmitt, L. M., 43b, 47b
Schneider, C. M., 124a
Schoeller, V. D., 70a
Scholder, A. P., 50a
Schott, G., 38b
Schraders, C. G., 18a
Schroeder, Y., 52b
Schroth, R. G., 78a
Schryver, G. F., 56b
Schulz, C., 21b, 27b
Schumacher, M. E., 55b
Schwartz, B., 124b
Schwartz, C. G., 107a
Schwartz, D. R., 81b, 95a, 115b
Schwartz, M. S., 107a
Schweisheimer, W., 35b, 119a
Schwier, M. E., 43b, 55b, 69b
Sclare, I. M., 107a
Scotland. Department of Health, 43b, 69b, 112a, 126a
Scotland. Department of Health. Nurses' Salaries Committee, 34a
Scott, D. H., 78a, 95a
Scott, J., 71a, 78a
Scott, K., 18a
Scott, R. B., 121a
Scott, R. J. E., 78a
Scott, W. C., 33a
Scott-Brown, M., 102a
Scottish Health Services Council, 63b
Scottish Health Services Council. Standing Nursing and Midwifery Advisory Committee, 68b, 71b
Seacole, M., 18a
Searle, C., 53b
Sears, W. G., 86a, 94a, 123b
Sehsuvaroglu, B. N., 2b
Seifert, V. D., 84a
Selbert, N., 95a
Select Committee on Registration of Nurses, 32b
Select Committee of the House of Lords on Metropolitan Hospitals, etc., 126b
Sellew, G., 1b, 63b, 66b, 67a, 102b
Sellon, P. L., 18a
Sellors, T. H., 125a
Selly Oak Infirmary, 131b
Senior, W. G., 88a
Senn, N., 27b
Sergeant, M., 18a
Seton, E., 18a

Severinghaus, A. E., 21b
Sevestre, R., 64b
Sewall, A. M., 104a
Sewall, M., 1b
Sewart, C. B., 36a
Seyffer, C., 47b, 53b, 69a
Seymer, L. R., 1b, 16b, 18b, 57a
Sgarra, A., 24a
Shackleton, A. D., 122b
Shadyside Hospital School of Nursing, 57b
Shafer, K., 94a, 132b
Shannon, A. M., 119a
Shannon, M. A., 90a
Shaw, H. F., 71a
Shear, H. J., 63b
Shee, W. A., 38a
Sheedy, J. P., 14b
Sheehy, M. M., 109b
Sheen, D., 43b
Sheen, E. M., 114b
Shelby, B., 128a
Sheldon, E. B., 59b
Shepard, K., 78a
Shepard, M. E., 89a
Sheps, C. G., 132b
Sherman, M., 109b
Sherrer, Q. M., 38a
Sherrod, H. H., 71b
Shestack, R., 123b
Shetland, M. L., 47b, 115b
Shields, C. D., 124b
Shimberg, B., 95a
Shockley, E. L., 107a
Shoemaker, Sister M. T., 6b
Sholtis, L. A., 49a, 120a
Shontz, F. C., 124b
Shortliffe, E. C., 132b
Shrimpton, C., 16b
Shryock, R. H., 2a
Shuter, G. P., 132a
Shyne, I. J., 127b
Sibley, A., 18a
Sibley, H., 38a
Siegal, S. E., 43b
Siegel, E. L., 81a
Silverman, S., 38a
Simmonds, F. A. H., 36a
Simmons, L. W., 52a
Simon, J. R., 59b, 70a, 82b
Simons, J. E., 10a
Simonson, R. E., 96a
Simpson, C. E., 10a
Simpson, H. M., 57b, 59b, 101a
Simpson, I. H., 106a
Simpson, M. A., 127b
Sinclair, A., 21b
Sindlinger, E., 110b
Singeisen, F., 81b
Singer, C., 6b
Sisler, G. C., 81b
Sister of Charity of Emmitsburg, Maryland, 1b
Sisters of Mercy, 1b
Sitler, D. W., 122b
Skaggs, L. S., 124a
Skellern, E., 70a, 105a, 121a, 121b, 124b
Skelley, E. G., 123b
Skimming, S., 10a
Skinner, C. E., 109a
Skinner, R. W., 79b
Slack, M., 114b
Slatterley, L. C., 4b
Sledge, M., 103b
Sleeper, R., 48a, 55b
Sloan, I. W., 17b
Sloane, A., 84b
Sloggins, M. L. C., 124a
Smellie, J. M., 103a
Smet, H., 53b
Smith, A. W., 10a
Smith, B. F., 87b
Smith, C., 18b
Smith, C. L., 56b, 78a
Smith, D. E., 86a

Smith, D. M., 29a, 50b, 55b, 63b
Smith, D. W., 33a
Smith, E. M., 23a, 78a, 101a
Smith, F. C., 30b
Smith, F. J., 91a
Smith, G. M., 128b
Smith, G. W., 71b, 96b
Smith, H., 89a, 107a
Smith, H. G., 92a
Smith, J., 18b
Smith, J. A., 18b
Smith, J. F., 78b
Smith, K. M., 44a
Smith, L., 10a
Smith, L. C., 55b
Smith, L. O., 23a
Smith, M. E., 8a
Smith, M. R., 78a
Smith, N., 38a
Smith, R. L., 53b
Smith, V. J., 131a
Smith, W. D. L., 99b
Smith, W. I., 99b
Smith, W. R., 78b
Smyth, M. J., 26a
Snitman, M. F., 88b
Sniveley, M. A., 18b, 47b
Snoke, A. W., 38a, 67a, 127a
Social Survey, 38a
Socialist Medical Association, 38a, 47b
Society for Promoting Christian Knowledge, 95a
Society for the State Registration of Trained Nurses, 3b, 29b, 30b
Society of Chartered Nurses, 30b
Soddy, K., 109b
Solomon, G., 118b
Solomons, B., 98a
Solon, J., 132b
Solon, J. A., 81b
Somerset, H. C. D., 103a
Somerset Nurses' Social Union, 51b
Somerville, C. E. M., 112a
Sommer, R., 107a, 109b
Sommermeyer, L., 86b
Sorsby, A., 131a
Soule, E. S., 18b
South, J., 125b
South African Nursing Council, 31b
South Australia. Parliament, 31a
South Australian Trained Nurses' Centenary Committee, 2a
South-East Metropolitan Area Nurse-Training Committee, 65b
Southard, S., 61b
Southern Regional Education Board, Atlanta, Georgia, 53b, 96a
Souza, L. E., 53b
Soyer, A., 10a, 18b
Spain, R. W., 80b
Spalding, E. K., 21b, 44a, 46b, 47b, 64b
Spalding, H. S., 27b
Spaney, E., 50b
Spann, F. P., 18b
Sparshott, M. E., 18b
Spectator, *pseud.*, 30b
Speer, T. V., 6b, 44a
Speller, S. R., 32b
Spencer, A. M., 86a
Speroff, B. J., 81b
Spieseke, A. W., 50b
Spohn, R. R., 72b
Springer, D. M. M., 124b
Squibbs, A. E. A., 44a, 123b
Squire, J. E., 123b
Stacer, H. J., 36a
Stafford, E. S., 118b
Stafford-Clark, D., 96a
Stainbrook, E., 7b
Stallard, H. B., 101b
Stamp, M., 34a
Standard, S., 61b
Stanford, E. D., 60a, 67a
Stanley, A., 28a
Stark, S. B., 81b

Starr, D. S., 63b
Statham, C., 81b
Statham, R. S. S., 98a
Stauble, W. J., 50b
Stauffacher, J. C., 59b
Stearns, L., 67a, 107a
Steele, K. M., 107a
Steer, F., 131a
Steffey, P., 70b
Steiner, E., 45b
Stephen, B., 16b
Stephen, Sister, 35b
Stephenson, D. D., 63b, 72a
Stephenson, E., 46b, 53b
Stephenson, G. E., 1b, 2a, 11a
Stern, E. M., 108b
Stern, E. S., 106b
Stern, W. E., 45b
Stevenson, A. G., 93a
Stevenson, D. M., 116b
Stevenson, E. A., 112a
Stevenson, I., 10b
Stevenson, J., 92a, 92b
Stevenson, L., 18b
Stevenson, N. M., 71b
Stewart, B. L., 84b
Stewart, D. D., 67b
Stewart, G. A., 99b
Stewart, I., 18a, 44a, 48a, 67a, 78b, 94a, 122b, 127a
Stewart, I. M., 12a, 15b, 16b, 18b, 41b, 44a, 55b
Stewart, N., 90b
Stewart, W. M., 35b
Sticht, V., 44a
Still, A. L., 18b
Stimson, J. C., 5a, 10b
Stiver, M. P., 28a
Stobo, E., 117a
Stockdale, M. G., 93b
Stocks, M., 6a
Stokes, G. M., 87a
Stokes, J. H., 88b
Stokes, K. R., 36a
Stoney, A. H., 2a
Stoney, E. A. M., 72b
Stonsby, E. V., 44a
Storer, H. R., 21b, 27b, 78b
Storey, M., 18b
Story, J., 24a
Stott, F. T., 132b
Stout, E., 53b
Strachan, E. J., 82a
Strand Union's Board of Guardians, 7a
Strang, R. R. S., 88b
Strayer, C. H., 50a
Street, M. M., 59a
Strong, R., 18b, 44a
Struthers, L. R., 117a
Stuart-Clark, A. C., 81b
Stubbs, T. H., 95b
Sturdavant, M., 79b
Sturges, O., 64b
Sullivan, C., 61b
Sullivan, C. M., 84b
Superintendents of Training Schools, 55b
Supply of Nurses Committee, 38a
Sutcliffe, I., 57b
Sutherland, D. G., 27b, 67b, 76a, 114b
Suttell, B. J., 72b
Sutter, R. A., 99b
Swanson, M., 117b
Swedish Nurses' Association, 121b
Swenson, R. P. S., 76b
Swift, A., 103a
Swire, M. E., 78b
Sykepieierskenes, S. I. N., 54a
Sykes, C., 100b
Symonds, P. M., 44a

Tabor, M. E., 16b
Taietz, P., 90a
Talley, C., 61b
Tasmania, *pseud.*, 22b

Tasmania. Parliament, 31a
Tate, B. L., 55b, 84b
Tatham, —, 26a
Taunton and Somerset Hospital, 131b
Tayback, M., 68b, 115b
Tayler, D., 44a
Taylor, A. M., 50b
Taylor, R. G., 103b
Taylor, S., 116b, 118b
Taylor, T. M., 34a
Teeney, L., 18a
Ten Group, 37b
Tener, M. E., 80a
Tennessee State Nurses' Association, 30b
Terenzio, J. V., 33a
Teresa, Sister, 51b
Terman, L. M., 117b
Territorial Commission on Nursing Education and Nursing Services, 23b
Territorial Force Nursing Service, 8a
Terrot, S. A., 10b, 18b
Texas Graduate Nurses' Association, 30b
Thatcher, V. S., 122a
Theodore, A., 36a
Thigpen, L. W., 122b
Thoburn, J. M., 5b
Thomas, B., 107a
Thomas, B. W., 129b
Thomas, D. L., 78b
Thomas, J. L., 50b
Thomas, M., 18b
Thomas, M. W., 77b, 78b
Thompson, A. M. C., 51b
Thompson, A. T., 78b
Thompson B. A. 78b
Thompson L., 117b
Thompson, M. E., 78b
Thompson, P. M., 34b
Thompson, W. G., 56a
Thoms, A. B., 4a
Thoms, E. J., 82a, 82b
Thomson, A. S., 95a
Thorek, P., 121b
Thorndike, A., 78b
Thorne, W. B., 30a
Thornu, I., 21b
Thorp, E., 92a
Thurman, H., 61b
Thurston, M., 18b
Thurston, V., 10b, 18b, 84b
Tibbitts, C., 114b
Tibbitts, H. G., 67b, 70a
Tiesselinck, J., 67a
Tiffany, F., 13a
Tindall, S. G., 19a
Tippetts, L. M., 19a
Tipple, D. C., 117b
Tobin, M. J., 35b
Todd, A. B., 19a
Todd, H., 44a
Todd, R. McL., 102b
Toddie, E., 88b
Tokuhata, G. K., 108b
Tollefson, D. M., 89b
Tolmon, J., 34b
Tomlinson, S. C. 23a
Toogood, F. S., 3b
Toohey, M., 94a
Tooley, S. A., 2a 16b 58a
Topalis, M., 106a
Topping, A., 126a
Toronto General Hospital. Training School for Nurses, 23a
Toronto. Nightingale School of Nursing, 58a
Toronto Western Hospital, 131b
Torrop, H. M., 71b 74b
Tourtillot, E., 50b
Tracy, M. A., 68b 78b
Tracy, S. E., 124b
Tracy, S. M., 36a
Traiforos, E., 19a
Trained Nurses' Association of India, 95b

Training School for Nurses, General Hospital, Toronto, Canada, 23a
Trasko, V. M., 100a
Treacy, J. M., 124b
Treacy, K., 19a
Treasure, E. H., 48a
Tregarthen, M., 65b
Tremo, I., 78b
Trenholme, L. I., 4a
Trevethick, R. A., 95a
Triggs, F. O., 46b
Trott, L. L., 29b, 95a
Trounce, J. R., 123b
Trowell, H. C., 95b
Trudeau, J., 63b
Tschida, E. M., 132b
Tschudin, M. S., 44a, 116b
Tudbury, M. A., 107a
Tudway, R. C., 124a
Tufts, M. H., 61b
Tupas, A., 2b
Turer, A., 57b
Turner, A. L., 129a
Turner, C. E., 16a
Turner, E. M. C., 19a,
Turton, M. A., 19a 24a
Tuttle, W. W., 85b
Twining, L., 7a
Tyson, J., 107a

Uber, W. J., 99b
Udell, F., 33b
Ullman, A., 81b
Ulster Hospital, Belfast, 131b
Union of South Africa. Senate and House of Assembly, 31b, 32a
United Hospital Fund of New York, 71a
United States. Communicable Disease Center, 86b
United States. Department of Health Education and Welfare, 68b
United States. Department of Labor. Bureau of Labor Statistics, 34b
United States. Department of National Health and Welfare, Research Division, 67a
United States. Department of the Army. Office of the Surgeon General. Technical Liaison Office, 5a, 27b
United States. Department of the Navy. Bureau of Medicine and Surgery, Nursing Division, 6b
United States. Division of Public Health Methods, 70a
United States. Division of Vocational Education, 71b
United States. Federal Civil Defense, 84b
United States. Federal Security Agency, 70a
United States. National Cancer Institute, 87a
United States. Office of Education, 38a, 71b, 72a
United States. Public Health Service, 27b, 44b 67b, 87b, 96a, 116a
United States. Public Health Service. Division of Nursing Resources, 60a, 70a
United States. Public Health Service and Commission on Chronic Illness, 81b
United States. Women's Bueau 34b
University of Manchester, 51a, 106a
University of Pennsylvania Hospital, 131b
(For other universities See: Alabama, Boston, Ibadan, Indiana, Liverpool, McGill, Missouri, New York State)
Upham, E. K., 102a
Uprichard, M., 22a, 28b, 60a
Urban Life Research Institute, 102b
Urbanic, D., 44b
Urey, B., 84b

Van Allyn, K., 38b
Van Blarcom, C. C., 98a
Vancouver General Hospital. School of Nursing, 58a
Vanderbilt University. School of Nursing, 54a
Van Kamm, A. L., 63b
Vannier, M. L., 78b
Vaughan, Sister R. H., 61b
Vennes, C. H., 124a
Verhonick, P. J., 65b
Vermont State Nurses' Association, 30b
Verney, R. E., 36a
Vestal, A., 67a
Victoria (Australia). Parliament, 31b
Victorian Order of Nurses for Canada, 30b, 78b
Victorian Trained Nurses' Association, 30b
Vincent de Paul, Saint, 19a
Vincent, E. L., 96a
Vines, H. W. C., 110b
Virginia, Sister, 84b
Visiting Nurse Association of Detroit, 30b
Vivian, M., 78b
Vlasto, M., 89a
Vodev, E. D., 56a
Vogel, M. A., 83a
Voysey, M. H. A., 78b
Vreeland, E. M., 45a, 60a

Wade, J., 19a
Wadham, M. A., 116b
Wagner, B. Q., 95a
Wagner, R. A., 79b
Wagner, S. P., 99b
Wahn, E. V., 31b
Wain, O. M., 72a
Wakeford, C., 11a
Wakeley, J. C. N., 121b
Wakely, C., 88b, 121b
Wald, L. D., 6a, 19a
Waldrum, A. F., 69a
Wales, M., 114b
Wales. Board of Health, 126b
Walker, F. H., 114b
Walker, J. B., 88b
Walker, L., 19b, 44b
Walker, R. E., 24a
Walker, V. H., 65b, 81b
Wallace, A. B., 119a
Wallace, A. J., 16b
Wallace, G. S., 54a
Wallace, R. E., 19b
Wallace, W. S., 44b
Waller, B., 119b
Wallinger, E. M., 102a
Walsh, J. J., 2a, 14b
Waltham Training Home and School for Nurses, Mass., 58a
Walton, A. M., 34b
Wandelt, M. A., 124b
Wansbrough, R., 122b
War Office, 5a, 44b
Ward, I., 5a
Wardroper, S., 19b
Warin, J. F., 85a
Warley Hospital, Brentwood, 131b
Warman, G. A., 38a
Warnock, R. B., 49b
Warrington, J., 98a
Warstler, M. E., 48b
Warwick, T., 125b
Warwick Hospital, 86a
Wartime Social Survey, 26a, 38a
Washburn, D., 51b
Washington State Nurses' Association, 31a
Washington State Nurses' Association. Joint Committee on Nursing Services, 69b
Waterer, J., 44b
Waterman, I. D., 56a

Waterman, T. L., 114b
Waters, I., 112a
Waters, M., 104a
Watkin, B. V., 34b, 44b, 82b, 83a, 127a
Watkin, P. J., 129b
Watkin, V., 22a
Watkins, A. G., 102b
Watkins, J. G., 23a
Watson, E., 100b
Watson, J. C., 124a
Watson, J. K., 78b, 79a, 122a
Watson, J. M., 92a
Watt, J., 60a
Watt, P. F., 5a
Way, H., 61b
Wayland, M. M., 67b
Wearn, E. M., 114b
Webb, D. E., 95a
Webb, J., 63b, 127a
Weber, H. J., 68b
Weber, S., 92b
Webster, R. C., 60a
Wedd, G. D., 84b
Weddell, D., 44b, 107a, 109b
Wedgery, A., 22a
Weed, W. W., 67b
Weeks-Shaw, C. S., 79a
Weil, T. P., 38a, 81b, 127a
Weiner, F. R., 26b, 33a
Weiner, L., 83b
Weiner, W., 88b
Weinschreider, M. M., 81b
Weir, G. M., 44b
Weiss, M. O., 107a
Weitz, R. D., 109a
Weitzman, D., 94a
Welch, J., 44b
Welham, S., 79a
Wellenkamp, J., 67b
Wellington Hospital, New Zealand, 131b
Wells, C., 118b
Wenden, M., 72b
Wensley, E., 114b
Werley, H. H., 84b
Werminghaus, E. A., 13b
Wessex Regional Hospital Board, 79a, 132b
West, C., 102b
West, G. M., 81b
West, J. P., 120a
West, J. S., 103a, 119b
West, M., 55a
West, M. M., 100a
West, R. M., 4a
West London Hospital, 132a
West Virginia State Nurses' Association, 31a
Westberg, G., 61b
Western Australia. Parliament, 31b
Western Infirmary, Glasgow, 132a
Western Interstate Commission for Higher Education, 44b
Western Ophthalmic Hospital, 132a
Westminster Hospital, London, 132a
Westminster Training School, 58a
Westmorland, J. E., 112a
Weston, E. M. A., 92a, 92b
Wheble, V. H., 86a
Wheeler, H., 5b
Wheeler, M. C., 79a
Wheeler, M. M., 100a
Whitaker, A., 131b
Whitby, L. E. H., 91a
Whitcombe, G., 129a
White, A. M. W., 26a, 128a
White, J. M., 79a, 86b
White, J. V., 19b
White, M. R., 116b
White, T. H., 79a
Whitfield, R. G., 98b
Whiting, J. F., 60a, 63b
Whiting, M. H., 101b
Whitlock, O. M., 100a
Whitney, F., 33b
Whitney, J., 13b
Whitney, J. S., 36a

Whitridge, J., Jr., 98a
Whitteridge, G., 131b
Whittet, T. D., 86a
Who's Who in the Nursing World, 11a
Whyte, V., 79a
Wickensheimer, V., 87b
Wickham, E., 98a
Widenbach, E., 98a
Widmer, C. L., 10b
Wiggins, V. L., 50b
Wild, E., 116b
Wilkie, C. B. S., 7a
Wilkins, E., 114b
Wilkinson, A., 2b
Wilkinson, D. S., 88b
Williams, B. C., 11b
Williams, D. M., 112a
Williams, D. R., 45b, 56a
Williams, F. A., 95b
Willliams, F. J., 123b
Williams, F. M., 78a
Williams, G., 30b
Williams, J., 12b, 109b
Williams, J. B., 81a
Williams, L. W., 79b
Williams, M. M., 22a, 44b, 54a, 100a
Williams, R., 79a
Williams, R. C., 50b
Williams, R. L., 110b
Williams, T. J., 18a
Williams, T. R., 22a, 44b
Williamson, A. G., 132a
Williamson, A. M., 19b
Willie, C. V, 63b, 114b
Willis, Sir F., 107b
Willis, I. C., 17a
Willis, L. D., 22a
Wills Eye Hospital, Philadelphia, Pennsylvania, 132a
Wilson, A. T. M., 71a
Wilson, D. M., 131b
Wilson, E., 120a, 130a
Wilson, E. C., 29a, 73a
Wilson, H. T. H., 35b, 85a
Wilson, I. G. H., 109b
Wilson, J. C. 92a
Wilson, K. J. W., 78a
Wilson, L., 45b, 50b, 96a
Wilson, M., 61b
Wilson, M. J., 84b
Wilson, R., 50b, 54a
Wilson, T., 7a
Windemuth, A., 132b
Windmuller, I., 115a
Windsor, A. E., 65b, 72a, 125b
Windsor Group of Hospitals, 119a
Wingent, R. M., 128b
Winmill, M., 19b
Winnipeg General Hospital School of Nursing, 58a
Winslow, C. E. A., 19b, 116b
Winter, K. E., 81b
Wintle, W., 17a
Winters, M. C., 92b
Wisconsin State Nurses' Association, 2a, 31a
Wise, P. M., 79a
Witney, F., 22a
Withington Hospital, Manchester, 132a
Witting, M., 112a
Witton, C. J., 86b
W. K. Kellog Foundation, 71a
Wofinden, R. C., 112a, 115a
Wohl, M. G., 82a
Wolcott, H., 71a
Wolf, L. K., 22a, 27b
Wolff, I. S., 62a
Wolff, L. V., 40b, 74b
Wolfson, B., 81b
Wolfson, T., 34b
Women Public Health Officers' Association, 115a
Wood, A., 110b
Wood, A. G., 98a
Wood, C. J., 7a, 22a, 23a, 24a, 56a, 62a, 72b, 79a, 102b, 112a, 128b

Wood, E. C., 87b
Wood, M. M., 46b, 83a
Wooden, H. E., 87b
Woodgate, M. V., 14b, 19a
Woodham-Smith, C., 17a
Woods, N. A., 117b
Woodward, H. L., 98a
Woodward, J., 66b
Woodward, J. J., 127a
Woolever, G. M., 79b
Woolf, M. S., 118b
Woollacott, F. J., 92a
Woolsey, A. H., 4a
Woolsey, J. S., 4a
Wootton, N. E., 30b
Worcester, A., 2a, 4a, 22a, 27b, 44b, 56a, 62a
Worcester Royal Infirmary, 132a
Workhouse Infirmary Nursing Association, 7a
World Health Organization, 22a, 31a, 44b, 54a, 70a, 115a
World Health Organization. Expert Committee on Nursing, 115a
World Health Organization. Expert Committee on Psychiatric Nursing, 107a
World Health Organization. Regional Office for Europe, 44b, 54a, 100a, 107a, 115a
World Health Organization. Regional Office for South East Asia, 68b
World Health Organization. Western Pacific Region, 45a
World Health Organization. Working Conference on Nursing Education, 45a
Wortabet, E., 24b
Wortham, E. D., 102b
Worthington, G., 27b
Worthy, E. J., 52a
Wren, G. R., 69b
Wright, F. S., 100a
Wright, M. J., 82b
Wright, W. R., 22a
Wulfsohn, N. L., 121b
Wyatt, H. T., 79a
Wyche, M. L., 4a
Wylie, W. G., 128b

Xavier Berkeley, Sister, 19b

Yankauer, A., 116a
Yanta, G. M., 72b
Yapp, C. S., 103a, 121b
Yeager, M. E., 118b
Yergen, L., 24a, 28a
Yingling, D. B., 101a
York, M. E., 55b
York County Hospital, 132a
York Education Committee, 48b
Yost, E., 11a
Youlden, E. F., 19b
Young, C. S., 11b
Young, E. H., 19b
Young, E. H., 95b
Young, H., 36a, 79a
Young, M. A., 23a
Young, M. L., 127a
Young, R., 115a
Young, V., 22a
Young, V. M., 77b

Zaboli, C., 83a
Zabriskie, L., 98a
Zaufas, I. E., 124b
Zboray, D. E., 63b
Zernay, J., 22a
Zimmerman, M. W., 82a
Zucker, E. M. M., 64b
Zurrer, G., 48a

INDEX 1961-1970

a, after page number denotes the left hand column of the page
b, after page number denotes the right hand column of the page

Aasterud, M., 60b
Abbott, M., 49a
Abbott, N. C., 131b
Abdallah, M. C., 80a
Abdellah, F. G., 6a, 55a, 86b, 88a, 158a
Abel-Smith, B., 6a, 177a
Abels, P., 144a
Abraham, A., 159a
Abraham, G. E., 45b, 55a, 72a
Abrahams, C., 109a
Abramovitz, A. B., 29a
Abramson, G. K., 50b
Abreau, X. A., 87b
Abstracts of efficiency studies in the hospital service, 177a
Achiwa, G., 1b
Ackner, B., 134b
Ackral, M., 142a
Acton Hospital, London, 180b
Adams, A. R. D., 115a
Adams, G. F., 109b
Adams, J., 44a
Adams, J. G., 170b
Adams, J. M., 88a
Adams, M., 116b
Adams, R. E., 85b, 86a
Adamson, E. I. O., 19b
Adebajo, S. O., 45b
Adler, S., 119b
Adranvala, T. K., 14a
Adriani, J., 157a, 168b
Agate, J. N., 109b
Agnes Karll Nurses' Association, 52b
Agnew, K., 180b
Aguilera, D. C., 60b, 134b
Ahad, M. A., 29a, 63a
Ahern, M. S., 125a
Ahlers, M. E., 125a
Aichlmayr, R. H., 6a
Aiken, L. H., 88a
Aird, I., 98a
Aish, A., 129a
Aitken, J., 181b
Akester, J. M., 151b, 153b, 154b
Akey, D. T., 161b
Alabama Board of Nursing, 29a
Albers, J., 107b
Alberta, Department of Health, 75a
Alberta. Nursing Care Survey Committee, 88a
Alberta. Nursing Education Survey Committee, 29a
Alberta. University. Committee on Nursing Education, 29a
Aldag, J. C., 11b
Alder, V. G., 166b
Alexander, D. M., 173a
Alexander, E. L., 76b, 163b
Alexander, F. M., 6a, 39a, 73a, 177b
Alexander, I. R. W., 155b
Alexander, M. E. F., 49a
Alexy, B. J., 121b
Alford, D. M., 88a
Aliapoulios, M. A., 99a
Allardice, J. T., 125a
Allen, B., 141b
Allen, C., 41b
Allen, D., 144b
Allen, G., 95a
Allen, J. C., 175a
Allen, L., 75a
Allen, M. G., 45a
Allen, R. W., 179b
Allen, V., 22b, 28a
Allen, W. H., 154b

Alley, J. A., 88a
Allgire, M. J., 174a
Allgood, J., 68b, 141b
Allick, H. D., 129b
Alodia, Sister M., 164a
Alonzo, B. S., 77b
Alsop, J. A., 168a
Altnagelvin Hospital, Londonderry, 179b
Altschul, A., 22b, 43b, 52b, 88b, 144a
Alyn, I. B., 45a
Ambler, M., 154b
American Association of Industrial Nurses, 125b, 127b
American Association of Industrial Nurses Journal, 18b
American Cancer Society, 98a
American College of Cardiology, 99b
American College of Surgeons, 164a
American Heart Association, 99b
American Hospital Association, 27b, 29a, 67a, 76a, 88b, 177b
American Hospital Association. Hospital Research and Educational Trust, 84a
American Journal of Nursing 2a, 22b, 87a, 102b
American Journal of Nursing Company. Educational Services Division, 29a
American Medical Association, 6a, 15b, 84a, 88b, 121b, 129a
American Nurses' Association, 15a, 15b, 19a, 19b, 20a, 22b, 29a, 29b, 50b, 52b, 54a, 55a, 60a, 60b, 63a, 63b, 74a, 76a, 80a, 81b, 84a, 84b, 85b, 87b, 88a, 88b, 89b, 90a, 90b, 91a, 92b, 93a, 95b, 99a, 99b, 101b, 104b, 110a, 111b, 115a, 117a, 118a, 118b, 125b, 132a, 132b, 133a, 134a, 134b, 135a, 135b, 137b, 139b, 141a, 148a, 151b, 152a, 156a, 156b, 157a, 160b, 161b, 162a, 162b, 164a, 166a, 169a, 174b, 175a
American Nurses' Association. Committee on Ethical, Legal and Professional Standards, 60a
American Nurses' Association. Committee on Research and Studies, 55a
American Nurses' Association. Committee on Standards for Geriatric Nursing Practice, 109b
American Nurses' Association. Council of State Boards of Nursing, 29b
American Nurses' Association. Division on Psychiatric-Mental Nursing, 134b
American Nurses' Association. Economic Security Unit, 19a
American Nurses' Association. Education Administrators, Consultants and Teachers Section, 29b
American Nurses' Association. Occupational Health Nurses Section, 121b, 125b, 156a
American Nurses' Association. Research and Statistics Unit, 20a, 141b
American Nurses' Association. Special Committee on Allied Nursing Personnel, 80a
American Nurses' Foundation, 131b, 151b
American Nursing Home Association, 171a

American Psychiatric Association. Committee on Public Information, 41a
Amroliwalla, F. K., 175a
Anderson, A. M., 6a
Anderson, B. E., 19b, 29b, 99b
Anderson, B. L., 164a
Anderson, C. J., 109b
Anderson, C. M., 130b
Anderson, D., 41b
Anderson, D. B., 134b
Anderson, E. H., 93a
Anderson, H. C., 112a
Anderson, J., 98a
Anderson, J. A. D., 129b, 154b
Anderson, K. C., 39a
Anderson, L. C., 76b, 81a
Anderson, L. D., 48b
Anderson, M. C., 47b, 63b, 88b
Anderson, M. H., 92b
Anderson, N. J., 129b
Anderson, O. W., 6a
Anderson, P. S. B., 42b
Anderson, R. M., 67a
Andreoli, K. G., 100a, 100b
Andrews, E. M., 106a
Andrews, J., 45b, 131b
Andrews, J. M., 81b, 142a, 142b
Andrews, J. T., 173a
Anello, M., 6a
Angrist, S., 88b
Angus, M. D., 22b, 50b
Ankers, E., 133a
Annan, G. L., 50b
Anning, S. T., 181b
Anstice, E., 6a, 98a, 109b, 131b
Anthony, C. P., 96a
Antoft, K., 98b
Anton-Stephens, D., 109b
Araneta, N. C., 45a
Archambeault, C. A., 161b
Archer Memorial Hospital of Lamont, 181a
Archibald, R., 88b
Archibald, R. McL., 121b
Arenillas, L., 116b
Argamaso, R. V., 106a, 168a
Arizona. Joint Committee to Study Nursing Needs and Resources, 25a
Arje, F. B., 142b
Armiger, B., 45a, 88b
Armitage, S., 161b
Arms, F. C., 2b
Armstrong, D. M., 86a
Armstrong, E., 74a
Armstrong, J. D., 158a
Armstrong, K. F., 4a, 96a, 97b, 164a
Armstrong, S. W., 134b
Arndt, C., 75a
Arnold, H. M., 104b, 109b, 162b
Arnold, L. M., 91b
Arnstein, M. G., 151b
Arrowsmith, R., 182a
Arwold, M. F., 6a
Asbury, G., 45b
Asher, P., 114b, 118b, 129b, 171a
Ashley, P. J., 109b
Ashurst, P. J. C., 103b
Ashworth, A., 107b
Ashworth, P. M., 86a, 179b
Ask, R., 63b
Asperheim, M. K., 171a
Asperilla, P. F., 76b
Aspinall, M. J., 85a
Associated Hospitals Board of Management, 36b

Association for the Prevention of Drug Addiction, 158b
Association of British Paediatric Nurses, 129b, 130a
Association of Canadian Hospital Administrators, 13a
Association of Hospital and Welfare Administrators, 179a
Association of Hospital Matrons, 15b, 68b
Association of Nurses of the Province of Quebec. Ad Hoc Committee on Nursing Needs and Resources, 77b
Association of Operating Room Nurses. Statement Committee, 164a
Association of Professional Nurses of the Province of Quebec, 20a
Association of Registered Nurses of Newfoundland. Committee on Nursing Service, 77b
Association of Supervisors of Midwives, 156a
Atkinson, E. J., 121b
Atkinson, W. J., 84a
Atty, L. M., 141b
Audette, A., 164a
Audric, J., 12b
Aufhauser, T. R., 131b
Augenstein, D., 170b
Auld, M. G., 23a, 77b, 95a
Austin, A. L., 1a
Australasian hospital directory and nurses' year book, 1963, 41a
Australasian Nurses' Association, 23a
Australasian Trained Nurses' Association, 16a
Australia. New South Wales, 20a
Avery, H., 113b
Avery, H. P., 121b
Awon-Khan, V., 74a
Axelrod, A. R., 98b
Ayd, F. J., 171b
Aydelotte, M. K., 6a, 23a, 67a, 76b
Ayers, R., 76b
Ayliffe, G. A. J., 166b
Ayres, S. M., 84a

Babich, K. S., 6a
Bach, W. G., 131b
Bachar, M. E., 61b
Badgley, R. F., 29b
Badland, S. G., 142b
Badouaille, M.-L., 14a
Baechtold, M., 14b
Bagenstose, M., 158a
Baggallay, O., 4a
Baggott, E., 11b, 81b, 88b, 134b, 141b
Bailey, A., 73a
Bailey, D., 148a
Bailey, D. E., 75a
Bailey, D. H., 145a
Bailey, H., 159b, 160a
Bailey, I. C., 86a
Bailey, J. T., 44a
Bailey, M., 158a
Bailey, R. E., 119b, 171b
Bain, B., 63b
Bain, W., 23a
Bain, W. H., 160a
Baker, A. Z., 170a
Baker, C. D., 154b
Baker, Sister M. E., 164a
Baker-Rogers, M., 110b
Baldwin, A. H., 134b
Baldwin, E. M., 130a
Baldwin, J. T., 13a
Balkonen, I., 134b
Ball, B. M., 164a
Ball, H., 119b
Ballantyne, W., 10b
Baly, M., 4b, 36b, 145b
Bame, K. B., 162b
Banfill, B. J., 13a
Banister, R. F. H., 6a
Banks, A. L., 150b

Banks, A. W., 73a
Banks, I., 40b
Bannister, D., 28b
Banu, A., 29b
Baptist Hospital, Nashville, Tennessee, 99b
Barabas, M. H., 67a
Barbados Registered Nurses Association, 13b
Barbata, J. C., 63b
Barbee, G. C., 19a
Barber, R. M., 109b
Barbus, A. J., 49a
Barckley, V., 98b
Bare, C. E., 45a
Barker, A. E., 23a
Barker, B. L., 67b
Barker, J. C., 134b
Barker, K. N., 171b
Barker, P., 134b
Barlow, M. L., 72a
Barlow, T. G., 162b
Barnard, D., 153b, 159a
Barnard, J. E., 119b
Barnard, K. E., 113b
Barnes, A. L., 117b, 180a
Barnes, E., 88b, 135a
Barnes, M., 45b
Barr, A., 22a, 93a
Barrett, J., 67a
Barritt, E., 52b
Barrow, N., 13b
Barry, A. C., 135a
Barry, H., 133b
Bartel, G. J., 73a
Barton, C., 4a
Barton, J., 84a, 88b, 144a
Barton, R., 59b, 88b
Barton, W. E., 135a
Bartscht, K. G., 77b
Basara, S. C., 133b
Basco, D., 156a
Bashford, A. J., 44a
Bassett, R. L., 48b
Bassey, P., 86a
Bassford P. A., 98b, 121b
Basu, S., 149b
Bateman, D. J., 115a, 115b
Bates, B., 62a, 154a
Batey, M., 142b
Batey, M. V., 49a, 55b, 59b, 61b
Batley, N., 52b
Batten, L. W., 109b
Battersea College of Technology, 43b
Battle, A. O., 55b
Bauer, M. L., 127b
Baum, J. D., 133b
Baumgart, A. J., 3a, 154a
Bavin, J. T. R., 115b, 116b, 151b
Bayer, A. E., 23a
Baynham, J. E., 164a
Baziak, A. T., 6a
Bazley, M. C., 135a
Beal, B., 12a
Beal, E., 135a
Beal, J. M., 164a
Beamish, R. M., 4a
Bean, M. A., 88b
Bean, W. B., 88b
Beattie, I. E., 154a
Beaudry-Johnson, N., 29b
Beavers, S. V., 170b
Bechtoldt, A. A., 102b
Beck, F. S., 6a, 14b, 55b, 80a
Beck, M. E., 170a
Becker, B. G., 81b
Beckhard, R., 67a
Bedside Nurse, 81b, 157a
Beeby, G. J., 141b
Beer, G. E., 164a
Beland, I. L., 63b
Belcher, H. C., 38b, 141a
Bell, A., 125b
Bell, H. S., 161b
Bell, K. K., 115b
Bell, S., 84a

Bellinger, A. C., 6a
Belote, M., 148a
Belsjoe, E. H., 80a
Belton, M. K., 168b
Beltran, H. G., 95a
Bendall, E. R. D., 6a, 16b, 23a, 36b, 43b, 44a, 55b, 63b, 67a, 68b
Bender, J., 55b
Benedikt, L., 81b
Benjamin, N., 39b
Benne, K. D., 55b
Bennett, B. A., 13b, 28a, 81b, 150a
Bennett, C., 50b
Bennett, H. J., 161b
Bennett, J. P., 161b
Bennett, K., 28b
Bennett, L. R., 6a
Bennett, M. H., 82a, 180b
Bennett, R. A., 19b
Bennett, T. R., 67a
Bennis, W., 55b, 75a
Benoliel, J. Q., 144a
Benson, M. C., 115a
Bentinck, C., 142b
Bentley, C., 82a
Benz, E. G., 76b
Benz, G. S., 174a
Beresford, C. C., 109b
Bergel, F., 98b
Bergeron, Sister R. M., 52b
Bergersen, B. S., 64a, 106b, 129a
Berggren, H. J., 46a
Bergin, M. A., 88b
Berglind, H., 75a
Bergman, R., 14a, 52b, 145b
Bergman, R. L., 6a
Bergman, V., 5a
Berita Jururawat, 46a
Berkerson, B., 172b
Berkowitz, N. H., 57b, 62a, 75a, 88b
Bermosk, L. S., 64a, 142b
Bernadette Poirier, Rev. Sister, 164a
Bernall, M. E., 61a
Bernard, J., 64a
Bernstein, L., 23a, 64a
Bernzweig, E. P., 19a
Berry, C. E., 29b
Berry, D. M., 98b, 164a
Berry, M., 168b
Berthold, J. S., 6a, 27a, 55b, 60a
Berzins, G., 77b
Berzon, F. C., 44a, 172a
Best, L. A., 55b
Besterman, E., 100a
Beswetherick, M. A., 29b
Bethea, D. C., 119b
Bethell, M. F., 130a
Bethune, S., 166b
Betschman, L. I., 164a
Betson, C., 133b
Bett, J. H. N., 100a
Bettice, D., 100a
Bettley, F. R., 103b
Betts, G. A., 162b
Beuker, K., 141b
Bevan, J., 41b
Bevan, P. G., 105b
Bevis, E. O., 95a
Bevis, G., 107b
Beyers, M., 65a
Beytell, J. H., 62a
Bhatia, B. D., 55p
Bhattacharya, A., 67b
Bickford, J. A. R., 142b
Bickerstaff, E. R., 118b
Biddle, H. C., 102a, 171b
Biddlecombe, A., 103b
Biddulph, C., 92b
Biden-Steel, K., 121b
Bidstrup, P. L., 121b, 122a
Bier, R., 110a
Bierer, J., 141a, 141b
Biggin, K. M., 46a
Bignall, J. R., 98b
Bignold, V., 29b
Bigue, C., 168a

Bilitch, M. J., 65a
Billings, G. A., 141b
Bilton, K., 153b
Bingle, J., 171b
Binkley, L., 77b
Bioastranautic Operational Support Unit, 79b
Birch, M. G., 106a
Birch, N. M., 42b
Bird, T. E., 60b, 84a, 135a, 142a, 174a
Birinyi, R., 149a
Birkbeck, L., 148a
Birmingham, D. J., 103b
Birmingham Regional Hospital Board, 92b, 177a
Bissonette, G., 29b
Bitzer, M. D., 47b
Black, B., 142a
Black, C., 29b
Black, E. E., 95a
Black, I., 148a
Black, M., 67b
Blackburn and East Lancashire Royal Infirmary, 181a
Blacklaws, D. M., 125b
Blackstock, C. R., 157a
Blainey, J. D., 108a
Blair, E., 96b
Blair, M., 122a
Blais, N., 29b
Blake, F. G., 130a, 132a
Blakeley, M., 122a, 125b
Blaney, L., 122a
Blansfield, M. G., 77b
Blaylock, E., 44b
Bleier, I. J., 82a, 119b
Blenkiron, C. H., 113a, 173a
Blishen, B. R., 77b
Bliss, M. R., 103b, 108a, 110a
Bliss, S. G., 151b
Bloch, M., 169a
Bloch, V. C., 157a
Blodgett, F. M., 151b
Bloom, A., 114b
Blumberg, J. E., 88b
Blumberg, M. S., 86a, 93a
Blume, D. M., 171b
Blundy, M. G., 174a
B.O.A.C., 128b
Bocock, E. J., 96a, 97b
Boddy, F. A., 150a
Bodenham, D. C., 98b
Bogash, R. C., 180b
Bogdan, A., 133b
Boguslawski, M., 177b
Bois, M. S., 108a, 168a
Boisvert, C., 100a
Bolam, R. F., 105b
Bolitho, H., 177a
Bolster, E., 3b
Bolton, W. B., 141b
Bompas, B. M., 29b
Bond, H. M., 122a
Bond, M. R., 105b
Bondy, D. M., 155b
Bone, A. I. C., 29b
Bone, M. R., 141b
Bonham, A., 23a
Bonham, D. G., 133a, 133b
Bonine, G. N., 130a
Bonnell, J. A., 122a
Bonnet, P. D., 29b, 54a
Bonney, V., 64a
Boorer, D., 2a, 11b, 23a, 50b, 60b, 67b, 83b, 106a, 125b, 135a, 142b, 150a, 154b, 174a, 177b, 178b
Boorer, H., 135a
Booth, C., 173a
Booth, H., 144a
Booth, S., 100a
Boozer, H. R., 30a
Bor, S., 103b
Bordicks, K. J., 88b, 164a
Borlick, M. M., 148a, 154a
Borrie, P., 103b
Borrow, M. L., 179b

Borsay, M., 118b
Bouchard, R., 98b
Boucher, C. A., 110a
Bouchier, I. A. D., 98b
Boucot, K. R., 125b
Boudreau, M. C., 101b
Boudreaux, M. C., 47b
Bourne, G., 113b
Bourne, J., 110a
Bourne, J. G., 160a
Bourne, L. B., 103b, 122a
Bourne, M. W., 23a, 75a, 77b, 177b
Bourton-on-the-Water Cottage Hospital, 181a
Bowd, D. G., 4b
Bowden, E. A. F., 64a, 75a
Bowe, E. J., 1b
Bowen, R. G., 104b
Bowler, K., 114a
Bowman, G., 18a
Bowns, B., 145b, 154a
Boyd, E., 52b
Boyd, V., 154a
Boydston, G. D., 21a, 79b
Boyland, E., 98b
Boyle, J. A., 171b
Boyle, R. E., 19a, 30a, 55b
Brackett, M. E., 88b, 148a
Bradbeer, T. L., 167b
Bradby, M. B., 160a
Bradley, D., 162b
Bradshaw, C. E., 71b
Bragdon, J. S., 47a
Brambilla, M. A., 164a
Brand, V. R., 52b
Brandt, E. M., 52b, 64a
Branson, H. K., 121a, 134a
Branstetter, E., 132a
Brasset, D. A., 182a
Bratton, J. K., 89a
Braun, H. A., 100a
Brazilian Nursing Association, 14b
Bray, R. E., 60b, 84a, 135a, 142a, 174a
Breckenridge, F. J., 169a
Bregande, B. J., 179b
Brennan, K., 30a
Brennan, K. S. W., 108b, 136b
Breslau, R. C., 164a
Bressler, B., 135a
Brester, M., 45a
Brewer, J. I., 113a
Brewin, P. H., 154b
Bricker, D. L., 160a
Bridgeman, G. J. O., 129a
Bridger, H., 125b
Bridges, D. C., 5a, 15a, 17a
Bridges, D. E., 62a
Brigden, R. J., 74a, 162b, 164a, 166b
Brigg, M., 156b
Briggs, L., 100a, 164a
Briggs, M. R., 41b
Brim, O. G., 89a
Brincklow, P., 59b
Bristol. United Bristol Hospitals, 54b, 181a
Bristow, A., 43b
British Columbia. Department of Health Services and Hospital Insurance. Division of Public Health Nursing, 84a
British Columbia. Department of Health Services and Hospital Insurance. Mental Health Services Branch, 30a
British Columbia. Hospital Insurance Service. Consultation and Research Divison, 75a
British Commonwealth Nurses War Memorial Fund, 16a
British Diabetic Association, 104b
British Hospital and Social Service Journal, 50b
British Hospital Journal and Social Service Review, 23a, 68b
British Medical Association, 18b, 89a
British Medical Association. Planning Unit, 86a

British Medical Journal, 84b
British Red Cross Society, 2b, 66b
British Tuberculosis Association, Joint Tuberculosis Committee, 151b
Brittain, G. J. C., 164b
Britten, J. D., 64a
Broadhurst, M. J., 12a
Broadley, M. E., 145b
Broadribb, V., 130a
Broadwell, L., 82b
Broatch, D. L., 105b
Brock, M., 148a
Brock, R. Lord, 164b
Brockbank, W., 1a
Brockhurst, R. J., 129a
Brockington, F., 49a
Brocklehurst, J. C., 103b, 110a
Brockmeier, M. J., 115b
Brockopp, G. W., 115b
Brodsky, I., 1b
Brodt, D. E., 6b, 30a, 64a, 67b, 93a
Broe, E., 6b
Brogan, M. M., 125b
Bromley, D., 130a
Bromley, R., 68b
Bromley Hospital, Kent, 181a
Brompton, A. W., 118b, 174a
Brompton Hospital, 86a
Brookes, B., 148b
Brooks, C., 151b
Brooks, E. A., 95a
Brooks, S. M., 102a
Broome, W. E., 45a, 96a, 97b, 161b, 164b, 166b
Browder, J. J., 30a, 52b
Brown, A. M., 107a, 170a
Brown, C., 15a, 69a, 88a, 157a
Brown, C. H., 105a
Brown, C. M., 101a, 170a
Brown, D. E., 145b
Brown, D. I., 135a
Brown, D. R., 80a
Brown, D. S., 67b
Brown, E., 95a
Brown, E. A., 64a
Brown, E. L., 64a, 67b, 80a, 89a
Brown, I. M., 22a
Brown, J. A., 60b
Brown, L. E., 87a
Brown, M. C., 50b
Brown, M. H., 42a
Brown, M. I., 55b
Brown, M. K., 98b
Brown, M. L., 122a, 125b, 127b
Brown, M. M., 135a
Brown, R. A., 75b
Brown, R. E., 30a
Brown, R. G. S., 12a
Brown, U., 75b
Brown, W. K., 75b, 80a
Brownell, K. O., 82a
Browning, E., 122a
Brownlowe, M. A., 84b
Browse, N. L., 102b
Bruckner, S., 64a
Brudenell, M., 98b
Brueggen, S. L., 122a, 129a, 156b
Bruhn, J. G., 26a, 34a
Brunclik, H. L., 23a, 27a, 27b, 38a, 45a
Brunel University. Hospital Organization Research Unit, 67b
Brunner, L. S., 64a, 164b
Bruno, P., 169a
Bryant, W. D., 79a
Bryant, Z., 148a, 150a
Bryden, E. G. M., 43b
Buchanan, B. B., 135b
Buchanan, P. C., 67b
Buckby, E., 47b
Buckle, D., 137a
Buckles, B. V., 142b
Budge, U. V., 52b, 135a
Budzyna, A. H., 6b, 55b
Bueker, K., 55b
Buerki, R. C., 89a
Buick-Constable, B., 6b, 18a

BIBLIOGRAPHY OF NURSING

Bulbulyan, A., 115b, 135a
Bull, M. R., 13b, 30a, 145b
Bullock, B. L., 101a
Bullock, M. W., 105a
Bullough, B., 1a, 1b, 6b, 40b
Bullough, V., 1a, 1b, 6b, 40b
Bulterijs, A., 170b
Bumbalo, J., 46a
Bunch, A. J., 50b
Bundle, N., 122b
Bunge, H. L., 55b
Burchill, E., 13a
Burd, S. F., 135a
Burdon, I. M., 96a
Burgeson, E. C., 128b
Burgess, A., 96a
Burgess, D. M., 162b
Burgess, R. E., 96a
Burke, J. F., 166b
Burke, J. L., 60b
Burke, M., 115a
Burke, N., 135a
Burn, J. L., 84b, 100a, 110a, 115b, 122b
Burn, J. M. B., 86a
Burnett, C. W. F., 120a
Burnett, M. K., 122b
Burnham, E., 29a
Burnside, I. M., 110a
Burr, J., 82a, 135a
Burrell, L. O., 86a
Burrell, Z. L., 86a
Burrows, K., 108a
Burston, W. R., 130a
Burt, M. M., 118b
Burtis, M.B., 118b
Burton, G., 46a, 60b
Burton, P. M., 151b
Burton, R. A., 23a
Burwell, D. M., 170b
Bush, C. H., 62a, 82a
Busby, E. R., 100a
Busby, J., 122b
Butcher, M. G., 82a
Butler, C., 89a
Butler, C. B., 30a
Butler, R., 54b
Butler, R. M., 89a
Butler, R. O., 169a
Butt, J., 158a
Butterworth, J., 154b
Buttimore, A., 155a
Button, D., 97a
Byatt, J., 151a
Bye, W. G., 61a
Byerley, E. L., 55b
Byers, V. B., 84b
Byrne, J., 80a
Byrne, M., 154a
Byrne, M. W., 154a

Cable, J. V., 114b
Cabot, E. E., 170a
Cabot, R., 34b
Cady, E. L., 83b
Cady, L. L., 175a
Cafferty, K. W., 39a
Caffrey, C. A., 125b
Caie, H. B., 171b
Caine, T. M., 135a, 142a
Cairney, J., 96a, 96b, 113a, 160a
Calderwood, C., 163a
Calender, T. M., 67b
Caliandro, G., 47b
Callander, R., 96b
Callin, M. E., 42b
Calnan, M. F., 110a
Cam, J. F., 86a
Cameron, F., 174a
Cameron, F. J., 4a, 4b, 6b, 28b, 30a
Cameron, J. D., 122b
Cameron, J. S., 108a
Camp, R. P., 135a, 141b
Campbell, D., 169b, 170b
Campbell, E. B., 6b, 67b, 81a
Campbell, I., 151a
Campbell, J., 52b
Campbell, K., 30a, 151b
Campbell, M., 67b
Campbell, M. A., 55b
Campbell, M. B., 169a
Campbell, N., 20a
Campbell, W., 141b
Campion, F. L., 93a
Canada. Royal Commission on Health Services, 23a, 30a, 32a
Canadian Hospital, 20a, 23b, 75b
Canadian Nurse, 36b, 49a, 93a, 129a
Canadian Nurses' Association, 6b, 13a, 16a, 20a, 30a, 41b, 55b, 56a, 75b, 78a, 115b, 145b, 148a
Canadian Public Health Association. Research Committee, 75b
Canadian Red Cross Society. National Nursing Committee, 150b
Cantlin, V. L., 164b
Cantrell, E. G., 104b
Cape, R. D. T., 110a
Carb, G. R., 39b
Carbol, K. L., 49a
Cardona, H., 129a
Carey, M. C., 78a
Carey, M. E., 170a
Caribbean Nurses' Organisation, 13b, 16a
Carini, E., 164b
Carleton, E. I., 135a
Carlson, C. E., 64a
Carnegie, M. E., 30a
Carnell, C. M., 104b
Carnevali, D., 56a, 61a, 64a, 71a, 85a, 175b
Carney, L., 168a
Carney, R. G., 104a
Carpena, E., 15a
Carpenter, H. M., 30a
Carpenter, M. F., 4a, 23b
Carr, A., 84b, 102b
Carr, A. C., 143b
Carr, A. J., 6b, 28a, 80a, 110b, 150a
Carrier, P. J., 110b
Carriker, D., 177b, 178a
Carrington, M., 21b
Carroll, M. C., 52b
Carruthers, B. M., 14a
Carson, N. A. J., 107a
Carson, R., 23b
Carstairs, V., 74a, 150a
Carter, B. S., 106a
Carter, E. W., 135b
Carter, G. B., 41a
Carter, L., 102b
Carter, L. S., 65a
Carter, M. L., 4a
Cartier, G.-E., 102b
Cartwright, A., 154b, 177a
Cartwright, F., 16b
Carver, M., 6b
Case Western Reserve University. Frances Payne Bolton School of Nursing. *See:* Frances Payne Bolton School of Nursing
Cashman, T., 1b
Caskey, K. K., 158b
Cason, J. S., 161b
Cassell, M., 171b
Cassem, N. H., 100a
Caswell, G., 44a
Catania, J. J., 23b
Cathcart, H. R., 30a
Cattell, W. R., 108a
Catnach, A., 47a
Catterall, M., 170b
Catterall, R. D., 176a
Cauffman, J. G., 156b
Cavell, E., 4a
Cedars-Sinai Medical Center. Department of Nursing, 100a
Cento, 30a
Central Council for District Nursing in London, 16a
Central Health Services Council, 74a, 89a
Central Health Services Council. Joint Sub-committee of the Standing Medical and Standing Nursing Advisory Committees, 74a, 164b
Central Health Services Council. Joint Sub-committee of the Standing Mental Health and the Standing Nursing Advisory Committees, 135b
Central Health Services Council. Standing Nursing Advisory Committee, 89a, 148a, 177b, 182b
Central Middlesex Industrial Health Service, 128b
Central Office of Information, 6b
Central Youth Employment Executive, 39b
Ceylon Nurses Association, 16a
Chadwick, D. L., 122b
Chaffee, E. E., 96a
Chai Keum Kim, 22a
Chalk, D. N., 6b
Chalmers, J. A., 120a
Chaloner, L., 132a
Chamberlain, E. M., 30a
Chamberlain, G., 98b
Chamberlin, R. W., 62a
Chambers, V., 43b
Champagnie, L. E., 22a
Chandra, J., 19a
Charbonneau, G., 6b
Chard, H. F., 125a
Chard, S. D., 125b
Charing Cross Group of Hospitals, 34b
Charing Cross Hospital, London, 86a, 181a
Charles Marie Frank, Sister, 84b, 93a
Charley, I. H., 4a
Charlotte, Sister M., 59b
Charter, D., 78a, 164b
Chartered Society of Physiotherapy, 114a
Charters, J. M., 173b
Chase, P. H., 62a
Chater, S. S., 39a, 52b
Chavasse, J., 36b
Chave, S. P. W., 122b
Chavigny, K. H., 100a
Cheadle, J., 135b
Cheetham, J., 161b
Chenery, J. L., 110b
Cheraskin, E., 96b
Cherescavich, G., 6b, 64a, 80a
Cherian, A., 52b
Chersterman, J. N., 120a
Chesney, D. N., 105a, 173a
Chesser, E., 158a
Chest and Heart Association, 100a, 157a
Cheung, P. L., 113b
Chew, D. C. E., 23b
Childers, E. D., 100a
Childress, G., 158b
Childs, E. M., 89a
Childs, P., 164b
Chino, S., 14a
Chinque, K. M., 107a
Chioni, R. M., 30b
Chisholm, A. S., 145b
Chisholm, G. D., 108a
Chisholm, M. K., 68b, 145b, 148b, 151b
Chittick, R., 1b, 6b, 43b, 49b
Chivers, R. J., 118b
Chivers, T. S., 154a
Cholmeley, J. A., 163a
Chomley, P., 6b
Chong, S., 100a
Chow, R., 86a, 88a, 164b
Choyce, D. P., 129a
Christenson, W. C., 78a
Christian Medical Association of India. Nurses' League, 30b
Christie, E. J., 125b
Christie, J. E., 166b

INDEX 1961-1970

Christie, L. S., 177b
Christman, L. B., 6b, 62a, 64a, 67b, 81a, 89a
Christopoulos, A. C., 142a, 177b
Christy, T. E., 4b, 5b, 49b
Church, R. E., 104b
Chutz, A., 162a
Ciardi, J., 7a
Cicatiello, P., 39b
Clack, B., 84b
Clack, J., 135b
Clain, A., 84b
Clampit, J., 13a
Clappison, G. B., 2b
Clare Marie, Sister, 30b, 86a
Claridge, M., 108a, 120a
Clark, A. L., 133b
Clark, B. F., 23b
Clark, D. F., 23b
Clark, D. H., 7a, 62a
Clark, G., 145b
Clark, J., 108a, 154a
Clark, J. A., 160a
Clark, J. A. P., 74a
Clark, J. F., 144a
Clark, L., 62a
Clark, M. A., 67b, 76b
Clark, N., 73a
Clark, W. S., 114a
Clark-Kennedy, A. E., 4a, 181b
Clarke, C. A., 120a
Clarke, E., 173b
Clarke, K. H., 84b
Clarke, M. K., 164b
Clarke, V. H., 43b
Clarkson, G., 160a
Clatterbridge Hospitals, 181a
Claus, K. E., 44a
Clayton, J. I., 157a
Cleavely, K. B., 166b
Cleghorn, T. E., 102b
Cleino, B., 47b
Cleland, V., 23b, 56b
Clement, A. J., 100a
Clements, G., 110b
Clemons, B., 164b
Cleveland, V. S., 6a
Cleveland University Hospitals, Ohio, 75b
Cleverdon, J., 169a
Clifford, J., 2b
Clissold, G. K., 45a, 46a
Clout, I. R., 145b
Clow, C., 131a
Clow, J. T., 155a
Clwyd and Deeside Hospital Management Committee, 89a
Coakley, J. M., 156b
Cobb, M. M., 147a
Cochrane, M. S., 4a
Cockburn, E O., 182a
Cocker, P., 166b
Cockerill, G., 170b
Coe. C. R., 30b
Coffin, M. A., 130a
Coffman, J. A., 144a
Cogan, E., 12b
Cognet, L., 5b
Cohen, H., 56a
Cohen, J. L., 106b
Cohn, H., 154a
Coker, N., 40b
Colardarci, A. P., 7a
Cole, A. C. E., 113b
Cole, J. W., 144a
Coleman, A. M., 145b
Coleman, D., 160a
Coles, M., 102b
Coles, R. R. A., 106a
Colledge, M., 75b
College of General Practitioners, 94b
(See also: Royal College of General Practitioners)
College of Nursing, Australia, 30b, 36b
Collett, S. W., 181a
Collie, A. W., 158b

Collier, C., 177b
Collier, L. H., 129a
Collins, J. A., 162a
Collins, S. M., 35b, 46a, 68b
Collis, W. R. F., 133b
Columbia University. Teachers' College, 40b, 166b
Columbia University. Teachers' College. Division of Nursing Education, 49b, 89a
Columbia University. Teachers' College. Institute of Research and Service in Nursing Education, 30b
Colver, A., 4b
Commission for Administrative Service in Hospitals, 75b, 78a
Commonwealth Caribbean Nurses, 16a
Commonwealth Medical Conference. Nursing Services Committee, 76b
Community of the Nursing Sisters of St. John the Divine, 16b
Conant, L. H., 30b, 56a, 56b, 61a, 130a
Concordia, Sister M., 50b
Cond, R., 71b, 178a
Conder, P., 30b
Condon, M., 132a
Condron, C. A., 121b
Confederation of Health Service Employees, 68b, 182b
Conference of Catholic Schools of Nursing, 30b
Congalton, A. A., 7a, 23b, 42a
Conlon, A. Y., 20a
Conn, V. S., 57b
Connell, A., 160a
Connor, J., 30b
Connor, R. J., 75b, 78a
Connors, H., 145b
Conover, C. L., 135b
Conroy, M. D., 168a
Consultative Council on the General Hospital Service, 177a
Conway, B., 171b
Conway, M. M., 80a
Cook, A. C., 171b
Cook, D. W., 174a
Cook, F. P., 20a
Cook, J. B., 118b
Cooke, E. M., 120a
Cooke, M., 179a
Cooke, M. A., 122b
Cooke, R. G., 114b, 164b
Cookson, J. S., 30b
Cooley, C. E., 122b
Cooley, D. A., 168a
Cooley, E. J., 133a
Coombes, D. B., 174a
Coombs, R. P., 64a
Cooper, B., 148a
Cooper, J., 61a
Cooper, P., 114b
Cooper, R., 67b
Cooper, R. G., 167b
Cooper, S., 110b
Cooper, S. S., 23b, 30b, 49b, 53a, 64a, 78a
Cope, H. J., 135b
Copeland, D. M., 13a
Copeland, O. E., 89a
Copeman, W. S. C., 114a
Corby, P., 110b
Corcoran, L. E., 113b, 151b
Cordiner, C. M., 28b
Corfmat, P. T., 116b
Cormick, G. W., 20a
Cornelius, D. A., 7a, 145b
Cormer, B., 134a
Corona, D. F., 40b, 95a
Corrado, V. P., 80a
Corrigan, M. J., 113b, 151b
Cortazzi, D., 141a
Corwin, R. G., 7a, 11b
Costello, C. G., 23b, 30b, 89a
Costonguay, T., 30b
Cotes, J. E., 170b

Couldrey, B. M., 174a
Coulson, M. E., 99a
Coulter, P. P., 23b, 40b, 73a, 76b
Council for the Training of Health Visitors, 154a
Council of Europe, 30b
Council on Occupational Health, Chicago, 126a
Court, J., 130a
Cove-Smith, R., 89a
Cowan, P., 177a
Cowie, A. V., 13b
Cox, E. V., 105b
Coye, D. H., 47b
Coyle, M., 56a
Crabtree, N. L., 106a
Craft, N. B., 86a, 179b
Cragg, C. E., 98b
Craig, J. B., 82a, 177a, 179a
Craig, J. S., 86a, 179b
Craig, W. S., 134a
Cramond, W. A., 110b
Cramp, B., 56a
Crandall, E. J., 39b
Crane, K. H., 75b, 78a
Cranstoun, J., 7a
Crassweller, P. O., 108a
Crawford, A. L., 135b
Crawford, M., 167b
Crawford, M. P., 67b, 177a
Crawford, R. L., 147a
Craytor, J. K., 47b, 98b
Creamer, B., 105b
Creelman, L., 148a
Creighton, H., 19a
Crichton, A., 67b, 177a
Crim, B. J., 172a
Crisp, E., 121a
Crispo, J. H. G., 20a
Critchley, D. L., 135b
Crockett, G. S., 88a
Croft, D. N., 173a, 173b
Cromwell, G. E., 156b
Cronin, E., 104a
Croog, S. H., 30b
Crookes, T. G., 23b
Cropper, C. F. J., 100a, 110b, 157a
Crosby, M. H., 130a
Cross, K. W., 23b
Cross, Y., 60a
Crotin, G. G., 19a
Crow, A., 144a
Crow, L. D., 144a
Crow, R. A., 130a
Crowley, D., 31b, 82a
Crowther, B., 83b
Crowther, H. A. H., 104a
Croxford, E. A., 120a
Crumpsall Hospital, 49b
Crumpton, E., 95a
Cubbin, J. K., 135b
Culbert, P. A., 101a
Cullinan, J., 23b, 56a, 173b
Culpan, P., 23b
Culver, V. M., 64a, 82a
Cuming, M. W., 78a
Cumming, E. E., 50b
Cumulative Index to Nursing Literature, 39b
Cundell, R., 135b
Cunningham, E. V., 41b
Cunningham, J. T., 4a
Cunningham, L. S., 64a
Cunningham, P. J., 41a, 130a, 146a, 151b
Curwen, M., 148b
Cusdin, S. E. T., 179b
Cust, G., 145b
Cuthbert, B. L., 61a
Cyriax, J., 114a

Dabritz, L., 132a
Dagsland, H., 7a
Dahlstedt, J. M., 64b
Dahlsten, A. M., 78a

BIBLIOGRAPHY OF NURSING

Dainton, C., 181a
Dake, M. A., 62a
Dakin, F., 66b
Dale, J., 4b
Dallas, N. L., 129a
Dally, P., 144b
Dalton, B. M., 23b, 142b
Daly, O. M., 179a
Damhacher, E., 175a
Dan Mason Nursing Research Committee, 23b, 82a, 89a
Dana, R. H., 64a
Danao, M. L., 30b
Dancer, M. E. G., 154a
Daniels, R. R., 93b
Dann, T. C., 84b
Darnell, L. M., 23b, 39b
Darrah, W. E., 152a
Darwin, J., 64b, 106a
Das, D. M. H., 19a, 42b
Dauk, C. S., 42b
Daveluy, D., 14b
David, H. P., 114b, 159b
David, J. D. P., 110b
David, O. D., 7a
Davidson, A., 164b
Davidson, J. S., 160a
Davidson, L. C., 68a
Davidson, R., 86a
Davidson, S., 130a
Davidson, T. W., 89b
Davie, T. B., 41a
Davies, B. M., 122b
Davies, D., 122b
Davies, J. B. M., 145b, 153b
Davies, J. O. F., 56a
Davies, M. K., 126a
Davies, P. M., 41a
Davies, R. P., 24a
Davies, T. I. H., 142b
Davio, E. L., 107a
Davis, A., 42b
Davis, A. E., 24a
Davis, A. J., 24a, 74a
Davis, B. M., 110b
Davis, C. E., 161b
Davis, F., 7a, 39b, 53a, 65b, 71b
Davis, K. G., 93b
Davis, M., 73a
Davis, M. E., 120a
Davis, M. L. C., 65a
Davis, N. C., 167b
Davis, P. E., 48b
Davis, P. R., 114a
Davis, R. W., 106a, 110b, 118b, 164b
Davison, R. L., 98b
Davison, T., 64b
Davitz, L. J., 84b
Dawber, T. R., 100a
Dawes, J., 122b
Dawson, I. M., 82a
Dawson, R., 135b
Dawson, W. B., 171b
Dawson-Butterworth, K., 100b, 110b
Day, P., 138a
Day, V. M., 167b
Dayton, M., 136a
Deacon, C. E., 135b
Deakin, B. M., 30b
Deakin, H. G., 157a
De Alcantara, G., 14b
Dean, D. J., 43b, 74a, 142a
Dean, W. B., 96a
Dearden, R., 132b
Dearden, R. W., 78a
DeChow, G. H., 39a
Deck, E. S., 89b
Deegan, M., 46a
Deeley, T. J., 173b
Degardin, C., 30b
De Garzon, E. C., 14b
de Gras, L. A., 142b
De Gutierrez-Mahoney, C. G., 164b
Deibel, A. W., 110b
de Kretser, A. J. H., 126a
de la Court, L. C., 28a

Delahanty, M. B., 177b
DeLaney, R. E., 106b
DeLargy, J., 110b
Delehanty, L., 108a
Delgardo, A., 4b
Deller, H. J., 68a
DeLora, J. R., 24a
DeMarco, J. P., 73a, 78a
de Marillac, L., 4a
DeMeyer, J., 86a
de Montfort, Sister M., 68a
Dempsey, M., 140b
Dempster, W. J., 108a
Denault, P. M., 119a
Denis, M., 31a
Denman, K. M., 46a
Denney, R. R., 174a
Dennis, L. B., 144b
Densen, P. M., 93b
Dent, M. J. W., 60a, 108a
Deocampo, Sister M. A. de J., 42b
Department of Employment and Productivity. See: Great Britain. Department etc.
Department of Health and Social Security. See: Great Britain. Department etc.
Department of Health for Scotland. See: Great Britain. Department etc.
de Pass, B., 145b
Derasari, A. J., 133b
Derr, S. D., 104b
Desainz, D., 145b
Desmond, Sr. M., 68a
de Stefano, G. M., 76b
Deuble, H., 149b
Devane, D. J., 160a
Devaneson, B. A., 44a
Devas, M. B., 110b
Devlin, H. B., 98b, 105b, 106a
DeVries, R. A., 92b
Dewar, J., 135b
Dewhurst, J., 135b
DeWolfe, A. S., 175a
de Young, L., 7a
Diack, L., 13a
Diament, M. L., 45a
Diamond, L. K., 30b, 56b
Dickens, M. L., 96a
Dicker, J., 123a, 135b, 136a
Dicker, K., 78a
Dickie, H. M., 84b
Dickoff, J., 40b, 56a, 64b
Dier, K. A., 80a
Diers, D., 56a, 142b
Dietrich, B. J., 68a
Diettert, G. A., 100a
Dietz, L. D., 1a
Dillman, E., 139a
Dillon, A., 149b
Dillon, D. C., 80a
Dilworth, A. S., 7a, 56a, 81a
Dineen, M. A., 40b
Dingleton Hospital, Melrose, 181a
Dipietro, M. H., 56a
Dismukes, L. M., 46a, 100b
Dison, N. G., 64b, 172b
District Nursing, 3a, 150b
Dithridge, E. H., 156b
Dittman, L., 116b
Dix, M. R., 106b
Dixon, N., 48b, 171b
Dixon, P. N., 146a
Dixon, W. M., 104a, 122b, 126a
Dlin, B. M., 108a
Dobbie, K., 162a
Dobson, M., 100b
Dock, L. L., 1a, 4a
Dodd, B., 166a
Dodd, I. A., 96a
Dodds, Sir C., 96b
Dodds, G. H., 41a, 113a
Dodenhoff, J. T., 90a, 138a
Dodge, J. S., 64b
Dodwell, B. I. R., 68b

Dolan, J., 1a
Dolan, M. B., 15b, 24a
Dolan, N., 100b
Dolch, E. T., 132a
Doll, R., 105b, 171b
Dolman, S., 100b
Dolton, W. D., 146a
Donabedian, A., 93b
Donaldson, F., 7a
Donaldson, J., 131b
Donelly, G., 142b
Donnan, S. G., 2a
Donner, G., 135b
Donovan, H. M., 89b, 177b
Donovan, J., 126a
Donovan, J. E., 80a
Dooley, J. W., 12b, 146a
Doran, W. T., 122b
Dornette, W. H. L., 169a
Dossetor, J. B., 168a
Dougherty, A. L., 106b
Douglas, E., 160a
Douglas, F. N., 171b
Douglas, L. M., 95a
Dowling, J. J., 162a
Downey, D., 136a, 152a
Downey, M. E., 75b
Downie, A. P., 122b
Downie, W. W., 114a
Downing, S. R., 108a
Downs, B., 153b
Downs, F. S., 56a
Downs, H. S., 105b
Doyle, M., 126a
Drage, E., 60a
Drane, J. W., 59a
Dransfield, G. A., 110b
Draper, P., 146a, 153b, 177a
Dreves, K. D., 7a, 40b
Drew, J. A., 93a, 93b
Drewery, J., 62a
Drillien, C. M., 134a
Driscoll, B., 146a
Driscoll, J. R. M., 19a
Drummond, E. E., 88b, 175a
Drummond, E. J., 29b, 31a, 41b, 43b
Dryden M. V., 7a
Duana, I., 50b
Dubiny, M. J., 41a
Ducas, D., 7a
Dudgeon, J. A., 120a
Dudgeon, M. Y., 89b
Duffy, W., 146a
Dugan, A. B., 64b, 68a
du Gaz, B. W., 85a
Duke, E. O., 1a
Dunbar, V. M., 46a
Duncan, A. C., 116b
Duncan, E. H. L., 112b, 153a
Duncan, K. P., 123a
Duncanson, M. B., 7b
Duncombe, M. A., 130a, 181b
Dundee College of Nursing, 54b
Dundee University, 128b
Dunham, P. E., 116b
Dunlap, L., 142a
Dunlap, M. S., 39a, 53a
Dunn, G. C., 102b
Dunn, H. W., 7b, 20a, 68a, 74a, 76b
Dunn, J. B., 64b
Dunn, M., 146a
Dunn, M. A., 93b
Dunsdon, E., 116b
Dunston, B. N., 56a, 120a
Duran, F. A., 136a
Durand, M., 105a
Durbin, F. C., 163b
Durdin, D. J., 7b
Durham, R. C., 93b
Durrant, C. W., 169a
Dustan, L. C., 7b, 31a, 44a
Dutcher, I. E., 96b
Dutton, A., 25a
Dwyer, J. M., 56a, 93b, 120a
Dyer, M. R., 103b

Eagen, Sister M. C., 78a
Earle, A., 136a
Easson, E., 173b
Easson, W. M., 89b
East London Hospital, 181b
East London Nursing Society, 2b
Easterly, J., 44b
Eastman, N. J., 120a
Easton, R. E., 14b
Eastwood, C. G., 46a
Eaton, E. S., 51a
Eckardt, R. B., 123a
Eckleberry, G., 61a
Eckels, J., 154a
Eckenfoff, J. E., 164a
Eckstein, H. B., 108a
Eddy, J. D., 100b
Ede, L., 19a
Edelson, R. B., 82a, 83a
Edelstein, R. R., 73a
Edelston, H., 120a
Edge, S. C., 64b
Edgecumbe, R. H., 93b
Edgeworth, D., 92b, 166b
Edinburgh, Royal Infirmary, 160a
Edmunds, C., 108a
Edson, E. F., 123a
Edwards, C. N., 39b
Edwards, G., 12a, 20a, 158a, 182a
Edwards, H. C., 105b
Edwards, J., 120a, 136a
Edwards, K. E., 126a
Edwards, L. G., 171b
Edwards, M., 164b
Edwards, M. M., 1a, 7b, 68a
Edwards, R., 106b
Edwards-Rees, D., 1a
Egerton, M. E., 98b
Ehrhart, A. M., 90b, 97b
Eichhorn, S., 31a
Ekdawi, M. Y., 123a, 136a
Elaine, Rev. Sister M., 164b
Elder, M. S., 159b
Elder, R. G., 89b
Elizabeth, Sister R., 110b
Elizabeth Garrett Anderson Hospital, 181b
Elkes, A., 59b
Elles, G., 62a
Elliott, J. E., 24a
Elliott, F. E., 31a, 179a
Elliott, J., 110b
Elliott, J. E., 38b, 56b
Ellis, C. R., 157a
Ellis, G. L., 64b, 87a
Ellis, J. R., 146a
Ellis, M., 169a
Ellis, R., 7b, 56b
Ellis, S., 171b
Ellison, R. R., 99a
Ellsworth, J., 136a
Ellsworth, R. B., 136a, 137b
Elson, R., 163a
Elwell, R., 115b
Elwood, E., 157a
Emens, A. E., 46a, 136a, 142b
Emers, J., 142b
Emerson, C. P., 64a, 164b
Emery, A. E. H., 114a
Emmanuel, S., 171b
Emory, F. H. M., 5a
Eng, E., 20a, 24a, 74a, 76b
Engberg, E., 174a
Engel, J., 82a
English Electric Leo Marconi Computers Ltd., 78b
Ennever, O. N., 146a
Ennis, H. G., 156a
Ensing, E. C., 7b, 80a, 170a, 180b
Epp, M. L., 158a, 158b
Eppink, H., 133b
Erasmus, C. A., 146a
Erickson, E. H., 41b
Erikson, F., 130a
Erith Technical College, Woolwich, 43b
Erlander, D., 170a

Erne, Sister M. J., 31a
Ernsberger, R. G., 15a
Errera, D. W., 162a
Errion, G. D., 136a
Espiritu, T. M., 31a
Etherington, A., 95a
Etzioni, A., 7b
Evagorou, D., 116b
Evans, C., 129a
Evans, D. S., 102b
Evans, F. M. C., 115b
Evans, M., 148b, 151a
Evans, P. J., 129a
Evelina Hospital, 181b
Everett, A. E., 99a
Ewell, C. M., 93b
Ewing, M. R., 84b
Exchaquet, N. F., 68a
Exton-Smith, A. N., 92b, 110b, 112a

Faddis, M. O., 89b, 110b
Fagerhaugh, S. Y., 136a, 175a
Fagin, C. M., 81a, 132a, 136a, 141b
Fahey, J. J., 73a
Fahey, P. M., 162a
Fahy, E., 31a
Fair, C. J., 107a, 129b
Fairley, G. H., 114b
Fairley, J., 148b
Fairweather, D. V. I., 120a
Falconer, M. W., 171b
Fall, M. B., 172a
Fallows, P. B., 84b
Fanning, W. W., 24a
Farberow, N. L., 115b
Farnham, S., 144b
Farnol, R. T., 82a
Farrar, G. E., 96a
Farrell, D., 132a
Farris, M. A., 145a
Farrow, R., 130a, 162a
Fasso, T. E., 62b
Faulkner, H., 111a
Faville, K., 39b
Fawkes, B. N., 7b, 31a, 56b, 69a, 82a
Feeley, E. McN., 100b
Fegan, F. J., 171a
Fegan, W. G., 102b
Fein, L. G., 31a
Feinstein, M. B., 171b
Feisel, K., 93b
Feiwel, M., 104a
Feldhusen, J. F., 27a, 27b, 42a
Feldman, H., 47b
Fell, A. V., 157a, 160a
Fell, J. H., 116b, 170b
Fell, M. R., 120a
Felstein, I., 111a, 158a
Felton, J. S., 11a, 126a, 127b
Fenn, L. J. S., 51a
Fennessy, C. M., 111a
Fensome, J. E., 31a
Fenton, M., 84b
Ferguson, J., 108a
Ferguson, L. K., 64a, 164b
Feguson, M., 56b, 148b
Ferguson, V., 24a
Ferlic, A., 7b
Fernandez, C. G., 68a
Fernie, W. W., 160a
Feroze, R. M., 159b
Ferrigan, M., 100b
Ferster, M. B., 97a
Feurtado, M., 123a
Feyerherm, A. M., 24a, 78a
Fieber, W. W., 160a
Fiedler, D. E., 95b
Fiedler, J. P., 165a
Field, M., 89b
Field, P. A., 31a
Field, W. E., 53a, 136a
Fielder, J., 175b
Fielder, R. E., 96a
Fielding, V. V., 95a
Fielo, S. B., 64b, 96b

Figueroa, M., 169a
Finch, J., 64b
Fincher, C., 24a
Fine, W., 111a
Finnegan, J. A., 165a
Fiore, M., 84b
Fisch, L., 106a
Fischer, B. H., 171a
Fischer, L. R., 115b
Fishbein, M., 126a
Fisher, A. M., 113a
Fisher, L. C., 162a
Fitch, G. E., 41a, 97a
Fitzgerald, A., 4a
Fitz-Gibbon, A. J., 89b
Fitzgibbon, M., 68a
Fitzpatrick, E., 120a
Fitzpatrick, G., 99a
Fitzpatrick, G. M., 113b
Fitzpatrick, K., 162a
Fitzpatrick, T. B., 57a, 91b
Fitzwater, J., 86a
Fivars, G., 31a, 56b
Flack, G., 155a
Flaming, K. H., 8b
Flanagan, J. C., 45a
Flandorf, V. S., 51a
Flatman, G. E., 173b
Flatter, P. A., 171a
Fleming, J. S., 100b
Fleming, M. O., 115a
Fleming, R., 141b
Fletcher, P. D., 31a
Fletcher, S. M., 172a
Fletcher, W. B., 155a
Flewett, T. H., 22a
Flick, J. A., 167a
Flint, R. T., 24a
Flitter, H. H., 24a, 26b, 34b, 35a, 41b, 134b
Flood, R. F., 78a
Florence Nightingale College of Nursing, Turkey, 54b
Florence Nightingale International Foundation, 16b, 17b, 19b
Florence Nightingale International Nurses Association Conference, 89b
Florentine, H. G., 156b
Flores, A. M., 84b
Floutz, V. W., 102a
Floyd, E. D., 142a, 177b
Flunder, D. J., 126a
Fly, O. A., 123a
Fogg, J., 171b
Fogt, J. R., 42b, 88b
Foley, J., 7b, 133b
Folta, J. R., 56b, 89b
Foo Chong Ah, 13a
Forbes, D. N., 13a
Forbes, F. A., 155a
Forbes, J. A., 111a
Ford, B., 154a
Ford, H. A., 133a
Fordham, M. E., 164b
Foreign & Commonwealth Office. See: Great Britain. Foreign etc.
Forman, A., 168a
Forman, A. M., 24a
Forman, J. A. S., 150b
Forrest, A. D., 136a
Forrest, C., 136a, 170b
Forrest, D., 130a
Forrest J., 82a, 96b
Forsyth, B., 170b
Fosberg, G. C., 2a, 95a
Foshay, A. W., 46a
Foster, J., 27a, 136a
Foster, R., 42b
Foster, S., 100b
Foster, V. L., 68a
Fourman, P., 96b
Fowler, E. A., 168b
Fowler, G. R., 135a
Fox, D. J., 7b, 30b, 31a, 44a, 56b
Fox, J., 119b
Fox, M. S., 106b

BIBLIOGRAPHY OF NURSING

Fox, R., 7b, 144b
Fox, S., 13a
Fox, Sir T., 159b
Frackelton, D. L., 39b
Frame, H. B. P., 136a, 141b
Frances, Sister M. A., 78a
Frances Payne Bolton School of Nursing, 56b
Francis, G. M., 99a
Francis, H. W. S., 155a
Francis, Sister J., 89b
Francis, P. C., 168a
Frank, C. M., 7b, 31a, 64b
Frank, E. D., 46a
Franklin, G., 110a
Franks, G. L., 68b, 69a
Franks, J., 152a
Fraser, J., 160a
Fraser, J. R., 45a, 164b
Fraser, M., 123a
Fream, W. C., 97a, 98a, 115a
Fredericks, M. A., 44a
Freed, E. X., 158b
Freedman, A. M., 158b
Freeman, H. E., 89a
Freeman, J. R., 68a
Freeman, M. G., 82a
Freeman, M. H., 129a
Freeman, R. B., 7b, 57b, 68a, 89b, 146a, 152a
Freeman, V., 148b
Frenay, M. A. C., 41a, 175b
French, J. G., 23b
French, R. M., 105a
French, T., 116b
Frerichs, M., 46a
Friend, P. M., 7b, 69a
Frisby, C. B., 28b
Fritz, E., 53a
Friz, B. R., 163b
Frommer, E. A., 132a, 133b, 136a
Frost, M., 89b
Frost, W., 146a
Fry, J., 100b, 150a, 155a
Fry, S., 165b
Frye, C., 108a, 108b
Fuerst, E. V., 31b, 46a
Fuhrer, M. J., 174a
Fujiki, S., 89b
Fulcher, J. M., 51a
Fulham Hospital, London, 54b
Fuller, D., 24a
Fuller, E. D., 46a, 100b
Funnell, E., 146b
Furfey, P. H., 66b
Fuszard, Sister M. B., 132a
Fyke, K. J., 75b, 78a

Gagnon, C., 16b, 146a
Gainsborough, H., 7b, 31b
Gaitz, C. M., 113a
Galbally, B., 86a
Galbraith, G., 73b
Galbraith, J. M., 62a
Gall, G., 51a
Gallagher, A. H., 31b
Gallaher, E., 150a, 153b
Gallaher, H. L., 123a
Gammon, O. M., 31b
Gander, D. R., 150a
Gans, B., 134a
Garb, S., 22a, 105a, 172a
Garcia, P. J., 56b
Gardella, F. A., 72b, 77a
Gardiner, G. O., 82b
Gardner, A. M. N., 84b, 168a
Gardner, A., 8a, 121b
Gardner, E. K., 86a
Gardner, R., 158b
Garland, G. W., 120b
Garland, H., 96a
Garland, P., 129a
Garland, T. O., 22a
Garner, G. S., 53a
Garnet, J. D., 104b, 120b

Garnham, P. D., 86a
Garretson, A. M., 43a
Garrett, S. A. G., 69a, 86b
Garrety, C., 116b
Garrow, C., 85a
Garvin, M., 24a
Garzon, E. C. de, 14b
Gascoyne, R. A., 13a
Gaston, R., 162a
Gauthier, L., 42b
Gazaway, R., 61a
Gear, H. S., 146a
Gearing, K. L., 165b
Gebbie, K. M., 155a
Geddes, J. D. C., 31b
Geis, G. L., 47b
Geister, J. M., 4a
Geitgey, D. A., 30a, 31b, 39a, 56b, 68a
Gelber, I., 158b
Gelfand, S., 142b
Gelman, S. J., 24a
General Nursing Council for England and Wales, 16b, 24a, 31b, 36b, 40b, 41a, 42a, 44a, 53a, 60a, 69a, 82b
General Nursing Council for Scotland, 142b
Gentry, B. A., 71b
George, J., 88a
George, V. M., 151a
Georgia Institute of Technology. School of Industrial Engineering, 68a
Georgopoulos, B. S., 8a, 81a, 89b, 93b
Gerard, M., 95a
Gerbie, A. B., 113a
Gerchberg, L. R., 31b
Germain, L. D., 68a, 76b
Germaine, A., 42b, 68a, 76b, 95a, 167a
German Nurses' Federation, 14a
Geronsin, J. R., 83b
Gerstein, A. I., 28b, 31b
Gettings, B., 3a, 69a, 155a
Getty, C., 136a
Ghei, P. N., 123a
Giannelli, S., 84a
Gibb, A. G., 106b
Gibberd, F. B., 173a
Gibbs, B. M., 84a
Gibbs, D. D., 114b
Gibbs, G. E., 108b
Gibson, J., 96b, 114b, 116b, 136a, 143a, 172a
Gibson, M., 130b
Gidseg, L., 115a
Gilbert, R., 146a
Gilbert, R. G., 13b
Gilchrist, M. I., 163a
Gildner, J. L., 62a
Giles, G., 51a
Giles, M. N., 80b
Gilhespy, M., 126a
Gill, W., 160a
Gillam, R., 8a, 31b, 40a, 73b
Gilles, H. M., 115a
Gillespie, C., 158b
Gillespie, W. A., 167a
Gillie, A., 150b
Gillies, D. A., 45a
Gillin, E. F., 126a
Gillis, L., 133a
Gilmer, L., 62a
Gilmore, M., 155a
Gilmore, R. F., 80b
Gilston, A., 100b, 169a
Ginsberg, F., 22a, 86b, 164b, 167a, 168a
Ginzberg, E., 8a, 20a, 24a, 78a
Gips, C. D., 85b, 132a
Girard, A., 8a, 15a
Girdwood, R. H., 8a
Gish, O., 24b
Given, B., 73b
Given, C. W., 73b
Glancy, J. E. McA., 142a
Glaser, W. A., 146a, 152a
Glasgow Retirement Council, 111a
Glasgow Royal Infirmary, 31b, 36b

Glatt, M. M., 158b
Glen, F., 59b
Glenister, T. W. A., 96b
Gliedman, M. L., 165a
Gloster Crusader Vending Limited, 178a
Glover, B. H., 136a
Glover, G., 76b
Glover, M. R., 181b
Gochoco, V. S., 52a
Godber, G., 120b
Goddard, H. A., 68b, 75b
Godden, G. M., 43b
Godfrey, J. M., 108b
Goldfarb, M., 76b
Goldfogel, L., 144b
Goldin, P., 64b
Goldman, M., 173b
Goldsborough, J. D., 144b
Goldsmith, R., 45a
Goldstein, J., 93b
Goldstein, L. S., 60b
Good, E. R., 167a
Good, S. R., 24b, 53a
Goodacre, R., 154a
Goodland, N. L., 8a, 24b, 64b, 89b, 100b, 172a
Goodman, L., 131b
Goodson, M. R., 31b
Goostray, S., 4a, 97b, 102a
Gordon, J. E., 18b, 24b, 40a, 182a
Gorham, W. A., 64b, 75b
Gorick, G. M., 85a
Gorrie, M. G., 152a
Gortner, S. R., 53a
Gorton, J. V., 142a
Gosnell, D., 56b
Gosney, K. G., 136b
Goswell, D., 31a
Gotsman, M. S., 102a
Gottlieb, M. I., 96b
Gough, M. A., 54b, 172a
Gould, M., 163a
Gould, M. E., 31b
Gourlay, D., 68b
Governale, G. N., 175a
Government Social Survey, 67a
Govoni, L. E., 172a
Gowan, M. O., 49b
Gowda, S. B., 163a
Gowell, E. C., 46a, 136b
Gowin, J., 165a
Gowland, W. P., 96b
Goyal, K., 53a
Gozzi, E. K., 62a, 130b
Grace, H. K., 123a
Grace, W. J., 100b
Gracey, M., 130b
Graffam, S. R., 64b
Graham, A. A., 152a
Graham, J. A. G., 152a
Graham, J. G., 118b
Graham, L. E., 53a, 93b, 100b
Graham, P., 116b, 130b, 136b
Grant, A., 120b
Grant, J., 102b
Grant, J. V., 68b
Grant, M. L., 168a
Grant, R., 44a
Grauhan, A., 8a, 49b
Graulou, R., 62b
Graveling, B., 114a, 173b
Gravelius, E. M., 40a
Graves, J., 48b
Gray, C. E., 96b
Gray, H. H., 120b
Gray, W. S., 44a
Grayson, G. A., 24b
Great Britain. Central Health Services Council. *See:* Central Health Services Council
Great Britain. Central Office of Information. *See:* Central Office of Information
Great Britain. Department of Employment and Productivity, 24b

Great Britain. Department of Health and Social Security, 53a, 69a, 148b
Great Britain. Department of Health and Social Security. National Nursing Staff Committee, 68b, 69a, 78a
Great Britain. Department of Health and Social Security. Social Science Research Unit, 155a
Great Britain. Department of Health for Scotland, 3a, 67a
Great Britain. Foreign and Commonwealth Office, 31b
Great Britain. Ministry of Health, 3a, 3b, 9b, 21b, 59b, 68b, 69a, 73b, 78b, 92b, 128b, 177a, 178b, 179b, 182b
Great Britain. Ministry of Labour. Central Youth Employment Executive. See: Central Youth Employment Executive
Great Britain. Ministry of Labour. Nursing Services Division, 24b
Great Britain. National Board for Prices and Incomes. See: National Board for Prices and Incomes
Great Britain. Parliament, 19a, 154a
Great Britain. Scottish Education Department, 44a
Great Britain. Scottish Home and Health Department, 3a, 3b, 6b, 27a, 37a, 68a, 128b, 148b
Great Britain. Scottish Home and Health Department. Scottish Nursing Staffs Committee, 72b
Great Britain. Welsh Office, 69a, 78a, 148b
Greaves, D. P., 129a
Green, A. P., 132a
Green, E. J., 37b
Green, G. H., 120b
Green, J., 136b
Green, M. D., 70a, 180b
Green, R. M., 92a
Green, W. M., 174a
Greenberg, B. G., 56b
Greenberg, R. C., 73b
Greene, J., 12a, 36b, 136b, 141a
Greene, M. C. L., 119b
Greene, R., 107a
Greene, V. W., 167a
Greenfield, R. L., 56b
Greening, P., 152a
Greenough, K., 93b
Greenwood, G. A., 178a
Gregg, E., 108b
Gregory, E., 136b
Greisheimer, E. M., 96a
Gremp, Z. von, 82b
Greville, R., 108b
Gribble, G., 39b
Gribbons, C. A., 99a
Griffen, G. S., 31b, 64b
Griffin, G. J., 46a, 48b, 90b
Griffin, H., 179b
Griffin, J. K., 90b, 120b
Griffin, L. M., 80b
Griffin, W. H., 35a
Griffith, J. R., 93a
Griffiths, J. C., 171a
Griffiths, S. H., 158b
Grillot, G. F., 102a
Grimwood, J. M., 175b
Grob, G. N., 182a
Grondin, P., 160a
Groomes, E. W., 178b
Grosicki, J. P., 93b, 108b
Gross, C. W., 106b
Gross, P. A., 75b
Grosvenor, P. A., 45b
Group, T. M., 146a
Group for the Advancement of Psychiatry. Committee on Therapeutic Care, 136b
Grove, E., 174a
Grove, W. A., 92b
Groves, M. D., 69a

Gruber, E. C., 29a
Gruendemann, B. J., 165a
Gruhl, V. R., 100b, 130b
Grun, J., 70a
Grundy, A. V., 170a
Grundy, F., 146b
Gruneau Research Limited, 8a
Gruhut, I., 42a, 96b
Guckian, J. C., 123a
Guild of St. Barnabas for Anglican Nurses, 60a
Guinee, K. K., 31b
Gulabani, L., 56b
Gumbley, C. N., 31b, 157a
Gunn, A. D. G., 22a, 80a, 102b, 105b, 108b, 111a, 120b, 155a, 158a
Gunn, I. P., 169a
Gunn, M., 136b
Gunter, L. M., 44a, 44b, 57a, 60a, 89b, 111a
Gunter, V., 171a
Gunzburg, A. L., 116b
Gunzburg, H. C., 116b
Gupta, A., 49b
Gurd, D. P., 129a
Guttman, Sir L., 114a
Guyot, H., 3b

Haas, J. E., 11b
Hacker, C., 3b, 84a
Hadley, B. J., 8a
Haffey, V. A., 136b
Hagan, F., 61b
Hagen, E., 70a
Hagerman, Z. J., 61a
Hahn, A., 100b
Haiduck, A., 72a
Haines, J., 173b
Haines, R. W., 96a
Hains, C. K., 153b
Hakerem, H. M., 133b
Haldane, J. D., 130b, 136b
Hale, R., 43b, 152a
Hale, S. L., 61a
Hale, T., 24b, 31b, 54b
Hall, A., 108b
Hall, B. L., 32a, 61a
Hall, C. M., 8a
Hall, E. D., 82b
Hall, G. C., 168a
Hall, I., 152a
Hall, J., 24b
Hall, L. E., 174a
Hall, M. E., 174a
Hall, M. F., 70a
Hall, O., 70a
Hall, T., 155a
Hall, V. C., 4a
Hallahan, J. D., 123a
Hallam, J., 126a
Hallas, C., 116b, 143a
Halliday, N. P., 100b, 134a
Halliday, R., 158b
Hallis, N. O. J., 176a
Halsey, F. Y., 57a
Halstead, H., 143a
Halstead, H. H., 64b
Hamil, E. M., 70a
Hamilton, C. M., 120b
Hamilton, D., 69a
Hamilton, D. I., 160b
Hamilton, G. L., 160b
Hamilton, P. M., 120b, 130b
Hamilton, T. S., 24b
Hamilton, V., 123a
Hamm, B. H., 143a
Hammersmith Hospital, London, 43b
Hammersmith Hospital, London. Royal Post-Graduate Medical School, 43b
Hanchett, E. S., 102a
Hancock, C., 141b
Handley, A. J., 102b
Handley, P. R., 116b
Hangartner, C. A., 32a

Hanham, H. J., 70a
Hankin, E., 167a
Hanley, J., 118b
Hannan, J., 82a
Hannigan, E., 179a
Hanron, J. B., 110a
Hansell, P., 182a
Hansen, A. C., 8a, 146b, 147b, 148b
Hansen, K. E., 75b
Hanson, G. C., 171a
Hanusz, P. P., 101b
Harbison, R., 148b
Hardin, C. A., 146b
Hardman, E., 70a
Hardman, F. G., 160b
Hardy, G. F. R., 69a
Hardy, M. I., 126b
Hardy, S., 111a, 155a
Hare, E. H., 115b
Hare, R., 97b
Hargest, T. S., 180b
Hargreaves, T., 105b, 107a, 120b
Hargreaves, W. A., 136b
Harlan, G. P., 181b
Harlow, F. W., 160b
Harlow, S. J., 48a
Harms, M. T., 27a, 41a, 46a
Harmuth, B., 144b
Harner, R., 146b
Harper, J. R., 86b, 132a
Harpman, J. A., 106b
Harris, A., 100b
Harris, A. M., 126a, 128a
Harris, C. F., 170a
Harris, H. E., 12a
Harris, L. E., 117a
Harris, R. M., 88a
Harrison, D. F. N., 99a, 160b
Harrison, G. G., 157a
Harrison, M., 111a
Harrison, P. H., 1a
Harrison, S. E., 28a
Harrold, J. M., 111a
Hart, A. L., 41a
Hart, A. M., 33a
Hart, E. W., 134a
Hart, F., 8a, 24b
Hart, F. D., 114a
Hart, G. S., 64b
Hart, J., 173b
Hart, L. K., 172a
Harte, M. B., 128b
Hartley, I. D., 100b
Hartmann, B., 78b
Hartnett, W. F., 89b
Hartsfield, S. L., 143a
Harty, M. B., 32a, 48b
Harvey, E. L., 41b
Harvey, J., 162a
Harvey, L. H., 44b
Harvey, R. H., 165a
Harvey, R. M., 106b
Haslam, O., 32a
Haslam, P., 89b
Hasler, D., 82b
Hasler, J. C., 148b, 151a
Hasselmeyer, E. G., 93b, 134a
Hassenplug, L. W., 32a, 46b, 49b, 57a
Hassler, R. A., 81b
Hastings, B., 46b
Hatcher, C. R., 160b
Hatcher, J., 97b
Hatt, F. M., 78b
Hattersley, F., 148b, 155a
Hatton, M. L., 147b, 149b
Hauer, R. M., 76b
Haugen, I. H., 148b
Haugland, B., 70a
Havener, W. H., 106b, 107a, 129a, 129b
Haward, L. R. C., 22b, 57a, 136b
Hawkins, E., 136b
Hawkins, J. L., 76b, 90a
Hawkins, R. B., 46b
Hawley, J., 57a
Hawley, K. S., 20a
Hawthorne, V. M., 123a

Hawthorne Experiment, 74a
Hay, S., 61a
Hayes, C., 148b
Hayes, E. J., 60a
Hayes, K. J., 155a
Hayes, M., 3b
Hayes, P. J., 60a
Hayes, W. J., 61a
Hayman, F., 15a
Haynes, I., 32a
Haynes, U., 117a
Hays, J. S., 61a, 90a, 136b
Hayter, J., 53a, 105b, 168a
Hayter, M., 111a
Haywood, S. C., 69a, 70a
Hazer, A., 158a
Healey, J. P., 24b
Healey, J. T., 126a
Health, 2b
Health Services Journal, 84a
Health Visitors' Association, 152a, 153a, 156a
Healy, H. T., 133a
Healy, K. M., 160b, 165a
Hean, L. M., 108b
Heartfield, M., 12b
Heathcock, R., 4a
Heaton, D., 158b
Hecht, A. B., 172a
Heckel, R. V., 130b, 144b
Hector, W. E., 32a, 35b, 46b, 47b, 48b, 53a, 64b, 65a, 104b, 113b, 114b, 179b
Hedricks, J. A., 53a
Hefetz, G., 126a
Heffner, W. W., 62b
Hehre, F. W., 120b
Heidgerken, L. E., 31a, 40a, 53a, 57a, 57b, 144b
Heimlich, H. J., 165a
Heinemann, E., 22b, 158b
Heinemann Training Services Ltd., 48a
Heller, A. F., 100b
Hellier, F. F., 104a
Helvie, C. O., 146b
Hemphill, R. E., 136b
Henderson, C., 70a, 90a
Henderson, J. E., 70b
Henderson, P., 156b
Henderson, V., 8a, 32a, 39b, 51a, 58b, 85a
Heneman, H. G., 20a
Henley, B., 112b
Henley, N. L., 162a
Henriksen, H. L., 126a
Henry, A. P., 148b
Henry, D. K., 75b
Henry, M., 16b, 32a
Henson, R. A., 118b
Herd, L., 111a
Herring, Sister C., 94a
Herrmann, J. B., 95b
Hershey, N., 19b
Herzig, N., 159b
Heslin, P., 45a
Hess, G., 136b
Hess, I., 57a
Hewes, A., 28b
Hewitt, H. E., 143b
Heyward, J., 179b
Hibbert, D., 75b, 80b
Hickey, J. T., 107a, 129b
Hickey, M. C., 169a
Hicks, J. B., 105a
Hicks, M. L., 118b
High Plains Baptist Hospital, Amarillo, Texas, 179b
Highnett, O. B., 82b
Highriter, M. E., 146b
Higson, J., 90a
Hilbert, H., 57a
Hilkemeyer, R., 118b
Hill, H., 159b
Hill, L. L., 24b
Hill, M., 70b
Hill, N. J. W., 117a
Hill, R. D., 24b
Hill, R. J., 71a
Hill, S. G., 20b, 69a, 178a
Hilleboe, H. E., 22b
Hiller, R. B., 130b, 148b
Hilliam, I. E. O., 111a
Hillsman, G. M., 98a
Hilton, A., 48b
Hine, C. H., 123a, 126a, 159a
Hines, P. A., 32a
Hirschfeld, A. H., 123a
Hirskyj, L., 99a, 102b
Hlohinec, E. M., 175b
Hoare, B., 69a
Hobbs, P., 99a
Hockey, L., 57a, 150a, 151a, 155a, 172a
Hodges, B. E., 117a
Hodgkinson, E., 69a
Hodkinson, L. J., 104a, 163b
Hodkinson, M. A., 28b, 85a, 111a
Hodgson, R. W., 97b, 109a
Hoff, F. E., 120b
Hoffman, C. P., 82b
Hoffman, M. J., 71b
Hoggins, D. E., 141b
Hohloch, F. J., 99a
Holden, D. E., 146b
Holden, H. M., 159a
Holder, B. J., 100b, 123a
Holder, S., 54b, 179a
Holderness, M. C., 169a
Holdsworth, J. N., 41a, 51a
Holdsworth, V. E., 65a
Holgate, P. D., 123b
Holland, S., 28b
Holliday, C. B., 172a
Holliday, J., 8a, 57a
Hollingsworth, E. B., 13a
Holmes, M. C., 65a, 96b
Holmes, M. J., 137a, 143a
Holt, K. S., 107a, 133a
Holt, P. J. L., 114a, 160b
Holtgrewe, M. M., 117a
Hommel, F., 120b
Honey, M., 100b
Hong Kong, Nursing Board, 32a
Honig, A., 130b
Hood, K. A., 181b
Hooper, J., 32a
Hooper, R., 165a
Hope, T., 167a
Hopewell, J., 108b
Hopkin, D. A. B., 165a
Hopkin, I., 139b, 143a
Hopkins, J., 130b
Hopkins, S. J., 105a, 168a, 172a, 175b
Hopkins, T. D., 3a, 22b, 137a
Hopkins, V. L., 59b
Hornback, M., 30b, 49a, 49b
Horsley, S., 115b, 118b, 119a, 137a, 146b
Horsman, H. M., 28b
Horton Hospital, Epsom, 74a
Hospital, 21b, 49b, 69a
Hospital Administration in Canada, 70b
Hospital Centre. *See:* King Edward's Hospital Fund for London. Hospital Centre.
Hospital Computer Centre for London, 78b
Hospital Management, 46b
Hospital Management, Planning and Equipment, 69a
Hospital Topics, 80b
Hospital World, 8a, 14b
Hospitals and Charities Commission for Nursing Aide Training Schools in Victoria, 80b
Houghton, M., 12b, 47a, 65a, 165a
Houliston, M., 137a
Howard, A. L., 155a
Howard, F. M., 32a
Howard, L. S., 126a
Howard, M. I., 32a
Howarth, W., 174a
Howat, H. T., 108b
Howe, A., 76b
Howe, J., 3a
Howe, P. S., 170a
Howell, J. P., 78b
Howell, T. H., 111a
Howells, L., 105a
Howkins, J., 99a
Howland, D., 88a, 94a
Hoyt, D. P., 45b
Hubert, Sister M. (A. M. Reinkemeyer), 10b, 26b, 36a, 50a, 58a
Hubner, P. J. B., 101a
Hudak, C., 101b
Hudd, J., 165a
Huddersfield County Borough, 128b
Huddleston, R. G., 179b
Hudson, E., 105b
Hudson, F. P., 107b
Hudson, H. H., 33a, 146b, 148a, 149b
Hudson, W. R., 6a, 23a, 71a
Hueper, W. C., 99a
Huff, M., 48b
Huffman, V., 75b
Hughes, D. M., 70b
Hughes, E., 167a
Hughes, J. P. W., 123b, 158b
Hughes, P. E., 57a
Hughes, T. A., 167a
Hughes, W., 28b
Hugo, C. M., 150a
Hulbert, C., 142b
Hulicka, I. M., 57a, 111a
Hulicka, K., 57a
Hull, E. J., 47b, 48a, 65a
Hults, M. S., 136a
Humble, J. G., 182a
Hume, B., 24b, 105b
Humenik, P., 106b
Humphrey, A., 78b
Humphreys, F. I., 3b
Hunn, V. K., 100a, 101a
Hunt, D., 128b
Hunt, J. E., 159b
Hunt, L. W., 90a
Hunt, P. J., 105a
Hunt, V., 46b, 66a
Hunter, C. B., 158b
Hunter, D. A., 155b
Hunter, M. H. S., 131a
Hunter, P., 137a
Hunter, W., 126b
Huntly, W. L., 146b
Huntsman, R. G., 103a
Hurley, H. P., 170b
Hurr, W. A., 111a
Hurrell, G., 181b
Hurst, T. W., 90a
Hurt, R. L., 165a
Husband, P., 130b
Hutchings, M. T., 108b
Hutchins, J., 123b
Hutchins, N., 48a
Hutchinson, D. A., 155b
Hutton, G. A., 94a
Hutton, J. M., 51a
Hutty, H. E., 24b
Hyams, D. E., 111b
Hyde, L., 70b
Hyde, N., 137a
Hymovich, D. P., 46b, 130b, 172a

Iafolla, M. A. C., 32a
Illing, M., 43b, 82b, 146b, 154a
Illingworth, C., 99a, 102b, 103a, 168a
Illingworth, R. S., 130b
Illinois League for Nursing, 24b
Illinois Nurses' Association, 24b
Illinois Study Commission on Nursing, 24b
Index of Opportunity in the Nursing Profession, 40a
Indiana University. Bulletin of the School of Education, 53a
Indiana University Medical Center, 90a
Ingalls, A. J., 133b
Ingbar, M. L., 76b

Ingles, T., 15a, 61a, 65a, 66b, 81b
Inglis, D., 111b
Ingram, J. T., 70b, 104a
Innis, M. Q., 32a
Institute of Hospital Administrators, 69a
Institute of Hospital Matrons of New South Wales and Australian Capital Territory, 8b
Interagency Council on Library Tools for Nursing, 51a
International Committee of Catholic Nurses, 16b
International Committee of the Red Cross, 60a
International Council of Nurses, 8b, 12b, 16b, 17a, 17b, 19b, 20b, 32a
International Council of Nurses. Florence Nightingale International Foundation, 16b, 17b, 19b
International Digest of Health Legislation, 32b, 80b
International Labour Organisation. International Labour Office, 128a
International Nursing Index, 39b, 51a
International Nursing Review, 32b
International Red Cross, 2b
International School of Advanced Nursing Education, Lyon, 32b
International Wool Secretariat, 85a, 180b
Intersociety Committee on Noise Exposure Control, 123b
Ioric, J., 120b
Ipswich and District Enrolled Nurse Training School, 54b
Irish Nurses' Organisation, 17b
Irven, I. D., 150a
Irvine, E. D., 111b
Irvine, M. B., 70b, 92b, 167a
Irvine, R. E., 111b
Irwin, C., 12a
Irwin, J. E., 51a
Isaacs, B. J., 47b, 48a, 65a
Isberg, R. A., 73b
Isbister, C., 132a
Ishiyama, T., 70b
Isler, C., 80b
Isola-Williams, C. A., 32b
Israel. Ministry of Health. Nursing Unit, 8b
Iu, S., 20b, 32a

Jack, A., 137a
Jackson, B., 140a
Jackson, F. E., 165a
Jackson, H., 160b
Jackson, M. M., 81a
Jackson, Q. M., 130b
Jackson, R. J. A., 120b
Jacob, R. E., 14b
Jacobowsky, N., 30b
Jacobs, D., 8b
Jacobs, E. M., 119a
Jacobs, J., 28b
Jacobs, L. M., 137a
Jacobson, J., 169a
Jacobson, J. H., 171a
Jacobson, M. D., 32b
Jacobson, S., 137a
Jacoby, N. M., 157a
Jacot, M., 12b
Jacox, A. K., 65a
Jaeger, M. A., 130b
Jahoda, M., 8b, 17a, 57a
Jamaican Nurse, 13b, 24b, 32b, 146b
James, A. R., 32b
James, D. E., 24b, 25a, 42a, 144b, 167a
James, D. G., 172a
James, F. R., 182b
James, I., 90a
James, M. J., 126b
James, P., 40b, 56a
James, P. M. C., 103b
Jameson, E. E., 8b, 76b

Jamieson, L. N., 35b
Jamieson, S. R., 113b
Jamieson, W. M., 113b
Jamison, S., 172a
Jane, R., 80b
Jansen, P. W., 146b
Jarman, B. M., 128b
Jarrett, L., 15a, 16a
Jarvis, D., 165a
Jarvis, J. M., 46b
Jayachandran, V., 32b
Jayawardena, Y., 25a, 32b, 59b
Jefferiss, D., 120b
Jeffery, I. J., 61b
Jeffries, I. J., 59b
Jelinek, R. C., 75b
Jenkins, A. C., 88a
Jenkins, M. M., 129b, 167a, 168a
Jenkinson, V., 57a, 62b, 78b, 95a, 101a, 151a
Jennings, M., 8b
Jenny, M. R., 65a
Jensen, D. M., 63b, 64a, 76b, 83b, 174a
Jensen, F. T., 78b
Jensen, M., 170a
Jerman, B., 132a
Jeschke, D. B., 45a
Jessee, R., 74b, 97b
Jeu, F., 146b
Jodias, J., 80b
Joel, A. L., 65a
Johannson, B., 75b
John, A. L., 137a
Johns, L. A., 162a
Johns, M. P., 172a
Johnson, A., 167a
Johnson, B. A., 165a
Johnson, B. D., 169a
Johnson, B. S., 144a, 144b
Johnson, D. E., 8b, 53b, 57a, 70b, 77a
Johnson, D. R., 126b
Johnson, E. A., 81a
Johnson, H., 79a
Johnson, J., 137a
Johnson, J. E., 57b, 90a, 142b
Johnson, M. A., 144b
Johnson, M. L., 117a
Johnson, M. M., 50b, 65a
Johnson, R. L., 8b
Johnson, W. L., 146b
Johnston, D. F., 2b, 82b, 90a, 113b
Johnston, G. W., 105b
Johnston, M. D., 28b
Johnston, M. E., 44b
Johnston, R. N., 99a
Johnstone, T., 143a
Joiner, J. P., 99a
Joint Committee to Study Nursing Needs and Resources in Arizona, 25a
Joint Working Party on Group Attachment, 156a
Jolly, C. R., 179a
Jonathan, M., 15a
Jones, B., 101a
Jones, B. E., 123b
Jones, B. R., 172a
Jones, C., 25a
Jones, G. K., 102b
Jones, K., 25a, 159a
Jones, L., 137a
Jones, M., 67b, 135b, 137a
Jones, M. C., 157a
Jones, N., 82b
Jones, P. E., 15a, 155b
Jones, R. E., 25a
Jones, T. A., 32b
Jordaan, P., 168b
Jordan, C. H., 20b
Jordan, R. M., 144b
Jordon, M., 41a
Joseph, M., 101a, 134a
Joshi, J. B., 111b
Joslin, E. E., 133b
Joule, J. W., 114b
Jourard, S. M., 45a, 46b

Journal of Practical Nursing, 86b, 99a, 148b
Judd, E., 113b
Jugoo, A. R., 14a
Junel, I., 128a

Kahn, J. H., 117a
Kakosh, M. E., 32b, 94b
Kalafatich, A. J., 130b
Kalkman, M. E., 137a
Kallins, E. L., 146b
Kalwinski, H., 137b
Kamalamma, S., 159b
Kaminker, B., 179b
Kane, A. H., 152a
Kane, M., 42b
Kaneko, M., 32b
Kansas Health Facilities Information Service, Inc., 25a
Kapadia, G. P., 21a, 21b
Kapke, K. A., 133a
Kaplan, A., 120b
Karlin, M. McC., 137b
Karminsky, D., 97b
Karnicki, J., 103a
Karnosh, L. J., 137b
Karvonen, M. J., 158a
Katajamaki, M., 13b
Katona, E. A., 105b
Katz, F., 143a
Katzell, M. E., 40a
Kaufman, E. S., 44b
Kaufmann, M. A., 90a
Kaunda, B., 54b
Kay, E., 8b
Keane, C. B., 65a, 82b, 172a
Kear-Colwell, J. J., 62a
Kearns, B., 85a, 157a
Keating, L., 133a
Keen, H., 105a
Keidan, O., 25a
Keim, D., 32b
Kelber, M., 8b, 70b, 74b
Kelleher, W. H., 157a
Keller, M. J., 44b, 123b, 126b, 128a
Keller, N. S., 46b
Kelley, A. J., 152a
Kellie, G. A., 14a, 132a
Kellogg Foundation, 49b, 86b
Kelly, C. W., 8b
Kelly, D., 120b
Kelly, D. E., 60a
Kelly, D. N., 20a
Kelly, E. A., 104a
Kelly, J., 126b
Kelly, K. J., 2a
Kelly, R. L., 56b
Kelsey, F. D., 137b
Kemble, E. L., 70b
Kemp, E., 25a
Kemp, I. W., 152a
Kemp, R., 111b
Kempf, F. C., 57b, 144b
Kempsill, C. D., 114a
Kendall, J. S., 115a
Kendall, K. K., 53b
Kenna, F. R., 172a
Kennedy, E. A., 151a
Kennedy, E. M., 150a
Kennedy, I. M., 13a
Kennedy, M., 137b
Kennedy, M. J., 90a
Kenneth, H. Y., 43b
Kenny, E., 4a
Kerchner, L., 147a
Kergin, D., 32b, 80b
Kernicki, J., 101a
Kerr, A., 163a
Kerr, M. E., 15a
Kessel, I., 130b
Kettle, E. S., 1b, 146b
Keveren, R. H., 48b
Kevill, G. A., 133a
Keyloun, V., 100b
Keysell, P., 106b

Keywood, O., 151a
Khan, M. P., 32b
Khoury, Y. G., 14a
Kibble, M. R., 14b
Kibrick, A. K., 25a
Kidd, D. E., 48a
Kidd, H. B., 137b
Kilander, V. C., 135b
Kilgour, O. F. G., 134b
Killam, L., 70b
Killby, M., 16b
Killen, B., 62b
Kilourie, C. W., 95a
Kim, H. T., 41a
Kimball, C. P., 160b
Kimball, L., 137b
Kimber, D. C., 96b
Kimber, P. M., 119a
King, C., 40a
King, E. S., 62b
King, H. M., 44b
King, I. M., 8b
King, J. M., 61a
King, J. S., 156b
King, M. J., 167a
King, M. P., 13b
King, P. E., 32b
King, V. M., 80b, 150a, 154b
King Edward's Hospital Fund for London, 25a, 59b, 69b, 70b
King Edward's Hospital Fund for London. Hospital Centre, 21b, 25a, 44b, 48a, 51a, 78b, 79b, 86b, 88a, 108b, 111b, 128b, 130b, 150a, 158b, 159a, 177a, 178a, 178b, 179a, 179b, 180a, 180b
King Edward's Hospital Fund for London. Nursing Recruitment Service, 35a
Kingsbury, V., 14b
Kingston Public Hospital, Jamaica, 32b, 181b
Kinnaird, L. S., 114a
Kinoy, S. K., 111b
Kinsella, C., 48b
Kinsinger, R. E., 48b
Kinsler, D., 137b
Kirk, G. M., 86b
Kirkham, I. L., 82b
Kirkpatrick, W. J., 61a, 137b, 143a
Kirkwood, E. C., 160b
Kirman, B., 107b, 117a
Kirwin, W. B., 42a
Kisseih, D. A. N., 12b
Kitchell, J. R., 86b, 101a
Kitchin, C. H., 178a
Kitzes, G., 105b
Kitzinger, S., 121a
Klachan, J., 137b
Klahn, J. E., 32b
Klaiman, R. R., 48a
Kleffner, F. R., 174a
Klein, M. A., 111b
Klein, M. K., 106a
Klein, M. W., 75a
Klocke, J. M., 103b
Klonoff, H., 32b
Klopper, A., 121a
Klugman, H. B., 111b, 170a
Klutas, E. M., 128a
Knabe, H., 126b
Knight, G., 115b, 160b
Knight, J., 78b
Knight, J. E., 25a, 178a
Knight, K. L., 123b
Knight, M. C., 128b
Knight, R. K., 157b
Knopf, L., 38a, 45a, 82b, 146b
Knowles, L. N., 51a
Knowles, M. S., 32b, 70b
Knox, S. J., 144a
Knudsen, E. T., 172a
Knudson, E. G., 40a, 147a
Koch, H. B., 65a
Koch, L., 137b
Koch, M. J., 83b

Koehler, M. J., 29a
Koehler, M. L., 48a
Koehler, V. J., 97b
Koinange, M. W., 12b
Kolthoff, N. J., 56b
Komorita, N. I., 60a
Kona, W., 51a
Korkis, F. B., 106b
Kornfeld, D. S., 86b
Kos, B. A., 101a
Kossoris, P., 108b
Kotlarsky, C., 148b
Kovacs, M., 46b
Kozier, B. B., 85a
Kramer, H., 157b
Kramer, J. R., 64a
Kramer, M., 8b, 62b, 65b
Kratter, F., 115b, 170b
Krenzel, J. R., 119a
Kretzer, M. L., 4b
Kriegel, J., 70b, 178a
Krister, J., 147a
Kron, T., 74b, 95a
Krueger, E. A., 48a
Krug, E., 172b
Kruger, D. G., 123b
Kruger, D. H., 20b
Kruse, M., 8b, 20b
Kucha, D. H., 70b
Kuchinsky, S., 51a
Kuenssberg, E. V., 155b
Kuhli, R., 126b
Kuhn, B. G., 33a, 77b
Kumagai, T., 82b
Kumar, B., 19b
Kupka, M. E., 137b
Kursteiner, P., 147a
Kurtz, R. A., 8b, 76a
Kushlick, A., 116b, 117a
Kuzucu, E. Y., 121a

Laeger, E., 75a
Lafave, H. G., 60b
La Flair, E. I., 48b
Laing, J. E., 162a
Lam, S. J., 163a
Lamb, A. M., 149a, 151a, 155b
Lamb, D. E., 111b
Lamb, D. W., 163a
Lamb, M., 70b
Lamb, M. C. N., 8b, 33a
Lambert, E. E., 128a
Lambert, K., 96b
Lamberton, C. J., 162a
Lambertsen, E. C., 8b, 9a, 25a, 25b, 33a, 41b, 46b, 57b, 59b, 61a, 65a, 70b, 71a, 75b, 78b, 86b, 90a, 94a, 144b
Lambrechts, W., 157a
Lamont, A. M., 33a
Lamont, D. J., 152a
The Lamp, 25b
Lancaster, A., 9a
Lancaster Moor Hospital, 181b
Lancet, 19b, 20b, 69a, 152a
Landauer, S., 13b
Landdeck, J. R., 94a
Lande, S., 40a
Landesberg, A., 137b
Lane, C., 101a
Lang, P. A., 80b
Langan, E., 165a
Langdon, L. M., 82b
Lange, B., 60a
Lange, C. M., 33a
Langhoff, H., 48b
Langley, L. L., 96b
Langton, B. M., 152a
Lantz, U., 144b
Lapping, A., 33a
Large, H., 101a
Largey, L. B., 160b
Larson, C. B., 163a
Larson, D., 162a
Larson, K. H., 85a, 90a, 143a

Larson, L. G., 71a
Larson, R., 137b
Lassers, B. W., 101a
Latham, H. C., 130b
Laurence, K. M., 133a
Laurie, M., 25b
Lawes, T., 140b
Lawn Hospital, 181b
Lawrence, J. G., 25b
Lawrence, R. D., 105a
Lawrie, R., 132b
Lawson, A. A. H., 115a
Lawson, D., 132b
Lawson, J. S., 25b
Lawson, M. G., 9a
Lawson, W. G. A., 137b
Lawton, U., 25b
Laycock, J., 128b
Layton, M. M., 46b
Leabeater, B., 138a
League of Red Cross Societies, 2b, 3a
Leahy, K. M., 147a
Leathart, G. L., 123b
Leavell, L. C., 96b
Leche, P., 119b
Ledingham, I. McA., 171a
Lee, A. S., 57b
Lee, C.M., 12a, 80b, 130b
Lee, D. M., 126b
Lee, E., 49b
Lee, J. A., 126b
Lee, J. M., 182b
Lee, R. M., 65a
Lee, W. R., 123b
Leeds General Infirmary, 181b
Leeds Regional Hospital Board, 78b
Lees, W., 92b
Lefave, H., 139a
Lefkowitz, A. S., 33a
Legault, J.-P., 108b
Lehmann, H., 103a
Lehr, L. W., 180b
Leib, E., 137b
Leicester Royal Infirmary, 78b, 179a
Leideritz, A. F., 33a
Leifer, G., 130b
Leininger, M., 33a, 57b, 65a, 137b
Leino, A., 40b
Leisten, D. P., 119a
Leitch, A., 137b
Leite-Ribeiro, M. O., 137a
LeMaitre, G. D., 165a
Lemin, B., 71a, 152b, 167a
Leminen, A., 9a
Lenburg, C., 87b
Lentz, E. M., 57b
Leonard, M., 105b
Leonard, R. C., 56a, 57b, 61b, 66b, 92a
Leone, L. P., 15a, 65b
Leonetti, A. N., 40a
Leopoldt, H., 137b, 138a, 142a, 174a
Lerch, C., 113b, 121a
Leslie, E. A., 117a
Lesnik, M. J., 19b
Lesparre, M., 25b
Lester, B. A., 48b
Lester, M. R., 146b
Lethi, Y., 9a
Letourneau, C. U., 59b, 62b, 71a, 180a
Leung, J. S. M., 165a
Leva, I., 42b
Leventhal, B., 71b
Levey, A. L., 97b
Levine, D. C., 165a
Levine, E., 25b, 33a, 55a, 78b, 88a, 97b
Levine, H., 65a, 171b
Levine, M. E., 4b, 9a, 65b, 90a, 172b
Levine, S., 89a
Levison, H., 103b
Levitt, E. E., 9a, 99a
Levy, A. H., 131a
Levy, J. M., 146b
Lew, Y., 33a
Lewis, B. J., 172b
Lewis, E. M., 4a
Lewis, E. P., 20b, 33a, 39a, 81a

Lewis, G. K., 61a, 143a
Lewis, I. C., 147a
Lewis, R. V., 115b
Lewis, T. D., 155b
Ley, P., 90a
Leyshon, G. E., 108b
Leyshon, V. N., 113b
Librach, I. M., 167a
Library Association, 51a
Liddell, D., 119a
Liley, A. W., 158a
Lin, P. M., 162a
Lindabury, V. A., 13b
Lindars, M. E., 149a, 151a
Lindberg, H. G., 154a
Lindeman, C. A., 42b, 57b
Linden, K., 48a
Lindquist, N. E., 79b
Lindsay, A., 133a
Lindsay, D. W., 154a
Lindsey, E. M., 152b
Lindsey, M., 9a
Lines, M. B., 152b
Linsky, A. S., 71a
Linville, C. H., 71a
Lipkin, G. B., 82b
Lippitt, G. L., 60a, 71a
Lipsey, S. I., 97b
Lisboa, J., 104a
Lister, D. W., 46b
Litin, E. M., 161a
Little, D., 174b
Little, D. E., 32a, 56a, 61a, 71a, 81b, 85a, 175b
Little, K., 159b
Livengood, L., 78b
Liverpool Royal Infirmary, 54b
Livesey, A., 28b
Llewellyn, E. M., 43b
Llewellyn-Jones, J. D., 33a
Lloyd, J. W., 160b
Lloyd, W. A., 12a, 69a, 69b, 142a
Lloyd, W. H., 111b
Lloyd-Davies, R. W., 108b
Lo Cascio, R., 145a
Lochore, M. S., 42b
Lock, J., 4a
Locke, J. T., 69b
Lockerby, F. K., 74b
Lockett, J., 117a
Lockhart, P., 174b
Loftin, E., 101a
Logan, D. L., 143a
Logan, W. W., 39a, 45b, 53b
London, P. S., 115a, 162a
London Hospital, 21b, 181b
Long, L., 33a
Long, S. E., 65b
Loomis, M. E., 90a, 138a
Lorber, J., 133a
Lord, A., 154a
Lord, W. J. H., 155b
Lore, A., 131a
Lorig, K. R., 9a
Los Angeles County General Hospital Coronary Care Unit, 61a
Loudon, N., 159b
Loughlin, B. W., 154a
Loughlin, T. M., 51b, 143a
Louise, Sister M., 165a
Love, R. J., McN., 160a
Loveland, M. K., 152a
Lovell, H., 3a
Low, M., 82b
Lowbury, E. J. L., 167a
Lowe, A., 53a
Lowe, M. L., 57b
Lowe, S., 59b, 61b
Lowery, M., 162a
Lowry, M. F., 163a
Lowry, M. V., 94a
Lowthian, P. T., 85a
Loy, L., 27a
Lucas, B. G. B., 169a
Luck, G. M., 71a
Luck, M., 160b

Luckman, J., 77a, 79b
Ludemann, R. S., 90b
Ludman, H., 106b
Ludwig, D. J., 78b
Lukens, L. G., 9a, 25b
Lum, J. L. J., 41a, 61a
Lunde, D. T., 168b
Lundgaard, M. J., 169b
Lundstrom, P., 121a
Lundy, J. S., 169b
Lunn, A. G. M., 174b
Lunn, J. E., 155b, 156b
Lunt, J., 90b, 151a
Luntz, G. R. W. N., 175b
Luschinsky, L., 121a
Luty, E., 1b
Lyle, M. R., 28b
Lyman, K., 33a
Lynch, M. D., 162a
Lynn, D. H., 75b
Lyon, G. G., 138a
Lyon, W. M., 151a
Lyons, B., 33a
Lyons, T. F., 25b, 78b
Lysaught, J. P., 47b

Maas, R. B., 123b
Maass, C., 4a
Macara, A. W., 150a
MacArthur, C. H., 138a
Macaulay, D., 138a
Macaw, K. D., 171b
Macbeth, R., 157b
McBride, M. A., 65b
McBrien, M., 138a
McCabe, Sister M. C., 51b
McCaffery, M., 46b
McCain, R. F., 65b
McCall, J., 111b
McCall, M. B., 28b
McCallister, J., 105b
McCallum, R. I., 123b
McCann, J. K., 123b
McCarrick, H., 25b, 54b, 84a, 86b, 163a
McCarthy, M., 173b
McCartney, R. A., 79a
McCatty, B. E., 123b
McCauley, J. M., 106b
McCauley, S., 126b
McClain, M. E., 97b
McClelland, R. M. A., 157b
McClure, L. M., 156a
McClure, M. J., 132b
McCluskey, J. A., 33a
McCormack, R. C., 147a
McCormick, W., 178a
McCullough, L., 156b
McCutcheon, M. I., 65b, 92b, 93a
McDermott, R., 159a
McDevitt, B. A., 60b
McDonagh, V. P., 154b
Macdonald, A., 104a
MacDonald, E. M., 132b
Macdonald, F. G., 90b
McDonald, F. J., 41a, 46a
Macdonald, G., 40b, 53b
MacDonald, J., 108b
Macdonald, R., 33b
Macdonald, R. R., 121a
Macdonald, S., 96a
Macdonell, J. A. K., 75b
MacDonnell, F., 4b
MacDougall, I. A., 156a
McDowell, W. E., 94a
McEwan, M., 152b
McEwan, R., 25b, 29a
McFadden, G. M., 80a
McFarland, B., 163b
McFarlane, J. K., 33b, 94a
McGee, J. E., 86b
McGhee, A., 90b
McGhie, A., 144b
Macginniss, O., 107b
McGinty, P., 74b

McGlothlin, W. J., 9a
McGovern, J. P., 123a
McGrath, M. E., 165b
McGregor, A., 155b
Macgregor, F. C., 9a, 57b
McGregor, G., 79a, 25b
McGregor, I. A., 168b
McGuigan, H. A., 172b
McGuiness, A. F., 31a, 77a, 138a, 143a
McGuinness, J. P., 159a
McGuire, J., 9a, 25b, 33b, 35b, 41b, 116a
Maguire, R. E., 153b
Mach, E., 80a
Machen, W. V., 71a
McHenry, R. W., 126b
Machey, D., 71a
Machin, D., 69b
McHugh, N., 85a
McIlwraith, P. L., 109b
MacInnes, D., 138a
McInnes, E. M., 4b, 5b, 182a
McIntosh, D. M., 33b
McIntyre, H. M., 81b
McIntyre, M. C., 86b
Mcintyre, P. H., 173b
MacIver, A. A., 36b
Mciver, H., 9a
McKay, J., 25b, 104a
McKay, R., 9a, 33b
McKee, G. K., 163a
MacKeith, R., 90b
McKelvie, P., 99a
McKenemy, A., 33b
MacKenna, R. M. B., 104a
McKenzie, B., 119a
McKenzie, F. L., 48a, 49a, 101a
McKenzie, H., 33b, 94a
Mackenzie, M., 77a
Mackenzie, M. D., 66a
Mackenzie, N., 9a
McKenzie, W., 106b, 160a
McKeown, D., 80b
McKevitt, R., 116a, 156b
McKibbin, B., 163a
Mackie, E. J., 8b, 76b
McKilligin, H. R., 134a
Mackintosh, E. M., 14b
McKnew, D. H., 44b
McKnight, E. T., 144b
Mackworth, J., 116a
McLachlan, G., 38b, 56a, 59a, 89a, 90a, 93a
Maclaggan, K., 9a, 33b
McLain, Sister M. A., 33b
Mclaren, C. G., 85a
McLaren, R., 103b, 110a, 112a
Mclaughlin, A. I. G., 123b
McLaughlin, H., 71a, 180a
McLaughlin, L., 105a
McLean, C. D., 54b
Maclean, D. M., 168b
McLean, M. D., 65b, 73b
McLemore, S. D., 71a
Maclennan, W. D., 162a
MacLeod, A. I., 9a
Macleod, E. B., 3a
MacLeod, H. M., 152b
McLeod, I., 33b
Macleod, V., 75b, 78b
Macleod, W. G., 138a
McLoughlin, M. J., 101a
McManus, R. L., 57b
McMillan, E. B. B., 152b
McMillan, I. K. R., 160b
McNabola, E. K. A., 155b
McNair, E., 71a
McNaught, A. B., 96b
Macnaughton, M. C., 121a
McNaughton, N., 126b
McNeil, H. J., 149a
McNicholas, E. L., 71a
McNicholls, J., 174b
McNulty, B., 90b
Macphail, A. N., 151b, 154b
MacPhail, J., 10b, 26b

McPhetridge, M., 42b
MacQueen, I. A. G., 152a, 152b, 158a
McQueen, R. J., 61a
McQuillen, F. A., 169b
Macrae, A. K., 178a
MacRae, I., 114a
McVey, F. A., 152a
Macvicar, J., 173b
McWalters, B. H., 90b
McWee, A. C., 53b
McWilliams, W., 138a
Maddison, D., 90b, 138a
Madland, L., 61a
Madsen, I. M., 178a
Maegraith, B. G., 115a
Magherafelt Hospital, Ulster, 93a
Maginn, R. R., 168b
Maguire, J. M., 167b, 168b
Mahar, I. R., 149a
Mahoney, A. B., 20b
Mahoney, R. F., 95b
Maillé, P., 178a
Maingot, R., 105b
Mair, J., 119a
Major, D. M., 9b, 33b, 40a, 46b, 57b
Major, K., 60a, 152b
Makhwade, K. M. I., 33b
Malaspina, H., 45b, 71a
Malcolm, M., 123b
Malcomson, K. G., 157b
Malkin, S. A. S., 9b
Mallon, M., 4b
Mallory, E., 61b
Malmi Hospital, Helsinki, 21b
Malone, M. F., 9b, 25b, 57b, 62a, 75a
Maloney, E., 138a
Malpas, J. S., 103a
M.A.M.E., 1b
Manaser, J. C., 61b
Manchester Area Nurse Training Committee, 33b
Manchester District Nursing Service, 2b
Manchester Regional Hospital Board, 51b
Manchester University, 49b
Mandin, J., 33b
Manfreda, M. L., 138a, 143a
Mangan, H. M., 65b
Manly, R., 14b
Mann, F. C., 89b, 93b
Mann, T. P., 130b, 134a
Mann, T. S., 162a
Manning, M., 117a
Mannino, S. F., 12a
Manoharan, A., 22b
Mansbridge, I., 155b
Mansfield General Hospital, 51b
Manthey, M., 65b
Marais, J., 12a
Marchesini, E. H., 71a
Marcus, A. M., 32b, 61b
Marcus, C. M., 108b
Marie, 1b
Marie Curie Memorial Foundation, 99a
Marino, B., 101a
Markham, J., 34a, 64b, 65b, 106a
Marks, A. E., 171a
Marks, F., 79a
Marlow, D. R., 131a
Marlow, H. L., 26a, 71b
Marmor, S., 102b
Marquand, C. J., 90b
Marram, G. D., 9b, 26a, 138a
Marrow, N., 169b
Marsden, J., 149a
Marsh, D. C., 26a
Marsh, G. N., 155b
Marsh, G. V., 43b
Marsh, N., 49b
Marsh, V. W., 180b
Marshall, D. G., 21b
Marshall, E. H., 152b
Marshall, J., 103a, 119a
Marshall, M. A., 135a

Marshall, M. J., 26a, 34a
Marshall, S., 97b, 107a
Marson, S. N., 34a, 48a
Martin, A. B., 39a
Martin, A. J., 168b
Martin, C. H., 142b
Martin, D., 144b
Martin, D. V., 138a
Martin, H. W., 61b
Martin, J., 62b
Martin, J. L., 82b
Martin, J. R., 34a
Martin, M., 79a, 101a, 138a
Martin, M. A., 119a, 165b
Martin, N., 174b
Martin, R. G., 82b
Martina, P., 37a
Marvin, J. T., 7a
Marwick, I., 138a, 143a
Mary Blaise, Sister, 62b
Mary Donald, Sister, 71b
Mary Elena of the Cross, 61b
Mary Paulina, Sister, 9b, 13a
Mary Suzanne, Sister, 71b
Mason, E. M., 152b
Mason, R., 60a, 129b, 152b
Matheney, R. V., 9b, 34a, 45b, 65b, 90b, 138a
Mather, H. G., 100a, 101a
Matheson, J. G., 171a
Mathew, G., 71b
Mathews, B. P., 57b
Mathews, R. C., 13a
Mathieson, J. B., 9b
Matic, V., 132b
Matsunage, G., 116a, 156b
Matteoli, R., 142a
Matthews, F., 154a
Matthews, J., 101a
Matthews, W. B., 114a
Matthias, A. M., 62b, 165b
Maudsley, R. H., 171a
Mauksch, H. O., 65b, 71b, 90b
Mauksch, I. G., 182b
Maule, H. G., 174b
Maureen, Sister, 90b
Mawson, S., 107a
Maxwell, R. M., 34a, 53b
May, A. R., 116a, 138a
May, L., 152b
May, P. R. A., 90b
May, R. E., 106a
May, W. T., 128a
Mayes, M. E., 80a
Mayes, N., 26a
Mayston, E. L., 148b
Mayuga, P. N., 147a
Mazzarella, M. C., 150a
Mead, B. P., 13a
Meade, D. M., 180b
Meadow, L., 83a
Mearns, A. G., 19b
Mechner, F., 48a
Medical College of Georgia, 68a
Medical Defence Union, 85a
Medical Officer, 152b
A Medical Officer of Health, pseud., 155b
Medical Practitioners' Union, 20b
Medical World Newsletter, 20b
Meehan, A. R., 162a
Meere, C., 160a
Meiklejohn, A., 126b
Meilicke, C. A., 71b
Meinhart, N. T., 85a
Melbin, M., 26a
Meldman, M. J., 116a
Mele, F. M., 27a
Mellings, M., 167b
Mellor, V., 137b
Mellow, J., 138b
Melnick, W., 124a
Melnyk, E., 104a
Melton, B. L., 181b
Meltzer, L. E., 86b, 101a
Melvin, J., 28b

Memorial Hospital for Cancer and Allied Diseases. Nursing Division, 99b, 165b, 173b
Mencel, Z., 154a
Mental Health Tutors Association, 53b, 143a
Menzies, I. E. P., 62b, 74b
Mercadante, L., 34a, 77a, 79a, 90b
Mercy Hospital, Pittsburgh, 95a
Mereness, D., 9b, 57b, 137b, 138b, 174a
Merivale, R. F., 144b
Merkel, R., 101a, 101b, 170a
Merry, J., 159a
Merskey, H., 138b
Merton, R. K., 9b, 15a, 62b
Mertz, H., 90b
Mesolella, D. W., 62b
Message, M. C., 73a
Metcalfe, J. T., 108b
Metheny, N. M., 96b
Metson, B. H., 117a
Metz, E. A., 45a, 56b
Metzner, C. A., 94b
Meurer, M. C., 99b
Meyer, B., 57b, 85a
Meyer, G. R., 71b
Meyer, H. L., 132b
Meyer, M. A., 26a
Meyer, P. F., 103a
Meyer, R. G., 119a
Meyer, R. H., 9b
Meyer, S. W., 165b
Meyers, M. E., 9b
Meyric-Hughes, J., 110b
Mezer, R. R., 138b
Mezzanotte, E. J., 165b
Michael, M. G., 164a
Michaels, R. G., 57b
Michaelson, M., 71b
Michell, B., 111b
Michelson, A., 133b
Michie, W., 160b
Michigan League for Nursing, 26a
Michigan Nurses' Association, 26a
Middleton, A. B., 138b
Middleton, B. M., 90b
Middleton, M. D., 160b
Midwives Chronicle and Nursing Notes, 69b
Mile End Hospital, London, 51b
Miles, B., 65b, 84a, 129b
Millard, R., 34a
Miller, A., 61b, 160b
Miller, B. E., 119b
Miller, C. L., 45a
Miller, D. I., 68a, 77a
Miller, D. M., 53b
Miller, H. J. B., 138b
Miller, I. C., 157b
Miller, J., 165b
Miller, J. M., 34a
Miller, M. A., 43a
Miller, N. F., 113b
Miller, S. J., 79a
Milliott, H. L., 29a
Mills, E. W., 4b
Millward, R. C., 69b
Milne, J., 84b
Milner, F. H., 96a
Mims, F. H., 45b
Minckley, B. B., 57b, 58a, 86b, 90b, 94a, 162b, 165b, 169b
Ministry of Health. See: Great Britain. Ministry of Health
Ministry of Labour. See: Great Britain. Ministry of Labour
Mink, G., 51b
Minnesota Board of Nursing, 26a
Minney, R. J., 181a
Minski, L., 138b
Mirenda, R., 170a
Mitchel, M., 26a
Mitchell, H. E., 62b
Mitchell, J., 111b
Mitchell, J. P., 108b

Mitchell, M., 17a, 74b
Mitchell, M. Le Q., 87a
Mizer, H. E., 98a, 159b
Mobbs, J., 131a
Mockett, M., 83a
Modell, W., 101b
Modern Hospital, 86b, 91a
Mok, A. L., 9b
Molbo, D. M., 113a
Moloney, Sister M. M., 14a
Monaghan, J. R., 34a
Monaghan, M. A., 51b
Moncrieff, A., 107b
Moncrieff, M. J., 163a
Moncur, S. D., 163a
Montag, M. L., 34a, 37a, 39a, 49b, 53b, 79a
Montford, A. A. W., 107b
Moon, W. R., 91a
Moore, B., 165b, 168a
Moore, J. S., 91a
Moore, L., 46b, 144b
Moore, L. F., 77a
Moore, M., 158b
Moore, M. A., 45b, 65b
Moore, S., 116a
Moore, W. K. S., 124a
Mooth, A. E., 71b
Moran, A., 165b
Moran, L. P., 83b
Morant, P. E., 124a
Moravec, D. F., 172b
Mordan, M. J., 64a
Mordaunt, V. L., 107b
Morgan, B., 26a
Morgan, B. D., 132b
Morgan, E. M., 93b
Morgan, G. A., 119a
Morgan, H., 93a
Morgan, W. F., 34a
Morison, L. J., 145a
Moritz, D. A., 45b
Morley, A., 86b
Morley, G. H., 168b
Morley, W. E., 143b
Morman, R. R., 45b
Moroney, J., 160b
Morpurgo, J. E., 51b
Morrice, J. K. W., 138b
Morris, D. G., 101b
Morris, I. H., 150a
Morris, J. E., 9b
Morris, M., 58a, 149a
Morris, M. L., 142b
Morris, P. A., 138b
Morris, R. P., 165b
Morris, W. M., 138b
Morrison, A. A., 1a
Morrison, A. W., 107a
Morriston-Davies, M., 162b
Morse, R. M., 161a
Morten, H., 41a
Mortensen, J. D., 100a
Mortimer, K., 86b, 87a
Morton, K., 51b
Morton, L. T., 51b
Morton, P., 43b, 49b
Morton, R. S., 176b
Morton-Mason, S. R., 143a
Mosby, C. V. & Co., 9b, 83a
Moser, D., 119b
Moser, D. H., 34a
Moses, D., 170a
Moses, D. V., 24a
Moses, E. B., 20b
Moss, B. J. L., 116a
Moss, F. T., 85a
Moss, H. J. L., 69b
Mottram, E. M., 155b, 156a
Moulson, F., 143a
Moulton, D. P., 147a
Mountford, P. A., 180a
Mountford, S. W., 174b
Mountjoy, P., 85a
Mousley, J. S., 165b
Mowry, L., 170a

Moynahan, E. J., 104a
Muecke, M. A., 91a, 143a
Muhs, E. J., 43a
Muir, M., 12b
Muirhead, I. E., 161a
Mullane, M. K., 34a
Mullard, K., 161a
Mullen, C., 137a
Muller, H. M., 61b
Muller, T. G., 46b
Mumby, D. M., 155b
Mumford, D., 152b
Mumford, E., 12a, 65b
Munck, H., 20b
Munday, L., 45b
Mungovan, R., 138b
Munro, A., 138b
Munro, D. D., 104a
Munro, L. B., 124a
Munro-Ashman, D., 22b, 104a
Munson, A. H., 51b
Muntz, J., 74b
Murdaugh, J., 147a
Murison, J., 117a
Murphree, H. B., 172b
Murphy, A. J., 124a
Murphy, C., 66b
Murphy, D. C., 126b
Murphy, J. F., 9b
Murray, A. V., 120b
Murray, I., 182a
Murray, J. B., 65b
Murray, M., 117a
Murray, R., 138b
Murray, V. P., 58a, 95b
Murrie, E., 163b
Musoke, A. S. B., 12b
Mussallem, H. K., 13b, 30a, 34a, 58a, 71b, 79a
Myers, E. N., 174b
Myers, R. S., 94a
Myles, E. L., 13a

Nadarajah, I., 181a
Nadel, L., 126b
Nadler, G., 94a
Naegele, K. D., 6b, 30a, 34a
Nagano, S., 14a
Nagele, M. F., 34b
Nahm, H., 9b, 10a, 27a, 34b, 53b
Nahmias, A. J., 168a
Naiman, H. L., 1a
Nairn, M., 114a, 152b
Naish, B., 162b
Nance, J. L., 45b
Napke, E., 172b
Nash, D. F. E., 165b
Nash, M. K., 26a
Nassen, A., 109a
Nast, M., 97b, 172b
Nation, M. B., 152b
National Association for Mental Health, 117a, 141b
National Association for Practical Nurse Education and Service, 98a
National Association for the Welfare of Children in Hospital, 132b
National Association of Chief and Principal Nursing Officers, 138b
National Association of Chief Male Nurses, 138b
National Association of Hospital Management Committee Group Secretaries, 69b
National Association of State Enrolled Nurses, 16b, 17b, 20b, 83a, 147a
National Association of Theatre Nurses, 17b
National Association of Theatre Nurses. West Riding Branch, 165b
National Board for Prices and Incomes, 20b, 21a
National Commission on Accrediting, 40b

National Federation of Licensed Practical Nurses, 60b, 81b, 83a, 95b
National Florence Nightingale Committee of Australia, 19b, 26b
National League for Nursing, 10a, 17b, 18a, 29a, 34b, 35a, 41b, 42a, 51b, 53b, 77a, 91a, 94a, 95b, 131a, 147a, 175b
National League for Nursing. Committee on Careers, 34b
National League for Nursing. Committee on Quality of Organized Nursing Service in Hospital. 65b
National League for Nursing. Department of Baccalaureate and Higher Degree Programs, 40b, 53b
National League for Nursing. Department of Diploma and Associate Degree Programs, 39a, 41b, 51b
National League for Nursing. Dept. of of Hospital Nursing, 66a, 77a, 94a
National League for Nursing. Department of Public Health Nursing, 149a
National League for Nursing. Division of Nursing Education, 51b
National League for Nursing. Interdivisional Council on Occupational Health Nursing, 128a
National League for Nursing. Measurement and Evaluation Services, 26a
National League for Nursing. Research and Studies Service, 34b, 35a, 54a, 54b, 79a, 174b
National Nurses' Association of the Netherlands, 111b
National Nursing Staff Committee. See: Great Britain. Department of Health and Social Security
National Society for Mentally Handicapped Children, 117a
National Tuberculosis Association. Nursing Advisory Service on Tuberculosis and other Respiratory Diseases, 175b
National Union of Public Employees, 26a
Nauen, C. M., 134a
Naylor, A., 163a
Naylor, P. N., 46b
Neal, M. V., 95b, 134a
Needham, R. C., 46b
Needle, A., 150b
Neelon, V. J., 171a
Nehren, J. G., 61b, 62b
Neill, G., 4b
Neill, J. O. C., 4b
Nelson, A. C., 131a
Nelson, E. M., 43a
Nelson, K. R., 91a
Nelson, M. M., 121a
Nelson, R., 2a
Nelson, S. L., 98a
Nemir, A., 156b
Nesbitt, L., 109a
Nether Edge Hospital, Sheffield, 22a
Nett, L. M., 157b
Neville, R., 111b, 139a
Newcastle General Hospital, 181b
Newcastle Regional Hospital Board. Cherry Knowle Hospital Management Committee, 79a
Newcomb, P., 103a
Newcombe, J., 163a
New England Council on Higher Education for Nursing, 35a
Newhouse, M. L., 104a
Newington, D. K., 152b
Newland, R. A., 66a
Newman, J. L., 109a
Newnham, W. H., 170b
New Plymouth Public Hospital, New Zealand, 181b
Newsom, B. H., 91a
New Southgate Hospital Management Committee, 26a

215

New South Wales. Hospitals Commission of New South Wales. Committee of Inquiry to Study Education of Nurses in New South Wales, 35a
New South Wales College of Nursing, 6b, 8a
Newton, E. J., 119a
Newton, K., 112a
Newton, M. E., 58a
Newton, N., 133b
New York State Nurses Association, 35a
New York State University. State Education Department, 26a, 39a, 49b
New York State University. State Education Department. Division of of Professional Education, 76a
New Zealand. Department of Health. Operational Research Unit, 61b, 131a
New Zealand. Department of Health. Research and Planning Unit, 61b, 111b, 163a, 165b
New Zealand Nurses' Association, 49b
New Zealand Nursing Journal, 20b, 85a, 139a
New Zealand Red Cross Society, 3a
New Zealand Registered Nurses' Association, 18a, 21a
New Zealand. Special Committee of Cabinet, 21
New Zealand Wool Board, 85b
Nicholls, M. E., 35a
Nichols, G. A., 35a
Nicholson, B. M., 80b
Nicolas, B., 10a
Nicoll, K. B., 114a, 163b
Nicoll, S., 174a
Nightingale, C. H., 172b
Nightingale, F., 1a, 4a, 4b
Nightingale Training School, London, 37a
Niles, A. McK., 51b
Nilo, E. R., 124a
Nishikawa, H. A., 66b
Nite, G., 101b
Nobbs, K. L. G., 112a
Noble, E., 128a
Noble, I., 4a
Noble, M., 10a, 74b
Noble, M. A., 117b
Nolan, B., 168b
Nolan, B. T., 90b
Nordmark, M. T., 66a
Norman, A. P., 157b
Norman, M. R., 171b
Norris, C. M., 10a, 61b, 66a, 71b, 139a, 169b
North, N., 24b
North Dakota Nutrition & Diabetes Workshop, 105a
North East Metropolitan Regional Hospital Board. Work Study Unit, 86b, 87a
North Eastern Regional Hospital Board, 79a
North Eastern Regional Hospital Board. Work Study Department, 71b
Northern Ireland. Parliament, 19a
Northern Ireland Hospitals Authority, 10a, 35a
Northern Nurses' Federation, 21a, 58a
Northwick Park Hospital, 180a
Norton, D., 58a, 85b, 112a, 180b, 182b
Norwood, R., 26a
Notman, A. G., 35a, 42a
Notter, L., 58a, 63a, 76a
Nuki, G., 114a
Nurses' Christian Movement, 145a
Nursing Clinics of North America, 61b, 71b, 91a, 101b, 107a, 131a, 162b, 167b
Nursing Education Through Multi-Sensory Approaches, 48a
Nursing Forum, 44b
Nursing Journal of India, 3b, 35a, 40a, 95b

Nursing Mirror, 18b, 19b, 35a, 66a, 69b, 71b, 83a, 91a, 95b, 101b, 107a, 126b, 152b, 153a, 162b, 163b, 180a, 180b
Nursing Outlook, 35a, 51b, 58a, 71b
Nursing Recruitment Service, 35a
Nursing Research, 51b
Nursing Studies Index, 39b
Nurse Teachers' Association, 69b
Nursing Times, 10a, 22a, 35a, 35b, 50a, 51b, 66a, 69b, 80a, 91a, 99b, 109a, 112a, 153a, 158a, 159b, 173b, 178b
Nussbaum, H., 10a, 17a
Nutting, M. A., 4b
Nylander, V. M., 12b

Oakes, J., 145a
Oakes, L., 41a
Obayan, M. N., 176b
Obcarskas, S., 140b
O'Brien, M. E., 126b
O'Brien, M. J., 83a, 156b
Obuchowski, M., 2b
O'Connell, P. E., 50a, 149a, 153a
O'Connor, A., 12b
O'Connor, D., 61b
O'Connor, F., 139a
O'Connor, K. J. R., 124a
O'Connor, R., 170b
O'Connor, V., 93a, 165b
Oden, G., 144b
O'Donnell, C. T., 129a
O'Flynn, M. E., 107b
Ogden, R. P., 35b
Ogg, E., 10a
O'Gorman, G., 143a
Ogston, D. G., 44b
Ogston, K. M., 44b
O'Gureck, J., 101b
O'Hara, F. J., 145a
O'Hara, J., 139a
O'Hare, B., 83a
Ohio Department of Health, 149a
Ohliger, J. F., 52b
Oiye, F., 39b
Okell, C., 131a
Old International Association, 10a
Oldmeadow, E., 80b
Olesen, V. L., 39b, 53a, 62b
Oliver, B., 3a
Oliver, S., 62b
Ollerenshaw, K., 10a, 26a
Olsen, M. P., 81b
Olson, E. V., 112a
Olsson, D. E., 73b, 178a
O'Malley, C. D., 66a, 71b
Onnembo, F., 141b
Ontario. Department of Health. Environmental Health Branch, 126b
Ontario. Department of Health. Research and Planning Branch, 149a
Ontario Hospital Association, 35b
Ontario Hospital Services Commission, 35b, 76a
Ontario Registered Nurses' Association, 73b
Oparinde, S. O., 153a
Oram, P. G., 58a
Orbell, A., 4a, 71b, 77a
Orgain, F., 128a
Orlando, I. J., 61b
Orleans, D., 94a
Ormerod, T. P., 105a
Ortelt, J. A., 94a
Osborne, O. H., 66a
Osburn, L., 4b
Oscar, M., 43a
Osmond, J. D., 162b
Ostlund, L. A., 44b, 62b
Owen, E. N., 119b
Owen, G. M., 152a, 153a
Owen, J. E., 14b
Owen, M. E., 2b
Owen, S. V., 42a

Owens, F. M., 124a
Owens, J., 159a
Oxford Area Nurse Training Committee, 35b
Oxford Regional Hospital Board, 44a, 79a, 91a, 179a, 180b
Oxford Regional Hospital Board. Operational Research Unit, 66a, 94a

Packard, H., 142a
Paetznick, M., 79a
Page, S. C., 174b
Pair, N., 58a
Palk, M. L., 43a
Pallin, E., 81b
Pallister, L. K., 180a
Palmer, H., 71b
Palmer, I. S., 50a
Palmer, M. E., 35b
Palmer, R. A., 115b
Pan American Sanitary Bureau. Regional Office of the W.H.O., 35b, 80b
Panayotova, Z. P., 147a
Pankratz, D. M., 40a
Pankratz, L. D., 40a
Pantall, J., 71b, 178a
Pape, R. H., 54a
Paplauskas-Macdonald, R., 168a
Paquette, A., 139a
Pardee, G., 79a
Pare, C. M. B., 172b
Pare, P., 145a
Parish, P. A., 155b
Park, W. D., 106a
Parke, P. C., 134a
Parker, B., 173b
Parker, C., 10a
Parker, D. J., 165b
Parker, E. R., 143b
Parker, J. M., 156b
Parkin, M. L., 51b, 52a
Parliament. See: Great Britain. Parliament
Parnell, J. E., 65a
Parnell, J. W., 167b
Parris, E., 83a
Parry, D. W., 172b
Parry, W. H., 103b, 106a, 112a, 124a, 147a, 155b, 167b
Parse, R. R., 39a
Parsonage, M., 119a
Parsons, H. M., 107a, 161a
Parthey Uller, M. T., 10a
Parton, I., 109a
Pask, E. G., 131a
Pask, M. M. F., 1b
Patel, N. B., 121a
Paterson, M. A., 35b
Path, F. C., 167a
Paton, A., 106a, 109a
Patrylow, S., 82b
Pattemore, W. R., 143b
Patten, M. E., 20b
Patten, M. K., 21a
Patterson, E. G., 117b
Patterson, H. R., 171b
Patterson, T. K., 91a
Patterson, W. G., 63b
Pattison, D., 4a
Pattullo, A. W., 113b
Paul, W. K., 139a, 144a
Paulina, Sister M., 9b, 13a
Paull, E. H., 17b, 35b
Paulley, J. W., 157b
Paulson, E., 79a
Payne, G. O., 26a
Payne, J. P., 169b
Payne, L. C., 73b
Payne, R. L., 145a
Paynich, M. L., 74b, 147a
Pazdur, H., 139a
Peacey, B., 3a
Peach, A. M., 113b
Peacock, J. H., 103a

Pearce, E. C., 66a, 97a, 145a, 165b
Pearman, E., 113b
Pearsall, M., 58a
Pearson, E., 60a
Pearson, J. B., 97a
Pearson, L., 91a, 115a
Pearson, P., 29a
Pearson, R. J. C., 162b, 182b
Peart, M. L., 35b
Peck, C., 14b, 139a
Peckham, A. H., 180a
Pedelty, K. M., 178a
Pederson, W. D., 26a, 28b
Peel, J. S., 172b
Peers, R. E., 69b
Peimer, S. C., 26a, 83a
Peitchinis, J., 25a
Pellegrino, E. D., 35b, 50a, 62b, 72a
Pelley, T., 1a
Pemberton, D., 124a
Pembury Hospital, 52a
Penfold, M. J., 165b
Pennington, G. W., 103a
Pennington, M., 93a
Pennsylvania Nurses' Association, 21a
Penny, M., 44b
Penrose, J. H., 163b
Pentecost, B. L., 101b
Pentz, M., 54a
Peplau, H. E., 91a, 139a
Pepperell, E. M., 178b, 179a
Pequegnat, D., 167b
Perchard, S., 139a
Percy, D. M., 91a
Perkins, E. W., 10a
Perrine, G., 101b
Perry, D. A., 86a
Perry, E. L., 72a
Perry, L., 53a
Perry, M. E., 139a
Perspectives in Psychiatric Care, 139a
Peschin, A., 169b
Peszczynski, M., 112a
Pesznecker, B. L., 143b
Peters, C., 132a
Peters, L., 54a
Petersen, S., 144a
Peterson, E., 10a
Peterson, F. K., 41b
Peterson, G. C., 72a, 91a
Petrie, P., 180a
Petrovich, D. G., 139a
Petrowski, D. D., 10a, 60a, 149a
Pettit, H. F., 143b
Pettus, M. A., 43a
Petty, T. L., 157b
Pétursdottir, M., 14a
Pfaltzgraff, R. E., 163b
Pfnister, A. O., 35b
Phaneuf, M. C., 94a
Philipp, E. E., 121a, 165b
Phillips, R., 148b
Phillips, T. T. B., 103a
Phinney, R. P., 143b
Piana, B. M., 35b
Pickworth, K. H., 155b
Picton, L. V., 72a
Piehler, P., 52a
Piepgaras, R., 35b
Pilkington, T., 117b
Pill, R., 132b
Pillai, A. S., 143b
Pillepich, M. K., 40b
Pinfield, I. N., 117b
Pings, V. M., 52a
Pinker, R., 177a
Pinneo, R., 101a, 101b
Pinsent, R. J. F. H., 155b
Piper, D. A., 80a
Pirnie, F. A., 43a
Pitman, A. J., 48b
Pitorak, E. F., 101b
Pittman, R., 147a
Plachta, Sister M. M., 145a
Plaisted, L. M., 163b, 174b
Planansky, K., 139a

Plank, E. N., 132b
Plant, J., 12a
Plant, J. A., 105b, 106a
Plapp, J., 29a, 35b
Platou, C. N., 26a, 28b
Platou, R. V., 10a
Platt, D. M., 91b
Platt, H., 36b
Platt, L. I., 99b, 113b, 124a
Player, D. A., 156a
Pleasants, I., 126a
Plein, E. M., 172b
Plein, J. B., 172b
Plessis, D. J. Du., 72a
Plotner, E. K., 170a
Plymouth Council of Social Service, 112a
Pohl, M. L., 46b, 47a
Poindexter, J., 170a
Poirier, W. A., 38b
Pol, M. L., 104b
Poland, M., 91b
Polar, J. F., 159a
Pole, K. F., 60b, 159b
Pollack, H. P., 50a
Polley, M., 109a, 161a
Pomeranz, R., 33b
Pomeroy, M. R., 131a
Ponte, M. L., 36a, 54a
Pope, C., 12a
Pope, J. L. W., 139a
Pope, R. A., 173a
Popiel, E. S., 54a, 166a
Popkin, D. R., 116a, 143b
Porowski, P. C., 168b
Porritt, J. L., 103b, 124a
Porter, D. L., 47a
Porter, E. K., 21a
Porter, I. A., 22b
Porter, P., 48a
Posner, E., 124a
Post, S., 36a, 43a
Posyniak, H., 22a
Pothier, P. C., 117b, 138b
Potter, J. M., 166a
Potter, M. C., 147a
Potter, T., 10a, 95a
Poulos, J., 116a
Pounds, F. J., 22b
Pounds, L., 130a
Pounds, V. A., 117b, 119a
Powell, A., 15a
Powell, C., 101b
Powell, E., 18a, 177a
Powell, F. L. A., 15a, 15b
Powell, M., 62b, 119a, 163b
Powell, M. B., 4a, 10a, 36a, 72a, 94b, 154a
Powers, E. F., 40a
Powers, M., 101b, 166a
Poynter, F. N. L., 181a
Pozz, L. W., 117b
Practical Approaches to Nursing Service Administration, 159a
Prange, A. J., 61b
Pratt, H., 10b, 63a
Pratt, R., 12a, 119a
Preece, S., 153a
Prentice, G. M., 166a
Prentice, W. E., 91b
Price, A. L., 36a, 66a
Price, E. M., 54a, 73b, 79a
Price, G. G., 63a, 97b
Price, W. R., 162b
Pride, L. F., 91b
Priestley, H. E., 181b
Primrose, R. B., 131a
Prince, G. S., 153a
Prince, R., 105a
Prince of Wales's General Hospital, Tottenham, 181b
Princess Muna College of Nursing, Jordan, 36a
Pringle, D. M., 85b, 133b
Pritchard, J. G., 112a
Psathas, G., 29a, 41b

Pueschel, S. J., 36a
Pugh, M. A., 65a
Pugh, W. T. G., 66a
Punshon, P. M., 58a
Puras, B., 65a
Purdy, F., 77a
Putt, A. M., 85b, 106a

Quade, D., 92b
Quarrell, E. J., 157b, 175b
Queen Alexandra's Royal Naval Nursing Service, 2b
Queen Victoria Hospital, East Grinstead, 181b
Queen's Home and the Queen Victoria Maternity Hospital, Adelaide, South Australia, 181b
Queen's Institute of District Nursing, 149a, 150b, 151b, 156b, 167b
Queen's Institute of District Nursing, Scottish Branch, 19b
Quigley, C. J. P., 117b, 180a
Quinn, S. M., 10b, 13b, 14b, 17a, 21a
Quint, J. C., 44b, 56b, 58a, 91b, 94b
Quittenton, R. C., 36a
Quixley, J. M. E., 120b

Rabin, B., 102a
Radcliffe Infirmary, Oxford, 181b
Radwanski, D. M., 128b
Rae, A. V., 10b
Rae, M., 112a
Rae, N. M., 101b
Rae-Grant, Q., 116a
Raffensperger, J. G., 131a
Raffle, P. A. B., 126b, 128b
Raheja, K. K., 139a
Raine, N. L., 48b
Rains, A. J. H., 66a, 161a, 162b, 166a
Rainsbury, J. P., 112a
Raja, G. L. P., 124a
Rajabally, J., 42a
Rajokovich, M., 117b
Ralla, E., 36a
Ralphs, D., 124a
Rambousek, E., 87a
Ramey, I. G., 119a
Ramos, P. G., 72a
Ramphal, M., 40a, 66a, 81b, 84b
Ramsay, A. M., 119a
Ramsay, E., 2b
Ramsden, G. A., 23b
Ramsing, Sister, B., 36a
Rangreji, D. S., 163b
Rann, S. E., 157a
Rao, A. S. P., 18b
Rao, K. S., 147a
Raphael, Sister M., 74b
Raphael, W., 91b
Rapier, D. K., 83b
Rasak, E., 128a
Rasmussen, E. H., 36a, 63a
Ratchford, P., 168b
Ratner, M., 66a
Raulston, J., 146b
Raven, K. A., 10b
Raven, R. W., 99b
Rawlinson, K., 148a, 156a
Rawnsley, P. A., 109a
Ray, R. M., 166a
Raybould, E., 16b, 52a, 63b
Rayner, C., 40a, 63a, 91b, 182b
Rayner, D. M., 80b
Raynes, N. V., 26b
Rea, J. N., 83b
Reade, T., 131a
Reading, S., 149a
Reddin, M., 133b
Redman, B. K., 26b, 48a
Redman, P., 72a
Redwood, D. R., 101b
Reed, D. A., 72a
Reed, F. C., 36a, 54a
Reeder, S. R., 120a

Rees, J. R., 116a
Rees, S., 173b
Rees, S. A. H., 3b
Reese, D. E., 26b, 54a
Reeves, K. R., 131a
Regina Elizabeth, Sister, 95a
Registered Nurses' Association of British Columbia, 36a
Registered Nurses' Association of Nova Scotia, 18a
Registered Nurses Association of Ontario, 8a, 21a, 35b
Rehm, D. A., 79a
Reich, T., 103a
Reid, A., 50a
Reid, F., 47a
Reid, H. E., 74b
Reid, J. J. A., 153a
Reid, M., 91b, 150b
Reid, W. H., 162a, 168b
Reinkemeyer, A. M. (Sister M. Hubert), 10b, 26b, 36a, 50a, 58a
Reiter, F., 81b, 94b
Reith, H. R., 145a
Remillet, J. G., 49a, 149a, 154a
Rennie, R. S., 124a
Rennoldson, M., 80b
Resnick, E. B., 120b
Restrepo, L. A., 14b
The Retreat, York, 181b
Reuell, V. M., 58a
Revans, R. W., 10b, 26b, 44a, 66a, 69b, 72a, 74b
Reynard, W. A., 127a
Reynolds, G. H., 45a
Reynolds, K. W., 106a
Reynolds, M., 101b
Reynolds, P. L., 83b
Rhodes, C. E., 126a, 127a
Rhodes, I. B., 166a
Rhodes, R. J., 158b
Riahi, A., 36a
Richards, I. D. G., 107b, 149a
Richards, M., 12b
Richards, P. R., 80a
Richards, S. F., 121b
Richardson, B., 69b, 142a
Richardson, D. K., 112a
Richardson, G. A., 88a
Richardson, S., 98a
Riches, H. R. C., 97a
Richman, A., 73b
Richter, F. S., 27a
Ricks, M. J., 169b
Riddell, A. G., 172b
Riddell, D. G., 36a
Riddell, D. M., 156a
Riddell, J., 151a
Riddle, J. T. E., 97a
Riddoch, M., 79a
Ridley, M., 85b, 167b, 172b
Riedel, D. C., 57a, 91b
Rifka, G. E., 14a
Riley, E. C., 107a, 124a
Riley, M., 139a
Rimmer, T., 72a
Rines, A. R., 36a
Ring, P. A., 161a
Risley, M., 181a
Ritchie, E. A., 139a
Ritchie, J. B., 117a
Ritchie, M., 101b
Ritson, E. B., 136a, 158b
Ritvo, M. M., 71b, 91b
Rivlin, S., 103a
Roach, E. G., 124a
Roaf, R., 163b
Roake, D. P., 133a
Robb, K., 36a
Robb-Smith, A. H. T., 181b
Roberts, D. E., 149a, 149b
Roberts, E., 12b
Roberts, G. W., 85b
Roberts, I., 153a
Roberts, L., 128a
Roberts, S. L., 101b

Roberts, T., 42a, 45b, 98a
Roberts, T. E., 96a
Roberts, W. L., 116a
Robertson, H., 112a
Robidoux-Poirier, H., 107a
Robinson, A. M., 139b, 143b
Robinson, C. H., 170a
Robinson, D., 132b
Robinson, E., 153a
Robinson, F. N., 157b
Robinson, J. M., 116a
Robinson, J. O., 109a
Robinson, J. R., 117b
Robinson, J. T., 139b
Robinson, K., 10b
Robinson, L., 91b
Robinson, M. E., 18b
Robinson, R. J., 134a
Robinson, S. C., 36a
Robinson, S. S., 76a
Robinson, W., 179a
Robischon, P., 145a, 147b
Robson, J. G., 169b
Robson, J. M., 172b
Robson, R. A. H., 23a, 26b
Roch, S., 61b
Roche, J., 95a
Roche, L., 124a
Rockwell, V. T., 167b
Rodil-Martires, C., 52a
Rodman, M. J., 172b
Roehm, M. M., 109b
Roemer, M. I., 91b
Roeschlaub, E. L., 49a
Rogan, J., 127a
Rogers, C. G., 139b
Rogers, E. P., 95a
Rogers, M. E., 10b, 36b
Rogers, P. J., 21a
Rogers, R., 10b
Rogers, W. H., 174a
Rohde, I. M., 159a
Rohrer, L. M., 119a
Rohweder, A. W., 66a
Roland, P. E., 107a
Rollin, H. R., 114b, 170b
Roper, N., 36b, 41a, 66a, 97a
Roper-Hall, M. J., 129b
Rorem, C. R., 10b, 93a
Roscher, C. L., 147a
Rose, Sister F., 36b
Rose, J. F., 106a
Rose, P., 63a
Rose, W. G. D., 139b
Rosen, A., 45b, 72a
Rosenbaum, M. J., 179a
Rosenberg, J. M., 172b
Rosenberg, M., 73b, 178a
Rosenheim, G., 121a
Rosenthal, S. R., 22b
Rosier, M., 97b
Rosin, A. J., 112a
Ross, A. D., 40a
Ross, C. F., 63a, 72a, 83b
Ross, D. S., 115a, 124a
Ross, J. K., 161a
Ross, J. R. W., 96b
Ross, J. S., 66a, 97a
Ross, S. G., 108b
Ross, V. M., 71b
Roswell, D., 117b
Rothberg, J. S., 60b, 64a, 174b
Rothnie, N. G., 161a
Rottkamp, B. C., 26b
Roualle, H. L. M., 99b
Rouslin, S., 134b
Routh, T. A., 81a
Routhier, W. R., 58a
Rowan, R. L., 73b
Rowe, A., 91b
Rowe, H. R., 26b, 34b, 41b
Rowe, J. W., 97a
Rowland, A. J., 151a
Rowland, G. T., 117b
Rowland, H. A. K., 115a
Rowsell, G., 21a, 36b, 50a

Roxburgh, R. A., 107b
Roy, Sister C., 10b
Royal Australian Nursing Federation, 18a, 19b, 26b, 36b
Royal Australian Nursing Federation. National Nursing Education Division, 139b
Royal Australian Nursing Federation, West Australian Branch, 114b
Royal College of General Practitioners, 155b, 156a (See also: College of General Practitioners)
Royal College of Midwives, 156a
Royal College of Nursing, 18a, 58a, 85b, 156a, 178a
Royal College of Nursing. Library of Nursing, 52a
Royal College of Nursing. Nurse Administrators Section, 83b
Royal College of Nursing. Occupational Health Section, 127a
Royal College of Nursing (Public Health Dept.), 153a
Royal College of Nursing. Working Party on Salary Structure, 22a
Royal College of Nursing and National Council of Nurses of the United Kingdom, 10b, 18a, 18b, 21a, 25a, 36b, 58a, 58b, 69b, 72a, 77a, 79b, 84a, 85a, 94b, 112a, 112b, 117b, 124b, 128b, 139b, 149b, 151b, 178a, 180a
Royal College of Nursing and National Council of Nurses of the United Kingdom. Hospitals Department. Intensive Therapy Nursing Group, 87a
Royal College of Nursing and National Council of Nurses of the United Kingdom. Nurse Administrators Section, 26b
Royal College of Nursing and National Council of Nurses of the U.K. Occupational Health Committee, 124b, 127a
Royal College of Nursing and National Council of Nurses of the United Kingdom. Ward and Departmental Section, 102a
Royal College of Nursing and National Council of Nurses of the United Kingdom. N. Ireland Board, 70a
Royal College of Nursing and National Council of Nurses of the United Kingdom. Scottish Board, 26b, 70a
Royal College of Nursing and National Council of Nurses of the United Kingdom. Welsh Board, 70a
Royal College of Nursing, Scotland, 42b
Royal Medico Psychological Association, 26b, 118a, 134b, 139b
Royal Society of Health Congress 1970, 149b
Royal Women's Hospital, Melbourne, 37a
Royle, G. C., 49a
Ruben, M., 129b
Rubin, A. P., 169b
Rubin, R., 10b, 66b, 120a
Rubin, S., 119b
Rubinstein, K., 129b
Rudd, T. N., 85b, 112b, 174b
Rudge, P. F., 72a
Rudick, E., 182b
Rummerfield, M. J., 124b, 173b
Rummerfield, P. S., 124b, 173b
Rumshevics, M., 5a
Runck, H. W., 74b
Runnels, H., 147a, 149b
Runyon, N., 136b
Rusell, J. G. B., 173b
Rush, H. C., 127a
Ruslink, D., 115a
Russaw, E. H., 159a
Russell, A. M. E., 108a

Russell, B., 64b, 181b
Russell, C. H., 178b
Russell, E. K., 5a
Russell, J. K., 121a, 133b
Russell, J. T., 169b
Russell, S., 91b
Russo, A. M., 127a
Rutherford, R., 72a
Rutherford, W. L., 72a
Rutledge, F., 156b
Ryan, J. R., 21a, 79b
Ryan, M., 156a
Ryan, T. M., 153b
Ryback, D., 29a, 44b
Ryburn, C., 132b
Rycroft, P. V., 129b
Ryder, M., 177a
Rykheer, G. M., 66b
Rykken, M. B., 142b
Rynbergen, H. J., 170a

Saathoff, D. E., 76a
Sabel, M. E., 174b
Sacharin, R. M., 131a
Sackett, H. G., 115a, 115b
Sackheim, G. I., 97b, 102b, 134b
Sahney, V., 94a
Sainato, H. K., 141b
Sainsbury, M. J., 139b
St. Andrew's Ambulance Association, 66b
St. Claire-Vernon, J., 107a, 118a
St. George's Hospital, London, 43b
St. Helen's Hospital, Hastings, 93a
St. John Ambulance Association, 66b
St. John's Hospital for Diseases of the Skin, 181b
St. Leonard's Hospital, Shoreditch, 182a
Saint Paul, Sister, 12a
St. Thomas's Hospital, London, 1a, 182a
St. Thomas's Hospital, London. Intensive Therapy Unit, 87a
St. Thomas's Hospital, London. Nightingale School, 37a
St. Vincent's Hospital, St. Louis, Missouri, 116a
Saleh, S. D., 26b
Salisbury General Hospital, 182a
Salmin, D., 37a
Salmon, B., 54a, 68b, 73b
Salmon, E. B., 37a
Salmon, G. B., 52b
Salter, M. E., 87a
Salter, R. H., 170b
Samater, H. N., 147a
Samson, E. G., 47a
Samuel, H. S., 104b
Sanazaro, P. J., 91b
Sandison, R. A., 139b
Sanford, N., 44b
Sangster, J. O., 153b
Sanner, M. C., 10b
Sant, E. G., 145a
Santo Tomas Nursing Journal, 147b
Sapeika, N., 172b
Sara, D., 115a
Saren, M., 77a
Sargeaunt, B. Z., 156a
Sasdi, M., 127a
Saskatchewan. Board of Nursing Education, 37a
Saskatchewan. Department of Public Health, 37a
Saskatchewan Registered Nurses' Association, 18b, 37a, 54a
Sata, L. S., 143b
Sataloff, J., 124b
Satchell, B. M., 116a
Sather, M. A., 131a
Saunders, C., 112b
Saunders, H. B., 166a
Saunders, M., 153a

Saunders, R., 73a
Saunders, W. H., 106b, 107a, 129a, 129b
Savage, C. R., 161a
Savage, W. W., 54a
Savich, D., 65a
Sawkins, E. M., 44a
Sawyer, H. P., 103a
Sawyer, J., 139b
Sawyer, J. R., 109a
Sax, S., 112b
Saxton, D. F., 97b, 172b
Sayanjarvi, R., 127a, 128a
Sayers, B. P. C., 109a
Sayers, L. A., 111b
Scahill, M., 131a
Scanlan, P., 14a
Schapira, K., 112b
Schatzman, L., 56b
Schechter, D. S., 79b
Schindall, H., 92a
Schlotfeldt, R. M., 10b, 26b, 37a, 54a, 58b, 61b, 63a, 94b
Schlotter, L., 109a
Schmahl, J. A., 66b
Schmalzried, G. L., 132b
Schmidt, J. E., 41a
Schmidt, M. D., 37a, 127a
Schmidt, M. S., 39a, 39b, 47a
Schmidt, W. H., 72a
Schmieding, N. J., 66b, 76a
Schmitt, J. A., 93b
Schmitt, L. M., 50a, 58b
Schmitt, M. H., 10b, 133b
Schmitt, Y., 102a
Schnee, B., 107b
Schneider, M., 27a, 121a
Schoen, E., 30b
Schoenberg, B., 143b
Schoenfeld, H., 27a
Schofield, D., 109a
Schofield, H., 49a
Schowalter, J. M., 79a
Schroeder, H. G., 166a
Schultz, R. M., 102b
Schulz, E. D., 182b
Schurr, M. C., 11a, 72a, 72b
Schurr, P. H., 161a
Schwabacher, H., 181a
Schwaid, M. C., 157b
Schwalm, M. E., 97a, 102b
Schwartau, N. W., 76a
Schwartz, B., 176b
Schwartz, D. R., 58b, 92a, 94b, 112b, 149a
Schweer, J. E., 37a
Schweisheimer, W., 161a
Schwenck, J. R., 102a
Schwier, M. E., 72b, 77a
Scopes, J. W., 103a
Scotch, N. A., 89a
Scotford, H., 11a
Scott, B. O., 103a
Scott, D., 145a
Scott, D. F., 166a
Scott, J., 153a
Scott, J. S., 158a
Scott, M. E., 157b
Scott, O., 104b
Scott, R., 154b
Scott, W. A., 42b
Scott Wright, M., 27a, 28a, 56b, 73a, 77b
Scottish Education Department. See: Great Britain. Scottish etc.
Scottish Home & Health Department. See: Great Britain. Scottish etc.
Scottish Hospital Centre, 58b, 180a
Scottish Hospitals Work Study Group, 76a
Scottish Nursing Staff Committee. See: Great Britain. Scottish Home and Health Department
Scully, N. R., 81b
Seacole, M., 5a
Seager, C. P., 139b

Seale, J., 11a
Seargeant, P. W., 106a, 115a
Searle, C., 1b, 12a, 37a, 72b, 147b
Searle, D. J., 109a, 112b
Sears, W. G., 97a, 114b, 173a
Seashore, E., 71a
Secor, J., 66b, 157b
Secor, S. M., 106a
Seedor, M. M., 48a, 48b, 105b, 166b
Seidl, F. W., 131a
Seidman, J., 21a
Seiler, H. E., 19b
Seivwright, M., 5a, 27a, 58b, 94b
Sell, I. L., 142b
Sellew, G., 66b, 131a
Sellors, P. J. H., 129b
Selmanoff, E. D., 90a, 178b
Semple, S. J. G., 157b
Sen, A., 27a
Seppelt, I. H., 112b
Seward, J. F., 72b
Seward, Sister J. M., 11a
Sewell, E. M., 43a
Sexton, D. L., 45b
Sexton, H. M., 95b
Seyffer, C., 58b, 72b, 81a
Seymour, C. A., 169b
Shackleton, A. D., 170b
Shade, D. A., 131b
Shafer, K. N., 66b
Shaldon, S., 109a
Shamess, D., 97b
Shanks, M. D., 37a
Shannon, A. M., 136a
Shannon, E., 87a
Shannon, I. R., 147b
Shapiro, F., 19b
Shapiro, M. B., 145a
Shapiro, S. G., 149b
Sharp, LaV., 102a
Sharp, L. J., 58b
Sharpe, D., 139b
Sharpe, M. E., 37a
Sharrock, R. L., 139b
Shaver, M. C., 52a
Shaw, A., 112b
Shaw, B. A., 85b
Shaw, H. J., 99b
Sheafor, M. M., 72b
Sheahan, J., 11a, 103a
Shears, L. W., 11a
Sheath, H. C., 50a
Shee, W. A., 180a
Sheen, E. M., 112b, 153a
Sheldon, E. B., 11a, 58b
Shelton, B., 86a
Shenning, M., 143b
Shepard, M. W., 92a
Shepherd, J. A., 106a
Sheps, C. G., 61b
Shepstone, A., 143b
Sherlock, B. J., 140a
Sherman, A. W., 127a
Sherman, R., 73b
Shetland, M. L., 37a, 40a, 47a, 50a
Shewchuk, M., 163b
Shield, B., 60b
Shields, H. P., 1b
Shillingford, J. P., 102a
Shneidman, E. S., 116a
Sholtis, L. A., 47a
Shone, 92a
Shoobs, D., 116a, 156b
Shope, J., 132b
Short, D. P., 2a
Shorthouse, M. A., 61b
Shrand, H., 131b
Shuck, W. H., 141b
Siegel, G. S., 124b
Siegel, H., 3b
Siegel, N. H., 92a
Sieggreen, M., 109a
Sierra-Franco, M., 170a
Siggins, C. M., 74b
Silverthorn, A., 104b
Sime, E., 37b

Simmonds, E. H., 149b
Simmons, J. A., 140a
Simmons, J. Q., 114b
Simmons, L. W., 11a, 58b
Simmons, P. H., 169b
Simms, L. L., 77a, 81b
Simms, M., 158a
Simon, G., 100b, 173a
Simon, J. R., 92a, 147b
Simon, P. L., 181a
Simonds, A., 47a, 166a
Simpson, H. M., 27a, 59a, 74b, 77a, 128a, 147b, 153a, 181a
Simpson, J., 174b
Simpson, K., 97a
Simpson, M. J., 37b
Simpson, N. L., 129b
Singer, P., 140a
Singh, S. P., 100b
Singleton, M., 76a
Sinkler, G. H., 140a
Sinnott, M. B., 124b
Sitler, D. W., 171b
Sitzman, J., 157b
Sivaraman, P., 123a
Sjoberg, K., 72b
Skaggs, K. G., 37b
Skeet, M., 14a, 23b, 89a
Skerry, W. J., 72b
Skinner, G., 66b
Skinner, J. E., 47a
Skipper, J. K., 11a, 61b, 65b, 74b, 92a
Skrimshire, M., 112b, 124b, 127a
Slack, M., 72b
Slaney, B., 124b, 125a, 127a, 128a, 128b
Slater, P., 92a
Slater, P. V., 37b
Slater, R. R., 162b
Slavinsky, A. T., 143b
Sleeper, R., 77a, 96b
Slocum, W. L., 23b
Smail, D. J., 135a
Smalley, H. E., 68a
Smellie, H., 59b
Smeltzer, C. H., 29a, 37b, 145a
Smith, A., 73b, 92a
Smith, A. B., 76a
Smith, A. J., 143b
Smith, B., 73b
Smith, B. C., 102a
Smith, B. J., 79b, 112b, 167b
Smith, B. L., 150b
Smith, C. A., 72b
Smith, C. S., 121a
Smith, D. B., 94b
Smith, D. M., 37b, 61b, 92a
Smith, D. W., 11a, 50b, 85b, 89a, 92a, 94b, 172b
Smith, E., 159b
Smith, E. J., 124b
Smith, E. M., 83b, 112b
Smith, E. S., 140a, 150b
Smith, F. E., 21a
Smith, G. L., 48b
Smith, G. M., 44b
Smith, J., 87a
Smith, J. D., 132b, 136b
Smith, J. L., 73b
Smith, J. M., 162b
Smith, J. P., 37b, 118a, 133b
Smith, J. W., 156a
Smith, K. M., 11a, 76a
Smith, M. C., 118a
Smith, M. E., 165a
Smith, P., 156b
Smith, P. M., 21a
Smith, R., 77a
Smith, R. A. G., 115a
Smith, S., 66b, 144a, 167b
Smith, S. B., 154a
Smith, S. E., 99b, 103a, 173a
Smith, V. L., 124b
Smithells, R. W., 121a
Smolens, J. B., 24a
Smoyak, S., 11a, 66b
Smyth, G. D. L., 107a

Snaith, L., 113b
Snavely, S. A., 73a, 78a
Snedden, B. M., 37b
Sneddon, I. B., 104b
Sneddon, J., 104b
Sneddon, R., 112b, 140a
Snellman, V., 5b, 66b
Snively, W. D., 96b, 97a
Sobel, D. E., 102a
Sobol, E. G., 147b
Society of Medical Officers of Health, 156a
Society of Occupational Medicine, 124b
Society of Registered Male Nurses, 12a
Sohn, D., 159a
Solomon, L., 11a
Solomons, G., 147b, 149b
Solosko, A., 166a
Sommer, R., 49a
Sorbie, C., 169b
Sorenson, G., 92a
Soriano-Cabrera, V., 47a
Sorsby, A., 129b
Sotejo, J. V., 77b, 154b
South African Nursing Association, 18b, 37b, 77b
South African Nursing Council, 18b
South African Nursing Journal, 37a, 171a
South Australian Journal of Nursing, 13a
South East Metropolitan Region. Greenwich and Deptford Hospital Management Committee, 180b
South Eastern Regional Hospital Board, Scotland, 181a
South West Metropolitan Area. Nurse Training Committee, 47a
South Western Regional Hospital Board, 66b
Southampton University, 43b
Southwood, J., 119b
Sovie, M. D., 101b
Spalding, E. K., 19b, 47a, 63a
Spalding, W. J., 151b
Spandau, M. M., 102a
Spark, M., 86b
Sparks, S., 33b
Spaziante, G., 76a
Speed, E. L., 74a
Speelman, A., 83b
Speers, R., 167b
Speller, S. R., 19b, 60b
Spelman, M. S., 90a
Spencer, C. S., 27a
Spencer, D. A., 118a
Spencer, G. T., 157b
Spencer, M., 83b
Spencer, V., 21a
Spensley, K. C., 24a
Sphire, R. D., 169b
Spicer, C. C., 158a
Spikantia, S. G., 170b
Spohn, R. R., 37b
Sporne, P., 85b, 105a
Spratt, I. H., 59a
Spriggs, C., 150b
Squire, J. E., 173a
Stacey, M., 132b
Stachyra, M., 140a
Stackpole, C. E., 96b
Stafford, N. H., 113a
Stage, T. B., 140a
Stahl, A. G., 27a, 79b
Standard, K., 147b
Standeven, M., 147b
Stanley, P. H., 161a
Stanley-Brown, E. G., 131b
Stanner, S., 138b
Stanton, A., 102a
Staton, E. E., 23a
Statts, H. A., 76a
Staupers, M. K., 11a
Stearns, N. S., 52a
Stedman's Medical Dictionary, 41a
Steed, M. E., 41b

Steel, V., 114b
Steele, M. L., 124b
Steele, R., 59a
Steele, S., 46a, 163b
Steele-Bodger, A., 124b
Stein, L. I., 140a
Stein, R. F., 37b, 44b, 62a, 178b
Steindler, F. M., 37b
Steiner, B. H., 79b
Stembridge, J., 124b
Stephen, C. R., 131b, 169b
Stephenson, E., 37b, 59a
Stephenson, J. B. P., 107b
Stevens, B., 27a, 101a
Stevens, L. F., 62a
Stevens, M. K., 63a, 113a
Stevens, V., 107b
Stevenson, N., 81a, 83b
Stewart, A. C., 3b
Stewart, D. R., 140a
Stewart, D. Y., 77b
Stewart, I. M., 1a, 5b
Stewart, M. A., 99b
Stewart, W. H., 11a, 15a
Stickel, D. L., 168b
Sticker, A., 4b
Stinson, S. M., 72b
Stobo, E. C., 116a, 156b
Stock, F. E., 175b
Stock, W., 60b
Stockmeyer, I., 81a
Stockwell, M. L., 66b
Stoker, M. G. P., 99b
Stokes, G. A., 140a
Stokes, O. J. J., 37b
Stone, R. M., 163b
Stone, V., 113a
Stones, P., 105a
Stones, R. W. H., 12a
Stoops, M., 37b, 44b
Storlie, F., 11a, 87a, 101b, 166a
Stotsky, B. A., 113a
Stoves, V., 124b, 127a, 128b
Strachan, D. W., 180b
Strachan, I. G., 131b
Strand, H. R., 41b
Strank, R. A., 81a
Stratford, D. O., 2a
Straub, A., 77a
Strauss, A., 87a
Stravino, V., 108a
Street, M. M., 27a
Streeter, J., 178a
Striegel, B., 127a
Stringer, J., 77a
Strong, P. G., 81b, 140a, 143b
Strulovici, N., 14a
Struthers, J. E., 153b
Struthers, J. N. M., 134a
Stryker, R. P., 37b, 54a, 59a, 179a
Student Nurses' Association, 24b
Stunt, C. L., 157b
Sturzl, J. A., 81b
Suarez, R., 140a
Subhadra, V., 149b
Suchinsky, L. W., 140a
Suddarth, D. S., 64a, 164b
Sudduth, A. G., 103b
Sugden, B., 161b
Sugden, J., 140a
Sullivan, C. M., 95b
Sullivan, J. D., 140a
Sullivan, J. J., 52a
Summerford, R. V., 102a
Summers, M., 127a
Sutherland, D. J., 3b, 21a
Sutton, A. L., 66b, 83b
Sutton, C., 132b
Suzanne Marie, Sister, 173a
Swain, V. A. J., 181b
Swansburg, R. C., 37b, 43a, 95b
Swanson, A. L., 81a
Sweeney, A., 140a
Sweeney, B. T., 149b
Sweeney, C., 113b
Swift, G., 156a

Swinney, J., 161b
Swyer, G. I. M., 159b
Sydow, G. von, 134a
Sykes, M. K., 171a
Sylvester, D. G. H., 27a
Sylvester, P. E., 97a
Symington, A., 140a
Symonds, S., 14a
Szentpetery, K., 147b

Tabler, M., 27a
Tabor, R. B., 52a
Taddy, Sister J., 132b
Tagart, R. E. B., 161b
Tagliacozzo, D. M., 90b, 92a
Tague, J. M., 72a
Tait, E. A., 170b
Tait, J., 143b
Tait, K. M., 83b
Talbot, J. A., 147b
Tan, N. C., 87a
Tanguay, J., 131b
Tansley, D. A., 99b
Tao-Chen Yu, 59a
Tarlinton, P., 11a
Tarrant, B. J., 74a
Tarry, C., 159a
Tarsitano, J. J., 166a
Tate, B. L., 27a, 29a, 38a, 45a, 45b, 82b, 94b
Tate, G. V., 85b
Tattersall, E. R., 38a
Taub, D. L., 26a
Tauber, I. J., 107b, 140a
Taverner, D., 97a, 173a
Taves, M. J., 11b
Taylor, C. D., 72b, 92a
Taylor, C. E., 24a
Taylor, C. M., 143b, 144a
Taylor, C. W., 27a
Taylor, D., 70a
Taylor, G., 98a
Taylor, J., 113a, 127a
Taylor, J. K., 27a
Taylor, M., 28b, 38b
Taylor, S., 166a
Taylor, S. D., 15b
Taylor-Young, S., 115a
Tayona, S., 1a
Tease, J. W., 120b
Telfer, A. B. M., 162a
Templeton, R. J., 27a
Tenney, D. A., 175a
Teplow, L., 124b
Terrazas, F., 113a, 141a
Terry, F. J., 174a
Testoff, A., 76a, 79b
Tewari, S. N., 113a, 173a
Tewinkle, M. B., 92a, 166a
Thigpen, L. W., 59a
This, L. E., 75a
Thomas, B. J., 131b
Thomas, D., 41b
Thomas, D. B., 8a, 146b, 147b, 148b
Thomas, D. H., 145a
Thomas, D. J., 151a
Thomas, E. B. J., 87a
Thomas, F. A., 74a, 140b
Thomas, J., 41b
Thomas, L., 50b
Thomas, L. A., 72b
Thomas, M. J., 29a
Thomas, S., 173a
Thomas, S. M. G., 124b
Thompson, A. M. C., 17a, 18a, 39b, 52a
Thompson, B., 119b
Thompson, E. D., 131b
Thompson, E. M., 66b, 82b
Thompson, G., 52a
Thompson, J., 13b
Thompson, J. D., 113a, 180b
Thompson, L. M., 11b
Thompson, M. C., 134a
Thompson, N. A., 131b

Thompson, T., 140b
Thompson, V. D., 38a
Thoms, E. J., 87a
Thomson, C. P., 140b
Thomson, C. W., 171a
Thomson, W., 22b, 99b, 115a, 124b, 173b, 177b
Thorne, M. E., 85b
Thorne, N., 104b
Thornton, M., 133a
Thorpe, A., 18a, 153b
Thorpe, E., 153b
Thurlow, J., 22b
Thurston, J. C. B., 171a
Thurston, J. R., 23a, 27a, 27b, 38a, 45a, 45b
Tibbs, T., 175a
Till, K., 163b
Timaru Hospital, New Zealand, 22b
Timmins, N. G., 38a
Timoney, R. F., 173a
Timothy, Sister M., 175a
Tims, N. S., 27b
Tindall, V. R., 103a, 121a
Tingle, J., 154a
Tobin, M. J., 59a
Todd, J., 140b, 151a
Tompkins, S., 27b
Tomlinson, R. M., 83b
Tomsett, V., 143b
Tonkin, D., 129b
Tonkin, R. D., 173a
Toohey, M., 114b
Toomey, L. C., 143b
Topalis, M., 138a
Topf, M., 75a
Tornyay, R. de, 49a
Toronto. Committee for Survey of Hospital Needs in Metropolitan Toronto, 27b, 38a
Toronto. Division of University Extension, 38a
Toronto General Hospital, 72b
Toronto University. School of Nursing, 38a
Torrance, J. T., 134a
Torrance, P. N., 38a
Torrens, P. R., 102a
Torrie, A., 116a, 153b
Torrie, P. J., 72b
Tosiello, F., 38a, 43a
Tovey, G. H., 103a
Townsend, N., 161b
Trail, I. D., 140b
Trained Nurses Association of India, 18b, 21a, 21b, 38a, 147b
Trasler, B. J., 150b
Travelbee, J., 66b, 140b
Treece, E. M., 45a
Treece, E. W., 83b
Tribou, M., 47a
Trick, K., 22b, 140b
Trigiano, L. L., 119b
Trimble, A. S., 161b
Trinidad and Tobago. Ministry of Health, 27b
Trites, D. K., 76a, 92a, 95b
Troop, E. H., 156b
Trounce, J. R., 173a
Trouten, F., 38a, 166a
Tryon, P. A., 85b, 92a
Tschudin, M. S., 38a, 58b
Tubbs, A., 140b
Tudor, L. L., 109a
Tumilty, E. M., 140b
Tunbridge, R., 128b
Tunis, B. L., 50b
Turer, A., 14b
Turk, H., 66b, 81b
Turner, F. W., 70a
Turner, W. J., 113a, 179a
Turner, W. K., 38a
Tutt, N. S., 118a, 144a
Twomey, Sister M. R., 163b
Tym, R., 162a
Tyman, B. M., 168b

Tyrer, F. H., 124b
Tyrrell, B., 166b

Uddoh, C., 38a
Ujhely, G. B., 62a, 140b, 145a
Ulin, P. R., 121a
Ullmann, L. P., 142b
Ullom, M. M., 83b
United Bristol Hospitals, 54b, 181a
United Kingdom Council for Overseas Student Affairs, 27b
United States. Bureau of Disease Prevention and Environmental Control, 99b, 125a
United States. Bureau of Labour Statistics, 21b
United States. National Center for Health Statistics, 27b
United States. National Institute of General Medical Sciences, 74a
United States. National Institutes of Health. Clinical Center, 107b
United States. Public Health Service, 27b, 35a, 94b, 102a, 147b
United States. Public Health Service. Department of Health, Education and Welfare, 54a
United States. Public Health Service. Division of Chronic Diseases. Diabetes and Arthritis Program, 105a
United States. Public Health Service. Divison of Hospital and Medical Facilities, 93a, 180b
United States. Public Health Service. Division of Nursing, 19b, 38b, 54b, 59a, 76a, 102a, 134a, 149b, 166b, 175a
United States. Public Health Service. Division of Occupational Health, 127b
United States Surgeon General, 73a
University of Arizona College of Nursing, 42b
University of California Extension, 116a
University of California. School of Nursing, 76a, 116a
University of Colorado. School of Nursing, 158a
University of Kansas Medical Center. Department of Nursing Education, 66a
University of Surrey, 43b
(For other universities See: Alberta, Brunel, Columbia, Dundee, Manchester, New York State, Toronto, Yale)
Unsworth, G. P., 140b
Uprichard, M., 11b
Urry, N., 140b
Useem, R. H., 144b

Vaill, P. B., 63a
Vaillot, M. C., 38b, 63a, 145a
Valentine, L. R., 114b
Van Aernam, A. B., 42b, 57b
Vancouver General Hospital, 182a
Van der Horst, R. L., 102a
Vanhoorne, M., 127b
Van Sant, G. E., 143b
Vaughan, V. C., 157b
Vaughan-Jackson, O. J., 114b
Vaughan-Richards, G. A., 38b
Vaz, D., 27b
Velazquez, J. M., 92a
Venger, M. J., 77b, 171a
Venus, A., 110b
Verhonick, P. J., 59a, 85b, 95b
Verrill, M. T., 150b
Veterans Administration. Department of Medicine and Surgery, 43a
Vevang, B., 118a
Victoria Hospital for Children, Chelsea, 182a

Victoria Infirmary, Glasgow, 182a
Viitala, M., 5b
Viljoen, J. F., 161b
Villegas, E. L., 45b
Vinall, R. P., 76a
Vincent de Paul, 5b
Vineberg, A., 161b
Vlok, M. E., 66b
Voda, A. M., 97a
Voelz, G. L., 125a
Von Matt, L., 5b
Von Schilling, K. C., 118a
Vreeland, E. M., 149b
Vreeland, R., 87a
Vyas, R. W., 12a

Waddicor, P. E. E., 91b, 150b
Waddy, F. F., 85b
Wadsworth, W. V., 140b
Waechter, E. H., 130a
Wagner, J. K., 113b
Wagner, S. P., 75a
Wain, O. M., 83b
Wakeley, C., 107b, 109a, 161b
Walano, D. A., 133b
Walcher, S. D., 119b
Wald, F. S., 66b
Wald, L. D., 5b
Walike, B. C., 170b
Walker, A. H. C., 134a
Walker, A. S., 107a
Walker, C., 149b
Walker, C. N., 39b
Walker, D., 149b, 151a
Walker, G. G., 125a
Walker, J. H., 156a
Walker, K., 162b
Walker, R., 140b
Walker, V. H., 90a, 94b, 178b
Wall, B. A., 170b
Wallace, A. G., 100a
Wallace, C. A., 157b
Wallace, C. M., 92a, 116a, 140b
Wallace, D. M., 109b
Wallace, M. A., 143b
Wallace, M. B., 27b, 38b
Wallace, S. A., 125a
Waller, M. V., 59a
Wallin, J., 95b, 147b
Walmsley, P. Y., 21b
Walsh, E. G., 114b
Walsh, J. E., 143b, 144a
Walsh, M. B., 95a
Walsh, R. C., 56b
Walsh, S., 27b
Walter, J. F., 97b, 172b
Walter Reed Army Institute of Research, 59b, 151b
Walters, E., 103b, 169b
Walton, A. M., 28b
Waltz, C. F., 154a
Wandelt, M. A., 59b
Warcaba, B., 44a
Ward, D. J., 140b
Ward, M. J., 13a
Ward, P. M., 113a
Wares, E., 173b
Warin, J. F., 156a
Wark, I. W., 27b
Warltier, A. W., 161b
Warren, B., 105a
Warren, C. P., 97a
Warren, D. de M., 179b
Warren, W., 141a
Wass, J. R., 166b
Waterhouse, R. A., 133a
Waters, N. W., 156a
Watkin, B., 3b, 21b, 31b, 38b, 54a, 73a, 79b, 92a, 115a, 178b, 181b
Watkinson, G., 106a
Watson, G., 118a
Watson, J., 162b
Watson, M., 38b, 121a
Watson, M. W., 48b
Watt, J. 19b

Watt, J. K., 160a
Watt, J. M., 131b
Wax, J., 59b
Wayne, D., 156b
Weakley, L. R., 153b
Weaver, M. E., 97b
Weaver, S., 118a
Webb, F. W. S., 103b
Webb, J., 178b
Webster, L., 70a
Weddell, D., 141a
Weddige, D., 49a
Wedgery, A. W., 11b, 12a, 54a, 81a
Weeks, K., 141a
Weeks, L. K., 93a
Weil, J. W., 74a
Weil, T. P., 74a, 94b
Weinberg, S., 131b
Weiner, H. N., 75a
Weinstein, A. S., 29a
Weir, T. W. H., 118a
Weiss, J. M. A., 67a, 94b
Weiss, M. O., 8b, 14a, 28a, 40b, 83b
Welbrock-Smith, J., 28a
Welch, J. D., 167b
Wellenkamp, D., 87a
Weller, B. F., 79b
Weller, M. F., 159b
Wells, P., 166b
Welsh Office. See: Great Britain. Welsh Office
Welter, M. L., 54a
Wenborn, J. K., 150b
Wenkert, W., 75a
Wensley, E., 92b
Were, V., 12b
Werley, H. H., 59b
Werner, A. M., 61b, 92b
Werner, J. A., 137a, 141a
Weschler, I. R., 73a
Wessell, M. A., 151b
Wessex Regional Hospital Board, 87a
Wessler, R. L., 62a
West, M. D., 83b
West, M. M., 125a
West, N., 54b
West, N. C., 67a
West, R., 125a
West, T., 12b
West, W. L., 175a
West Cumberland Hospital, 179a, 179b
Westbrook, G. M., 178b
Western Council on Higher Education for Nursing, 38b, 59b, 79b, 95a
Westley, B. H., 49a
Westminster Hospital, 182a
Westminster Hospital. Wolfson School of Nursing, 54b, 55a
Weyman, J., 103b
Whaley, K., 114b
Whaley, P. J., 59b
Whatley, E., 133a
Wheble, V. H., 97a
Wheeler, A. M., 141a, 175a
Wheeler, D. V., 87a
Wheeler, R. H., 175a
Wheldon, M., 63a
Whitaker, A., 113a
Whitaker, E. W., 62b
Whitaker, J. G., 11b
White, B. J., 127b
White, D., 13b
White, D. K., 166b
White, D. T., 38b
White, E. L., 118a
White, G. D., 46b
White, H. J. O., 168b
White, J. H., 28a
White, K. C., 28a
White, K. L., 92b
White, L. S., 98a
White, M. A., 47a
White, P. D., 119b
White, R., 73a, 125a, 127b
White, R. P., 92b
Whiteford, L. J., 43a

Whitehead, E., 109b
Whitehead, J., 70a, 79b
Whitehead, J. A., 141a
Whitehead, S. L., 109b
Whiteley, J., 156b
Whiteside, J. E., 67a, 166b
Whiting, J. F., 59b
Whiting, L., 59b
Whitlam, V., 141a
Whitley, N. N., 134a
Whitner, W., 134a
Whittaker, C. B., 143a
Whittall, K., 87a
Whittington Hospital, London, 28a
Whittow, M., 65a, 173a
Whyte, B. B., 42b, 47a, 48b, 49a, 64b, 167b
Wiebe, A. M., 163b
Wiedenbach, E., 11b, 47a, 67a
Wieland, G. F., 28a, 75a
Wiener, A. D., 125a
Wiens, A. N., 73a
Wignall, E. W., 113b
Wijesinghe, O. B., 142a
Wilbur, D. L., 28a
Wilbur, M. B., 28a
Wilcox, F. W., 125a
Wilcox, J., 49a
Wild, A. A., 174a
Wild, R., 79b
Wilkie, E. E., 147b, 150b, 153b, 154b
Wilkins, F., 4a
Wilkins, P. S. W., 113a
Wilkinson, A. W., 134b
Wilkinson, D. S., 104b
Wilkinson, L., 127b
Wilkinson, M., 175a, 90b
Wilkinson, M. A., 141a
Wilkinson, M. G., 38b
Wilkinson, P., 52b
Wilkinson, R., 103a
Will, H. E., 67a
Willcock, H. D., 67a
Willcocks, A. J., 26a, 179a
Williams, B., 121a
Williams, B. L., 121b
Williams, C. E., 129b
Williams, D., 73a
Williams, D. I., 109b
Williams, E. M., 15a
Williams, E. V., 52b, 127b
Williams, G., 121b, 168b
Williams, G. W., 92b
Williams, H., 13a
Williams, H. M., 38b, 154b
Williams, I. D., 154b
Williams, J. D., 141a
Williams, J. E., 170a
Williams, J. I., 11b
Williams, M., 2b, 125a
Williams, M. A., 81b
Williams, M. H., 157b
Williams, M. M., 47a, 59b, 125a, 128b, 161b
Williams, R., 5b
Williams, R. F., 98a
Williams, R. M., 50b, 118a
Williams, S., 11b
Williams, S. R., 170a
Williams, W., 175a, 179b
Willingham, J., 166b
Willington, F. L., 113b
Willis, F. N., 101b
Willis, J. H., 159a
Willis, T., 121b
Wills, V. E., 100a
Wilmarth, M. G., 181a
Wilmore, S. B., 118a
Wilmshurst, M. K., 175a
Wilson, A. B., 92b, 150b
Wilson, A. B. K., 175a
Wilson, A. H., 147b
Wilson, A. V., 13b
Wilson, C., 45a
Wilson, C. T., 28a, 170b
Wilson, F., 158a, 166b

Wilson, H. T. H., 104b
Wilson, J. S. P., 22b
Wilson, K. J. W., 38b, 50b, 66a, 97a
Wilson, L., 79b, 181a
Wilson, M., 113a, 148a
Wilson, M. E., 98a
Wilson, P. D., 125a
Wilson, W. L., 38b
Wiltshaw, E., 99b
Wing, J. K., 141a
Wingate, D., 115a
Wingert, P., 131b
Winner, H. I., 98a
Winsor, T., 67a
Winston, M. E., 163b
Winter, C. C., 109b
Winters, M. C., 62a
Winwood, R. S., 114b
Wirth, A., 2b
Wloch, N., 70a, 141a
Wofinden, R. C., 148a
Wohl, M. T., 119b
Wolfe, H., 28a, 79b
Wolfer, J. A., 161b
Wolfer, J. W., 27a
Wolff, I. S., 118a
Wolff, L. V., 31b, 46a, 70a
Wolford, H. G., 47a
Wolfson, W., 145a
Wolfson School of Nursing, Westminster Hospital, 54b, 55a
Wollen, W., 118a
Wollowick, A., 11b
Wood, B. G., 133a
Wood, H. L. C., 114b
Wood, J. J., 49a
Wood, M., 162b
Wood, S., 109b
Wood, T., 118a
Wood, V., 38b, 45a, 47a
Woodall, L., 181b
Woodard, E., 2b
Woodfall, R. E., 118a, 118b
Woodman, M. M. L., 127b
Woodmansey, A. C., 141a
Woods, B., 104b
Woods, J., 127b
Woods, M. F., 92b
Wood-Smith, D., 168b
Woodward, H. L., 121b

Woodward, M. H., 109b, 133a
Woodward, P., 153b, 159b
Wooldridge, P., 67a
Woollaston, M. E. F., 141a
Woolley, A. S., 47b
Worcester State Hospital, Massachusetts, 182a
Worgan, M., 159b
World Health Organization, 11b, 14a, 15a, 43a, 81a, 116a, 148a
World Health Organization. Pan American Sanitary Bureau, 35b, 80b
World Health Organization. Regional Office for the Eastern Mediterranean, 11b
World Health Organization. Regional Office for Europe, 45b, 81a, 131b
Worledge, C. B., 49a
Worley, E., 173a
Wormald, E. G., 28b
Worrall, O., 166a
Worsley, J. L., 141a
Wreford, B. M., 128b, 129a
Wren, G. R., 93a
Wright, B. J., 125a
Wright, F. H., 130a
Wright, F. K., 109b
Wright, J. A., 126a, 159a
Wright, M. J., 79b
Wright, M. S., 27a, 28a, 56b, 73a, 77b
Wright, M. W., 118b
Wright, R. D., 11b
Wright-Warren, P., 150b
Wulfsohn, N. L., 166b
Wurm, R., 28a
Wyatt, G. M., 123a
Wygant, W. E., 145a
Wylie, N. A., 180b
Wyndham, L., 4b
Wythe, B., 85a

Yale University. School of Nursing, 39b
Yalom, I. D., 113a, 141a
Yates, E. L., 3b
Yates, H. W., 141a
Yates, W. L., 15a
Yeatman Hospital, Sherbourne, 182a
Yeaworth, R. C., 121b

Yeoman, W., 114b
Yeomans, N. T., 142a
Yett, D. E., 28a
Yokes, J. A., 102a
Yost, E., 4a
Young, E. G., 77b
Young, E. H., 63a
Young, J. P., 28a, 79b
Young, L. S., 73a
Young, N. A., 74a
Young, R., 77b
Young, Z., 163b
Yourman, J., 77b
Yu, P. N., 102a
Yunek, M. J., 121b
Yun-o, L., 43a
Yura, H., 95a

Zabriskie, L., 120a
Zaccaria, J. S., 45a
Zachariah, A., 11b
Zachary, M. C., 75a, 99b, 113b, 124a, 127b
Zagornik, A. D., 46a
Zalba, S. R., 144a
Zambia Nurse, 37a
Zarraga, M. G., 19b
Zderad, L., 38b, 141a
Zeitz, A. N., 39b
Zeitz, L., 112b
Zeman, F. D., 113a
Zerbe, R. A., 92b
Zilm, G., 171a
Zimmer, J. G., 178b
Zimmerman, A., 21b
Zimmerman, C. E., 85b
Zimmerman, E. D., 39b
Zinberg, N. E., 38b
Zipes, D. P., 100a
Zix, L. G., 73a, 177b
Zodiacal, C. P., 38b
Zohman, L. R., 84b
Zoldos, A. J., 96a
Zschoche, D., 87a
Zubkoff, H., 79b
Zuck, D., 121b, 170a
Zugsmith, G., 129b
Zuidema, G. D., 106a
Zwemer, A. J., 30b

SOUTH BANK UNIVERSITY LIBRARY